S0-ASO-095

PHARMACEUTICAL DOSAGE FORMS

PHARMACEUTICAL DOSAGE FORMS

Parenteral Medications

In Two Volumes
VOLUME 2

EDITED BY

Kenneth E. Avis
Goodman Professor and Chairman
Department of Pharmaceutics
College of Pharmacy
The University of Tennessee, Memphis
The Health Science Center
Memphis, Tennessee

Leon Lachman
Lachman Consultant Services, Inc.
Garden City, New York

Herbert A. Lieberman
H. H. Lieberman Associates, Inc.
Consultant Services
Livingston, New Jersey

MARCEL DEKKER, INC. New York and Basel

Library of Congress Cataloging-in-Publication Data
(Revised for vol. 2)

Pharmaceutical dosage forms, parenteral medications.

Includes bibliographies and index.
1. Parenteral solutions--Collected works.
2. Pharmaceutical technology--Collected works.
I. Avis, Kenneth E. II. Lachman, Leon.
III. Lieberman, Herbert A.
[DNLM: 1. Infusions, Parenteral. 2. Technology, Pharmaceutical. WB 354 P536]
RS201.S6P49 1984 615'.191 84-7056
ISBN 0-8247-7084-6 (v. 1)
ISBN 0-8247-7085-4 (v. 2)

MARCEL DEKKER, INC.
270 Madison Avenue, New York, New York 10016

Current printing (last digit):
10 9 8 7 6 5 4 3

PRINTED IN THE UNITED STATES OF AMERICA

Preface

The reception accorded the first volume of this two-volume set on parenteral medications has confirmed our belief in the need for a comprehensive, authoritative treatise on the current technology associated with the development, manufacture, and quality control of parenteral medications and associated medical devices. The dramatic technological advances that have taken place in this field during recent years have resulted in the need for a thorough, organized, and current reference on this subject area. The favorable reviews and personal comments received have confirmed the value of the first volume.

With the availability of Volume 2, a complete coverage of the subject area is now provided. This second volume includes a thorough treatment of the subject of sterilization, a subject recognized as the processing key for achieving a sterile product. Confirmation of the effectiveness (validation) of the process is discussed at length. Included are a chapter on the formulation of large volume parenterals and three chapters on primary packaging components, that is, glass, plastic, and rubber. This volume contains a comprehensive chapter on the problems associated with particulate matter in injectable preparations. Another chapter deals with environmental control and its evaluation. The concepts and practices of quality assurance and an expansive chapter on regulatory matters are also in this text. An in-depth treatment of the subject of medical devices describes the manufacture, quality control, quality assurance, and associated regulations in a manner not found in other textbooks. The final chapter is a unique treatment of parenteral products in the hospital setting, presenting the distinctives of hospital practice. The material presented in this chapter will help industrial pharmacists appreciate how their products are utilized in the hospital and hospital pharmacists to better comprehend the significance of the standards practiced by industry for preparation of products of the quality required for safe use in the patient.

The contents of the first volume, with its discussion of the administration of parenteral medications, factors associated with biopharmaceutics, preformulation, formulation, processing of parenteral products and facility design, provide a combination of topics which, with Volume 2, complete a comprehensive treatment of the highly specialized and demanding processes and standards required for the preparation of parenteral dosage forms of drugs.

The editors believe that, because of the outstanding qualifications of the authors who have written the individual chapters, these two volumes present an authoritative textbook and reference not available elsewhere. The qualifications of the authors assembled for these two volumes are truly impressive. The extended time interval required for the completion of these two volumes was due in large measure to the heavy commitments of these authors in their fields of expertise. Therefore, the editors wish to express their particular appreciation to each of the authors who have given so much of their time and energy from already full schedules to make these two volumes possible. Their forbearance with our demands for meeting of deadlines and refinements of manuscripts is deeply appreciated. Special appreciation is extended to Brenda Richey, Dr. Avis' secretary, for her expert assistance in the preparation of the index for both volumes.

The favorable response to Volume 1 encourages us to believe that the two volumes together meet a need for a useful and complete set of textbooks for students and practitioners alike in this challenging, specialized field.

Kenneth E. Avis
Leon Lachman
Herbert A. Lieberman

Contents

Contributors

Frank R. Bacon, M.S.* Chief Surface Chemist, Engineering and Research Department, Glass Container Division, Owens-Illinois, Inc., Toledo, Ohio

Jonas L. Bassen, M.S.† Consultant, Bowie, Maryland

Floyd Benjamin, M.S.‡ Vice President, Quality Assurance and Regulatory Affairs, American McGaw, American Hospital Supply Corporation, Evanston, Illinois

Carl W. Bruch, Ph.D.§ Vice President, Quality/Regulatory Affairs, Skyland Scientific Services, Inc., Belgrade, Montana

Patrick P. DeLuca, Ph.D. Professor and Associate Dean, College of Pharmacy, University of Kentucky, Lexington, Kentucky

Levit J. Demorest, B.S.¶ Consultant, Quality Assurance Systems, Danville, California

Franco DeVecchi, P.E. Chairman of the Board, Veco International, Inc., Farmington Hills, Michigan

---

Current affiliations:
*Consulting Chemist, Associated Technical Consultants, Toledo, Ohio
‡Vice President, Scientific Affairs, Kendall McGaw Laboratories, Inc., Santa Ana, California
§Vice President, Quality Assurance/Regulatory Affairs, St. Jude Medical, Inc., St. Paul, Minnesota
Former affiliations:
†Director, Division of Industry Liaison, Bureau of Drugs, U.S. Food and Drug Administration, Washington, D.C. (Retired)
¶Quality Assurance Product Manager, Quality Assurance Department, Cutter Laboratories, Berkeley, California (Retired)

Samir A. Hanna, Ph.D. Vice President, Quality Assurance, Industrial Division, Bristol-Myers Company, Syracuse, New York

Raymond W. Jurgens, Jr., Ph.D.* Section Manager, Pharmaceutical Sciences Department, American McGaw, American Hospital Supply Corporation, Irvine, California

Julius Z. Knapp, M.S. Principal, R&D Engineering Associates, Somerset, New Jersey

John W. Levchuk, Ph.D. Associate Professor of Pharmaceutics, College of Pharmacy, The University of Tennessee, Memphis, The Health Science Center, Memphis, Tennessee

Bernard T. Loftus, B.S.† Consultant, Fairfax, Virginia

Frank J. Marino, M.S.‡ Division Manager, Regulatory Affairs and Quality Assurance Department, American McGaw, American Hospital Supply Corporation, Evanston, Illinois

Robert J. Nash, Ph.D. Manager, Quality Development, The West Company, Phoenixville, Pennsylvania

Larry R. Pilot, J.D. Attorney, McKenna, Conner & Cuneo, Washington, D.C.

Edward J. Smith, Ph.D. Vice President, Research, Health Care Products Group, The West Company, Phoenixville, Pennsylvania

Donald D. Solomon, Ph.D.§ Research Scientist II, Research and Development, American McGaw, American Hospital Supply Corporation, Irvine, California

David H. Wayt, M.S.¶ Manager, New Product Development, Sets and Devices R & D, Abbott Laboratories, North Chicago, Illinois

K. Lim Wong, Ph.D.** Section Manager, Analytical and Material Research, American McGaw, American Hospital Supply Corporation, Irvine, California

---

Current affiliations:

*Assistant Director, New Product Development, Diagnostic Products Division, Mallinckrodt, Inc., St. Louis, Missouri

‡Corporate Consultant, Microbiology, Corporate Quality Assurance Department, Abbott Laboratories, North Chicago, Illinois

§Senior Research Associate, Research and Development, Deseret Polymer Research, Warner-Lambert, Dayton, Ohio

¶Operations Manager, New Systems Technology, Abbott Diagnostics, Abbott Laboratories, North Chicago, Illinois

**Manager, Analytical Laboratories, Semiconductor Product Division, Rockwell International Corporation, Newport Beach, California

†*Former affiliation:* Director, Division of Drug Manufacturing, Bureau of Drugs, U.S. Food and Drug Administration, Washington, D.C. (Retired)

Contents of Pharmaceutical Dosage Forms: Parenteral Medications, Volume 1

edited by Kenneth E. Avis, Leon Lachman, and Herbert A. Lieberman

Contents of Pharmaceutical Dosage Forms: Tablets, Volumes 1-3

edited by Herbert A. Lieberman and Leon Lachman

VOLUME 3

PHARMACEUTICAL DOSAGE FORMS

1

Industrial Sterilization

A REVIEW OF CURRENT PRINCIPLES AND PRACTICES

Frank J. Marino* and Floyd Benjamin†

American McGaw, American Hospital Supply Corporation, Evanston, Illinois

I. INTRODUCTION

Millions of products are being sterilized annually by the drug and medical device industries. Although the concept of sterilizing products is not new, the shift of primary responsibility to the pharmaceutical industry for this is fairly recent and has occurred simultaneously with the advent of mass-produced pre-prepared drugs and disposable devices. In meeting this responsibility, the industry has developed increasingly more stringent standards for sterility acceptance of its products. In this effort the industry is now spending millions of dollars annually to assure product sterility. To produce a sterile product, manufacturers must give careful consideration to a variety of factors, systems, and technical information.

The objective of this chapter is to present basic information about the various factors and systems that are applied by industry in the manufacturing of sterile products. Industrial sterilization is based upon a mixture of disciplines that draw upon expertise from technical knowledge in many areas to obtain an acceptable degree of effectiveness as well as understanding of the limitations of the process. Persons responsible for carrying out sterilization procedures must be completely aware of the principles and practices currently employed in the industry. Therefore, it is essential to proceed with a discussion of common terminology.

II. PRINCIPAL DEFINITIONS

A. Sterility

In the classic sense, sterility is defined as complete freedom from all viable microorganisms. The process of sterilization, however, can be

---

**Current affiliation*: Abbott Laboratories, North Chicago, Illinois
†*Current affiliation*: Kendall McGaw Laboratories, Inc., Santa Ana, California

explained as a probability function, because of the logarithmic order of microbial death and the less than absolute methods for confirming sterility.

At times, the term "sterile" is inappropriately used, such as a synonym for products that are merely disinfected or pasteurized. A tendency exists to believe that a product is sterile if all detectable pathogenic microorganisms are eliminated. For example, an antibacterial agent may be added to a product to effect "sterilization." However, due to varying resistance to the sterilization process, some microorganisms may survive the process and not readily be discernible using traditional methods of microbial recovery.

The data compiled by Avis, given in Table 1, illustrate the varying resistance of different spores to moist and dry heat. The Council on Pharmacy and Chemistry of the American Medical Association attempted to clarify the meaning of "sterility" by stating that the terms "sterilize," "sterile," and "sterilization," in a bacteriological sense, "are not relative and to permit their use in a relative sense not only is incorrect, but opens the way to abuse and misunderstanding" [1]. Since the determination of sterility is vulnerable to errors and limitations in the systems used for confirmation, *sterility* is best defined as the complete freedom from all viable microorganisms within specified limits of probability.

B. Aseptic Technique

Aseptic technique refers to the procedures by which microorganisms are intentionally excluded from a manufacturing area, article, or person. However, the term is often used somewhat rigidly, referring to the precautions taken to prevent the access of microorganisms to an environment that could cause pathological infection.

C. The D Value

The rate at which microorganisms are killed may be expressed kinetically. Kinetic death rates, when plotted on logarithmic paper, permit their expression in terms of D values (the time required to destroy 90% of the bacterial cells or spore population under a given set of conditions). The D value is generally noted according to the specific sterilizing conditions; for example,

Table 1 Times Required for Lethal Effect on Bacterial Spores by Thermal Exposure

	Moist heat time (min)			Dry heat time (min)		
Organisms	100°C	110°C	121°C	120°C	140°C	170°C
B. anthracis	5–15	–	–	–	180	–
C. botulinum	330	90	10	120	60	15
C. welchii	5–10	–	–	50	5	–
C. tetani	5–15	–	–	–	15	–
Soil bacilli	>1020	120	6	–	–	15

Source: From Ref. 2.

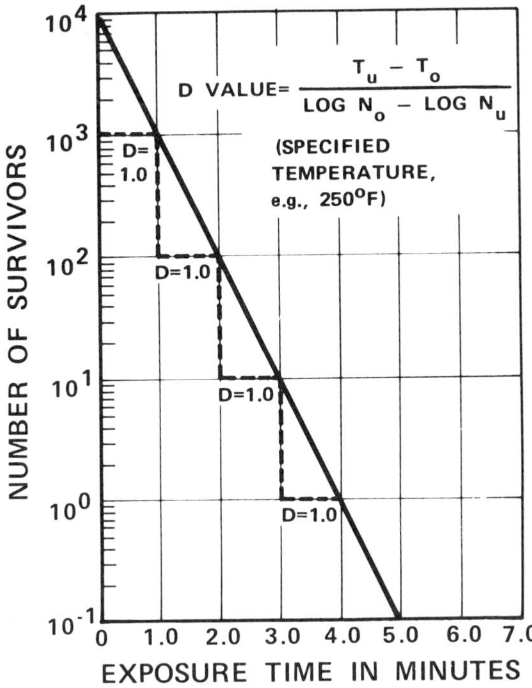

Figure 1 Thermal death kinetics D value.

D_{121} is the time required to reduce a population of cells (vegetative or spores) by 90% (one log) when exposed to a moist heat temperature of 121°C. D values are frequently used in describing the effectiveness of a sterilization process, such as the number of D values achieving a desired reduction of a microbial population in a sterilization process. For example, the notation 12D* indicates the reduction of a microbial population by 12 logs or a theoretical kill of 10^{12} microorganisms. Figure 1 shows the D values obtained from test data. The general equation of the straight line survivor curve is

$$\text{D value} = \frac{T_u - T_o}{\log N_o - \log N_u}$$

where

N = microbial population

N_o = initial number

N_u = surviving population

*12D has traditionally been applied to canning processes in the food industry. The designated D value of *Clostridium botulinum* is used as the standard.

T_o = initial exposure time

T_u = resultant time to destroy 90% of the initial population

D. The Z Value

Z value is defined as the temperature difference (degrees Fahrenheit or Celsius) causing a 10-fold change in the D value. The Z value may be derived from the formula

$$Z = \frac{T_x - T_o}{\log D_o - \log D_x}$$

where:

D_o = D value at the initial temperature T_o

D_x = D value at the subsequent temperature T_x

Z values are commonly derived from thermal reduction time curves in which D values are plotted on semilog paper against their corresponding temperature (see Fig. 2). The Z value is then determined as the temperature change required to traverse one log cycle [3].

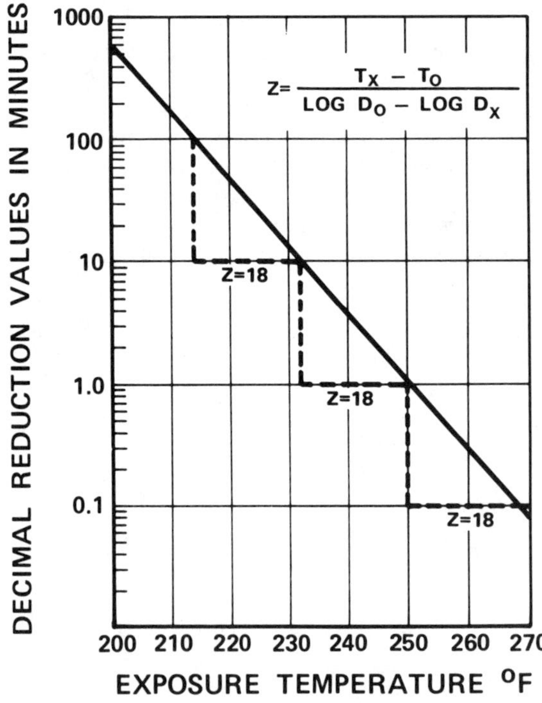

Figure 2 Thermal death kinetics Z value.

Typical Z values for moist heat-resistant spores (e.g., *Bacillus stearothermophilus*, ATCC 79330)* is 18°F (10°C). The accumulation of lethality at sterilizing temperatures below 250°F will be slower than with an organism with a similar D_{250} value and a larger Z value. Since routine 250°F sterilization processes are for the most part convection heated, a biological system with a Z value less than 18°F represents a greater challenge to the sterilization process. For example, the following heat survival times were found in different experiments: 284°F, 15–60 min; 302°F, 10–25 min; and 230°F, 10–15 min [4].

The destruction times were 5 min longer in each case than the figures cited. The slope or Z value of the destruction curves approximated from the results on many organisms is of the order of 40–75; with the consequence that, starting from the reference point, considerable increase in temperature must take place to appreciably reduce the destruction time [3].

E. The Q_{10} Value

The term Q_{10} is a temperature coefficient, which is the ratio of microbial death rate at a certain temperature to the rate at a temperature 10°C higher. This value is commonly used as an expression of microbial death kinetics, to which, from a practical sense, the Z value is not very applicable. For example, a Z value of 100°F for ethylene oxide sterilization is generally too large for the temperature processing ranges typically employed (i.e., 70–150°F) in ethylene oxide sterilization cycles.

Q_{10} values may vary, however, due to changes in certain sterilization parameters, e.g., gas concentration and temperature ranges. For example, in ethylene oxide sterilization, a Q_{10} value with 440 mg/liter of ethylene oxide gas typically was found to be 3.2 between 25 and 40.6°C and for 880 mg/liter of ethylene oxide gas, 2.3 between 25 and 33.4°C [3]. However, as the gas concentration increased (e.g., 1500 mg/liter of ethylene oxide), the Q_{10} value approached a value of 1.8 between 25 and 60°C [4].

F. The F_o Value

The term F_o value is defined as an equivalent sterilizing time (in minutes) of exposure to a saturated steam environment of 121°C. It is an integrated value derived from the typical formula

$$F_o = \int_{t_0}^{t_1} L\,dt = \int_{t_0}^{t_1} 10^{(T(t)\;-121)/Z}\,dt$$

where

L = lethal rate = $10^{(T(t)\;-\;121)/Z}$ dt

t = time variable

t_0 = initial process time

t_1 = final process time

---

*ATCC refers to the official American Type Culture Collection Number, 12301 Parklawn Drive, Rockville, Maryland 20852.

$T(t)$ = time-dependent temperature variable (°C)

Z = the temperature difference to cause a 10-fold change in lethal rate. For the calculation of F_o, $Z = 10°C$ is assumed.

The F_0 value is commonly used as a description of sterilization effectiveness in the pharmaceutical and food industries. It provides an integrated approach of minimizing heat exposure to heat-sensitive products, without compromising the reliability of their sterility. This is accomplished by integrating temperatures at less than 120°C during the heat up and cool down phases of the process and equating these integrated values to time at 121°C.

For illustration, Figure 3 displays the relationship between the process time t and the solution container temperature $T(t)$. The container temperature did not show as rapid an increase in attaining temperature because of density, as well as variations in viscosity. The curve of lethal rate L, in minutes at 121°C per minute for the solution container during the entire process period, is shown in Figure 4. The F_0 value is evaluated by integrating the area under the curve of lethal rate ½-min intervals over the time interval from t_0 to t_1. The cumulation of lethality or F_0 value is displayed in Figure 5.

G. Packaging

One final variable that affects Et0 sterilization is packaging. The unit package should include materials that allow rapid permeation of moisture, air, and gas. The best candidates are Tyvek and paper. Polyethylene is also permeable to Et0 and to moisture upon the addition of Et0.

H. Exposure Time

Once process parameters have been established, an appropriate industrial exposure time must be determined. To do this, the Et0 sterilization resistance of microbes in or on a given product type should be evaluated. The ability to sterilize a product can be determined in two ways: (a) by evaluating the effect of the product's physical characteristics on sterilizability, and (b) by the resistance of the product's normal microbial flora.

First, the sterilization time or D value can be determined for a given product containing standard bioindicator spores in the most difficult to sterilize location. The relative resistance of this device can be compared with other product types, and the most resistant product selected. The D value for the bioindicator spores in the most resistant product can be related to the total process by applying a desired log reduction factor.

Second, the resistance and levels of the product's normal microbial flora, or bioburden prior to sterilization, should be evaluated.

I. Thermal Death Time and Thermal Chemical Death Time

Thermal death time (TDT) and thermal chemical death time (TCDT) are sterilization expressions. These terms typically refer to the times to kill a specified microbial population distributed uniformly among replicate samples, upon exposure to a thermal or a thermal-chemical sterilizing

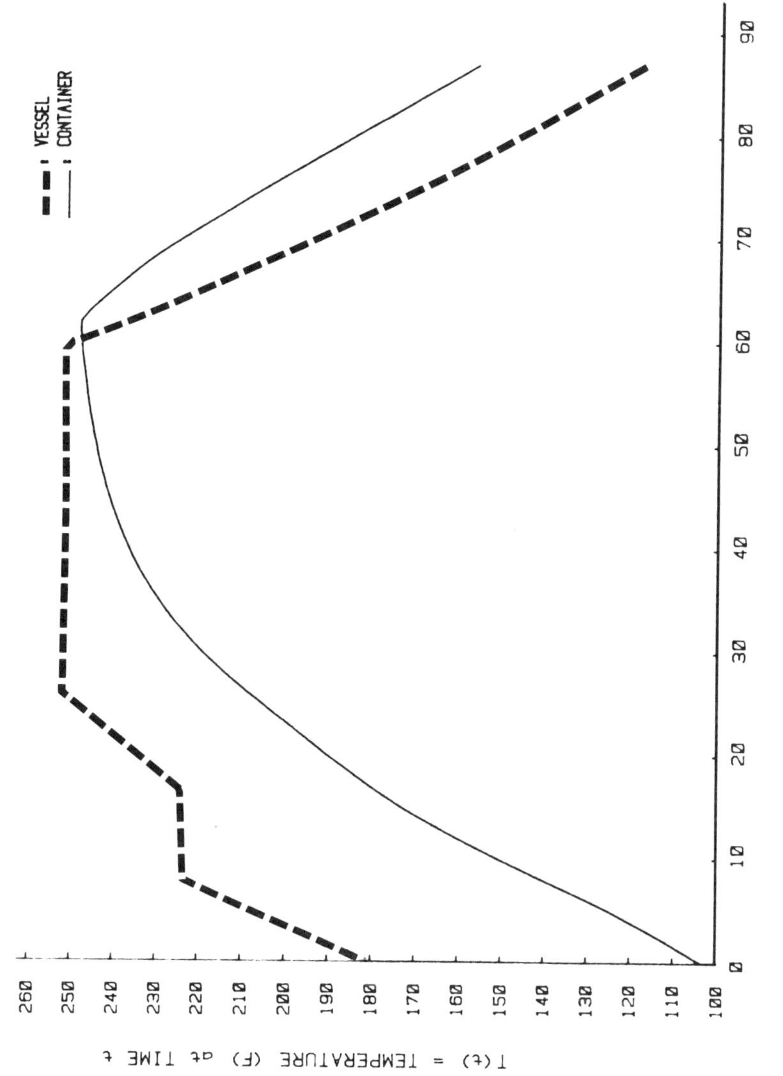

Figure 3 Typical temperature profile.

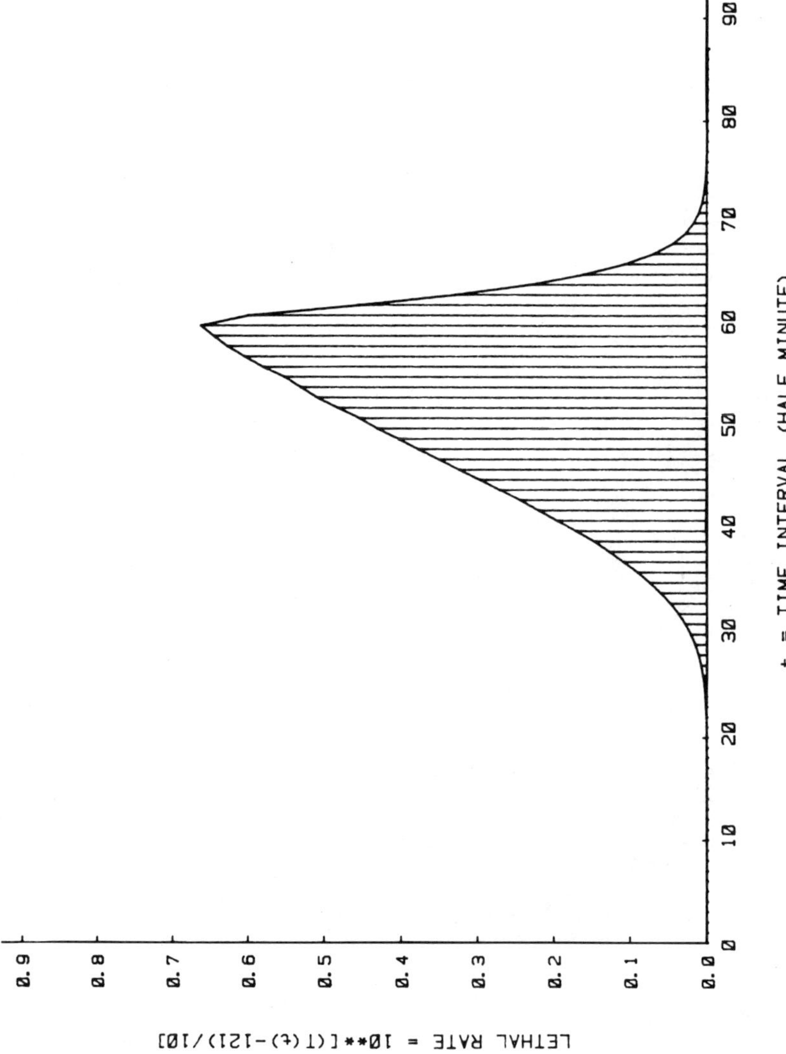

Figure 4 Typical lethal rate (F_o/min).

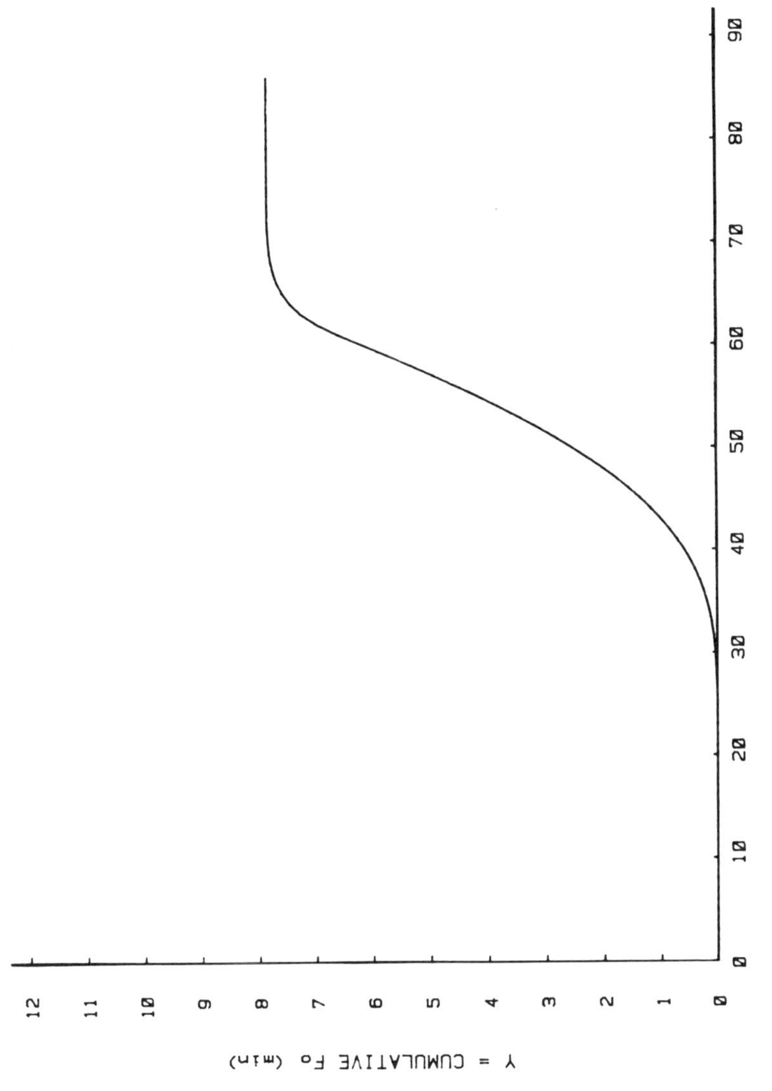

Figure 5 Typical cumulative F_o.

agent (e.g., saturated steam or ethylene oxide) under specified conditions.

Typical TDT and TCDT values reported for highly resistant spores to steam and ethylene oxide sterilizing media are 15 min at 121°C and 120 min at approximately 500 mg/liter ethylene oxide gas concentration, 54.4°C and 60% relative humidity (RH), respectively.

J. Principles of Microbial Resistance

One of the most important requirements for sterilization is the determination of microbial resistance to any sterilization technique. Sterilization process parameters are developed from this determination. Due to its importance, certain principles of microbial resistance are of interest, such as (a) the mathematical expression of microbial death, (b) the definition of microbial death, and (c) the mechanism of microbial death [5].

Mathematically, microbial death appears to follow a first-order, logarithmic rate. Such a phenomenon allows expression of microbial death in mathematical terms. It also becomes a basis for describing sterilization effectiveness of different processes.

In general, a logarithmic order of death is described by a straight line, when the logarithm of the number of bacterial survivors following exposure to a sterilizing agent is plotted versus increments of time (see Fig. 1). There are some exceptions to this phenomenon. For example, some spore populations upon initial exposure to sterilizing agents, such as steam, may actually increase in number due to a phenomenon called activation. Other populations may contain a few extremely resistant cells, causing tailing of the curve.

The definition of microbial death is, for all practical purposes, the inability of microorganisms to reproduce. This definition does not necessarily mean that the microorganisms are actually dead, for certain metabolic reactions and growth characteristics may continue to persist even though microorganisms may not be capable of reproducing. The definition is very important because it reflects the technological state of the art, applied to sterilization in a practical sense. It is also important to recognize that a "sterile" product is one that has been confirmed as such within the framework of this definition. Additionally, it is noteworthy that when certain microorganisms are "dead," chemical substances may still persist (in the form of endotoxins), which could cause a pyrogenic response.

Although the phenomenon of the logarithmic order of death is not yet fully clear, the mechanism of death is often considered to be a severe interaction of the sterilizing agent with critical protein or nucleic acid in the cell; for example, (a) with ultraviolet light, death appears to be due to the formation of thymine dimers on the same DNA strand; (b) with heat, it is proposed that hydrogen bonds are broken in DNA; and (c) in ethylene oxide, alkylation of amine groups on nucleic acids may be responsible for death [3].

K. Sterilization Assurance

Sterilization assurance is an expression of the reliability of having achieved sterility, normally without adversely affecting the quality or stability of the material being sterilized. This assurance is generally achieved by following established standards.

Although the goal of sterilization is the destruction of all bacteria, a certain probability of bacterial survival always exists. The important question is, what level of probability of bacterial survival is acceptable, or how sterile should the product be, or what is the Sterility Assurance Level (SAL)? The answer to this question may arise from economic and scientific considerations. The accepted industry standard today is a probability of 10^{-6} contaminated units. The econimic approach to this question may be very complicated. For example, an increase in process safety may result in an adverse effect on product quality or impact on productivity. A benefit-risk evaluation then must be made. Scientific consideration of the question may encompass such things as deviations from an idealized logarithmic death curve, the homogeneity of heterogeneity of the microbial population, or certain recognized, general limiting factors for a specific sterilization method (i.e., protection of microorganisms from the sterilizing agent due to an encrustation by organic materials, such as blood). A number of conditions exist that may affect the assurance of sterilization.

1. *Deviations from Specifications*

Critical sterilization parameters may be significantly out of specification. For example, the importance of relative humidity to ethylene oxide sterilization is such that humidity of less than 30% may cause failure of the process.

2. *Variation in Handling and Loading a Sterilizer*

The procedure employed (i.e., loading of a sterilizer) may be significantly different than demonstrated to provide effective sterilization. For example, it is recognized that linens or gowns in an autoclave should be positioned in such a manner as to allow free permeation of steam and removal of air. This means that every fiber or particle of any porous article undergoing sterilization will absorb an amount of moisture from the steam in exact proportion to the amount of heat absorbed by the article.

Assume for analysis a simple package consisting of 10 pieces of muslin cut into 10-in. squares and wrapped together without folding. If this pack were placed in the sterilizer flat side down, air within the pack would have to pass through 10 layers of muslin, plus the cover, in its down passage. The resistance of the dry pack will be increased by the moisture of the steam in contact with the outer layers, further retarding the evacuation of air. If the same pack is now placed in the sterilizer vertically (on edge), even though the pack may be wrapped fairly tightly, there will remain minute spaces between layers through which air can gravitate toward the bottom with comparative freedom. Figure 6 shows that 33 min of exposure at 250°F (121°C) would have been adequate for sterilization of the pack when placed on edge in the sterilizer. Industry places a great deal of emphasis on loading configuration. Substantially more than 30 min exposure for sterilization may progressively affect product quality [3].

Steam will not give up its heat except through the process of condensation. Steam will give up that heat to a nonporous article by conduction of heat absorbed by the exterior surfaces, thereby heating the interior without imparting any moisture. A typical example is a tightly stoppered glass bottle containing solution.

In time, the container-closure system would become heated to the temperature of the steam, but it could receive none of the moisture of the steam. To overcome this problem, closures for liquid containers should be designed to allow moisture to penetrate during the sterilization cycle,

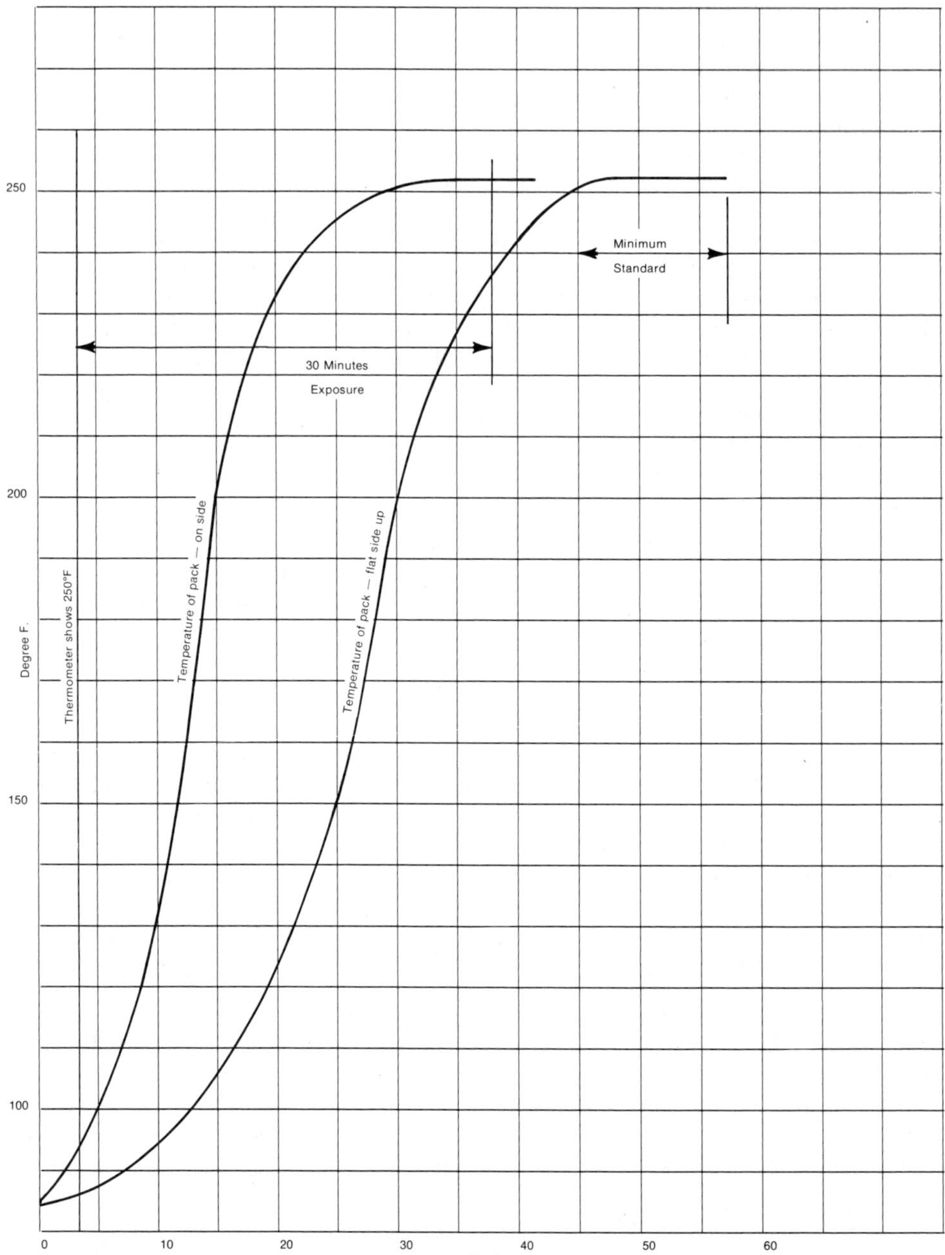

Figure 6 These two curves show load temperatures attained with the pack in different loading configurations. With the pack flat side up, 50 min exposure is required for sterilization. When the pack is placed on edge in the sterilizer, 33 min exposure is required to meet the minimum standard for sterilization. (From Ref. 10.)

or moisture added to the closure prior to assembly, or the closure component be presterilized (e.g., by radiation or ethylene oxide).

The sterilization of liquids in containers, flasks, or test tubes involves a different use of steam than is required for the sterilization of dry goods. In solution sterilization, the process is a matter of absorbing heat from the steam. The solution, if aqueous, contains the necessary moisture to generate steam within the container. The time required for heating the contents of the container governs the exposure period. This will vary with the size and shape of the container, the volume of liquid, the thickness of the container walls, the heat conductivity of the containers, and the closure system used. Measurements to determine the time required for a given container of solution to attain a temperature of 250°F (121°C) are usually made by means of a thermocouple and recorder.

Thermocouple probing of a lot of closure is difficult and will affect heat and moisture penetration. As a result, reliance is placed on destruction of a biological indicator in the closure to demonstrate the efficacy of a sterilization cycle. One method that can be used to demonstrate that a sterilization cycle will inactivate a bacterial spore challenge in the closure is fractional exposure [4]. In this method, closures are inoculated with bacterial spores and the units are randomly placed throughout a full sterilizer load. Following each of the various preselected fractions of the sterilization exposure time, the inoculated units are analyzed for the number of surviving spores. It can be assumed that the biological spore challenge has the same or greater heat resistance than the bioburden of the closure. The spore log reduction of the bacterial spore challenge is then related to the closure bioburden to ensure the cycle time is adequate for sterility assurance. Once the cycle time for the closure has been determined, a corresponding F_0 value in the solution for that cycle time can be established for routine sterilization of the container-closure system.

There are a number of methods for evaluating the integrity of container-closure system, including both biological and physical methods. The type of method depends on the closure system used [5].

Common errors in solution sterilization can often be avoided through a clear understanding of the operating cycle. Process modifications are designed to maximize the lethality effect of the cycle without distortion or damage to the product and/or container-closure system.

3. *Demonstrated Sterility Factor*

The sterility factor (margin of safety) is the probability of a contaminated unit surviving a sterilization process. It is typically based on the method and the type and number of product units to be sterilized. For example, because of numerous critical parameters for ethylene oxide sterilization versus moist heat sterilization, a greater probability of a contaminated unit for EtO sterilization should be expected than for moist heat (for further discussion, see Sec. III).

4. *Size of the Sterility Test Sample*

The sterility test sample may not demonstrate a low level of probability of microbial survivors if the method of testing is inadequate. For example (Table 2), if a lot contains 3.4% contaminated units and 20 units are tested for sterility, 50% of the time no nonsterile units will be detected (i.e., the test will pass). To detect contamination at a 95% confidence level on a

Table 2 Nonsterile Units That May Be Present in a Lot and *Not* Be Detected with a Given Sample Size

Sample size[a] Total units tested	Probability of sample containing *no*[b] nonsterile units		
	0.5 (%)	0.05 (%)	0.005 (%)
10	6.7	25.9	41.1
20	3.4	13.9	23.3
30	2.3	9.5	16.2
40	1.7	7.2	12.4
60	1.1	4.9	8.5

[a] United States Pharmacopeia XIX, Mack Publishing Company, Easton, PA.
[b] FDA Device Compliance Program Evaluation Report Fiscal Year (7324.04). Percentage of nonsterile units in a lot.

20-sample test, approximately 14% of the lot must be contaminated. This type of statistic indicates a need for establishing sterilization process specifications that assure a minimum level of probability of survivors. (For further discussion, see Sec. X.) A judgment on the interpretation of sterility test results must extend beyond simple microbiological aspects (i.e., growth or no growth upon sterility testing).

III. OVERVIEW OF STERILIZATION PROCESSES

The reliability of sterility for any product, material, or substance is dependent upon the sterilization method selected. Sterilization can be achieved by delivering sufficient quantities of any sterilizing medium, such as moist heat, dry heat, irradiation, or chemical agent (e.g., ethylene oxide, formaldehyde, hydrogen peroxide). However, it must be recognized that each sterilization process has its specific limitations. No universal method exists to encompass all products, materials, and substances.

The number of usable sterilization methods are few due to the inherent problem that any agent capable of destroying all types of microorganisms, including resistant spores, may not be compatible with the product or material to be sterilized. The major factors determining the utility of a sterilization method are (a) its compatibility with the product, material, or substance being sterilized; (b) the acceptability of the packaging; (c) the penetration of the agent to remote areas that may contain viable microorganisms; (d) a high level of lethal activity resulting in the need for only low quantities of the sterilizing agent; (e) relative inexpensive; (f) a high degree of safety and low toxicity; (g) simplicity; (h) time required for the process; and (i) its adaptability to in-line processing [3]. Comparison of the four most commonly used sterilization methods is made in Table 3.

Table 3 Comparison of Characteristics of Sterilization Methods

Factor	Moist heat	Dry heat	Ethylene oxide	Radiation
Material compatibility	Stable to moisture and heat	Stable to heat	Resistant to chemical alkylation	Resistant to radiation and ozone
Packaging	Highly permeable to moisture and air, resistant to heat and vacuum stress	Tolerant to heat	Highly permeable to gases, resistant to pressure changes	Resistant to deleterious self-propagating radical and chemical reaction
Penetration	Permeable to moisture and air	Highly time dependent	Permeable to EtO, air, and moisture	High penetration obtained with ^{60}Co, moderate penetration with accelerated electrons
Reliability	Good	Excellent	Good	Excellent
Cost	Low consumable cost and moderate initial capital cost	Low consumable cost and low initial capital	Moderate consumable cost and moderate initial capital cost	Considerable consumable cost and high initial capital cost
Safety requirements	Moderate	Low	Moderate to elaborate	Very elaborate
Toxicity	Low	Virtually none	High	Low

Source: From Ref. 21.

A. Moist Heat

Moist heat may be classified as a physical sterilizing agent, generally subdivided into four types of processes, that is, saturated steam, steam-air mixtures, prevacuum high-temperature steam, and superheated steam. For convenience, this discussion will be directed at saturated steam; however, in order to fully appreciate the physical and thermal properties of moist heat sterilization, it is important to note the differences in application.

Saturated steam is convenient, reliable, and well established as a sterilizing agent. Its mechanism for destroying microorganisms is thought to be denaturation of critical protein material essential for the growth and/or reproduction of microorganisms. Saturated steam has a high level of lethal activity and will destroy all types of microorganisms, including highly resistant spores, within 15 min at 121°C (15 psig). For more details on its mode of action and process principles, please refer to references on sterilization [2,3,5,6].

It is relatively inexpensive, compared with other sterilizing agents. Two advantages of saturated steam sterilization are its simplicity (requires monitoring only time, temperature, and pressure) and speed. One of the major disadvantages of saturated steam is that it is not compatible with many materials that are heat and/or moist heat sensitive. An inherent problem is the inability of saturated steam to penetrate certain packaging materials, very dense materials, and certain nonpolar materials, such as fats, greases, and oils. In saturated steam sterilization, the removal of air is extremely important, since air can become a barrier to diffusion of water vapor if it is entrained in a load of material.

Saturated steam has been used for the sterilization of numerous materials, including parenteral aqueous solutions, bacteriological media, surgeon's gloves, fermentation tanks, glassware, stainless steel instruments and utensils, hospital operating packs, and processing equipment.

Saturated steam sterilization is generally carried out as a batch process in a pressure vessel, commonly referred to as an autoclave. Autoclaves must be designed and tested to conform to American Society of Mechanical Engineering (ASME) Codes.

A typical profile of an industrial sterilization cycle is shown in Figure 7.

Steam-air mixtures do not provide the high temperatures that are typically characteristic of saturated steam. The resulting effect may be the principal reason for process failure. To determine the maximum temperature of a specific mixture of steam and air, apply the following formula.

$$P_1 = P_0 \frac{30 - V}{2} \qquad \text{from Dalton's law of gaseous pressures}$$

where:

P_1 = absolute pressure in pounds per square inch, the temperature of which is the desired factor (determine this by consulting steam tables in engineer's handbook)

P_0 = absolute pressure applied to the sterilizing chamber = gauge pressure plus 14.7 lb

V = the degree of vacuum applied to the sterilizing chamber in inches of mercury

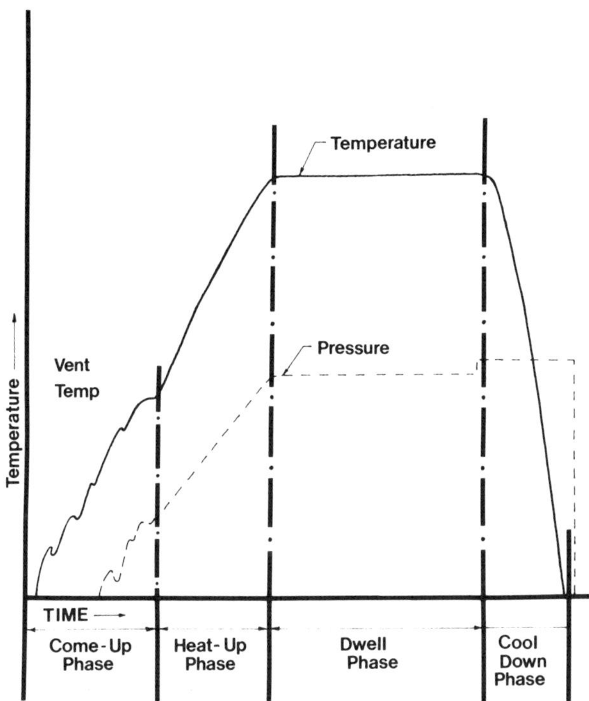

Figure 7 Typical industrial steam sterilization cycle profile.

Superheated steam is typically formed by passing saturated steam over a heated surface. The term "specific heat" is used to indicate the excess of the temperature over the temperature of saturation. This difference in temperature is called the degrees of superheat. Superheated steam does not increase the pressure of the steam. Instead, the steam is dried and will not condense until the temperature is lowered to its saturation point. Therefore, the dried-out steam does not contain the high moisture content necessary for effective sterilization.

Prevacuum steam sterilization consists of the use of a vacuum pump in conjunction with a condenser system to remove air and increase the efficiency of steam penetration during initial charging of the chamber with steam. Observations showed prevacuum to be consistent in the range of 15 ± 1 mm absolute in a period of about 4 min. Total sterilizer time can be reduced to one-quarter or less of the time required by conventional methods (e.g., saturated steam under pressure without use of prevacuum).

B. Fractional Sterilization

Fractional sterilization, which later became known as Tyndallization, was actually the forerunner of the nonpressure steam sterilizer (devised by Robert Koch and associates in 1880–1881). The process of Tyndallization still has use, especially in the sterilization of heat-sensitive materials, by steaming for 30 min on 3 consecutive days.

C. Dry Heat

Dry heat sterilization is generally applied to heat-tolerant materials (e.g., metal, glass, grease, and oils). Dry heat has been used to destroy not only microorganisms but also pyrogens. It is considered one of the most safe and reliable sterilization methods. More recently it has been applied in spacecraft sterilization. A typical dry heat temperature is at least 320°F (160°C) [5].

The mechanism of activity of dry heat was considered to be an oxidative process; more recent evidence indicates that it may be due more to the loss of moisture and its denaturizing effect on proteins [7]. It is conceivable that these two theories may be reconciled with one another by postulating that the target material may or may not be affected by loss of moisture during the process, depending on its previous and current microenvironment, and if no moisture is present at all, then the mechanism may be oxidative. It should be noted that, generally, dry heat microbial survivor curves (conversely, curves describing the rate of destruction of a microbial population) do not always fit a perfect logarithmic first-order rate model. Thus, dry heat sterilization processing time and/or temperatures may become much more excessive compared with other sterilizing methods. The level of dry heat lethality and penetration is dependent upon the energy supplied. If there is a sufficient quantity of heat energy, dry heat can penetrate and destroy any microorganism, eventually. This behavior prompted the National Aeronautics and Space Administration (NASA) to employ dry heat for numerous spacecraft componentry. The method is relatively simple—good heat circulation about the product load being sterilized is essential.

1. *Dry Heat Resistance*

The resistance of bacterial spores to dry heat temperatures was established by Koch and Wolffhugel [8] over 100 years ago. These early findings clearly demonstrated that the spores of *Bacillus anthracis* required a temperature of 284°F (140°C) for 3 hr in order to ensure their destruction. From these data and other information obtained in more recent studies, it can be concluded that an exposure to dry heat at 320°F (160° C) for 60 min is approximately the equivalent of an exposure to moist heat at 250°F (121°C) for 10–15 min.

It is of special importance to note that the microbial action of dry heat is markedly influenced by the nature of the fluid or substance surrounding the organism. In the presence of organic matter, such as a film of oil or silicone, the organism is definitely protected or insulated against the action of dry heat. This factor can be emphasized by pointing out the case of surgical instruments, which, if properly cleaned prior to heat treatment, may be sterilized in 1 hr at 320°F (160°C). If silicone treated, an effective sterilization cycle of 4 hr exposure, or greater, at 320°F (160°C) would be required to attain the desired sterility assurance level.

2. *Requirements for Dry Heat Sterilization*

Due to the variety of factors involved in a dry heat sterilization process, effective sterilization cycles will vary. The characteristics of the material undergoing sterilization must be known. For example, with such materials as glassware, it becomes possible to employ a high temperature for shorter periods of time than with sterilizing powders, which may undergo physical or chemical change unless the temperature is maintained below the critical point of the substance. Attention also must be given to the manufacturing, packaging, and loading of the sterilizer.

D. Radiation

Radiation is a recently developed sterilizing agent. Although several types of radiation exist, the most reliable types utilized for sterilization are ^{60}Co and accelerated electrons. Radiation sterilization appears to have advantages for select materials, but it seems unlikely that it will be widely applicable. The major concerns in radiation sterilization are product damage (e.g., disruption of chemical bonds), high initial capital cost, and process safety. As a method of destroying all types of microorganisms, it is highly reliable, demonstrating excellent lethal activity. It has a high level of penetration through most materials. ^{60}Co generally has a greater penetration ability than accelerated electrons. This is dependent upon the energy source and type of material; for example, ^{60}Co radiations can penetrate as much as 2 ft of water, but a typical accelerated electron may penetrate only 1 in. of water.

Sterilizing conditions are generally described in terms of radiation dose (megarads). One megarad is equal to 10^6 rad. A typical sterilizing dose is 2.5 Mrad. A dose less than 2.5 Mrad is permissable providing bioburden determinations and resistance studies are performed.*

Radiation sterilization, although not universally accepted, has been applied to foods, pharmaceuticals, medical disposable items, cosmetics, and drugs. Among its most reliable and proven uses have been the sterilization of sutures, plastic hypodermic syringes, and disposable hospital packs (i.e., gowns).

1. *Dosimetry*

Dosimetric procedures are the primary means by which radiation processes are controlled. There are two basic dosimetric systems currently in use in monitoring large gamma sterilization facilities: red acrylic-plastic dosimeters and radiachromic film dosimeters. Both chemical indicators, when properly calibrated, give readings within 5% of the delivered dose. Dosimetric determination is typically carried out as follows.

The cycle time for the irradiator is determined by placing a number of dosimeters in a homogenous "dummy" material of similar density and effective atomic numbers as the product. With the irradiation chamber completely filled with product or dummy material, the dosimeters are passed through a typical irradiation cycle. The red acrylic dosimetry (RAD) system or equivalent determines the cycle time to give a nominal dose at a position of minimum dose. Factors governing the maximum-minimum dose

---

**Process Control Guidance for Gamma Radiation Sterilization of Medical Devices*, Association for the Advancement of Medical Instrumentation (March 1985). This recommended practice contains guidelines for processing medical devices through gamma radiation facilities and recommendations for establishing process specifications.

ratio vary with each facility design. Means of focusing on this ratio include the number of passes the product makes by each side of the source, the distance of the product from the source, the shape and size of the source rack, the distribution of the source in the rack, and the uniformity of exposure to each side of the product carrier.

2. *Biological Indicator for Radiation Sterilization*

Bacillus pumilus spore preparations have been studied extensively as biological indicators for radiation sterilization. The Ethicon, Inc., strain E601 was characterized and deposited with the ATCC and was assigned the number 27142.

Figure 8 depicts typical shapes of dose-survival curves obtained when populations of pure cultures of microorganisms are exposed to increasing graded doses of high-energy radiation. The following key points are evident.

a. With increasing radiation treatment, the fraction of viable cells progressively decreases.
b. The rate of decrease can vary over the dose range.
c. At relatively high radiation doses, the fraction of cells surviving the process approaches zero.
d. Such curves are reminiscent of those generated from the simple negative exponential function [9].

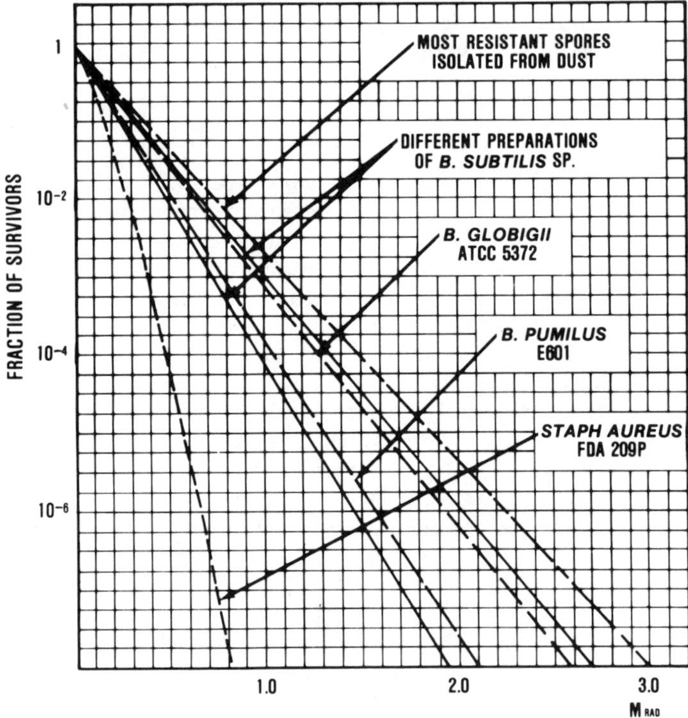

Figure 8 Inactive curves for various dried bacteria and spores.

$$y = Ae^{-kx}$$

in which A and k are constants. On taking logarithms, the equation transforms to the linear expression

$$\log_e y = \log_e A - kx$$

The curve describes the behavior of microbial populations on an item initially possessing 10^6 organisms of a given type. Over the measurable range of survivors (to one viable organism), the slopes are constant and their numerical values a measure of the response of the organisms to the treatment. Below one viable organism, where estimates of numbers of survivors are impractical, the curves are extrapolated, giving levels of survival that are represented as fractional numbers of viable organisms [9].

A wide range of decimal reduction values of *B. pumilus* have been reported in the literature. D_{Mrad} values (the amount of dose that will reduce a population by 90%) as low as 0.12 to slightly greater than 0.3 have been published.

With more information becoming available on process reliability and reproducibility of the irradiation process and the increased recognition that physical-chemical dosimeters are more accurate than biological preparations, continuation of routine use of biological indicators on product sterility testing becomes an important issue in irradiation treatment.

E. Ethylene Oxide

Ethylene oxide is a highly reactive, alkylating, toxic, flammable, and explosive chemical agent that is commonly employed for sterilizing myriad medical disposable devices. This method has been used in other sterilizing applications also, but to a lesser extent than for sterilizing medical disposable devices. Compared with the other sterilizing agents previously discussed, ethylene oxide sterilization is very complex.

The mechanism by which ethylene oxide kills microorganisms has been linked to its chemical activity as an alkylating agent [6]. According to the alkylation theory, ethylene oxide replaces labile hydrogen atoms with hydroxyethyl ($—CH_2CH_2OH$) groups, thus blocking many reactive groups needed in essential metabolic reactions.

The death of microorganisms by ethylene oxide sterilization is directly dependent upon relative humidity, gas concentration, temperature, and exposure. The importance of these parameters on the death of microorganisms is briefly described as follows.

a. Relative humidity is necessary to the ethylene oxide sterilizing effectiveness. Kaye and Phillips [6] demonstrated that the microbicidal action of EtO was 10 times faster at 28 than at 97% RH. Maximum activity of spores on paper carriers was at approximately 33% RH, and on nonhygroscopic carriers was about 45–50% RH, as reported by Gilbert et al. [10]. However, Kereluk et al. [11] demonstrated varied activity of EtO on both porous and nonporous surfaces as relative humidity varied. Gilbert et al. [10] and Ernst and Shull [12] demonstrated that EtO activity was minimal when spores were desiccated and that relatively high humidities were required to reduce the resistance of desiccated spores.

b. Gas concentration was reported by Phillips and Kaye [13] to have a proportional concentration-time effect on the death of spores. They reported that doubling the gas concentration reduced the sterilizing time by one-half at temperatures below 37°C. Ernst and Shull [12], however, demonstrated that the kinetics of EtO sterilization changed from first-order to a zero-order activity level at ethylene oxide concentrations above 1000 mg/liter. However, the effectiveness of gas concentrations in excess of 500 mg/liter is influenced to a large extent by chamber temperature and the ability of the heated chamber to maintain ethylene oxide in a vaporized state.
c. Temperature was demonstrated by Phillips and Kaye [12] to reduce the sterilizing exposure time by one-half with each 30°F rise in temperature. Ernst and Shull [14] demonstrated that the activity of ethylene oxide increased approximately 2.74 times (a temperature coefficient) for each 18°F (10°C) rise in the temperature range of 41–98.6°F (5–37°C).
d. Exposure time is a variable depending upon the gas concentration, relative humidity, and temperature, as briefly described above.

To verify proper sterilization parameters, control of the following factors is critical for sterilizer effectiveness.

A slight elevation of temperature assists permeation of the gas and provides a means of obtaining a desired level of lethality throughout the sterilization chamber. Temperature control is also important in controlling pressures produced by a given volume of gas. If a reduction in temperature occurs, the gas will condense and lose its biocidal effect. On the other hand, if the chamber is controlled at a specific temperature range and more gas is introduced, an increase in sterilizing efficiency of the ethylene oxide occurs. Care should be taken, however, to assure that excessive increases in gas concentration are accompanied by an appropriate increase in temperature in order to maintain the gas in the vapor state at the higher pressure levels; otherwise, the gas will tend to condense on surfaces.

The moisture content of the microbial cell is another important factor in gaseous sterilization. Gilbert et al. [10] demonstrated that excessive drying of bacterial cells will result in a nonuniform reaction to ethylene oxide, and to rehydrate, direct contact with water is necessary. In view of this property, moisture distribution and permeation should be controlled at approximately 50% relative humidity (40–70% is the optimum range) to minimize the potential for production of desiccated spores.

Effective processing systems must also be designed to minimize the possibility of gas stratification. Less than optimal conditions will also influence the efficiency of sterilizing with the gas [10].

Besides its wide use in sterilizing medical disposable items, ethylene oxide has been applied to heat-sensitive pharmaceuticals, cosmetics, drugs, and foods (e.g., spices and herbs).

One of its main disadvantages is the potential for toxic residues to be left in products and materials that have been sterilized. The three most common toxic residues of importance are ethylene oxide and two of its reaction products, ethylene chlorohydrin and ethylene glycol. There is considerable concern by the Food and Drug Administration regarding the mutagenicity and toxicity of these compounds. In a general sense, ethylene oxide toxicity is basically equivalent to ammonia; however, its additional reactivity and mutagenicity require that elaborate safety precautions be taken with the use of this sterilizing method [13].

IV. PROCESS SELECTION

Selection of a sterilization process is an important consideration for any manufacturer or processor of sterile products. Because millions of product units may be sterilized per year under a single standard or slightly modified process, a sterilization problem may affect many products. It is important, therefore, to select and validate a sterilization process with as much information as possible before proceeding to a large-scale sterilization operation.

Sterilization is employed in numerous fields, such as food processing, pharmaceuticals, cosmetics, fermentation, medicine, laboratories, hospitals, and space exploration. Yet even with the wide application, the number of different sterilizing processes are relatively few.

To derive the best results, the selection of a sterilization process should be approached systematically. In this approach a variety of factors should be carefully considered: the type of product to be sterilized, characteristics of product packaging, inherent process considerations, economics, regulatory requirements, safety considerations, disciplines required, technology, facility and space requirements, toxicological effects, degree of simplicity, and processing time.

As an example, several ethylene oxide sterilizing cycles can be used in the medical or hospital field. These cycles differ somewhat from those employed in industry in that they are designed specifically for hospital usage in commercially available sterilizing equipment. Figure 9 best exemplifies

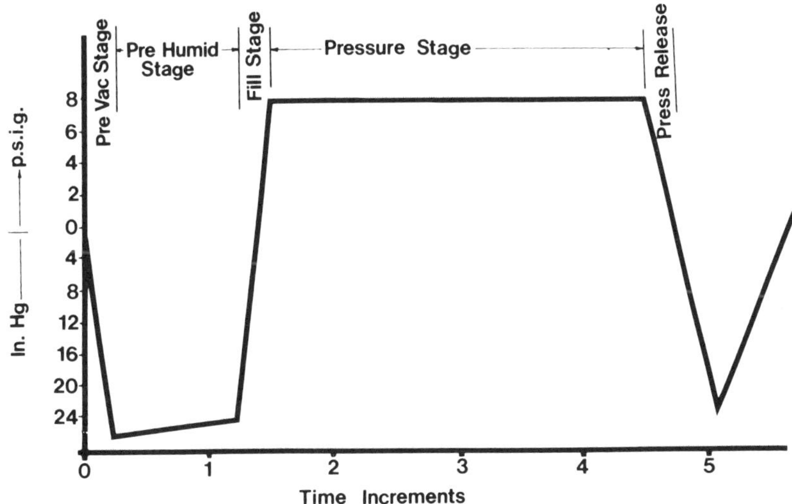

Figure 9 Typical industrial EtO (Cry-Oxide) sterilization cycle.

a typical gas mixture that can be used by both hospital and industry with minimum equipment variation. In operation, the initial vacuum is pulled to a level of 25–26 in. Hg. This is followed by a prehumidification dwell with the relative humidity controlled in the range of 50–60% RH at a temperature near 125–130°F. The vessel is then charged with pretreated gas, in this case the 12:88 (12% ethylene oxide–88% dichlorodifluoromethane) sterilant mixture. The net pressure increase is approximately 21 psi, reaching a final exposure pressure near 8.5–9.5 psig. This is equivalent to a minimum EtO concentration of approximately 530–650 mg/liter [12–14].

A. Product Considerations

In all sterilization processes, a minimum of two goals must be ultimately achieved and/or reconciled: achievement and maintenance of product quality characteristics (e.g., chemical purity and strength, functionality, physical dimensions, and packaging integrity), and attainment of product sterility (e.g., destruction of microbes on and in the product). The achievement and/or reconciliation of these two goals is not always an easy task. For example, sterilization of heat-labile solutions, such as antibiotics and vitamins may be adversely affected by typical moist heat processes designed to destroy the more heat resistant type of microorganisms (e.g., *Bacillus stearothermophilus* spores). Sterilization of greases and oils by typical moist heat processes will fail to destroy all bacteria, because moisture cannot permeate the material. Sterilization of certain plastic materials (e.g., polypropylene) by radiation may result in discoloration or loss of strength of the plastic. Ethylene oxide treatment of antibiotics (e.g., penicillin) may result in loss of antibiotic potency because of chemical reactions. Ethylene oxide sterilization of some plastic materials may result in critical levels of toxic residues [14].

B. Packaging

The following are keys in selecting a suitable packaging material for gas sterilization:

a. The packaging material must be permeable enough for ethylene oxide and moisture to enter the package (and air escape) and sterilize the contents within the desired cycle time; the penetration rate must be uniform. Productivity requirements make short cycles (high porosity rates) desirable.
b. The packaging material must be impermeable to bacteria and other contaminants.
c. The packaging material must not be deformed or porosity altered by pressure variations during vacuum cycles.

Films of polyethylene, polypropylene, nylon, polyvinyl chloride, and paper may be reasonably suitable for use with ethylene oxide. However, aluminum foil is completely unacceptable because it is not permeable to ethylene oxide gas. Nylon, although acceptable, generally requires longer sterilization time than other materials. All plastic films used for wrapping should be evaluated on their ability to allow reasonable permeation of ethylene oxide gas, moisture, and air before and after sterilization [14].

Table 4 Packaging Materials for Articles to Be Sterilized

Material	Nature	Type of product	Thickness or grade	Suitable for: Steam	Suitable for: Dry heat	Suitable for: EtO gas
Muslin	Textile	Wrappers	140 thread count	Yes	Yes	Yes
Canvas	Textile	Wrappers	—	Yes	No	Yes
Kraft	Paper	Bags	30–40 lb	Yes	No	Yes
Glassine	Coated paper	Envelopes, bags	30 lb	Yes	No	Yes
Parchment	Paper	Wrappers	Patapar 27-2T	Yes	No	Yes
Crepe	Paper	Wrappers	Dennison wrap	Yes	No	Yes
Cellophane	Cellulose film	Tubing, bags	Weakly sterilizable	Yes	No	Yes
Polyethylene	Plastic	Bags	1–3 mils	No	No	Yes
Polypropylene	Plastic	Film	2–3 mils	—[a]	No	Yes
Polyvinyl chloride	Plastic	Film, tubing	1–3 mils	No	No	Yes
Nylon	Plastic	Film, bags	1–2 mils	—	No	Yes
Polyamide	Plastic	Film, wrappers	1–2 mils	—	No	Yes
Aluminum	Foil	Wrappers	1–2 mils	No	Yes	No

[a]Not recommended; difficult to eliminate air from packs.
Source: Ref. 3.

Permeability is one of the most important criteria. Not only must the sterilant be able to permeate the package, but the packaging material must have sufficient breathability to permit release of toxic residues (e.g., ethylene oxide residual gas). Additionally, the porosity and bond strength (the seal, or bond, between two packaging substrates) must be adequate enough to maintain package integrity.

For steam sterilization, certain types of paper material (e.g., Kraft and parchment paper) are reasonably acceptable. Plastic materials, such as nylon and polypropylene, are not generally suitable because air and steam do not effectively permeate. Nylon, however, because of its high permeation to water vapor, may be inappropriate because of potential large loss of the container contents through vapor permeation outward during and after sterilization.

For typical dry heat sterilization processes (e.g., 160–180°C for 2–4 hr), aluminum foil, Mylar, glass materials, and stainless steel are suitable. Under less severe temperature conditions but at longer exposure times (e.g., 125°C for 24 hr), certain plastic materials, such as polycarbonate and polypropylene, may be appropriate [15].

In radiation sterilization, in which the penetration power of electrons and gamma rays is high, a large variety of packaging materials are suitable. The main difficulty here lies with physical or chemical incompatibilities (e.g., discoloration of glass and certain plastic materials, such as polypropylene and polyvinyl chloride). Radiation-resistant grades of these plastics, however, are available.

To confirm the suitability of a packaging material, the material should be preliminarily qualified by subjecting it to a sterilization process and prolonged exposure (e.g., storage stability) after sterilization to preselected environmental cyclic conditions, in order to determine packaging acceptability. See Table 4 for typical packaging materials used in sterilization.

V. PROCESS CONSIDERATIONS

Although a sterilization process may be appropriate, in general, for a specific type of product and packaging material, inherent questions must be answered, such as the volume and quantity of product to be sterilized and the capacity of the process equipment.

In general, all sterilization processes are dependent upon loading configuration, positioning, and density.

A. Typical Sterilization Loading Considerations

1. *Ethylene Oxide*

The load should be geometrically designed to provide for circulation and permeation of gases. For example, space should be provided between walls of the sterilizer and the product load, between pallet loads, and between cartons. This is especially important in degassing of ethylene oxide after sterilization is complete. Additional space may be required for postaeration cabinets or rooms. A postaeration cabinet or room is a confined area in which products are quarantined and gas residues are allowed to degas, generally under controlled temperature or airflow conditions.

During this period, samples of product are analyzed for the presence of ethylene oxide by gas chromatography.

2. *Moist Heat*

The load should be positioned in a manner to allow for complete removal of air. This is particularly important in a gravity air displacement process cycle. Additionally, problems may occur with small loads in which pockets of air may occur. This latter condition can be overcome with an initial high vacuum.

3. *Dry Heat*

The individual units in the load should be as small as possible to permit heat penetration. Also, the chamber should be loaded to permit free circulation of heated air.

4. *Radiation*

For electron accelerators, packages to be irradiated must be placed within the zone of the electron beam where irradiation is uniform and concentrated. For all irradiation types, the more closely together the material is placed, the greater is the output. For example, the penetration of electron rays through certain dense materials may become a potential limiting factor. In order to achieve better results, in this case, an increase in energy and/or exposure time would be required.

B. Economic Considerations

All sterilization processes bear some costs. In general, sterilization costs can be divided into three general areas: initial capital costs for equipment and facilities, consumables, and operation costs.

Steam sterilization is the most economical and convenient form of sterilization. Initial capital cost for steam sterilization-related equipment may appear to be costly because of the need for safety-coded pressure vessels, expensive controls, and safety alarms. However, in comparison with other sterilization processes, such as ethylene oxide and radiation, its initial capital cost is generally much lower. Currently, the most expensive (initial capital) process is radiation. In the case of cobalt 60 facilities, elaborate safety precautions and facilities (e.g., thick-walled concrete chambers) are costly. The least expensive process (initial capital) is likely to be for dry heat sterilization. However, due to the high temperature required, its application and use in industrial facilities is limited because of potential adverse effect on product due to high heat (e.g., 160–170°C or higher) [16,17].

Ethylene oxide and radiation sterilization systems are highly cost competitive. The deciding factors on choice of system may well rely on volume, density of the product, sterilizing dose, and gas mixture. Another important point to consider is product and package compatibility. The investment in research labor hours to convert product formulations to allow use of an alternate sterilizing system could eliminate further consideration. The various gas mixtures shown in Table 5 are typical and will differ in cost depending on the carrier system and ethylene oxide concentration.

Table 5 Ethylene Oxide Mixtures Used in Gaseous Sterilization Procedures

Mixtures	Manufacturer	Type of container (net wt.)
Ethylene oxide–carbon dioxide		
Carboxide	Union Carbide Corp.	
10% ethylene oxide	Linde Division	30
90% carbon dioxide	New York, N.Y.	60
Oxyfume Sterilant-20	Union Carbide Corp.	
20% ethylene oxide	Linde Division	30
80% carbon dioxide	New York, N.Y.	60
Steroxide-20	Castle Ritter Pfaudler Corp.	
20% ethylene oxide	Rochester, N.Y.	60
80% carbon dioxide		

Ethylene oxide—fluorinated hydrocarbons		
Cry-Oxide	Ben Venue Laboratories Bedford, Ohio	20-oz disposable cans
11% ethylene oxide 79% trichloromonofluoromethane 10% dichlorodifluoromethane		
Benvicide	The Matheson Co. East Rutherford, N.J.	Metal cylinder
11% ethylene oxide		16
54% trichloromonofluoromethane		100
35% dichlorodifluoromethane		270
Pennoxide	Pennsylvania Engineering Co. Philadelphia, Pa.	
12% ethylene oxide		25
88% dichlorofluoromethane		140
Steroxide-12	Castle Ritter Pfaudler Corp. Rochester, N.Y.	20-oz and 36-oz disposable cans
12% ethylene oxide 88% dichlorodifluoromethane		

Source: From Ref. 3.

Operational costs for various sterilization processes may be identified: wages (operator skill level), power requirements (e.g., electricity), utilities (e.g., water and steam demand), and maintenance support (frequency of electromechanical failures). Operational costs are not always easily quantified; however, they should be carefully analyzed.

Because of the important aspect of the economics factor in sterilization process selection, manufacturers of sterilizers and suppliers of consumables should be consulted for advice on the costs before choosing any process.

C. Regulatory Considerations

All sterilization processes are governed by regulatory requirements to some degree. The type of regulatory requirement is generally dependent upon the type of product (e.g., drug, food, or device), and the sterilization processor (e.g., manufacturer or hospital).

The drug and device industry specifications for sterilization processes are set to some extent by the official compendium, the United States Pharmacopeia (USP), since it describes minimal acceptance criteria for sterility testing and biological indicator systems for all sterilization processes. In the hospital field, sterilization processes are the responsibility of hospital staff, although accrediting associations may identify standards to be met for accreditation.

Sterilization processes generally employed in the food, cosmetics, devices, and drug industries are controlled to a large extent by the Food and Drug Administration (FDA) through Good Manufacturing Practices (GMP), which describe minimal acceptance criteria for qualification and performance of sterilizers.

Further, the FDA is charged with the responsibility of seeing that drug, food, devices, and cosmetics are safe and efficacious for their intended use. Since a sterilization process may have an impact on this requirement, its approval may be required by the FDA. Regulatory requirements in regard to sterilization are always prone to changes. Because of this concern, a survey of current and potential future regulatory requirements should always be conducted before selecting and accepting a process.

D. Safety Requirements

The hazards associated with equipment installation and handling of sterilizing agents require the application of specific safety requirements and/or operational limitations that will minimize the potential hazardous conditions that exist. For example, all steam sterilizers built in the United States should be constructed according to the Pressure Vessel Code established by the American Society of Mechanical Engineers. Ethylene oxide sterilizers intended for use beyond 15 psig should conform to this code. Further, in the case of ethylene oxide sterilization, provisions should be made to maintain ethylene oxide environmental air levels within acceptable limits required by the Occupational Safety and Health Administration (OSHA).

In the case of radiation, facilities (Fig. 10) must be constructed to minimize the potential possibility of exposure to harmful levels of radiation.

All interlocks in the plant control room (radiation) should be designed to be "fail-safe"; safety interlocks and devices to ensure personnel protection are as follows.

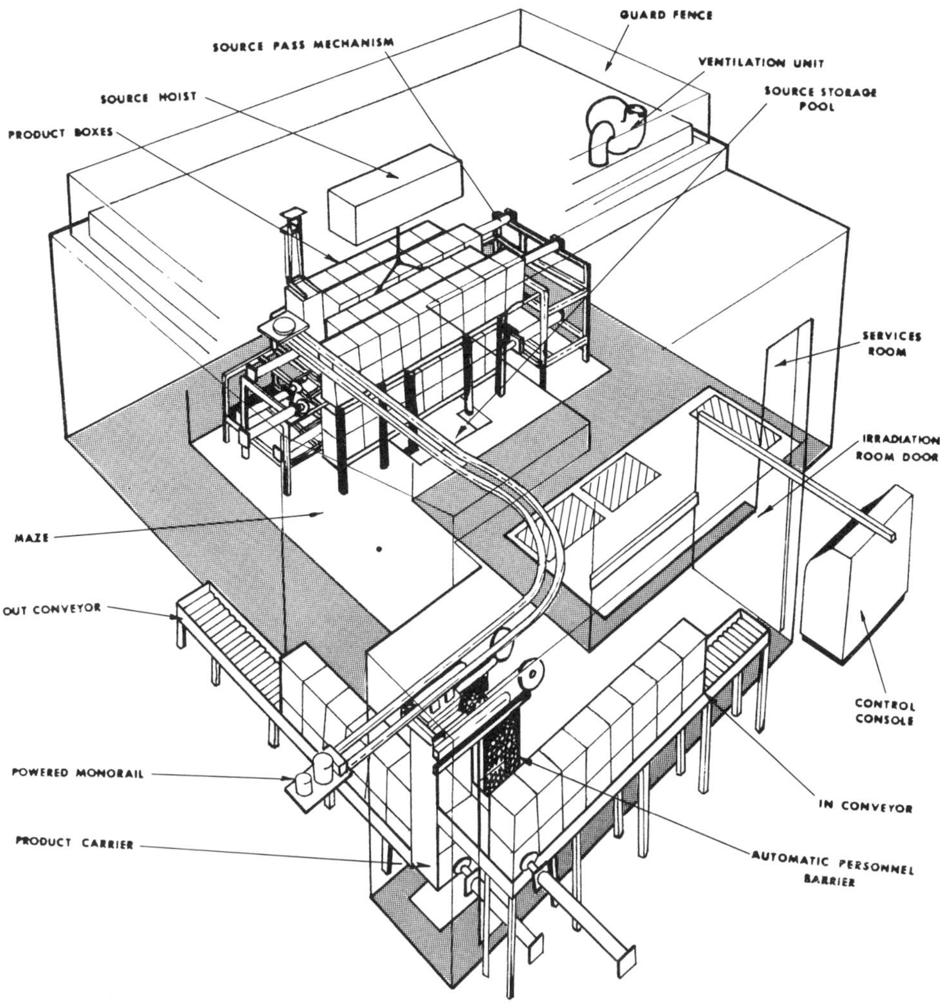

Figure 10 Medical products irradiator with variable box system. (Courtesy of Atomic Energy of Canada, Ltd., Ottawa, Canada.)

a. The safety door at the entrance to the access maze should be electrically interlocked with the source so that the source cannot be raised if the door is open, and conversely, the door cannot be opened if the source is exposed.
b. A 90-sec safety delay timer is located in the irradiation chamber. This allows the operator to walk out of the chamber, close the door, and start operations at the control panel within the prescribed delay period. This ensures that personnel cannot inadvertently be shut inside.
c. To ensure operation by authorized personnel, a master control switch key is retained in the possession of the plant operator and only issued to others with the operator's knowledge and consent.
d. Pilot lights on the control panel indicate the source position.

e. In the event of compressed air failure when the source is in the irradiate position, the source will automatically lower to the off position in the storage pool.
f. In the event of any malfunction of the source pass mechanism, the plant automatically shuts down and the source returns to the off position.
g. Air exhausted from the irradiation chamber is filtered to permit a periodic check for the presence of radioactive contaminants.
h. The source operating mechanism is constructed to give the source maximum physical protection with a minimum possibility of sticking or jamming.
i. The source automatically returns to the storage position in the event of power failure to prevent overexposure or uneven exposure of the product. Operation will recommence if the power failure is less than 30 sec in duration.
j. The ventilation system removes ozone formed by the radiation inside the irradiation chamber.

E. Discipline or Training Requirements

In general, all sterilization processes require an interdisciplinary investigation and effort (e.g., engineering, microbiology, chemistry, and physical support). Because sterilization is the complete absence or removal of all microorganisms, the role of the microbiologist is very important in determining and validating the effectiveness of a sterilization process and to establish the minimal criteria by which it can be accomplished (e.g., determination and verification of critical sterilizing process parameters). The role of the engineer is to develop, acquire, and establish the equipment and materials by which sterilization can be effectively performed. The chemist's role is generally one of product formulation to withstand the adverse conditions of different sterilization processes (e.g., high heat, chemical residues, and radiation damage) and the determination of toxic residues or product chemistry after sterilization.

Although each sterilization process is different, similar tests are performed to verify sterilizer performance. For example, in radiation sterilization, mapping studies are performed using sterilization containers fully loaded with product in which dosimeters (physical or chemical indicators capable of energy transfer by radiation) are appropriately placed throughout the load to determine penetration of energy and profile measurements of radiation of product or material being irradiated.

F. Data Analysis

Evaluation of sterilization processes and equipment is performed by analysis of documentation data. This analysis may be simple, for example, requiring a sample comparison of programmed process parameters to actual parameters or a simple review of data to determine if it fits within preestablished limits (i.e., ±1°C temperature range in a saturated steam environment). Analysis of data, however, may be more complex, requiring statistical analysis, such as t tests for determination of significant differences in process data monitored at different probe sites within the same sterilizer load. Figure 11 shows an example of mean F_0 values at specific locations along the vertical axis of a 1-liter glass container. Analysis of

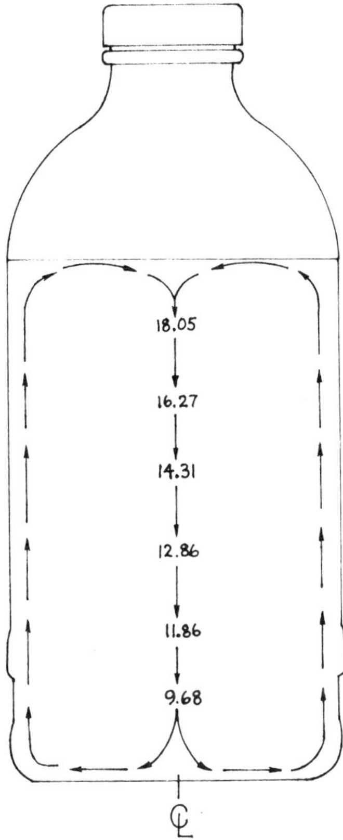

Figure 11 Glass container cold spot mapping. Toroidal thermal pattern for solution during convective heating. Mean F_o values at specific locations along the vertical axis of a 1-liter glass container of 50% dextrose.

container cold spot data to determine slowest to-heat characteristics and eventual process probe control locations may be established as follows.

For each container, calculate, $F_i = F_o$ from container location i and $F_c = F_o$ from control location in the same container: $\Delta F_i = F_i - F_c$

where

ΔF_i = mean of ΔF_i

sd_i = standard deviation of ΔF_i

n_i = number of pairs in the comparison of location i and the control location

Calculate t statistics for each location i as follows:

$$t_i = \sqrt{\frac{n_i \; \Delta F_i}{sd_i}}$$

The t statistics converts the difference in F_o between the control location and the test location to a standardized unit. If values of t_i are all positive, then the control location is to be designated as "container cold spot" location. Otherwise, the location i with the smallest t_i will be designated as the "container cold spot" location.

VI. PROCESS SPECIFICATIONS

Preliminary sterilizer studies indicate the absolute minimum standards of time and temperature throughout all portions of the sterilizer load to accomplish effective sterilization. These minimum conditions plus additional time factors to compensate for product heat up and cool down constitute a process specification. On the basis of the established specification, the process is monitored for conformance.

Due to the various factors considered, the selection and acceptance of the sterilization process requires an in-depth analysis and review of the type of discipline, personnel, and training required prior to undergoing a sterilization development program.

A. Technology

The selection of a sterilization process is dependent upon application and technical readiness. For example, steam sterilization is an old and proven art that has been supported by reasonable technological advances to make it one of the more convenient, effective, and accepted sterilization processes. Radiation and ethylene oxide sterilization, however, more recently developed methods, suffer the inherent problem that insufficient information, equipment, or material may be readily available. For example, among experts in the sterilization field it is recognized that radiation affects all materials. That is, all substances absorb energy from ionizing reactions. The absorbed energy excites the molecule. The process of excitation and ionization of a polymeric molecule may lead to ozone generation, polymerization, cross-linking scission, and double-bond formation. All these reactions may occur in an irradiated sample; however, one reaction usually predominates. Additives, stabilizers, and antioxidants will alter these effects and render materials compatible to radiation.

B. Facilities and Space Requirements

Prior to the selection of any sterilization process, careful review of facilities and space requirements should be made. Several factors should be considered, one being the installation of the sterilizer (e.g., size and weight of the working and power module).

Too often, sterilizers are selected and purchased without determining how they will be transported, located, and installed in a manufacturing facility or laboratory.

Other factors to be considered include the electrical, water (steam), air, and space requirements for operation. For steam sterilizers, boiler capacity must be equated with steam demands for operation. For ethylene oxide sterilization, additional space may be needed to precondition the product with moisture and heat prior to loading the product in the sterilizer and an aeration room to accelerate the degassing of ethylene oxide from the product after sterilization. For radiation sterilization (e.g., cobalt 60), additional space must be available for construction of thick concrete walls to minimize harmful radiation levels for human operators.

C. Equipment

A sterilizer consists of specialized and unique equipment specifically designed for its intended use. It may vary from a small portable laboratory type to a large bulk-sized unit for industrial application. It may range in degree of sophistication from inexpensive simple plastic disposable self-contained units to high-cost, intricate, and elaborate vessels utilizing microprocessor controls and monitoring instrumentation with computer analysis. The advancing technology of sterilization has brought forth new concepts in the design, construction, and control of sterilizing equipment.

D. Relationship to Total Manufacturing or Operational Process

Prior to selecting or designing any sterilization equipment, the determination of the relationship of sterilization to the total manufacturing process should be made. This requires analysis of information on the organizational structure and sterilizing needs of different departments and groups.

In large-scale industrial manufacturing facilities, sterilization may be viewed by production as the final bottleneck in production output, whereas the quality control department may view the process as one of its major responsibilities, because of the claim of product sterility. This latter responsibility is also handled by regulatory groups and quality assurance departments in a large manufacturing operation. Overall, engineering consideration for equipment and its design may be typically reflected by a number of factors, which are summarized in Table 6. Each of these factors plays an important role in assuring proper installation and the degree of process control necessary to maintain an effective sterilization program.

E. Specifications

Most commercially available sterilizers for hospital and industrial laboratories, central supply, and nursing departments or for small office use already are pre-established with a set of specifications. Because of the specialized purpose and the large scale of operation, most industrial stabilizers are, to a certain degree, custom-made, and must be specially described by specifications.

Basic specification information for ethylene oxide sterilizer equipment components typically may consist of the items identified in Table 7. Similar information would be required for other types of sterilizers.

In preparing specifications for a sterilizer, it is essential to discuss the details with vendors to assure final compliance and availability of equipment or components. Once the specifications have been established, it can then become the responsibility of the designated purchasing agent to handle the actual final negotiations and compliance to the specifications.

Table 6 Typical Engineering Considerations for Industrial Sterilizer Equipment and Design

Effectiveness/efficacy of sterilization method

1. Bacteriological kill safety factor
2. Product/packaging physical, chemical, and biological evaluation studies
3. Regulatory requirements
4. Premarketing studies of processed product

Costs and operational considerations

1. Estimated equipment cost/delivery time
2. Accessory equipment cost/delivery time
3. Total cost of system/delivery time
4. Operational costs
    - Consumable cost/cycle
    - Preliminary total estimated cost/cycle
    - Process/system demand (i.e., cycles/day)
    - Consumable demand (i.e., weight or energy storage)
    - Power requirements
    - Water demands
    - Air demand
5. Supervisor/technician skill direct and indirect (support) required
6. Hazard/safety to personnel
7. Reliability/maintainability
    - Frequency of electromechanical failures
    - Average time of repair failures
    - Maintenance skill levels required
    - Average costs to repair failures
8. Mobility
    - Working module
        - Size
        - Weight
        - Components
    - Power module
        - Size
        - Weight
        - Components
    - Space requirements

Table 7 Typical Basic Specification Information for Industrial Ethylene Oxide Sterilizer

1.0 Equipment specifications

- 1.1 Sterilizer chamber dimensions equal to load needs, pressure strength, stainless steel construction
- 1.2 Closure (door): automatic double doors or manually operated, interlock mechanisms, dimensions
- 1.3 System integrity: engineering test runs, checks for leaks, process qualification
- 1.4 Operator control: training manuals, operating procedures
- 1.5 Evacuation subsystem: water-sealed vacuum pump, Venturi pump
- 1.6 Chamber circulation: fan for gas distribution and absence of stratification or manifold system for effective introduction of steam
- 1.7 Heating systems: jacketed, floor heating by conduction
- 1.8 Process control: establish set points, reliability testing
- 1.9 Filters: particulate or bacterial retention, location
- 1.10 Instrumentation: computerized data acquisition, retrieval, and reduction systems

2.0 Sterilization cycle phase selections

3.0 Operation and maintenance

- 3.1 Operator instructions: operating manual and process specifications
- 3.2 Drawings: equipment, electrical and systems requirements
- 3.3 Maintenance procedures: full maintenance work, such as filter and steam trap servicing, gaskets, sticky valves
- 3.4 Calibration procedures
- 3.5 Recommended spare parts: pumps, switches, heat exchangers

4.0 Equipment guarantee

5.0 Applicable code design compliance intent

F. Installation and Facilities

In the installation of sterilizers, specific instructions, drawings, and specifications should be prepared by qualified engineering personnel. For commercially available hospital or laboratory sterilizers, this information is generally supplied with the sterilizer in the operation manual or specification sheet. For larger industrial sterilizers that are either custom designed or assembled in-house, a qualified engineer should be assigned the responsibility for carrying out this task. It is important that a detailed plan be prepared, in order to complete the job of installation effectively.

An important aspect of facility installation is in meeting insurance requirements. For example, facilities using 100% ethylene oxide gas in their sterilizer must be constructed with blowout walls and ventilation systems for removing potentially explosive levels of the gas. Radiation sterilizers require radiation shields (i.e., 6-ft concrete walls) of specified materials and dimensions to meet regulatory criteria.

In addition to the type of construction materials, the facility must meet specific sterilizer placement criteria so that maintenance personnel are able to service the sterilizer periodically after installation. In the interest of preventive maintenance, it is typical practice to locate a sterilizer through a wall. This is done so that it will allow easy access to sterilizer equipment in an area not directly in contact with the operator, which, if allowed to be freestanding in the room, may offer some interference in the operation of the sterilizer and the ability to conduct daily care of sterilizer equipment.

G. Processing Hardware

Proper selection of basic hardware, accessories, instrumentation, and controls is essential to the development of a relatively problem-free sterilization-processing routine for any contaminated product. Variables that should be considered include compliance with mechanical, electrical, and safety codes; component and instrument reliability; and ease of maintenance, repair, and modification.

1. *Basic Sterilizer Characteristics*

Cylindrical and rectangular ASME code-approved pressure vessels represent two basic designs for the containment of pressurized sterilizing agent. The rectangular design is generally preferred because of greater economy of chamber space. In either case, however, the pressure vessel shell used can be jacketed or nonjacketed. Jacketed vessels are utilized more often because they allow better assurance of uniform thermal characteristics as well as greater options for controlled cooling of vessel contents. Chamber door closing is achieved by means of manually operated or power-operated doors that must meet rigid safety codes. Other basic elements common to typical sterilization processes include temperature controllers and recorders, pressure gauges and recorders, timers, safety devices, door-lock mechanisms, abortive systems, and controlled electronic elements, such as microprocessors, in conjunction with computer control are becoming more widely used for demonstrating reliability and reproducibility of repetitive sterilization systems.

2. *Sterilizer Installation Qualification*

A number of steps should be carried out during hardware installation and qualification before start-up of process validation. Two important steps in this phase of the sterilization program are as follows.

a. Completion of a series of calibration procedures, which should be performed on all control instrumentation so that all control devices will accurately and reliably control the process. This information should be documented, recorded, and repeated on a periodic basis.
b. Routine inspection by qualified engineers to ensure that preventive maintenance programs are followed. This procedure will assist in maintaining the integrity of the system(s) to function as designed and also reduce hardware malfunctions and cycle failures in routine operations.

After control instrumentation has been calibrated, empty-chamber studies are carried out to verify and validate with documentation and records that there is reasonable similarity of heat distribution in the chamber during the entire sterilization process. There should also be indication of good reproducibility and uniformity throughout the chamber that will contain the product.

Another factor that has recently received considerable attention is the facilities employed for the removal of sterilant residuals from exposed materials. This is primarily a concern of ethylene oxide sterilization. Normally, the rate at which sorbed gases dissipate from exposed goods is dependent upon the nature of the material and the conditions under which the products are stored following exposure.

Methods of aeration other than allowing exposed materials to stand at room temperature have been explored. These include the subjection of gas-sterilized articles to multiple vacuums in a chamber and allowing fresh, filtered air to enter the chamber after each vacuum or exposing the sterilized materials to forced circulation in a ventilated area. The final judgment on required aeration times and the facilities needed to effectively remove diluent gases from each gas-sterilized article should be based on a set of laboratory studies before any manufacturing studies are done in the manufacturing environment.

Support facilities for sterilizers must be considered. For ethylene oxide, moisture preconditioning and poststerilization aeration rooms are generally needed in industrial facilities. In general, for all sterilizers, staging areas and poststerilization quarantine areas are employed. In order to guarantee separation of nonsterile and sterile material, fences and gates may be used.

VII. PROCESS DEVELOPMENT

Development of a sterilization process includes consideration of all important conditions that are required to be sure that the material processed receives a sufficient lethal dose of the sterilization medium. To be sure that this is achieved, tests must be performed. The types of tests vary, depending upon the type of sterilization method selected and the application of the process. However, in general, these tests include parametric studies, product evaluation, and equipment performance and repeatability. Studies of these parameters generally define the purpose and objectives, the procedure, the evaluation of data, the collection of data, documentation, and approval of the studies. In establishing process parameters, engineering testing is a key activity.

A. Parametric Studies

These are tests performed to measure and evaluate basic sterilization parameters, such as temperature and pressure and their rate of change for moist heat sterilization; gas concentration, pressure, temperature, and humidity and their rate of change for ethylene oxide sterilization; temperature and time and their rate of change for dry heat sterilization; and ionizing radiation intensity and its penetration for radiation sterilization.

Product evaluation varies with the sterilization method; however, physical and functional tests after sterilization are always applicable. For example, when radiation impinges on a plastic molecule, it may be broken into fragments. The free radicals formed by the resultant energy may form free radicals and cross-link to form new plastic entities. In a similar fashion, the effect of various ethylene oxide parameters on variations in the chemical formulation, dimensions, and manufacturing assembly procedures may all interact with the sterilization process and result in a product or package that differs from the product as designed and intended for use. Other evaluations may include inspection of product materials for crazing of plastics, kinked tubing, collapsed drip chambers, dilation of tubing, decrease in strength of binding agents, and others. There are no limits on the extent of the effect of a sterilization process on the product. Process performance testing will, however, limit any incompatibility. But, as a means of further verification, a program should be designed to evaluate acceptability of product routinely after sterilization.

B. Microbiological Criteria

Since sterilization in the classic sense is defined as the complete destruction or removal of all viable microorganisms, but in the reality of processing must be considered in terms of a probability function, microbiological criteria are indispensable in the development of any sterilization process. This section will consider microbiological criteria commonly utilized in developing and verifying sterilization processes.

1. *Bacterial Death Kinetics*

As previously discussed, bacteria exposed to a sterilizing agent are generally killed at a first-order rate. To gather this information on a practical level requires bacteria to be exposed to a selected sterilizing condition, at various increments of time, and number of survivors be assessed. With the information obtained, it is possible to mathematically analyze the effectiveness of a process. Additionally, the resistance and levels of the product's normal microbial flora, or bioburden, prior to sterilization require evaluation.

2. *Bioburden or Presterile Microbial Load*

The terms "bioburden" or "microbial load" refer to the total number and types of microorganisms in the load of product prior to sterilization. The development of any sterilization process must begin with a qualitative and quantitative determination of these microorganisms. This information combined with that of the resistance of these microorganisms to a sterilization process is essential for establishing effective sterilization cycle parameters.

The quantitative determination of the bioburden starts with an accurate and reliable method of recovering bacteria from the product. For precision, the method of choice usually is membrane filtration. One technique utilized consists of washing a nonliquid product with sterile saline or phosphate buffer and passing the wash solution through a sterile 0.45 μm membrane filter. If the product is a solution, it may be passed through a sterile 0.45 μm membrane filter. To determine the total number of microbes present on these filters, the filters must be aseptically placed on suitable culture media, such as Soybean Casein Digest Agar Medium for bacteria and Mycophile agar for isolation of fungi. Recovery media for microorganisms may be incubated at 30–35°C for mesophiles and 55–60°C for thermophiles. For fungi, the preferred incubation temperature is 20–25°C. Quantitative determination of the number of bacterial spores is generally performed by heating the wash solution or liquid product at 80°C for 20 min, to destroy all vegetative (nonspore) forms prior to filtration.

Once a total number of microorganisms has been determined from a large number of samples and from several typical batches of product loads prior to sterilization, a quantitative bioburden can be estimated. This may be done in several different ways. For example, one "worst case" situation is to multiply the total number of product units that comprise a batch to be sterilized by the highest number of microorganisms observed in the determination per product unit. Another example is to multiply this total number of units of product by the average number of microorganisms counted, or by the highest number of bacterial spores within three standard deviations (99.7% confidence). The latter approach may be applied when bacterial spores are considered much more resistant than vegetative microorganisms. In steam sterilization, resistant spores may be up to 100,000 times more resistant than vegetative bacteria [18].

A qualitative determination of bioburden may consist not only of determining and evaluating the types and resistance of microorganisms on the product but also the characterization of microorganisms with respect to their ability to resist sterilization due to environmental factors, such as water activity, organic encrustation, and desiccation (for further background, see Sec. V). Further, seasonal and other environmental variables may affect both the qualitative and quantitative bioburden.

3. *Probability of Survivors*

This terminology denotes a mathematical description of the full bacteriological effectiveness of any particular sterilization process. It indicates the statistical chance of a bacterial survivor from a process. As stated earlier, the death of bacteria in a sterilization process follows a first-order reaction. The mathematical formula for determining the probability of a survivor of a sterilization process is typically described for saturated steam sterilization as

$$N_b = \log^{-1}\left(\log N_o + \log r - \frac{F_o}{D_{121}}\right)$$

where:

D_{121} = time to kill 1 log or 90% of a population of the most heat resistant product isolate obtained from bioburden and microbial kinetic studies

N_o = highest initial microbial population in the product at zero time of exposure

r = number of product units in the sterilizer load

N_b = probability of a survivor from a contaminated product load

This formula is provided to demonstrate the method of calculation of probability of survival for a given steam cycle; it is a mathematical description, in either time mode or kill mode, of the degree of safety achievable with a sterilization process.

In industry, when large numbers of items are sterilized at one time, the effectiveness of the sterilizing process is sometimes expressed in terms of the margin of safety by which a given load of processed product will be sterilized. The determining of margin of safety is based on calculations made from data obtained from death rate kinetic curves and determining bioburden resistance of typical organisms found on the product. The following illustrates the method of calculation of process margins and safety.

Process safety margin (PSM) may be expressed as percentage of additional F_o over the necessary lethality required (time mode) or additional microbial log reduction (kill mode).

Time Mode

$$PSM_x = \left(\frac{\text{process } F_o}{t_x} - 1\right) \times 100\% = \left(\frac{\text{process } F_o}{D_x \log N_x} - 1\right) \times 100\%$$

where:

x = specified microorganism

t_x = time (in F_o unit) required to kill microorganism x

D_x = D value for the microorganism x

N_x = population or maximum allowable level of the microorganism x in the load

BI = biological indicator

I = bioburden isolate

For example,

$$PSM_{BI} = \left(\frac{9.87}{1.22 \times \log 10^8}\right) \times 100\% = 102\%$$

implies the PSM is 102% over the lethality required for BI challenge.

$$PSM_I = \left[\frac{9.87}{0.146 \times \log (1.5 \times 10^4)} - 1\right] \times 100\% = 16088\%$$

or 161 times

implies the PSM is 161 times over the lethality required for product bioburden.

Kill Mode

$$PSM_x = \frac{\text{process } F_o}{D_x} - \log N_x$$

For example,

$$PSM_{BI} = \frac{9.87}{1.22} - \log 10^4 = 4.09$$

(additional 4.09 log reduction in BI) and

$$PSM_I = \frac{9.87}{0.0146} - \log (1.5 \times 10^4) = 671$$

(additional 671 log reduction in bioburden isolate).

4. *Biological Indicator Systems*

The only true means of determining sterility is by the use of a living microorganism, since the organism typically selected as a biological indicator is susceptible to the sterilization conditions required for its destruction. Selection requirements are based on degree of resistance relative to other organisms to the process, stability, growth characteristics, and reliability of the system in reacting to the variables of the process (i.e., time, temperature, moisture, and gas concentration).

The usual method of preparing a biological control is to impregnate a paper strip, cloth, or some other material with a culture of bacterial spores of known concentration. Often the test organism is directly inoculated into product to reflect in the most accurate way the resistance of the indicator in product. The biological control is placed, clearly identified, in the load of materials in various locations prior to exposure. Following exposure, the control is aseptically removed or transferred to suitable culture medium and incubated at the optimum temperature of the indicator organism. If growth has not occurred in a minimum of 7 days, the articles sterilized are considered sterile.

The most commonly used test organism is *Bacillus subtilis* var. *niger* (ATCC 9273) for ethylene oxide and dry heat sterilization, *B. stearothermophilus* (NCA 1518, ATCC 7953) or nonpathogenic *Clostridium sporogenes* (PA 3679) for moist heat, and *B. pumilus* (E601) for irradiation sterilization [19].

It is important that the population of cells or spores bear a close relationship to the probable level of contamination on the articles to be sterilized and that the selected population be considered with a liberal margin of safety in mind. It has been proposed that the normal contamination in clean and room-dried articles ranges from a few hundred to 25,000 bacteria of various species [15]. On this basis, a biological control should contain a substantially higher population of organisms to provide a factor of safety.

5. Chemical Indicators

Chemical indicators are also available as indicators of sterilization treatment. These include special types of indicator tapes that change color in the presence of ethylene oxide or temperatures of about 250°F; chemically impregnated paper disks enclosed in paper or plastic envelopes, which change color when exposed to ethylene oxide; and chemically treated paper strips that contain bacterial spores in addition to a chemical indicator. However, it must be mentioned that indicators that undergo a color change are subject to a number of weaknesses. For example, ethylene oxide sterilization is dependent on a set of conditions that are critical in attaining effective sterilization. If any one of the conditions is varied (e.g., temperature of exposure), the indicator would be inaccurate as a monitoring device.

In radiation sterilization, chemical indicators are designed to change color and can be measured spectrophotometrically to indicate that the material exposed to the radiation source was given the radiation dose designed for the process.

6. Lethality Factor

An expression denoting by some factor the quantity of sterilizing condition(s) achieved is called the lethality factor. For saturated stem, the lethality factor is most often represented as an F_0 value, such as 15 min at 121°C. In radiation, the lethality factor is expressed as the dose in megarads (e.g., 2.5 Mrad). For ethylene oxide, a typical thermochemical death time is 4 hr exposure to 40–60% RH at approximately 130°F and 600 mg/liter EtO. Although lethality factors are generally expressed for convenience in terms of some physical value, they can similarly be expressed in microbiological terms, such as the number of logarithms of spores inactivated by a process. For example, in the food industry, inactivation of at least 10^{12} spores of *C. botulinum* is a commonly accepted lethality factor [19].

In summary, the establishment of process parameters is basic to any effective sterilization process. In industry, these process parameters are generally provided to a production department as minimum criteria that must be met. In a practical sense, the establishment of process parameters from a microbiological perspective can have as the objective either to reach a survivor probability of $<10^{-6}$ of a contaminated unit in a load or have an overkill based on the empirical approach of 12D-value reductions of the most resistant bacteria to the applicable process, such as *B. stearothermophilus* (ATCC 7953). For example, if a bioindicator in a device had a D value of 24.3 min, the demonstrated 6 log reduction represents a sterilization effect equivalent to 146 min. Yet, in about 59 min, the normal flora will theoretically be reduced 10^{-6}, a probability based on its known maximum D value and level.

C. Instrumentation for Process Control

Proper instrumentation is essential for both the development phase of a sterilization process and for its control. In order for a process variable to be controlled or utilized, it must be possible to successfully measure the variable.

Instrumentation permanently installed on a steam sterilizer used during test runs or during sterilizer validation will be used to generate production process data. A production monitoring instrument list is shown in Table 8 and illustrates the type of data recorded during the validation. However, several temperature probes would be used and the channels scanned and data recorded every 30 sec; additionally, a number of critical parameters may be monitored every 6 sec.

Operation of a sterilizer consists of creating a sequence of conditions within the chamber under manual or automatic control. Most sterilizer manufacturers develop and build sterilizers with automatic control mechanisms. Sterilizers equipped with automatic control mechanisms overcome many of the problems and inaccuracies occurring with manual operation. The instrumentation described in Table 8 allows automatic timing and recording of key phases of the sterilization process. The controllers assist in programming a cycle suitable to the product being sterilized.

For normal production, a sterilization operation report will be generated, as shown in Table 9. This report will normally be printed upon completion of a production cycle.

D. Calibration

Metrology is defined as the science of precision and accuracy of measurements. Basic considerations for a metrology program as applied to sterilization are accurate and reliable instrumentation, calibration of instruments to National Bureau of Standards recognized standard, frequency of calibration, documentation of calibration, and a system control for recalibrating instruments periodically.

To check the calibration of a temperature recorder, a test thermometer of known accuracy and a well-agitated constant temperature bath are required.

Remove the temperature probe from the process. Place it in the agitated temperature bath with the test thermometer as close to it as possible. The temperature of the bath should be approximately equal to the midpoint of the range. Allow approximately 5 min before comparing the temperature indication of the recorder with that of the test thermometer. If the temperature indicated by the recorder does not agree with that indicated by the test thermometer, adjust the recorder using the micrometer screw provided.

Data acquisition and reduction refers to a system to collect data, change it into meaningful units, store the data, and process the data. Basically, a data acquisition system can be classified into three categories: manual, semiautomatic, and automatic. A completely manual system would consist of a technician recording the data by hand, changing the units as applicable, storing the data on paper, and processing the data by hand calculations. A fully automatic system is diagramatically shown in Figure 12. Data are fed onto floppy disks for recording and storage, processed by a computer, and fed back to the technician according to a preselected format. A semiautomatic system uses data from three separate sources—a mercury thermometer in the vessel, a circular chart for pressure, and a multipoint automatic recorder for vessel temperature, product control temperatures, and product-vessel temperature differential—all of which are collected and evaluated by a technician.

Table 8 Sterilization Production Monitoring Instrument List

Parameter	Sensor		Output units
	Type	Range	
Vessel pressure	Transducer	0–50 psig	psig
Process water temperature	Resistance temperature device	100–300°F	°F
Vessel process temperature	Resistance temperature device	100–300°F	°F
Temperature set point	Controller output	100–300°F	°F
Pressure set point	Controller output	0–50 psig	psig
Process water flow	Transducer	0–1600	gpm
Cooling water flow	Transducer	0–	gpm
Airflow	Transducer	0–	CFM
Steam supply	Transducer	0–200 psia	psig
Heat exchanger	Transducer	0–100 psia	psig
Water level	Transducer	0–75 in.	in. H_2O
Steam valve	Potentiometer	0–100	%
Vent valve	Potentiometer	0–100	%
Pressure valve	Potentiometer	0–100	%
Mix valve	Potentiometer	0–100	%
Heat exchanger discharge temperature	Copper constantan (type T)	260°F	°F
Cooling water	Copper constantan (type T)	260°F	°F
Cooling water	Copper constantan (type T)	260°F	°F
Vessel temperature	Copper constantan (type T)	260°F	°F
Product temperature	Copper constantan (type T)	260°F	°F
Vessel temperature 2	Copper constantan (type T)	260°F	°F

Table 9 Sterilization Quality Control Report

Sterilizer no. 4 Date 11/26/80 Lot no. J0P122B

Card-O-Timer card no. 01-4-G-1000-1000-01-05 Catalog no. S2120

Start time 08:07:30 Stop time 09:04:54 Duration ______

Mercury thermometer 252.0 °F Vapor pressure 16.2 psig Time 08:12:30

Product Glass Size 1000 ml Fill 1000 ml

Production probe calibration code 1 4 1 2 ______

Vessel performance parameters

Product temperature @ vent close/ exposure step (plastic)	191.7	°F
Vessel temperature @ vent close	231.6	°F
Elapsed time above 250°C	18.0	°F
Maximum exposure step process temperature	252.2	min.
		251.8 °F Avg.
Minimum exposure step process temperature	251.7	°F
Thermometer correlation temperature	251.8	Pressure 15.9
Maximum exposure step process pressure	16.1	
Minimum exposure step process pressure	15.8	
Maximum product temperature	250.5	°F
Maximum cool-down product/ vessel ΔT	42.7	
Maximum cool-down process pressure	17.9	
Minimum cool-down process pressure	17.4	

Pilot bottle F_o

Bottle 1	Total	10.03
Bottle 2	Total	9.68
	Avg.	9.86

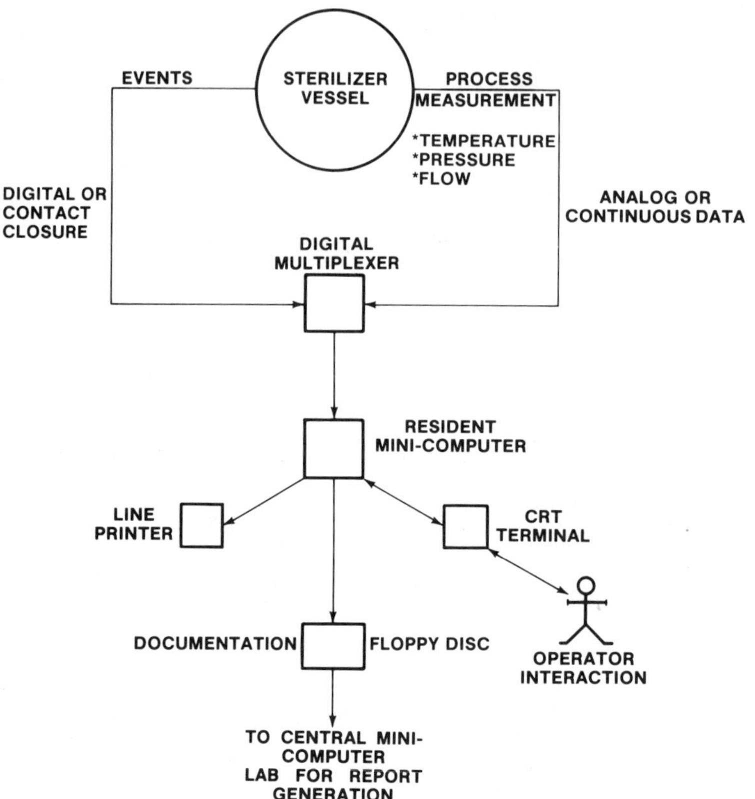

Figure 12 Instrumentation and data collection (development or production vessels).

VIII. VALIDATION OF PROCESS AND EQUIPMENT

To fully demonstrate and verify the effectiveness and reproducibility of a sterilization process and equipment, a series of tests and studies must be conducted. These tests and studies, collectively, are commonly referred to as a qualification or validation process. A brief discussion of each step of the validation process follows.

A. Biological Validation

A measurement and verification of sterilization effectiveness and lethality can be validated by biological indicators. This test is commonly performed by seeding and challenging a sterilizer and its process, under fully loaded conditions, with biological indicators. Upon completion of the processing, the biological indicators are assayed for survivors, in accordance with pre-established procedures. The results of this testing are then analyzed, and an indication of sterilization effectiveness and lethality can be deduced. In qualification of a process and equipment, biological validation must consist of more than one test, usually three consecutive tests.

Some of the key elements in a biological validation program are the number, type, and challenge level of the biological indicator organism, process parameters to be evaluated, location of biological indicators in a load, resistance of the biological indicator, recovery conditions of the biological indicators data, and analysis and interpretative criteria.

Figure 13 shows a typical steam sterilizer and Figure 14 a group of steam sterilizers with the process control panel on the mezzanine, as would be used in such studies. In general, the requirements for a biological validation program are more rigorous than those applied on a routine basis.

B. Process Control and Equipment

The effectiveness of a sterilization process in providing assurance of product sterility is determined by an extensive and well-developed validation and control program. At the onset of validation, engineering checkout and engineering test runs are performed for a critical and confirmatory establishment of process control and equipment. The results of these studies provide the basis for a description of the cycle profile and the specific sterilization parameters to be programmed in order to assure uniform and reproducible results on a cycle-to-cycle basis. Verification of the uniformity and reproducibility of the process is demonstrated through a series of performance tests. Upon completion of each test series, the data are statistically analyzed utilizing a computerized process control and data acquisition system.

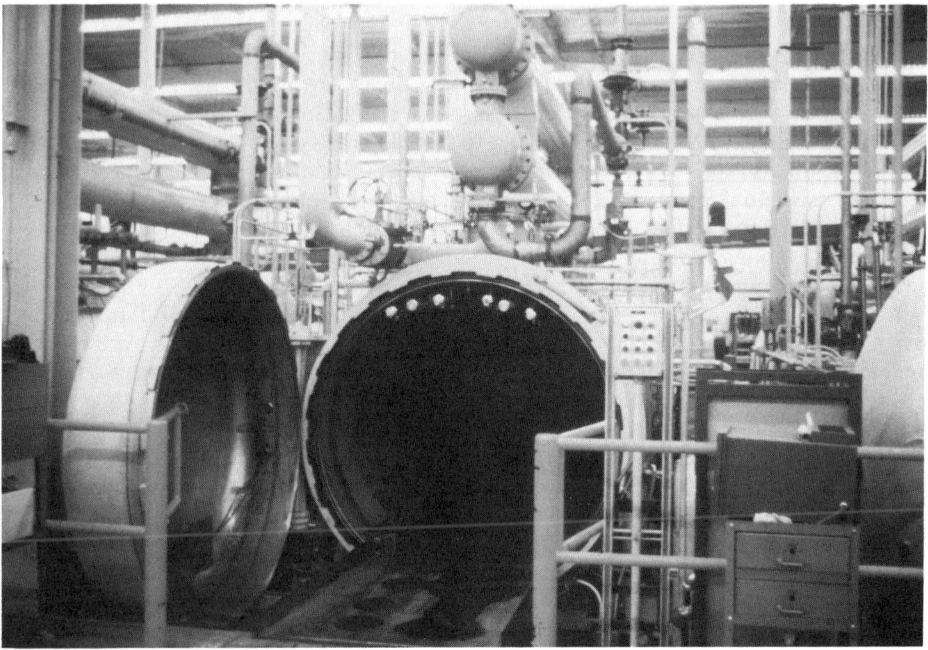

Figure 13 A steam sterilizer with steam headers inside and at top of chamber. View also shows heat exchangers (top) for process water used in sterilizer cycle.

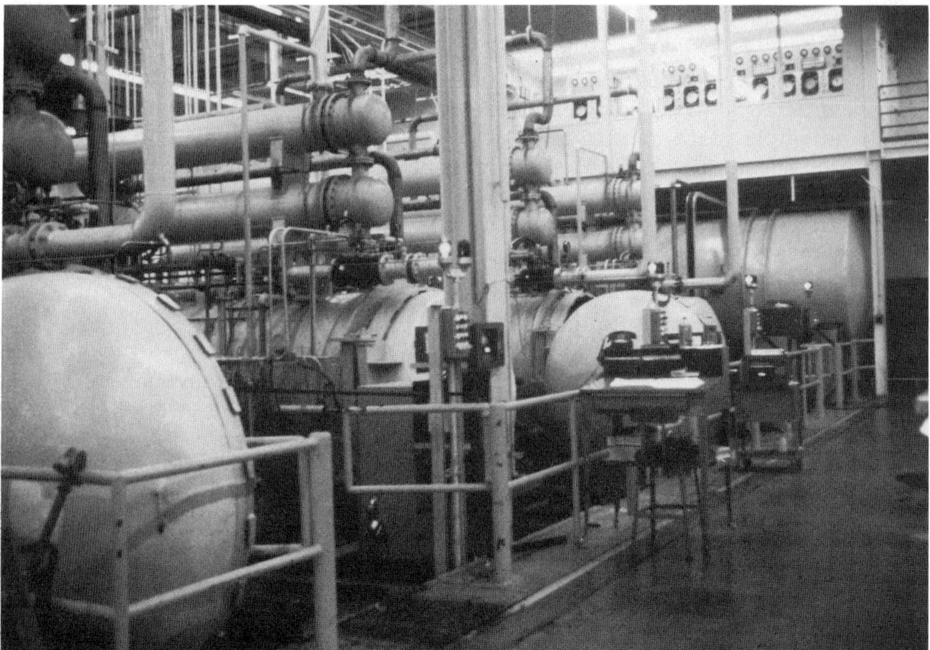

Figure 14 A group of steam sterilizers showing process control panel in top background.

Figure 15 shows a typical computer room, where the acquired validation data are analyzed, and Figure 16 shows a computer program board developed from the validation data for sterilizer operation.

The data system consists of the following subsystems. (a) Thermocouples used as sensors for temperature measurement are copper-constantan (type T) premium grade. The physical and EMF characteristics of these thermocouple assemblies are defined by specification and verified by actual test of each thermocouple at 250°C against an ASTM thermometer and highly accurate platinum resistance probe. (b) The data acquisition system for steam sterilization consists of all the hardware, procedures, and documentation necessary to assure accurate measurement of the output of individual sensors located in the sterilization system. (c) For moist steam sterilization to be effective, the following parameters are supplied (upon completion, sterilization process specifications are established):

Come-up. At the initiation of the cycle, the first parameter to be studied is the rate of rise of vessel temperature at close of vent. During this portion of the cycle, tests are conducted to demonstrate the efficiency of air removal. If the vessel has not been effectively evacuated (of air), there will be no material difference in density between the air pockets within and around the product and the air that has fallen to the areas below the product. These air pockets will remain in the load and greatly retard the penetration of steam.

Heating time is the time required for the entire load of product to reach the selected sterilizing temperature after the vent is closed. During

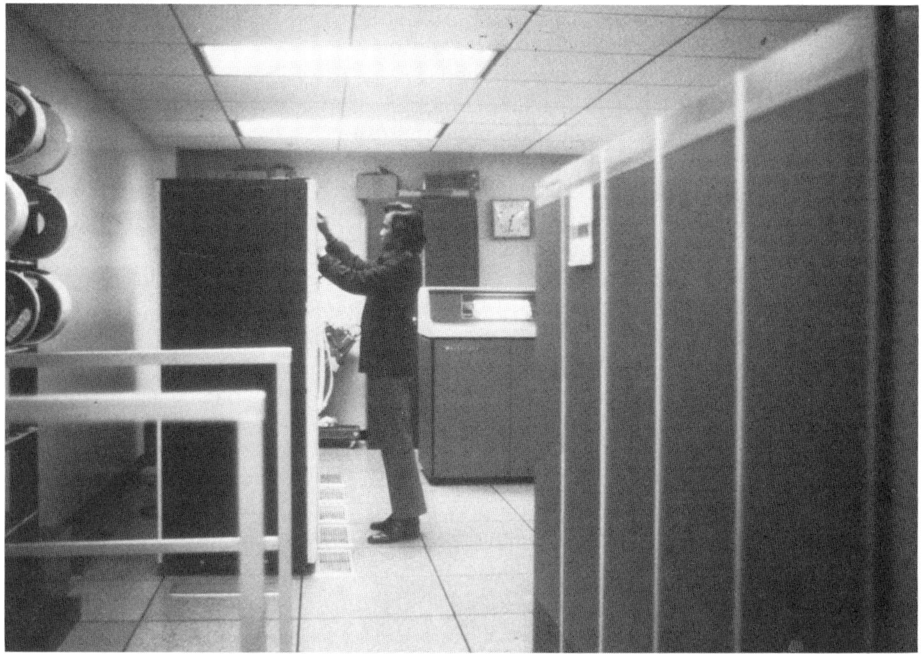

Figure 15 Computer room accommodates reduction and analysis of process validation data.

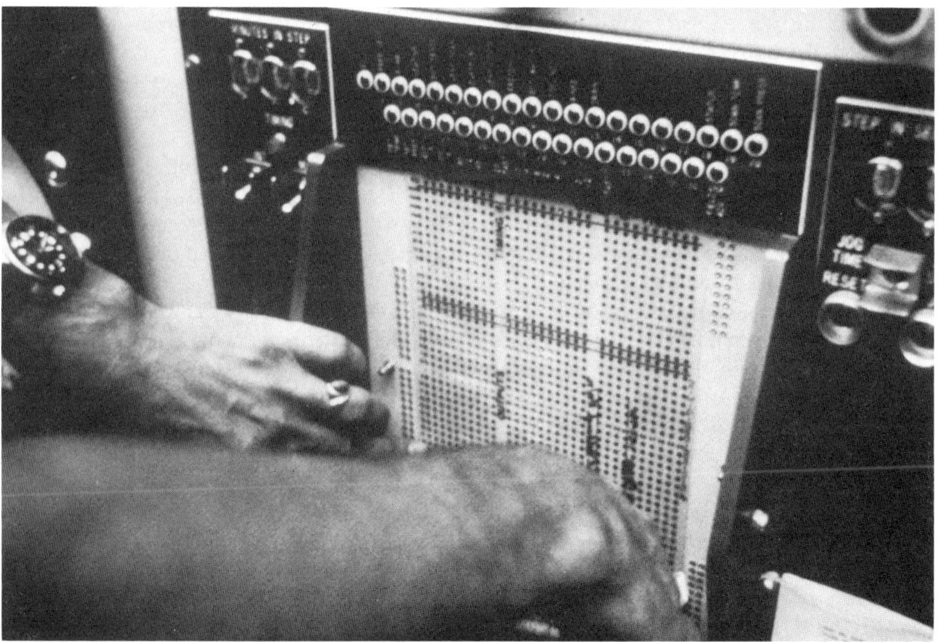

Figure 16 Close-up view of computer program developed for sterilizer cycle operation and control.

this phase of the cycle, the product being sterilized will absorb moisture and heat from the sterilizing medium.

Exposure time is the total time required for achieving sterility of the product being sterilized (F_0). Exposure criteria of time and temperature are based on biological considerations, including the destruction of the indicator organism.

Cool down is the time required to return the product being sterilized to as close to ambient temperature as is practical before removal from the sterilizer. It is also controlled to prevent product damage.

Product cold spot is the coldest spot in the product load during the sterilization process. For glass containers, this has been found to be very near the bottom of the container in the geometric center.

Vessel cold spot is the coldest spot in the vessel and is defined as the location of the container with the lowest heat history.

The program for qualifying the sterilization operation is designed to challenge the equipment and procedure used in the manufacture of product in compliance with good manufacturing practices. The functional operating parameters of the sterilization operations are routinely monitored, recorded, and maintained.

IX. HEALTH PHYSICS

Residuals associated with the sterilization process, such as ozone from radiation sterilizers, heat from ovens and autoclaves, and chemical vapors from ethylene oxide sterilizers, must be considered. Reports [14,15,16] in the literature have shown, for example, that certain goals for animal diets are adversely affected when subjected to ethylene oxide or high radiation doses, resulting in chemical changes in the constituents of the foods. Residual ethylene oxide in sterilized plastic tubing has been reported [16,17,18] to cause hemolysis of blood through the tubing in heart-lung surgery.

It has been the experience of many health care companies and professional personnel in recent years to conduct preliminary evaluations to determine the effect on product materials and on animal systems and, if necessary, provide changes in the manufacturing process to reduce the potential for problems.

Most of the residual products noted above can be determined by chemical methods in materials exposed to the sterilization process, or in the atmosphere where sterilization occurs. However, the exact quantities of these products cannot always be measured due to the insensitivity or the inability of current analytic methods to measure trace quantities of these compounds.

> Manufacturers are encouraged to develop procedures for sterility assurance that have been validated and appropriate for the particular circumstance and the nature of the product through GMP. Such procedures should be established and documented for each product in each manufacturing establishment.
>
> FDA should increasingly assess the adequacy of sterility assurance in manufacture, in NDAs and in inspections for conformity with current GMPs on the basis of appropriately validated

sterilization procedures, rather than on the results of final finished sterility tests [20].

ACKNOWLEDGMENT

The capable assistance of Wayne Rogers in various phases of this work is gratefully acknowledged.

REFERENCES

1. American Medical Association, *Report of the Council of Pharmacy. JAMA* 107:37–38 (1936).
2. K. E. Avis, Sterilization. In *The Theory and Practice of Industrial Pharmacy*, 2nd ed. (L. Lachman, H. A. Lieberman, and J. L. Kanig, eds.). Lea & Febiger, Philadelphia, 1976, pp. 567–585.
3. J. J. Perkins, *Principles and Methods of Sterilization in Health Sciences*, 2nd ed. Charles C. Thomas, Springfield, Illinois, 1970.
4. R. A. Caputo, T. E. Odlag, R. L. Wilkinson, et al. Biological validation of a steam-sterilized product by the fractional exposure method. *J. Paren. Drug Assoc.*, 33:214–221 (1979).
5. J. T. Connor, in process verification of closure-seal integrity. *J. Paren. Drug Assoc.*, 37(1):4–19 (1983).
6. S. Kaye and C. R. Phillips, The sterilizing action of gaseous ethylene oxide. *Am. J. Hyg.*, 50:296–306 (1949).
7. W. G. Murrel and A. D. Warth, Composition and heat resistance of bacterial spores, Spores III. *Am. Soc. Microbiol.*, 1–24 (1965).
8. R. Koch and G. Wolffhugel, Untersuchungen über die Desinfection mit hesser Luft. *Mitt. Kaiser L. Gesund*, 1:301–321 (1881).
9. P. B. Deasy, E. Kuster, and R. F. Timoney, Resistance of *Bacillus subtilis* spores to inactivation by gamma irradiation and heating in the presence of a bactericide. *Appl. Microbiol.*, 20:455 (1970).
10. C. L. Gilbert, V. M. Gambill, D. R. Spiner, R. K. Hoffman, and C. R. Phillips, Effect of moisture in ethylene oxide sterilization. *Appl. Microbiol.*, 12(6):496–504 (1964).
11. K. Kereluk, R. Gammon, and R. S. Floyd, *The Effects of Moisture on the Sporicidal Activity of Ethylene Oxide*. Society for Industrial Microbiology, Columbus, Ohio, 1968.
12. R. S. Ernst and J. J. Shull, Ethylene oxide gaseous sterilization. II. Influence of method of humidification. *Appl. Microbiol.*, 10:338 (1962).
13. C. R. Phillips and S. Kaye, The sterilizing action of gaseous ethylene oxide. II. Sterilization of contaminated objects with ethylene oxide and related compounds. *Am. J. Hyg.*, 50:280–288 (1949).
14. R. R. Ernst and J. J. Shull, Ethylene oxide gaseous sterilization. I. Concentration and temperature effects. *Appl. Microbiol.*, 10(4): 341 (1962).
15. I. J. Pflug and R. G. Holcomb, Principles of thermal destruction of microorganisms. In *Disinfection, Sterilization, and Preservation*, 2nd ed. (S. S. Block, ed.). Lea & Febiger, Philadelphia, 1977, p. 939.
16. G. L. Gilbert, V. M. Gambill, D. R. Spiner, R. K. Hoffman, and C. R. Phillips, Effect of moisture in ethylene oxide sterilization. *Appl. Microbiol.*, 12(6):498 (1964).

17. C. F. Schmidt, Thermal resistance of microorganisms. In *Antiseptics, Disinfectants, Fungicides, and Chemical and Physical Sterilization*, 2nd ed. (G. F. Reddish, ed.). Lea & Febiger, Philadelphia, 1957, pp. 831–884.
18. D. J. Finney, *Statistical Method in Biological Assay*. Hafner, New York, 1952.
19. C. O. Ball and F. C. Olson, *Sterilization in Food Technology*. McGraw-Hill, New York, 1957.
20. *Pharmacopeial Forum*, 6(4):357 (1980).
21. K. Kereluk and R. S. Floyd, *Ethylene Oxide Sterilization—A Current Review of Principles and Practices*. American Sterilizer Co., Erie, Pennsylvania, 1969.

2

Formulation for Large Volume Parenterals

Levit J. Demorest*

Consultant, Quality Assurance Systems, Danville, California

I. INTRODUCTION

The United States Pharmacopeia provides the following definition for large volume parenterals (LVPs): "Where used in this Pharmacopeia, the designation Large-Volume Solution applies to an Injection that is intended for intravenous use and is packaged in containers holding 100 ml or more."

The Food and Drug Administration has recommended that a broader definition be adopted:

> "Large Volume Parenteral" means a terminally sterilized aqueous drug product packaged in a single-dose container with a capacity of 100 milliliters or more and intended to be administered or used in man. It includes intravenous infusions, irrigating solutions, peritoneal dialysates and blood collecting units with anticoagulant. The term "large volume parenteral" does not include any biological drug product subject to section 351 of the Public Health Service Act (42 U.S.C. 262) [1].

This definition recognizes that there are some circumstances, other than intravenous administration, in which sterile fluids are used and failure to maintain microbiological standards would represent a risk to the patient.

The National Coordinating Committee for Large Volume Parenterals, a group representing manufacturers, users, regulatory agencies, and health care professionals, used a broader definition [2], similar to that of the FDA.

Commercial production of LVPs has grown from a small beginning in the 1930s to a specialized and major segment of the pharmaceutical industry. Early production consisted of only a few formulations packaged in half-liter

---

*Former affiliation: Cutter Laboratories, Berkeley, California (Retired)

and liter glass containers. Over 500 million units of LVPs were sold in 1983, and the users were offered numerous formulations in glass and in semirigid or flexible plastic containers, sized from 100 to 1000 ml [3].

Formulations have been developed to

a. Supply the water, electrolytes, and simple carbohydrates needed by the body
b. Act as the vehicle for infusion of drugs that are compatible in the solution
c. Supply nutritional requirements when the nutrients cannot be taken orally
d. Provide solutions to correct acid-base balance in the body
e. Act as plasma expanders
f. Promote diuresis when the body is retaining fluids
g. Act as dialyzing agents in patients with impaired kidney function

Recent years have seen an increase in the number of amino acid formulations that provide nutritional support and the use of lipid emulsions to supply calories and essential lipids. There are specialized solutions for renal support, hepatic support, and the newborn.

Intravenous (IV) administration provides a route that permits quick dispersion of large amounts of fluids and drugs throughout the body in order to achieve a rapid therapeutic effect. The rate of infusion can be controlled to establish and maintain the desired levels; IV pumps may be used when the administration rate must be controlled very precisely. Intravenous administration, however, bypasses protective mechanisms of the body, and the onset of adverse reactions, which may come about from many causes, can be as rapid as the beneficial effects. The National Intravenous Therapy Association (NITA) and the Centers for Disease Control (CDC) have developed recommendations for procedures to be followed during IV therapy [4]. The procedures are designed to minimize undesired reactions.

II. CONCEPTS OF FORMULATION

A. Physiological Parameters

The physiological parameters of an LVP formulation are limits on those characteristics of the solution that impart some effect on the biochemistry of the body.

Some constituents that are basic to the sustenance of life in the human organism can be influenced by IV therapy. These are water, electrolytes, carbohydrates, amino acids, lipids, and micro-nutrients such as vitamins, minerals, and trace elements.

The living cell, the body's basic unit, is bathed in tissue fluid kept constant in composition by the interaction of many processes, some of which are outside the scope of this chapter. Alteration in the amount or composition of tissue fluids can cause significant physiological derangements. Such imbalances may occur as a major or minor feature of illness, trauma, or surgical procedures. Under such circumstances it is necessary to anticipate and correct deficits and imbalances by administration of suitable fluids.

Table 1 Electrolyte Content of Fluid Compartments

Electrolytes	Intravascular (mEq/liter)	Interstitial (mEq/liter)	Intracellular (mEq/liter)
Cations			
Sodium (Na^+)	142	145	10
Potassium (K^+)	4	4	160
Calcium (Ca^{2+})	5	5	2
Magnesium (Mg^{2+})	2	2	26
Total	154	156	198
Anions			
Chloride (Cl^-)	102	115	2
Bicarbonate (HCO_3^-)	27	30	8
Phosphate (HPO_4^{2-})	2	2	120
Sulfate (SO_4^{2-})	1	1	20
Organic acids	6	7	—
Protein	16	1	48
Total	154	156	198

The body fluids, named for the compartments in which they are found, are intravascular (within the blood vessels), intracellular (within the cells), and interstitial (within the space between cells). Extracellular fluid is the total of intravascular and interstitial fluids. The fluids consist of water containing a mix of electrolytes, neutral solutes in a wide range of high and low molecular weights, and undissolved substances. The composition of each fluid differs, yet a chemical balance is maintained in each fluid. Approximate figures for the electrolytic composition of body fluids are shown in Table 1.

Extracellular fluid is characterized by high concentrations of sodium and chloride ions. The intravascular fluid contains a much higher concentration of protein than is found in interstitial fluid because the large plasma protein molecules are not diffusable. The retention of protein anions on one side of the semipermeable membrane causes a redistribution of the anions which are permeable, in order to maintain chemical balance [5]. As a result, the concentration of other anions is lower in intravascular fluid than in interstitial. The following section on tonicity will provide explanations of the movement of solvents and solutes through membranes and the restrictions on such movement. Intracellular fluid is characterized by very high concentrations of potassium, phosphate, and protein.

An LVP formulation must be developed to ensure that desired levels of the solution are administered in a therapeutically active and available form.

In order to obtain the desired response, the physiological intent of the formulation must be considered and the physiological, chemical, and physical properties of the formulation defined. The formulator must understand the biochemistry of the body and the chemistry of the ingredients of the solution because it is through their interaction that the result is achieved. These factors are discussed in the section to follow.

B. Formulation Parameters

1. *Physiological*

Body fluids rapidly exchange both water and electrolytes between the cells and extracellular compartments, maintaining equilibrium within and between the compartments. The movement of solvent and solute through the semipermeable membranes that separate the compartments is called osmosis. If the concentration of solutes in adjoining compartments differs, water moves very rapidly into the compartment with the higher concentration in the effort to establish equilibrium. Simultaneously, disassociated solutes diffuse at a slower rate to the compartment with the lower concentration. Because some components of the fluid cannot move through the semipermeable membrane, the fluid in the compartment must make adjustments to maintain its own ionic equilibrium (mentioned previously with respect to the difference in the ions contained in extracellular and interstitial fluids).

The resistance to unrestricted movement between compartments is defined as osmotic pressure and is expressed as osmoles per kilogram (Osmol/kg) or, more conveniently, milliosmoles per kilogram. (mOsmol/kg). Osmolarity values of dilute solutions can be calculated and their levels expressed as milliosmoles per liter (mOsmol/liter) by using the formula

$$\text{mOsmol/liter} = \frac{\text{gm/liter of solute}}{\text{mol. wt. of solute}} \times 1000 \times \text{no. of ions}$$

Sodium chloride, for example, has a molecular weight of 58.5 and forms two ions, Na^+ and Cl^-, in solution. The osmolarity of 0.9% Sodium Chloride Injection would be calculated as mOsmol/liter = 9/58.5 × 1000 × 2 = 307.7, rounded to 308. Table 2 lists the osmolarity of commonly used LVPs.

An immediate concern of introducing large amounts of fluid into the body system is that of maintaining the "tone" of the living body cells. Red blood cells (RBC) circulate in blood serum, which has an osmolarity of 306. Using osmolarity as a measure of tonicity, one would expect no physical change in the RBC if 0.9% Sodium Chloride Injection, with an osmolarity of 308, were infused into the vein. This is the case, as can be demonstrated by putting RBC into the 0.9% Sodium Chloride Injection and microscopically examining the cells for physical change. No changes result, and the solution is termed isotonic. If RBC are placed in a hypertonic solution, for example 20% dextrose (1010 mOsmol/liter), the water in the cell will diffuse out, causing the cell to shrivel. Conversely, RBC placed in a hypotonic solution, such as 0.45% sodium chloride (154 mOsmol/liter), will swell due to the flow of water into the cell and, if the effect is great enough, may rupture. For this reason, Water for Injection (WFI), which has no solids, despite its name is never injected alone. Table 3 shows the relationship between osmolarity and tonicity.

Tonicity, as defined by numerical calculation, is only one consideration that must be taken into account and it must be used with judgment. For example, a solution of 1.85% urea is isotonic but quite unsuitable for

Table 2 Osmolarity of Common LVPs

Solution	Mol. wt. (g)	Concentration (g/liter)	No. ions formed	Milliosmoles per liter	Tonicity
Plasma				306	Isotonic
Sodium chloride	58.5	9.0	2	308	Isotonic
		4.5	2	154	Hypotonic
Dextrose (hyd.)	198	50.0	None	252	Isotonic
		200.0	None	1010	Hypertonic
Dextrose-sodium chloride					
Dextrose	198	25.0	None	126	
NaCl	58.5	4.5	2	154	
			Total	280	Isotonic
Dextrose	198	50.0	None	252	
NaCl	58.5	2.0	2	68	
			Total	320	Isotonic
Ringer's injection					
NaCl	58.5	8.6	2	294	
KCl	74.6	0.3	2	8	
$CaCl_2$	111	0.33	3	9	
			Total	311	Isotonic
Lactated Ringer's					
NaCl	58.5	6.0	2	205	
KCl	74.6	0.3	2	8	
$CaCl_2$	111	0.2	3	5	
Na lactate	112	3.1	2	55	
			Total	273	Isotonic

Table 3 Osmolarity—Tonicity

Osmolarity (mOsmol/liter)	Tonicity
>350	Hypertonic
329–350	Slightly hypertonic
270–328	Isotonic
250–269	Slightly hypotonic
0–249	Hypotonic

administration at the rate isotonic solutions are normally infused; it can cause hemolysis as well as upset the body's nitrogen balance. A solution of amino acids, which is hypertonic at about 850 mOsmol/liter, may be life sustaining and the problems of tonicity can be overcome if it is introduced slowly into a large vein where there is ample blood volume to assure dilution. Hypertonic and hypotonic solutions can be used if administered slowly. The rates of shift of water into or out of the vascular system are determined by the rate of administration, rate of diffusion of the solute, and tonicity of the solution.

2. *Physicochemical*

Solubility

Most of the solutes used in LVP solutions are extremely soluble relative to their therapeutic concentrations. This means that solubility is rarely a consideration during formulation, and once in solution, the ingredients remain dissolved under normal storage and handling conditions. There are occasional reports of crystallization in highly concentrated solutions, such as mannitol; this is caused by a reduction in solubility when the bottle is cold and the crystals go back into solution readily when the bottle is warmed. The solubility of mannitol is 13 g per 100 ml water at 14°C; the package inserts for mannitol solutions caution the user that concentrations over 15% may show a tendency to crystallize.

In some cases, as with amino acid or high-concentration dextrose solutions, the temperature of the water for injection is elevated during mixing. Although the ingredients are soluble at lower temperatures, minimizing the preparation time reduces the time the solution is exposed to ambient microorganisms. The order in which ingredients are added to the mix tank may have an effect on how rapidly the mix is completed or whether it can be completed. Suby's solution G provides an example of order of mixing. Each 100 ml contains 2.65 g citric acid monohydrate, 0.808 g sodium citrate dihydrate (tribasic), and 0.384 g anhydrous magnesium oxide. Citric acid must be the first ingredient added to the mix in order to lower the pH; otherwise the magnesium oxide, which is essentially insoluble in water, will not go into solution. In general, solubility only becomes a consideration when the LVP is used as a carrier for other drugs.

Control of pH

The pH of a formulation must be considered from the following standpoints: the effect on the body when the solution is administered, the effect on stability of the product, the effect on the container-closure system, and the possible degradation of drugs that are added.

The pH of blood serum is normally 7.35–7.45, and the immediate effect of intravenously introducing fluids outside this range depends on the buffer capacity of the solution, determined by the amount of weak acids or bases that are part of the formulation. The solution is rapidly diluted in the bloodstream, and the body's buffering system can maintain the proper pH level when high or low pH LVPs are administered, although it does so less easily if the solutions are highly buffered. The proximity of the vein wall to the point of undiluted flow of solution makes the wall susceptible to irritation from solutions with high or low pH. This is one reason that injection sites are changed frequently during prolonged IV therapy.

Solutions with pH values approaching or over 7.0 accelerate glass attack and must be packaged in Type I glass. Since this glass is resistant to attack by alkaline solutions, it is used to prevent the pH from rising even higher. Other problems associated with degradation of the glass surface, such as the formation of glass flakes in the product, can be avoided by the use of Type I glass.

Vehicles

Water for Injection, USP, is the vehicle used for all large volume parenterals. All ingredients are dissolved, and the resulting aqueous solution is clear and generally colorless. The intravenous fat emulsion, an LVP that may be administered alone or in combination with amino acid and dextrose solutions for total parenteral nutrition therapy, is the exception. Essential fatty acids, egg phospholipid, glycerin, and Water for Injection are homogenized to produce a stable emulsion with fat particles approximately 0.5 μm in size.

Physical Parameters

The sensitivity of a solution when exposed to light and changes that might occur during exposure to extremes in temperature is determined during the developmental phase of a formulation. Certain vitamin solutions require protection from light, for example in the form of an amber bottle or an opaque unit carton. Solutions with high concentrations of dextrose or combinations with dextrose that have a tendency to develop slight discoloration with age will do so more rapidly if stored at high temperatures. The physical parameters that are defined for a solution are stated on the labeling and packaging inserts.

Packaging Parameters

The chapters on containers and closures in this text provide detailed information about the characteristics of materials available for packaging parenteral medications. New or modified plastics, elastomers, or surface treatments for glass are reported routinely from the research departments of the suppliers of the items. Out of this research, as well, comes development of potential applications. The formulator of LVPs would look with interest at polyvinyl chloride resins that do not contain DEHP (diethyl hexyl phthalate) as a plasticizer; fat-containing fluids, such as fat emulsions, extract DEHP from the plastic. Rubber closures of new formulations or improved coatings that have the potential for reducing particle levels or extractables would be subjected to the screening process. Reports that Type I glass treated with sulfur dioxide makes the glass surface less reactive would be carefully examined. The point of this, for the LVP formulator, is to take maximum advantage of the technical resources offered by the supplier. The supplier's laboratories can be particularly helpful during the early screening process. If the supplier is given basic information about the formulation, such as ingredients, pH, and proposed sterilization cycle, the number of candidates suitable for a particular application can be reduced to the few that seem to have the best potential for success. Additionally, some suppliers may conduct studies of the formulation in contact with materials they have recommended. The manufacturer of the LVP will have to conduct the final studies needed for support of the new drug application (NDA), but time will have been saved and unnecessary costs avoided.

As studies begin for extractables and degradation, any processing steps to which the packaging materials will be subjected must also be studied. Cleaning components before initiating tests is a basic step; however, the researcher should not be misled by high particle counts that may result from insufficient cleaning. Failure to remove, for example, a mold release agent that would be removed by normal cleaning or failure to extract an extractable that does not show up until later in the development process may occur if the cleaning in the laboratory does not duplicate normal process cleaning. Failure to treat the materials as they will be handled in the production process—or as nearly as it can be stimulated at this stage—may result in unreliable data.

The supplier of packaging materials also may have helpful suggestions about physical design features that will contribute to better handling on filling and packaging lines. Glass containers, for example, are less subject to damage from impact and thermal shock if designed to minimize residual stress points. Changing a radius at the bottom of the container may improve flow of the molten glass during molding and reduce stress; changing the point of impact between containers can reduce breakage rates and potential damage. Slight changes in the outer diameter of the plug of a stopper might be necessary because of differences in durometer and compression set between the current and proposed elastomers. Design features may promote the "company image" and provide convenience for the customer but must, above all, maintain the solution free from microbiological contamination and result in a product that is functional at the point of use.

Items that have been handled carefully in the production plant will move through various transport and storage conditions until the expiration date. The outer packaging must protect the units during this period, which may include several years of less than ideal handling by shippers and other handlers. High-burst-strength corrugated cardboard boxes with partitions inside to provide separation between containers are commonly used as outer packs. Additional corrugated pads inside the box will provide cushioning if the container is dropped; the partitions not only separate the contents but provide support when the boxes are put on pallets and stored in high stacks in warehouses.

3. *Stabilization of LVPs*

Added Substances

Chelating agents, buffering agents, and antioxidants, commonly added to parenteral medications, are rarely used in LVPs. By their nature and use, LVPs introduce large amounts of fluid and chemicals into the body. The active ingredients are present for a therapeutic effect, and although present in only very low percentages, added substances might, in total, have an effect on the patient who receives many bottles of solution during the course of treatment. Any substance that is added must be shown to be necessary for maintaining effectiveness of the product and must not be harmful to the patient. Steps taken by the producer during selection of ingredients and packaging materials and during processing generally obviate the need for substances to be added to the final product.

Such metals as iron, copper, or calcium, which are bound by chelating agents to form a soluble compound or to form a compound that will precipitate during a purification step, are present in only minute quantities in the ingredients of LVPs. The active ingredients, such as salts and sugars, as well as the acids and bases used to adjust pH, are the product of well-defined chemical processes and the quality is specified in the compendia or formulation specifications. Buffering agents are not added as such, although weak acids and bases, which are used to adjust pH, can add to the buffering capacity of the solution.

Antioxidants, such as sodium bisulfite or sodium metabisulfite, are part of some LVP formulations. They are added to protect the active ingredients from the action of oxygen in the solution or headspace of the container. The presence of oxygen, even very small amounts, can accelerate color formation or degradation of such products as 5% Dextrose in Lactated Ringer's or amino acid solutions. In lieu of the addition of an antioxidant, which might be added in concentrations of up to 0.1%, processing to displace the oxygen with an inert gas, usually nitrogen, may be done during mixing and filling operations. If both nitrogen and an antioxidant are used, the use of nitrogen will reduce the amount of bisulfite needed to protect the product during its shelf life. If nitrogen protection alone does not prevent color formation, the investigator must conduct experiments to bracket the amount of antioxidant needed. Based on the results from previous work with similar formulations, maximum and minimum amounts will be determined and added for the first tests of a proposed formulation. Data from successive tests will indicate how much to raise the minimum and lower the maximum until the desired result is achieved. The goal is to protect the product using the minimum amount of antioxidant.

C. Electrolytes, Carbohydrates, and Nutritionals

Examples of LVP formulations typical of the category, along with characteristics relating to the parameters that have been described in the previous sections, are shown in Tables 4, 5, and 6. They are only a few of the many formula variations that represent the basic theme of each grouping.

1. Electrolyte Solutions

Each 100 ml of Sodium Chloride Injection, 0.9%, contains 0.9 g sodium chloride in water for injection (Table 4). It will correct extracellular fluid and electrolyte losses from such causes as vomiting and diarrhea. If heart and kidney functions are normal, it can be administered very rapidly, up to 2000 ml/hr, in cases of extreme need.

Each 100 ml of Multiple Electrolyte Injection contains 0.526 g sodium chloride, 0.368 g sodium acetate, 0.502 g sodium gluconate, 0.037 g potassium chloride, and 0.030 g magnesium chloride hexahydrate in Water for

Table 4 Electrolyte Solutions

Solution	0.9% Sodium Chloride Injection	Multiple electrolyte		Lactated Ringer's Injection	
		plain	with 5% dextrose	plain	with 5% dextrose
pH	6.0	7.3	5.6	6.5	5.1
mOsmol/liter	308	294	553	273	524
Calories per liter	0	0	170	9	179
Anti-oxidant	No	No	Yes	No	No
Buffering capacity	Low	Low	Low	High	High
Light protection	No	No	No	No	No
Container[a]	G/P	G	G	G/P	G/P

[a]G = glass, P = plastic.

Table 5 Carbohydrate Solutions

Solution	5% Dextrose Injection	10% Fructose Injection	10% Invert Sugar Injection
pH	4.8	3.8	3.9
mOsmol/liter	252	555	555
Calories per liter	170	400	400
Anti-oxidant	No	No	No
Buffering capacity	Low	Low	Low
Light protection	No	No	No
Container[a]	G/P	G	G

[a]G = glass, P = plastic.

Injection. This solution has an ionic composition very similar to that of normal plasma; note that it is isotonic and the pH is close to that of extracellular fluid. The addition of potassium helps overcome potassium deficiencies that may develop due to stress in the hospitalized patient. The gluconate serves as a precursor to the bicarbonate ion and the acetate is metabolized rapidly to provide an alkalinizing effect. The addition of dextrose, 5.0 g per 100 ml, provides calories to the patient; this ingredient causes a downward shift in pH and rise in osmolarity. Sodium bisulfite, 0.03 g, is added to prevent discoloration during sterilization and storage. The multiple electrolyte injection is an example of a solution that must be packaged in Type I glass because of its high pH, 7.3.

Each 100 ml of Lactated Ringer's Injection contains 0.60 g sodium chloride, 0.03 g potassium chloride, 0.02 g calcium chloride, and 0.31 g sodium lactate (anhydrous) in Water for Injection. The lactate ion in this solution is metabolized in the liver to glycogen, which becomes carbon dioxide and water, requiring the consumption of hydrogen ions; the result is an alkalinizing effect. Again, the addition of dextrose, 5.0 g per 100 ml, is for the caloric value and results in lower pH and higher osmolarity.

Electrolyte solutions make it possible to maintain or, in the case of specific clinical disorders, bring about the balanced levels of water and electrolytes required for proper body functioning. The many combinations of electrolytes that have been formulated and are sold commercially reduce the need for the hospital pharmacist to "tailor" a solution for individual patients.

2. *Carbohydrate Solutions*

A standard solution that provides a source of water for hydration and carbohydrate calories is 5% Dextrose Injection (Table 5). The dextrose is metabolized rapidly, and the water moves into other body compartments. If it is necessary to replace large losses of body water the injection can be administered, the patient's condition permitting, at a rate as high as 8–10 ml/min. Higher concentrations of the dextrose injection provide more calories without overloading the body with water.

A 10% Fructose Injection may be used in most conditions in place of glucose or invert sugar solutions. Fructose has been shown to be a better glycogen former than dextrose and is metabolized better than glucose under stress conditions. It is a better "nitrogen-sparer" than glucose and can be administered rapidly with less loss by renal excretion.

Invert sugar is an equal mixture of dextrose and fructose and is formed by the hydrolysis of sucrose. The fructose portion of 10% Invert Sugar Injection possesses the advantages that have been cited.

Each of these carbohydrates may be combined with electrolytes to provide for specific needs that are indicated by a patient's blood chemistry. Some of the commercial solutions available, in addition to those listed, are

2½% Dextrose and 0.45% Sodium Chloride Injection
2½% Dextrose and 0.9% Sodium Chloride Injection
5% Dextrose and 0.2% Sodium Chloride Injection
10% Dextrose and 0.9% Sodium Chloride Injection
10% Invert Sugar in 0.9% Sodium Chloride Injection

Table 6 Solutions for Nutrition

	8.5% Amino Acids Injection	10% Intravenous Fat Emulsion
pH	6.6	8.0
mOsmol/liter	850	280
Calories per liter	—	1100
Antioxidant	Yes	No
Buffering capacity	Moderate	Low
Light protection	Yes	No
Container	Glass	Glass
Total nitrogen (g/liter)	13	—
Ratio of amino acids (essential/total)	0.48	—

3. *Nutritional Solutions*

For proper nutrition an individual must have an intake of carbohydrates, amino acids, and fatty acids, along with trace minerals and vitamins. Carbohydrate and amino acid solutions have been available as injections for a number of years and can supply part of the patient's nutritional needs. Problems of toxicity, stability of the emulsion, particle size, and formation of free fatty acids had to be overcome before fat emulsions became viable products. Successful commercial production of fat emulsions that could be administered intravenously made it possible to provide the additional calories and essential fatty acids needed to implement total parenteral nutrition (TPN) for the patient unable to take food enterally (Table 6).

The first fat emulsion, which had been developed and used in Europe for many years, was released in the United States in 1975. At the time of its introduction, soybean oil supplied the fatty acids, the shelf life of the product was 18 months, the product required storage at 2–8°C, and there were warnings not to add other substances to the emulsion.

The value of well-designed investigations of stability, compatibility, and formulation modification is reflected by the products now in the market. Safflower oil as well as soybean oil provides the fatty acids, package inserts state the maximum storage temperature is now 25 or 30°C, depending on the manufacturer, and guidelines for the addition of trace minerals as well as mixing with dextrose and amino acid injections have been established.

The fat emulsion listed in Table 6 has a formula in which each 100 ml contains 10 g soybean oil, 1.2 g egg yolk phospholipids, 2.25 g glycerin, and Water for Injection. Sodium hydroxide is used to adjust the pH to approximately 8.0. In the soybean oil, the major fatty acids are linoleic (50%) and oleic (26%), with palmitic, linolenic, stearic, myristic, arachidic, and behenic acids making up the remainder. The egg yolk provides a mixture of naturally occurring phospholipids; the glycerin and Water for Injection are necessary for formation of the emulsion. Size of the fat particles is controlled to about 0.5 μm; this permits infusion without the complications associated with larger particles. The emulsion is opaque, so the visible signs of incompatibility with additives might be concealed, although breaking of the emulsion or fatty acids floating on the surface can be seen. The user should adhere to the guidelines and limitations for mixing that are listed in package inserts.

When purified, crystalline L-amino acids became available, it became possible to combine precise amounts of those desired in a formulation. Complete amino acid solutions provide the eight essential and ten nonessential amino acids. Studies of blood serum levels of amino acids in normal individuals have established the ranges of each that is present and provide the basis for formulation. Each manufacturer of these solutions has particular combinations of amino acids that have been shown to be effective. An essential amino acid cannot be converted to another acid and must be used by the body to fill a need for that particular one or be broken into uric acid. A nonessential acid may be used if needed, metabolized to another nonessential acid that is needed or converted to uric acid. When amino acids are administered parenterally, adequate calories must be provided concurrently to bring about synthesis of proteins; high-concentration dextrose injection or fat emulsion provides the source of calories. Concentrations of amino acid solutions vary from 3.5 to 11.5%; the total nitrogen available is the sum of that contributed by each amino acid. The number and quantity of amino acids in a formulation will vary depending on the body deficiency the solution is meant to remedy. With some amino acids, however, there are limitations on the amount that will go into solution because the presence of other amino acids has an effect on solubility; the formulation of amino acid solutions is difficult because of this interaction and changing behavior. The ratio of essential amino acids to total amino acids in solutions now available varies between 0.39 and 0.66, depending on what is included in the formulation.

D. Stress Testing

Stress testing, testing after exposure to exaggerated conditions, is done throughout the developmental process and is designed to establish "safety factors." The data obtained from chemical, microbiological, biological, and physical tests, when compared with the results of tests on samples prepared under normal conditions, provide additional assurance that a safe and effective product will reach the market. Stress testing may take many forms.

Materials that will be in contact with the solution are subjected to extractions that far exceed the normal surface-volume ratios; the extracts are used for chemical, physical, biological, and toxicity testing. The first step in qualifying an immediate container or closure would be the development of tests that establish the identity of the component. These tests, which should be performed on several batches from the supplier, will also provide a measure of variation between batches, e.g., the durometer readings of rubber closures or melt flow index of plastic compounds, and later become part of the acceptance criteria for incoming shipments. Tests for plastic and rubber are listed in USP XXI (page 1235); in addition, the LVP manufacturer may prepare concentrated extracts for tissue culture tests, a screening test for direct cell effects, and tests in rodents for the LD_{50} dosage, the dosage lethal to 50% of the test animals. The identity of the material extracted can be established chemically, quantified, and, with the results of the biological tests, related to its effect on humans.

The sterilization cycle is challenged by seeding solutions in their final container with heat-resistant microorganisms. The level of organisms used is high enough to establish, by testing after sterilization, that the possibility of a survivor is one in a million. Similar challenges are performed at locations that may reach sterilizing temperature at a time that differs from that of the solution; the interface between a closure and container is representative of such a location. Filled containers are sent through two or three sterilization cycles and then checked for physical or chemical change. The data can be used to support procedures that define the action to be taken in the event of an equipment malfunction or power failure during the sterilization cycle.

Drop tests of the filled containers in their overpack demonstrate the protection afforded during rough handling. One such test is a 5-ft drop of the container with either the top, bottom, or side as the point of impact; an assessment of the resultant damage can be made.

Thermal shock tests, internal pressure tests, and impact resistance tests are measures of how well a glass container will withstand the rigors of sterilization and subsequent handling. The procedures for these tests are given in manuals that are available from the American Society for Testing Materials (ASTM). The tests are conducted by the glass suppliers on a scheduled basis; the LVP manufacturer may not have the equipment needed and will have to work with the supplier in order to get test results.

Alternating cycles of low and high temperatures provide information about how the solution and container react to adverse storage conditions. Such an evaluation may become part of the initial stability evaluation or the subject of a special stability study.

Stress testing programs should be well defined and documented so that reliable data are obtained. A protocol should be prepared for each test and, at the least, include the purpose of the test, the test method, and the rules for interpretation of the data that are generated. The same data can become part of a submission for a new drug application.

E. Stability Evaluation

The labeling for LVPs must bear an expiration date. As with other drugs, the establishment of an expiration date is to assure the product meets the standards of identity, strength, quality, and purity at the time of use. The period of time between release for distribution and the expiration date is called shelf life or market life, and during this period the LVP must meet all the specifications established for the product. The testing, which is done to establish the expiration date and continued to support the date, must be part of a company's ongoing stability program. The total stability program includes initial studies, proposed product studies, new product studies, established product studies, and special studies.

Initial studies are done on a laboratory scale, generally under extreme test conditions, to screen the formula and proposed packaging. Although the data may not be precise and the test conditions not representative of conditions of real exposure, such testing serves to differentiate between the unsuitable and the promising in a search for the optimum. The intent of such a study is to force degradation, if it is going to occur, to occur in a short time.

Storing samples at 50°C and testing monthly during a 3-month period, for example, will provide preliminary information about the suitability of the combination of solution, container, and closure. If the container is glass and there is a rise in pH level or particle count, the appropriate action would be to examine the results attained after reducing or buffering the initial pH of the solution or changing to a more resistant glass, Type I rather than Type II. Weighing solutions in plastic containers before and after storage will provide information about loss of content due to moisture vapor transmission (MVT); an increase in assay values of the ingredients is also an indicator of MVT. The solution should be tested for levels of any known or anticipated degradation products, as well as leachables identified during the early screening process. A change in color or formation of degradation products could indicate the need for an antioxidant in the formula or the use of an inert gas, such as nitrogen, for protection of the product during processing. Light sensitivity can be determined by placing samples in a light cabinet where they are exposed to a specified number of lumens and comparing the results of tests for color and degradation with the results from samples that have been shielded from light. Autoclaving at 121°C for 60 min will provide information about the stability of the product during sterilization; changes in pH, assay values, particulate levels, and color should be examined to determine if they are acceptable.

A study on proposed products involves stability testing on premarket batches. The data may be used to establish initial expiration dating, support an NDA submission, or be part of the decision-making process that determines whether to proceed with the new product. The batches, which are scaled up in size, may be prepared in a pilot plant or production facility. Care should be taken that all processing steps are well defined and are as close as possible to those that will be used later. The study must be designed carefully and be covered by written procedures that include processing parameters, statistical criteria, storage conditions, and test methods. An adequate number of batches must be tested to provide statistical validity of the proposed expiration dating. A typical study would include both accelerated and shelf storage samples. The accelerated study samples, stored at 30, 40, and 50°C, would be tested as they go into storage and at 30-, 60-, and 90-day intervals. The samples at ambient temperature would be tested at time of initial storage and at 30 days, 60 days, 6 months, and 1 and 2 years. Federal regulations for current good manufacturing practices state that if accelerated testing is used to establish an expiration date, it must be followed by actual shelf-life testing to verify the dating.

New product testing is the next stage of the stability program. The samples for this testing come from batches produced in the manufacturing plant and are representative of the approved product being released to the market. The data generated will either confirm that the premarket and production batches are consistent or, if appropriate, bring about a revision of the original dating. The first three batches of a new product undergo both accelerated and shelf-life testing.

As additional batches are manufactured, the LVP becomes an established product and stability testing must continue. Testing done on these products demonstrates consistency, and the data may be used to support or extend the dating period. The shelf life for such LVPs as electrolyte solutions can be as long as 5 years. Others, such as amino acid or dextrose solutions, may have only 2- or 3-year dating. At this stage, fewer batches are tested, and during interim test periods, all the specification tests need not be run. Initial and final test points must include testing for all release requirements; interim tests may include only a tracking of degradation products or indicators of change, such as pH, in addition to assays of the ingredients.

Changes occur, and when they do a revised product study is initiated. The following might be expected to affect the stability properties of the product:

Source or process for an ingredient
Changes in the manufacturing process
Packaging materials in direct contact with the product
Modifications in the formula
Package size changes
Changes in the sterilization cycle

A statement of what type of change requires initiation of a revised product study should be part of the protocol for the stability program.

Special studies are conducted to answer specific questions about the product, manufacturing processes, or conditions outside the control of the manufacturer. Such studies would be done to support labeling information about storage conditions, maximum and minimum temperatures, or the necessity to prevent exposure to light. Stability of the solution when the packages are stored upside down, when other drugs are added, and when the user asks questions about a particular circumstance of use are all part of the special studies program. The data obtained from such studies would be compared with that from previous work in order to answer the questions that were raised.

Stability studies will encompass many aspects: physical (change of color or formation of a precipitate), chemical (change in pH or assay), microbiological (there are no antimicrobial agents in LVPs), or the packaging, which must be nonreactive and protect the solution during the shelf life. Each study must be well documented. Stability reports are reviewed within the company as part of a decision-making process or quality assurance program; they are subject to review by Food and Drug Administration investigators. In May 1984, the Food and Drug Administration announced availability of a Draft Guideline for Stability Studies for Human Drugs and Biologics. The guideline describes the kind of data and information the FDA considers desirable and acceptable in demonstrating the stability of drug products. The information that should be included in a stability report for LVPs is shown in Table 7.

A well-developed and well-executed stability program can prevent the manufacturer from being surprised by unexpected consequences as well as assure compliance with applicable regulations.

F. Processing Conditions Affecting Formulation of LVP

Processing of LVP is described in detail in Chapter 7, Volume 1 of this textbook, but some aspects of water quality, filtration, and sterilization must be re-emphasized as they relate to LVP formulation.

Water for injection is the main ingredient of an LVP formula. Produced in large amounts by distillation or by reverse osmosis, the water must be tested frequently to assure that it is of the quality specified in the USP. Equally important is the monitoring of the quality of the water going into

Table 7 Content of Stability Reports

General product information
1. Name of the drug and drug product
2. Dosage form and strength
3. Labeling and formulation
Specifications and test methodology
1. Physical, chemical, and microbiological characteristics and prior submission specifications (or specific references to NDA or USP)
2. Test methodology used (or cited by reference) for each sample tested
3. Information on accuracy, precision, and suitability of the methodology (cited by reference)
Study design and study conditions
1. Description of the sampling plan, including
Batches and number selected
Containers and number selected
Number of dosage units selected and whether tests were done on individual units or composites
Time of sampling
2. Expected duration of the study
3. Conditions of storage of the product under study (light, temperature, humidity)
Stability data/information
1. Lot number (research, pilot plant, production) and manufacturing date
2. Analytical data and source of each data point, e.g., lot, container, composite. Pooled estimates may be submitted if individual data points are provided
3. Relevant information on previous formulations or container-closure systems should be included
Data analysis and conclusions
1. Documentation of appropriate statistical methods and formulas used in the analysis
2. Evaluation of data, including calculations, statistical analysis, plots, or graphics
3. Proposed expiration dating period and its justificiation
4. Release specifications (establishment of acceptable minimum potency at the time of release for full expiration dating period to be warranted)

the still. A breakdown of water treatment processes or faulty processes, either at the water source or production plant, can result in feeding the still water that will have a carryover to the distillate. Failure to pass the pyrogen test because the endotoxins from heavily contaminated feedwater pass through the distillation process, or high conductivity readings may result.

The USP requires that an LVP must contain no more than 50 particles per milliliter that are equal to or larger than 10 μm and no more than 5 particles per milliliter that are equal to or larger than 25 μm in effective linear measurement. Particle generation from any source to which the solution will be exposed must be identified and controlled. Likely sources are air, processing liquids and gases, or components. Each source may contribute only a few particles but in combination can have a significant effect on the quality of the solution. Emphasis should be placed on reducing the generation of particles as well as effective filtration of liquids and gases at the point of use in the process.

LVPs are terminally sterilized, that is, sterilized after the solution is filled and sealed in its container. The sterilization methods generally used are steam under pressure, hot water immersion, or hydrostatic pressure. Strict adherence to sterilization cycle parameters (time at temperature) that have been demonstrated to achieve sterility is necessary.

Sterility is mandatory, but as the cycle is established other factors must be considered. The product that goes into the sterilizer is the solution in its container-closure system; the process it undergoes is the primary impact on stability, affecting initial values that will then follow normal kinetics. Advanced knowledge of a solution's characteristics, perhaps gained from a similar solution or the same formulation in a different size of container, helps during cycle development by providing a starting point for the work that is to be done.

The type of container, size of container, and solution have an effect on the cycle. Plastic containers, for example, are flexible and permeable. Air overpressure inside the sterilizer must be adjusted during the cycle to counteract the internal pressure in the container in order to avoid distortion. The air that prevents distortion also can enrich the oxygen content of the solution and airspace in the container; the result is that 5% Dextrose in Lactated Ringer's develops more color in plastic than in glass. Amino acids are particularly susceptible to oxygen and are currently packaged in glass. Glass containers are rigid and impermeable but are subject to breakage due to thermal shock if the temperature differentials between the content of the bottle and sterilizer are excessive. The rate of heat up or cooling must be carefully controlled to avoid thermal shock. During sterilization of product in glass containers, the air overpressure in the sterilizer prevents lifting of the closure, which may be brought about by the internal pressure of the bottle. Cycle adjustments must be made for container size; smaller sizes have more surface available per unit volume than larger sizes and may be used as worst case samples for studying the effects of heat history.

Cycle parameters may be developed utilizing a worst case approach. Sterility of the product can be demonstrated by the microbial challenges discussed previously; sterilize at the proposed minimum temperature minus 1 degree Celsius for the minimum time. Stability may be shown by evaluating product that had been sterilized at the proposed maximum temperature plus 1 degree Celsius for the maximum time. A simple solution of electrolytes would not change and would be forgiving of an "overkill" cycle of high temperature for a long time, but the container or closure might not and could very well respond by discharging more extractables or distorting. With some solutions, a few minutes added to the time that is actually needed to achieve sterility can make the difference between a colorless, sparkling solution and one that is slightly off color, lacking "elegance."

The sterilization cycle must balance the required sterility with a functional and effective product in the market; this is possible if all factors are considered during cycle development.

G. Admixture Considerations

After an LVP formulation is developed to bring about a physiologic response, and it has been demonstrated by laboratory and clinical studies that the result is achieved without risk to the patient, the LVP may be considered safe, effective, and approved for use. The formulator, however, must be aware of the additional role that the LVP may play, that of being the vehicle to transport other drugs the physician may prescribe to remedy concurrent conditions.

Of all LVPs infused, 70–80% are estimated to be admixed with one or more drugs [6]. The number of new drugs and possible combinations is increasing steadily. The choice of the drugs, the LVP, and the suitability of the combination falls to other members of the health care team—the physician, the pharmacist, and the nurse.

Manufacturers of LVPs may anticipate certain usage patterns of drugs and combinations of drugs, conduct appropriate compatibility and stability studies, and cite the results in the direction sheet for the product.

Any LVP solution that was originally packaged in glass and is changed to a plastic container is considered to be a new drug. The manufacturer must receive approval of a new drug application before the product can be released for marketing. One of the conditions for approval of the NDA is a submission that reports the results of an investigation of the compatibility with certain drugs that may be added regularly to the parenteral delivery system. Drugs that must be studied are shown in Table 8 [7].

The manufacturer of the proposed product in a plastic container and representatives of the Food and Drug Administration normally agree on the protocol for the compatibility study before the investigation is initiated. Resolution of questions in advance of the laboratory work helps assure the acceptability of the data, speeds up the work, and minimizes costs. Points of discussion might include whether "family" grouping (same or similar ingredients but different concentrations) of products is acceptable. If a group is defined, it may be possible to determine which particular product in the group represents a worst case product on which testing will be done. The worst case would generally be the solution with the highest concentration, in a package for which the surface-volume ratio is the greatest. The data generated from such a product, if it demonstrates compatibility, can be used without further work to conclude the other family members are compatible; if the data demonstrate incompatibility, additional studies must be conducted. Given the number of drugs that must be studied, approximately 40, and the number of products in plastic in which each must be studied, numbering in the hundreds, it is obvious why some consolidation is necessary.

Compatibility data developed by a manufacturer of an LVP in plastic apply only to that manufacturer's particular combination of plastic formulation used in the container and LVP production process; a significant change

Table 8 Drugs to Be Tested for Compatibility with LVPs in Plastic Containers

Aminophylline	Isoproterenol
Amphotericin	Kanamycin
Ampicillin	Levarterenol
Calcium gluconate	Lidocaine
Carbenicillin	Lincomycin
Cephalosporins	Magnesium sulfate
Chloramphenicol	Metaraminol
Chloramphenicol sodium succinate	Methicillin
Clindamycin phosphate	Methotrexate
Cyclophosphamide	Methyldopa
Cytarabine	Oxacillin
Diphenhydramine	Oxytocin
Erythromycins	Penicillin G
Fluorouracil	Potassium chloride
Gentamicin	Sodium bicarbonate
Heparin	Sodium chloride
Hydrocortisone sodium succinate	Tetracyclines
Insulin	Vitamins, single-entity and multiple

in container or processing may bring about the need for repeating the study. Data developed by one manufacturer cannot be used by another producer because of the differences cited above.

An additive study would, as a minimum, include the following requirements:

a. Develop and use an analytic method specific for the additive in the presence of degradation products.
b. The additive concentration in the LVP should be at the maximum encountered in normal hospital practice.
c. The initial concentration in the sample must be no less than 90% of the target value.
d. Store admixtures at ambient temperature for up to 24 hr.
e. Test at 0 and 24 hr for assay of the additive, pH, and visual examination against a black-and-white background for color and evidence of precipitate.
f. Conduct an intermediate visual examination at 6 hr.
g. Any assay of less than 85% at 24 hr will be reassayed at 0, 4, 8, and 24 hr to determine at what point the potency dropped.
h. Controls will be run using LVP in glass containers.

The rule for interpreting the findings could be: If the concentration of the additive is less than 85% of the quantity present at 0 time or there is evidence of precipitation, the admixture is judged as not medically acceptable.

Examples of incompatibilities and explanations are

Erythromycins: The LVP solutions have pH values below 6; the additive is known to be unstable at a pH lower than 6.0.
Insulin: Incompatible in solutions containing sodium bisulfite. Sodium bisulfite is capable of reducing the disulfide bonds in the additive.
Thiamine HCl: In solutions containing sodium bisulfite, the assay is below 85% at 24 hr. Thiamine HCl is compatible in other IV solutions. It is reported that both oxidizing and reducing agents degrade thiamine.

The phenomenon of incompatibility occurs when the LVP and drugs produce, by physicochemical means, a product that is unsuitable for administration to the patient. Physical incompatibility may be detected by a change in the appearance of the solution, such as the formation of a precipitate, a haze, a change of color, or the breaking of an emulsion. Subtle incompatibilities, such as a change in pH or drug concentration, may not result in a visual change or may not become evident until a later time.

Instability occurs when an LVP product or admixture is modified due to sorption or such storage conditions as time, light, or temperature. The modified product may not be suitable for administration, and unless the combination has been studied in the laboratory, the only clue to a stability problem may be failure to get the expected clinical result.

The parameters of tonicity, pH, solubility, and added substances, which were considerations in the design of the LVP formulation, also must be considered in a different context when drugs are added to the solution. The drug product may contain solvents, preservatives, stabilizers, buffers, and other ingredients that, when added to the LVP, can result in instability and compatibility problems. Sodium benzoate, a preservative in some drugs, precipitates as benzoic acid when added to an LVP with an acidic pH. Copper, a trace metal needed by the body, can cause precipitation in amino acid solutions. The pharmacist must be knowledgable of the ingredients in the LVP and in the drug product and possible incompatibilities when preparing admixtures.

Stability of the combination must be maintained after mixing and during infusion if the desired result is to be achieved. Stability problems may be caused by pH, solubility, sensitivity to light or temperature, absorption, or chemical incompatibility. Stability may also be related to time, and this is one reason that it is recommended that admixtures not be stored for prolonged periods.

One example of the role of pH would be that of ampicillin B in dextrose solutions. Unless the pH of the dextrose solution is greater than 5.0, the combination is incompatible. The monograph for Dextrose for Injection allows a pH range of 3.5–6.5. When the pH of 5% Dextrose in Lactated Ringer's Injection is below 5, some nerve-blocking agents, such as succinylcholine, will precipitate from solution.

Chemotherapeutic drugs and vitamin preparations generally should be protected from light.

Sodium bisulfite, an ingredient added to some LVPs to reduce degradation caused by oxidation, may be present in only the quantity needed for protection of the solution during sterilization and shelf life. It may not be present in sufficient quantity to provide protection from the air that may be introduced to the container during admixing or storage in plastic containers.

The order of introduction of drugs to the LVP may either highlight or mask visible incompatibilities. If a drug is incompatible at a given pH and the pH of the LVP must be adjusted, the pH should be adjusted before the drug is added. A fat emulsion, white and opaque, masks reactions that might be visible in a clear solution, and the package insert cautions not to add electrolytes directly to the emulsion.

III. FORMULATION DEVELOPMENT

The idea for an LVP formulation to fulfill a specific need may be developed and result in a safe and therapeutic drug or it may meet its end as a discontinued project. In either case, the decision of whether to continue work or terminate the activity is made as the proposed product moves through a long checklist of questions to be asked and answered, of activities to be completed. The list is dynamic and may change during the course of the project as new information becomes available, new regulations become effective, or unanticipated problems surface. For example, what must be done when the formulator cannot obtain the plastic resin that has been qualified from the original source? Are changes required when the proposed regulations for Current Good Manufacturing Practice for Large Volume Parenterals become effective? Does the latest edition of the USP impact the project? The scope of a development project can vary from the relatively straightforward modification of a current formulation to the very complex production of a new solution in a new container in a new plant. In either event, there should be a method for tracking progress, anticipating problems, minimizing delays, and keeping the project within the budget that has been established. Checklists, a matrix, or critical path analysis all serve this function, and the choice of which to use may depend on the complexity of the development project. The examples that follow are typical, though oversimplified, and serve as the basis for discussion of the concept and merits of each approach to development.

A. The Checklist

The checklist provides reminders that certain tasks or activities are scheduled to be performed. In the context of procuring an ingredient for a formulation, the model checklist might be

a. Establish specifications for the ingredient.
b. Develop test methods for the ingredient.
c. Prepare purchase specifications for the ingredient.
d. Order the ingredient.
e. Receive, identify, and sample the ingredient.
f. Test samples of the ingredient.
g. Approve or disapprove use of the ingredient.

This is a simple and useful way of defining what is to be done, as well as provide some sense of the order in which the tasks are to be performed.

Obviously, the purchasing agent cannot order the ingredient until specifications are available to send to the supplier. The list can be expanded to accommodate as many ingredients as are required and can help prevent something from being overlooked, for example, the test method for one of the 18 amino acids in the formula.

Although checklists may be developed and used by individuals or small groups as a tool to track progress, if the complexity of the project increases, with the involvement of many groups and the coordination of their efforts, checklists alone will not suffice.

B. The Matrix

Forming a matrix is a step toward improved communication and coordination among the involved groups (see Fig. 1). During development, the product will have phases: laboratory (research), pilot plant, and production. Each of these phases deals with elements that are related to the product—how it will be manufactured and released for distribution. An overlay of internal (company policies) and external (government regulation or customer considerations) factors that must be met, along with involvement by staff functions associated with the project, add another dimension to what otherwise would be a straightforward matrix.

Visualize the numbers in the matrix as cells representing large blank spaces to be filled with questions to be answered, tasks to be assigned, and activities to be performed. There must be a free flow of data and information between adjoining cells as answers are generated or the total project will suffer because each scaleup of operations as the formulation moves from laboratory to production plant identifies associated problems as well as demonstrates the ability to process larger batch sizes. For example, chemicals were readily available and easily handled for the mix that was prepared in the laboratory as well as larger quantities used for the batches in the pilot plant. However, production requires procedures for the receipt, testing, storage, and movement of truckload quantities of chemicals that, all the while, must be identified and their status controlled. The technician in the laboratory filled the containers manually, the pilot plant used a filler at a line rate of 10 containers per minute, but the production plant must use a filler that will fill accurately at 200 containers per minute. Something

CONSIDERATION	PHASE		
	Laboratory	Pilot Plant	Production
Final Product	1	6	11
Components	2	7	12
Plant and Equipment	3	8	13
Processing	4	9	14
Tests and Controls	5	10	15

Figure 1 Development matrix.

of little concern in one phase may be a major problem in another phase. If communications lag, breakdown or empathy is lacking for the viewpoints and needs of other team members, the development effort can be seriously hampered. A small, random sample of bits from some of the cells will illustrate both content and interaction. The cells relate to each other horizontally and vertically; the key cell is cell 1 because it is in the laboratory that the product is defined. Obviously, processing parameters cannot be defined nor production begin until the laboratory work is completed.

Cell 1. Is the formula new or a revision; has it been tried before? Conduct a search of the literature. What is the appropriate package: glass, plastic, or both? How many batches must be in the accelerated stability study in order to reach a valid conclusion? A minimum of three batches must be put on stability test. Is the product toxic? Conduct safety tests and tissue culture tests. Are there side effects? Conduct animal tests. Do the test results indicate that a second source can be qualified as an alternate supplier of the chemical? Is the antioxidant really needed in the formula; what will be the effect on stability if it is removed? Will more stability studies be required? Determine the permissible tolerances from nominal values. Should the pH be adjusted so the product will be more useful in admixing? Study the effect of higher pH values. Finalize the product specifications. Publish the formula sheet; publish test requirements and limits.

Cell 4. A decolorizer, activated charcoal, is in the formula. This affects cell 9: the membrane filters will not clog if the mix goes through a prefiltration step. Cell 14 is affected by cells 4 and 9.

Cell 14. There has not been charcoal in a formula for years; during the remodeling of the mix area 2 years ago the bank of prefilters was removed. If a better grade of the chemical that causes color is used, will it not do away with the need for charcoal? Is the charcoal really necessary in the first place? The only possible time that reinstallation of the prefilters can be scheduled is during the next vacation shutdown.

Cell 15. The control laboratory does not have the equipment to perform the assay according to the procedure that was sent. It would require $12,000 and 6 month's delivery. Is not there another way? Cell 5 reports: No, four other methods have been tried and only this one gives the reproducibility needed. It is part of the NDA submission.

Cell 7. Where is the sodium gluconate? It is needed in order to run the preproduction stability samples. The answer from cell 2: Sodium gluconate has not been ordered; there is no purchase specification. Responding to a query from cell 2, cell 1 states: The specifications for sodium gluconate were sent to Documentation 3 weeks ago; check there.

The matrix has helped the development effort; there is increased awareness of what others are doing, dialog between groups and individuals, and an improved sense of timing. The problem in the last example in the matrix points to the need for a better definition of timing for the actions. There are a multitude of activities occurring within a company at any given time, and those that are performed to support the formulation development project represent only a few of many to be done. Individuals must be given specific deadlines within the matrix; otherwise they will determine their own priorities and the development effort will be delayed.

C. The Critical Path

Critical path analysis might at first seem complicated; it is not nearly as complicated as trying to reach the end of a development project that is not well coordinated. During the long time required for a complex development there are many opportunities for a loss of continuity; there may be personnel changes, other projects are started, and the daily work must go on. Critical path analysis with periodic reporting provides a common reference for all who are associated with the development effort as well as a method for monitoring whether activities are proceeding according to schedule.

The starting point for the small path we will develop begins by collecting checklists, which were discussed previously, from the department heads of the laboratory, purchasing, and the pilot plant. Our objective is to produce stability samples in the shortest possible time, without such problems as the one seen in a previous example when an ingredient was not ordered. As each list is gathered, the person providing it should estimate the time it takes to complete each activity on the list. The activities are rearranged and coded as answers are given to the following questions:

What activities must be completed before this one can start?
What activities can be done while this one is being done?
What activities cannot start until after this one is done?

Activities, coded to show starting and ending event numbers, are shown in Table 9 and are formed into a network in Figure 2. The following definitions will be useful in following this discussion.

Event: Points in time, theoretically of no duration, at which an activity is started or completed. Events are represented by circles in the network; the numbers in the circle are for reference.

Activity: An element that consumes time and/or resources. In the network it is represented by arrows that connect events.

Dummy activity: A constraint that indicates an activity cannot begin until another, which may not be in the direct line, has finished.

Critical path: The particular sequence of activities in the network that imposes the most rigid time constraint to accomplishment of the end event; the longest time path between start and end. It is indicated by a heavy black line.

The network shown in Figure 2 provides a graphic description of the activities listed in Table 9. The network flows from left to right. The numbers above the lines represent the duration of the activity. Numbers above the circles represent the accumulated time along a path, the expected time at which an event will finish. The numbers below the circle represent the latest allowable time an event can start without causing the end event to be late; numbers below the circle are calculated by subtracting activity times, beginning at the end point and working backward through the network. Note that the numbers at top and bottom of events on the critical path are the same; when the numbers are not the same, the difference between them represents slack time, the amount of delay that can be tolerated. All activities leading into an event must be completed before the next activity can start.

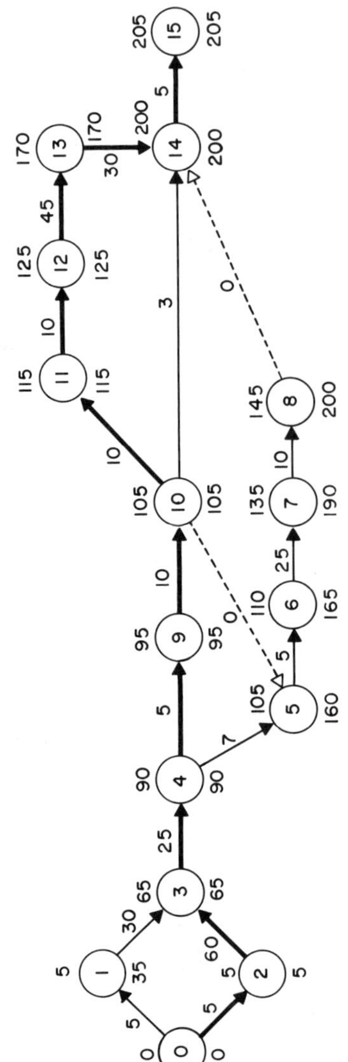

Figure 2 Critical path network.

Table 9 Network and Table for Critical Path Analysis

Events, start to finish	Activity	Days duration
0–1	Approve studies of container	5
0–2	Approve studies of solution	5
1–3	Select container	30
2–3	Determine solution characteristics	60
3–4	Evaluate solution-container combination	25
4–5	Provide specifications	7
4–9	Submit proposal to management	5
9–10	Management approval for development	10
10–5	Dummy	0
10–11	Determine equipment required in pilot plant	10
11–12	Buy equipment for pilot plant	10
12–13	Receive and install equipment	45
13–14	Validate equipment	30
5–6	Purchase ingredients and components	5
6–7	Receive ingredients and components	25
7–8	Test, approve ingredients and components	10
8–14	Dummy	0
10–14	Order ingredients and components for use	1
14–15	Manufacture stability samples in pilot plant	5

Examination of a few points in the network will illustrate the logic and principles of its construction. Event 3, the start of the evaluation of the solution-container combination, cannot start until both activities leading into it have been completed. The accumulated finish time at event 3 through the path 0 to 1 to 3 is 35, following path 0 to 2 to 3 the accumulated time is 65. Since 65 is the earliest possible time that the activities leading into event 3 can be finished, 65 is entered above the circle. Number 105 rather than 97 is above event 5 because the dummy line prevents it from starting before the activities leading into event 10 are completed; no purchases can be made until management has approved the project. The 160 below event 5 is obtained by subtraction beginning at event 15; the difference of 55 indicates that purchases can be delayed for a considerable amount of time without affecting the total time for completion of the project.

With the table and network at hand, the development coordinator can begin to make observations and determine whether there are trade-offs that will reduce the total time for completion of development. Will assigning more laboratory workers to this project reduce the time needed to characterize the solution? Does the prospect of management approval look good enough to risk starting the determination of equipment need earlier; there is the possibility of saving 10 days. How much time might be saved by having the equipment that is ordered shipped by air rather than truck? Can some validation activities be done simultaneously with production of the samples?

The individuals responsible for activities provide the coordinator with information about starting times and completion times; periodic progress reports are issued. The critical path may change because some activity is late getting started or is not finished on time. Computer programs ease the compilations and calculations needed for reporting, and such programs are available at reasonable cost. Costs and labor requirements, as well as time, may be followed using critical path technique.

In summary, the choice of whether to use a checklist, a matrix, or a critical path to guide the development depends on such factors as company size, resources available, and complexity of the project. Organizationally, when the product begins to move from the research stage, formulation development assumes management of the project. Whether development is for modification of an existing product or the multimillion dollar effort to bring a new product to the market, the same questions have to be asked and the answers generated in a systematic, technically sound, and businesslike manner.

IV. SOLUTION QUALITY

The release for distribution of a newly developed LVP is more than a simple acknowledgment that the batches have passed the specified tests. Initial production lots establish the quality level of the product and reflect the quality of all the development and manufacturing actions. If the quality level is acceptable in the market, the new challenge to the manufacturer is to maintain that level in subsequent production. Two steps help make this possible: (a) maximum use of data developed during routine tests and (b) control of changes.

Failure to meet a specification is followed by an investigation and determination of the cause in order to prevent recurrence. A systematic review of available data might have prevented the failure. Data from routine tests can be summarized, plotted, converted to averages and percentages, or used in any way that is appropriate to identify differences and trends. An increase in the percentage of containers discarded because of particles seen in the solution should prompt an investigation of component cleaning procedures and the filtration and handling systems, which were designed to minimize particles. Prompt action based on the level of visible particles probably will result in reducing levels of subvisual particles and avoid rejections because USP subvisual particle levels are exceeded. An increase in the percentage of lots that require retest for pyrogens would bring about an investigation to determine whether the problem in general or related to one product; appropriate action would follow. Detecting significant trends of rising or declining test values, even though individual test results are within specification, and following up to determine the cause are ways to prevent gradual erosion of a quality characteristic.

Control of changes in ingredients and components, processes, procedures, and tests is mandatory. The purchasing department, for example, should not have the sole authority to buy from an unknown, unqualified vendor in an effort to reduce costs. An unauthorized increase of the speed at which containers are filled may take the speed beyond the level at which equipment was validated. Proposed changes should be examined to assure they will accomplish the intent of the change. The effect on other operations should be carefully assessed before a change is implemented. A change control procedure should clearly delineate the individuals responsible for review and approval but should not be so cumbersome that it stifles progress. Inadvertent changes that may get into the system as a result of not following approved procedures or from suppliers who change their processes can often be identified by the data analysis mentioned previously.

The effort to bring an LVP from concept to realization is long, difficult, and costly. Failure to maintain the quality level of the product that reaches the user, by actions within the company, can result in unnecessary effort and cost.

V. SUMMARY

The safe and effective large volume parenterals now in use were formulated in response to advances in the state of the art of many scientific disciplines and technologies. Considering the regulatory constraints of today as well as the rate of advancement of both knowledge and technology, it is interesting to speculate what the LVPs of the future may be.

Amino acids, dextrose injection, and fat emulsion combinations in a single container may be available as a mixture ready for injection, thus eliminating the admixing now required. New products may evolve as products from biotechnology are combined with LVPs. Microencapsulation techniques may protect some drugs that are now incompatible in certain LVPs, releasing them only when the solution is infused; this would make it possible to commercially produce combinations with a long shelf life. The ambulatory patient at home may be wearing an LVP that is being dispensed with a precision that equals that of the electronic controllers now used in the hospital setting.

The future holds promise for many exciting developments in the way large volume parenterals are formulated and used.

REFERENCES

1. Current Good Manufacturing Practice in the Manufacture, Processing, Packing or Holding of Large Volume Parenterals, *Fed. Regist.*, 41(106) (June 1, 1976).
2. Recommendations of the National Coordinating Committee on Large Volume Parenterals, American Society of Hospital Pharmacists, 1978.
3. *Hospital Supply Index, Product Analysis 1B*:1743, IMS America, Ambler, Pennsylvania, 1983.
4. NITA, *J. Nat. Intravenous Ther. Assoc.*, 15(1), (1982).
5. *Parenteral Solutions Handbook*. Cutter Laboratories, Berkeley, California, 1978.
6. A. L. Plummer, *Principles and Practice of Intravenous Therapy*, 2nd ed., Little, Brown, Boston, 1975, p. 3.
7. Parenteral drug products in plastic containers, *Fed. Regist.*, *43* (58562) (Nov. 15, 1978).

3

Glass Containers for Parenterals

Frank R. Bacon*

Owens-Illinois, Inc., Toledo, Ohio

I. INTRODUCTION

Glass containers provide the producers of parenteral solutions with a number of advantages.

a. They have excellent chemical resistance to interaction with the contents, and they neither absorb nor exude organic ingredients.
b. Glass is impermeable. With proper closure, entry or escape of gases (e.g., water vapor) is negligible.
c. Glass containers are easily cleaned in preparation for filling, because of their smooth surfaces.
d. They are transparent, facilitating inspection of the contents.
e. They are rigid, strong, and dimensionally stable. They resist puncture. They will hold a vacuum. They can be heated to 121°C for stream sterilization or to 260°C for dry sterilization without deformation.
f. They can be easily assembled with administration devices.

This chapter discusses the nature of glass, the pharmacopeial specification of types of glass, the varieties of glassware used in parenteral packaging, the manufacture of glass containers, and their chemical and mechanical performance.

II. THE NATURE OF GLASS

Commercial glass is an inorganic product of fusion that has cooled to a rigid condition without crystallizing. In essence, it is a rigid liquid. Within broad ranges of suitable ingredients, it is infinitely variable in composition.

**Current affiliation:* Associated Technical Consultants, Toledo, Ohio

Ordinary containers, windows, and numerous other items of glassware are made of soda-lime-silica glass. In a simplified view, silica (SiO_2) derived from sand provides the structural backbone of this material. Soda (Na_2O) derived from soda ash reacts with silica to fuse the mass at attainable temperatures. The product, a true glass, will dissolve in water. The addition of CaO or CaO and MgO derived from lime assists the fusion, but its most important effect is to give the resulting glass water resistance. The effective proportioning of these, plus minor ingredients, particularly alumina (Al_2O_3), is responsible for the chemical durability and other desirable properties of familiar glassware.

It is useful to visualize the structure of glass as a partially arranged and partially disorganized mixture of atoms. Oxygen atoms are present as negatively charged ions. Most other atoms are in the form of positively charged ions. The electrostatic attraction of oppositely charged ions is a major force binding the atoms together in an impervious, rigid body. Figure 1 shows the relative sizes of these ions in comparison with game balls and their relative abundance in representative soda-lime and borosilicate glasses. The four oxygen ions surround each silicon ion in a tetrahedral array. Most oxygen ions lie between two silicon ions, but occasionally "nonbridging" oxygen ions are associated with but one silicon ion. The array of silicon and oxygen ions forms a partially random three-dimensional network. This is the strong backbone of the material. Boron and aluminum ions occupy sites similar to those of silicon. Nonbridging oxygen ions have an excess negative charge. So do arrays of four oxygen ions coordinated with B^{3+} or Al^{3+} ions. Excess negative charges are balanced by neighboring sodium and calcium ions. The monovalent sodium ion is freer than others to diffuse among appropriate sites about the network. Thus we have a picture of oxygen ions packed together with network-forming elements, principally silicon ions, tucked in interstices in a manner that conforms to restrictions of bond angle, valence, and size and with the network modifiers Na^+ and Ca^{2+}, among others, creating and balancing the negative charge of somewhat randomly oriented discontinuities.

A structural continuum lacking internal phase boundaries that would reflect radiation and the absence of components that would absorb a significant amount of radiation in the visible spectrum result in the transparency of familiar glassware. Ingredients can be incorporated that absorb selectively and give rise to glass that is transparent but colored. An interaction of iron and sulfide ions produces amber. Chromium and iron ions produce green, and cobalt ions produce blue. It is the property of transparency that makes possible visual inspection of the contents of sealed glass containers for suspended matter and filling level.

Photochemical reactions in packaged products are usually triggered by ultraviolet or short-wavelength visible radiation. As shown in Figure 2, amber containers exclude a large fraction of this radiation while still passing sufficient long-wavelength visible radiation to permit visual inspection of the contents. Green and blue containers are much less effective in absorbing ultraviolet and short-wavelength visible radiation. They provide only a moderate improvement over colorless glass containers, termed "flint" in the trade.

Although soda-lime glass containers have a high level of chemical durability, appropriate borosilicate glass compositions can be used to make containers that are about 10 times better in this general respect. These glasses also have a much lower thermal expansion. This gives improved

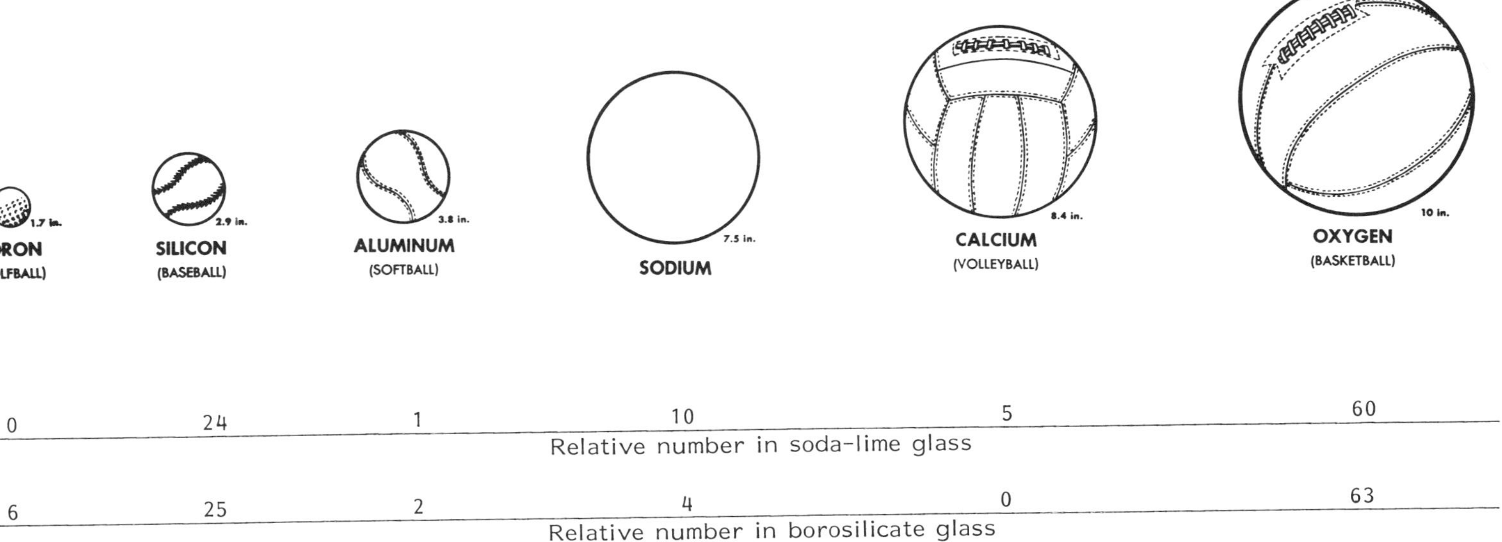

Figure 1 Principal ions in glass with relative size indicated by comparison with game balls.

Table 1 Representative Container Glass Compositions

Weight (%)	Soda-lime Type II, III, or NP			Borosilicate, Type I				
	Blown		Tubing flint	Blown		Tubing		
	Flint	Amber		Flint	Amber	Flint	Flint	Amber
SiO_2	73.0	71.9	67.7	68.5	66.4	80.4	70.6	69.2
B_2O_3	—	—	1.5	12.9	9.4	12.9	11.2	10.4
Al_2O_3	1.8	1.9	2.8	6.0	5.7	2.6	6.6	5.4
CaO	10.7	10.6	5.7	1.2	1.7	<0.05	0.5	0.4
MgO	0.4	0.8	3.9	<0.1	<0.1	<0.05	0.2	0.3
BaO	—	—	2.0	2.5	1.2	—	2.2	2.1
Na_2O	13.5	14.1	15.6	8.3	7.2	4.0	6.1	6.0
K_2O	0.3	0.3	0.6	0.5	1.0	—	2.5	2.3

TiO_2	0.02	0.04	—	—	—	—	—	2.8
Fe_2O_3	0.04	0.1	0.05	0.05	1.3	0.06	0.06	1.0
FeO	0.01	0.2	—	—	—	—	—	—
MnO	—	—	—	—	5.8	—	—	—
SO_3	0.2	0.01	0.2	—	—	—	—	—
S^{2-}	—	0.02	—	—	—	—	—	—
Cl^-	—	—	—	0.2	0.3	0.05	0.1	0.2
Thermal expansivity[a]	88	90	93	56	59	32	55	54
Powdered glass test[b]	7.0	7.6	8.0	0.6	0.7	0.3	0.3	0.4

[a]Thermal expansivity is given as units of length per 10,000,000 units per °C for the range from 0 to 300°C.
[b]Powdered glass test values are given as milliliters 0.02 N H_2SO_4.

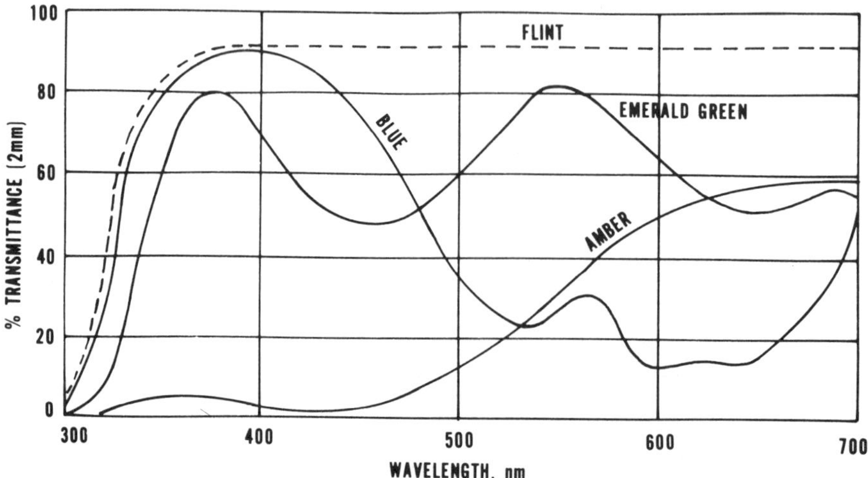

Figure 2 Light transmission of typical soda-lime container glasses. Ultraviolet radiation occurs below 400 nm. Visible light occurs from 400 to 700 nm.

resistance to the thermal shock that occurs when a container is suddenly heated or cooled.

Table 1 gives the chemical composition of typical soda-lime and borosilicate container glasses together with properties discussed in other parts of this chapter.

Glass is strong and rigid. In consequence, it is dimensionally stable. It does not yield to stress but is susceptible to brittle fracture if overloaded. Because of the high intrinsic strength, fracture of glassware is usually initiated in surface flaws. The design and handling of glass containers must take these facts into account.

III. USP-NF GLASSWARE SPECIFICATIONS

A. Chemical

The NF V, which became official July 1, 1926, was the first compendium containing chemical specifications for glassware. Development over the years has led to the specification of the four types of glassware shown in Table 2. Types I, II, and III are used for parenteral products. Type NP is intended for nonparenterals. Within each type, containers with a range of glass compositions are available, illustrated in part in Table 1. The USP XX recommends one or more types of glassware as desirable for packaging about 275 parenteral solutions or irrigations that are subjects of a monograph. There are about 175 additional monographs describing sterile solids for injection, antibiotics, biologics, radioactive injections, insulin preparations, and a few others for which no type suggestion is made. Table 3 shows the kinds of products that are packed in each of the four types.

A brief outline of the tests upon which the specifications are based follows. Attention to detail, particularly in the preparation of high-purity

Table 2 USP-NF Specification of Four Types of Glass

Type	General description[a]	Type of test	Size[b] (ml)	0.02 N acid (ml)
I	Highly resistant, borosilicate glass	Powdered glass[c]	All	1.0
II	Treated soda-lime glass	Water attack	⩽100 >100	0.7 0.2
III	Soda-lime glass	Powdered glass	All	8.5
NP	General-purpose soda-lime glass	Powdered glass	All	15.0

[a]The description applies to containers of this type of glass usually available.
[b]Size indicates the overflow capacity of the container.
[c]The USP XXI (page 1235) also stipulates that the extract solution obtained by application of the water attack at 121°C test to Type I containers shall not contain more than 0.1 ppm arsenic.
Source: From the USP XXI (1985), page 1234, reproduced by permission of U.S. Pharmacopeial Convention, Inc.

Table 3 Typical Uses of Glass Containers by Type

Type	Products packed
I	SVPs of all kinds regardless of pH; LVPs that are mildly alkaline or when high thermal shock resistance is important
II	LVPs; especially intravenous solutions and irrigating solutions; also anticoagulants, human blood, and its components, diagnostic preparations; a few SVPs; these parenterals are usually neutral or acidic
III	SVPs that have been demonstrated to be unharmed by packaging and storage in ordinary soda-lime glass; mostly solutions or suspensions in vegetable oil or sterile dry powders to which water for injection is added at the time of use; several neutral aqueous products
IV	Cough syrups, elixirs, tinctures, extracts, creams, salves, lotions, tablets, capsules, other dry products

water as set forth in the USP, is essential to obtain reproducible results in these tests.

1. Powdered Glass Test

In this test, containers are crushed to yield 10 g of grains that pass a no. 40 sieve but are retained on a no. 50. The crushed grains are exposed to the action of 50 ml of high-purity water at 121°C for 30 min in an autoclave. The resulting extract solution is titrated to the methyl red end point with 0.02 N sulfuric acid. The volume of acid required is recorded. This volume is a measure of the alkaline ingredients of the glass that have been extracted during the test.

The powdered glass test result is an indicator of the intrinsic chemical durability of a glass. The chemical resistance of containers tends to parallel the resistance of the glass as indicated by this test. Types I, III, and NP are specified in terms of this test. Thus, Type I containers comply with specifications for Type III and Type NP as well, and containers that meet the Type III specification necessarily also qualify as Type NP.

The National Bureau of Standards supplies Standard Reference Material 622 (a soda-lime glass) and 623 (a borosilicate glass) certified as to the typical value obtainable in the powdered glass test [1]. The SRM 623 is a typical Type I glass, and SRM 622 is typical of glasses that meet the Type III as well as the Type NP specification.

2. Water Attack at 121°C

In this test, glass containers are rinsed and filled to 90% of overflow capacity with water, suitably covered, and autoclaved at 121°C for 60 min. After removal from the autoclave, a 100-ml portion of the resulting extract solution is removed from one or several containers and titrated to the methyl red end point with 0.02 N sulfuric acid. The volume of acid required is recorded as the test result.

As will be explained below, Type II containers owe their exceptional chemical durability to an internal surface treatment carried out at the time of manufacture. This benefit is not reflected by the powdered glass test. Hence, Type II containers are specified by this bottle-surface test.

3. Type I Glass Containers

It can be seen in Table 1 that the borosilicate glass is relatively low in Na_2O. This and the relatively high Al_2O_3 content are primarily responsible for the superior chemical durability. This glass has superior resistance to alkaline products particularly because of the high Al_2O_3 content. The most important function of the B_2O_3 is to act as a nonalkaline flux to facilitate the melting of the low-Na_2O glass. Type I glass is used to make blown containers. In the form of tubing, it is used to make vials, ampuls, syringe bodies, and parts for large volume parenteral (LVP) administration sets. Some small volume parenterals (SVPs) are sold in disposable one-trip glass syringes or cartridges.

4. Type II Glass Containers

These are made of commercial soda-lime glass that has been dealkalized on the inside surface at the time of manufacture to obtain a great improvement in chemical resistance. The process employed to dealkalize the surface is known as sulfur treatment. Typically, sulfur dioxide is introduced as newly formed bottles pass from the forming machine to the annealing lehr. This reacts at the surface of the glass to form sodium sulfate. Cold bottles may be treated by introducing sulfur or a sulfur compound, such as sulfuric acid or ammonium sulfate, and reheating into the annealing temperature range, around 550°C or above. For treatment with SO_2, the reaction goes as

$$SO_2 + \tfrac{1}{2}O_2 + Na_2O \text{ (from the glass)} \longrightarrow Na_2SO_4 \quad (1)$$

Hydrogen ions from ambient moisture probably play a part, first forming sulfuric acid at the glass surface from which hydrogen ions exchange with sodium ions of the glass.

$$SO_2 + \tfrac{1}{2}O_2 + H_2O \longrightarrow H_2SO_4 \quad (2)$$

$$H_2SO_4 + Na\cdot\text{glass} \longrightarrow Na_2SO_4 + H\cdot\text{glass} \quad (3)$$

The ion exchange proceeds by diffusion within the glass. Simultaneously or subsequently H_2O escapes from the glass, providing the net effect represented in Equation (1) [2]. The depth of dealkalization is suggested by the amount of sodium sulfate formed on the surface of the glass. Typically, the amount of sodium in the sulfate deposit is equal to that in a layer of glass several tenths of a micrometer thick. Evidently a sodium concentration gradient is formed in the glass from near zero at the surface to the concentration in the bulk glass at a depth of perhaps a micrometer. The containers are delivered with a haze of sodium sulfate present. The haze is rinsed away when they are washed before filling, actually increasing the efficiency of cleaning. Not only does this process reduce the abundance of sodium ions available at the surface for reaction with a liquid product, but the chemical stability of the altered surface is greatly enhanced and the extraction of all glass components by the contents of the container is suppressed.

Dealkalization can also be carried out with other acidic gases. Chlorine or hydrogen chloride, for example, leads to the formation of sodium chloride instead of sodium sulfate. In a different method of treatment, hot bottles coming from the forming machine are exposed to a jet of gas consisting of fluorohydrocarbon and air. There is no visible product of the reaction, and the mechanism by which chemical resistance is enhanced is uncertain [3]. These methods are not in common use for parenteral containers at present.

As indicated in Table 2, two limits are set on the concentration of alkaline material in the water attack at 121°C test, one for containers having an overflow capacity of 100 ml or less and a lower limit for containers having an overflow capacity of more than 100 ml. This is close to the dividing line between SVPs and LVPs. (The Food and Drug Administration considers LVPs to have an actual product volume of 100 ml or more.)

The commercial use of dealkalized glass containers to package intravenous solutions dates back to the 1930s. Particularly in the large size range, they provide effective inert containment at moderate cost.

5. *Type III Glass Containers*

These are untreated soda-lime glass containers that must meet an intermediate limit in the powdered glass test. Most flint glass containers do, in fact, meet this limit. The USP recommends the use of Type III containers for a number of injectable preparations that have been found to be unharmed by storage in untreated glass. These are generally small-volume preparations for which the containers are presterilized and filled under aseptic conditions with sterile product. It is desirable to sterilize them by dry heat. In this process, water-rinsed containers are mounted in covered racks and heated to 160°C or more for several hours. Water evaporates from the surface of containers before the temperature can exceed 100°C. Autoclave sterilization of empty untreated containers involving exposure to saturated steam at 121°C for 20 min, by contrast, produces significant attack on the inside surface, leaving alkaline alteration products on that surface. When such bottles are filled with an aqueous product, the alkaline material dissolves at once and siliceous insoluble matter sometimes sloughs into the product.

6. *Type NP Glass Containers*

These containers, deemed generally suitable for nonparenteral products, meet the least restrictive specification. In fact, Types I, II, and III meet the Type NP specification also. Some colored and a few flint containers comply with Type NP but not Type III. Frequently these containers will yield test results that exceed the Type III test limit by only a small margin. Whenever a drug product is known to be adversely affected by material from untreated soda-lime glass containers, the use of Type I or Type II containers is strongly recommended.

B. Physical

1. *Light Protection*

The USP recommends the use of a light-resistant container for many different products. Generally, the USP requires that a light-resistant container should not pass more than 10% of the incident radiation at any wavelength between 290 and 450 nm. However, parenteral containers of 50 ml or less capacity are permitted higher penetration according to their size and manner of sealing (USP XXI, page 1233). This provision is made because thinner walls are used for smaller containers and a desirable compromise is made between maximum light protection and ease of visual inspection of the contents. Compliance can be checked by measuring the transmission in this range of a section of the container representing average wall thickness.

A colorless glass container can be made light resistant by enclosing it in an opaque covering, such as heavy paper or cardboard, but then the label on the container must state that the opaque covering is required until the contents have been used.

Blown amber glass containers that meet this specification are available in all types of glass. Although the use of amber Type II containers is unusual in human medicine, they are used in packaging many veterinary serums. A typical light transmission spectrum of soda-lime amber at 2 mm, a thickness representative of many blown containers, is shown in Figure 2. The absorption of ultraviolet and short-wavelength visible radiation is caused by an interaction of sulfide and iron ions.

Type I ampuls and vials made from tubing are available in amber glass meeting the above specification. The thickness of the sidewalls of tubing-made containers increases substantially with size. Here the absorption is due to an interaction of iron with manganese or titanium.

2. *Permeation*

Parenteral containers must have a hermetic seal. This requires a reliable mating and fastening of the closure to the glass container. To attain this, the opening of the containers, known as the "finish," must conform accurately to the intended design and be free of surface irregularities in the sealing zone. Procurement specifications must clearly designate the dimensional tolerances permissible.

3. *Capacity*

The USP XXI (page 1139), specifies that single-dose parenteral containers shall hold no more than 1 liter and that multiple-dose parenteral containers shall hold no more than 30 ml unless otherwise specified in the individual monograph on the packaged preparation. The large single-dose containers usually hold intravenous solutions. Irrigation solutions may be packed in larger than 1-liter units. The composition of irrigations and the manner of processing are similar to those of some LVPs.

IV. THE MANUFACTURE OF GLASS CONTAINERS

A. Melting

Container glass is melted in large refractory furnaces at around 1500°C. The glassmaking raw materials are mixed together and continuously introduced into the furnace along with cullet (recycled glass), which facilitates melting. The clear molten glass produced is continuously supplied to forming equipment. Glass composition is controlled by periodic chemical analysis and accurate proportioning of the raw materials. Control is verified in many operations by a daily check on a composition-sensitive property of the glass produced, such as density. It can be checked with extreme precision by the sink-float method [4] in which a heavy organic liquid is adjusted in temperature until its density exactly matches that of an annealed glass specimen. In the seal test sometimes used, a small glass rod is drawn and flame sealed to a standard rod and cooled under defined conditions. The resulting stress pattern at the weld as seen by polariscopic examination (explained below) indicates a close match or a deviation from the intended composition.

Homogeneity of the glass produced is checked by polariscopic examination of the finished ware. When a beam of polarized light is passed through glass, any stress causes a change in the plane of polarization. If the beam is viewed through an analyzer positioned to polarize in a plane perpendicular to the plane of polarization of the incident light, regions of stress appear as contrasts in brightness (or differences in color if a tint plate is used). Ring sections cut from the body of the container are often immersed for viewing in a liquid whose refractive index is close to that of glass. This almost eliminates reflections at the glass surfaces and enables one to observe stress more clearly. Inhomogeneity results in "cords" (elongated regions in which composition differs from the matrix glass). Since deviations in composition cause variations in thermal expansivity, the cords generate internal stress that cannot be relieved by annealing. The result is abrupt, streaky patterns in the polariscope. A practical degree of homogeneity is needed. Depending on severity and location, cords may detract from the practical strength of the containers produced.

B. Forming and Processing

Containers are formed by blowing and by automatic lampworking of tubing. (Lampworking is the trade term for working glass in an open flame.) Both Type I borosilicate and Types II, III, and NP soda-lime glass containers are made by both processes. Most blown containers are made of soda-lime glass. However, most of the blown containers used for SVPs and most tubing-made containers are of borosilicate glass.

1. Blown Containers

The most widely used blowing equipment is the IS (individual-section) machine. The manner in which containers are formed on this machine is represented schematically in Figure 3. Gobs of molten glass are extruded from the "feeder" and caught in a blank mold where the finish (mouth) and a parison are formed. Held by the finish, the parison is transferred to a blow mold where it is inflated with air to conform to the mold cavity. When the glass has chilled to a rigid condition, the container is placed on a moving belt and conveyed to the annealing lehr. At this stage, the temperature is usually above 500°C.

Annealing consists in reheating as necessary into the annealing range, then cooling in a controlled fashion so that all parts of the new container are at nearly uniform temperature and contract uniformly as they pass from a temperature high enough that stresses are immediately relieved, to a temperature at which stress relief can no longer occur in a reasonable length of time. From that point, the lehr continues cooling the ware to room temperature. The state of annealing is determined by polariscopic observation of the relative annealing stress present in finished containers. Annealing stress is represented by relatively broad zones of contrast in brightness or color in the polariscopic image [5]. These zones are oriented to structural features of the container, such as bottom and sidewall. Complete absence of annealing stress is not desirable or practically attainable, but a good degree of annealing is required.

At the cold end of the lehr, the ware is inspected both visually and mechanically (Fig. 4) for physical defects and then packed for shipment.

Sulfur treatment of blown soda-lime containers is carried out by injecting the treating agent, typically SO_2 gas, into the containers before they enter the annealing lehr. The effectiveness of treatment is largely determined by the sodium gradient established in the surface zone of the glass, and this is influenced by the time-temperature history of the container while it is in contact with an effective concentration of SO_2 during the high-temperature part of the annealing process. Temperatures should be sufficient to permit rapid diffusion of sodium ions but not so high that the ware is deformed. Some variation is inevitable in temperature across the lehr through which as many as 20 rows of bottles are passing. Nevertheless, it is necessary to hold the temperature at all points within a suitable range.

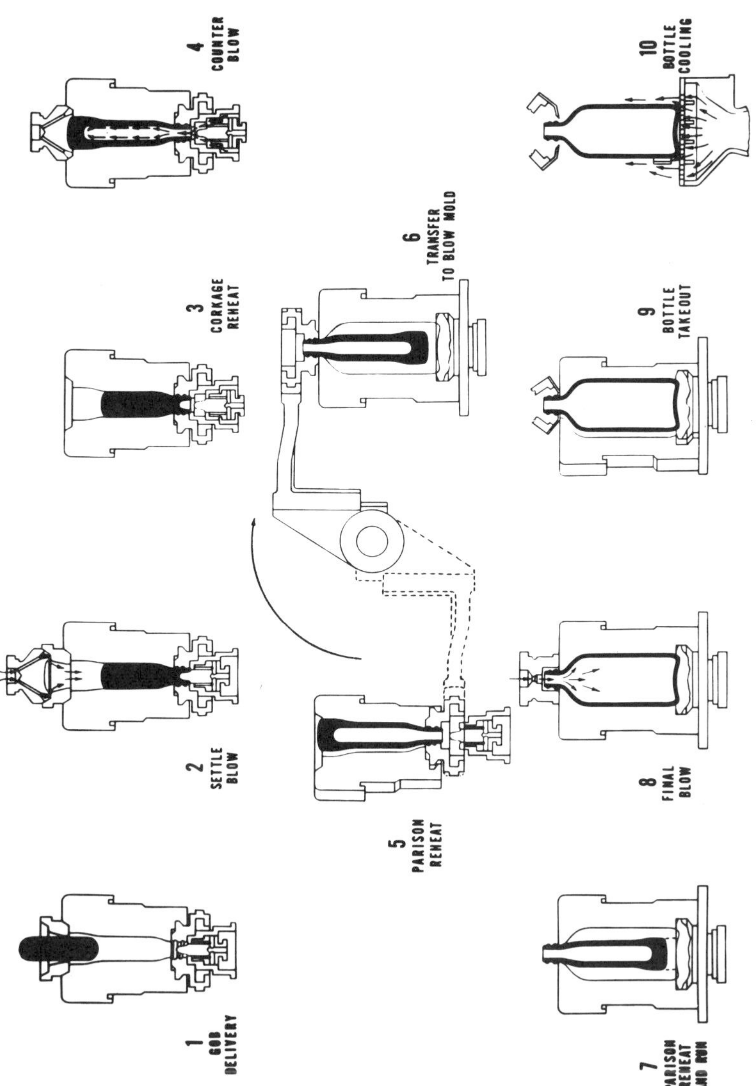

Figure 3 IS machine blow-and-blow forming process. Solid black sections represent glass, molten as the gob is delivered to the blank mold at (1) and rigid as the container reaches station (10).

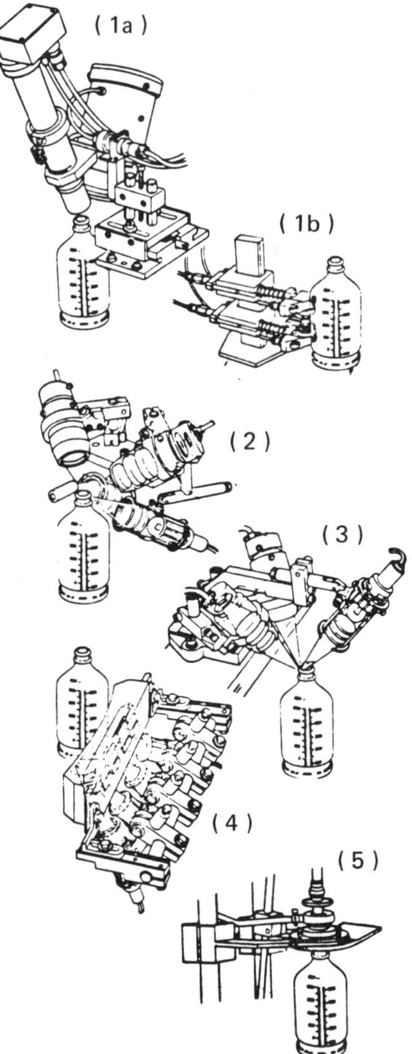

Station 1a: Optical gauge inspects sealing surface for blisters and irregularities.
Station 1b: Ratiofrequency gages measure thickness around the body at two levels.
Station 2: Optical gauge inspects finish for vertical checks (small surface cracks).
Station 3: Optical gauge inspects finish for horizontal checks.
Station 4: Optical gauge inspects bottom bearing area for checks.
Station 5: Plug gauge detects undersize necks, ensures compatibility with filling tubes.

Figure 4 Automatic selection. LVP bottles pass from station to station of intermittent-motion rotary machine, rotating on their own axis at the first four stations. Defectives are rejected from the production line.

Periodically, samples of treated and annealed bottles are taken from representative locations, e.g., right, left, and center rows, and tested to assure compliance with the USP Type II specification. If treatment is substandard or marginal, all ware that may be affected is retreated off-line by adding a treating agent, e.g., ammonium sulfate, to each bottle and reheating into the treating range. Samples of the retreated ware are then tested.

In addition to the inspection of all containers on the production line, representative samples of finished ware are checked by a quality-assurance laboratory for thermal shock resistance [6], state of annealing [5], dimensional conformance, capacity, and visual imperfections.

2. Tubing-Made Containers

The Danner process of tubing production is illustrated in Figure 5. Within a heated chamber on the end of the furnace, a stream of viscous molten glass flows onto the surface of an inclined refractory tube that is slowly rotating. The glass spreads evenly as it flows to the end where glass tubing is drawn off. The diameter and wall thickness of the resulting tubing are controlled by the rate of glass flow, the temperature in the Danner chamber, the amount of air introduced through the back end of the refractory tube and the rate of drawing imposed by a traction device operating

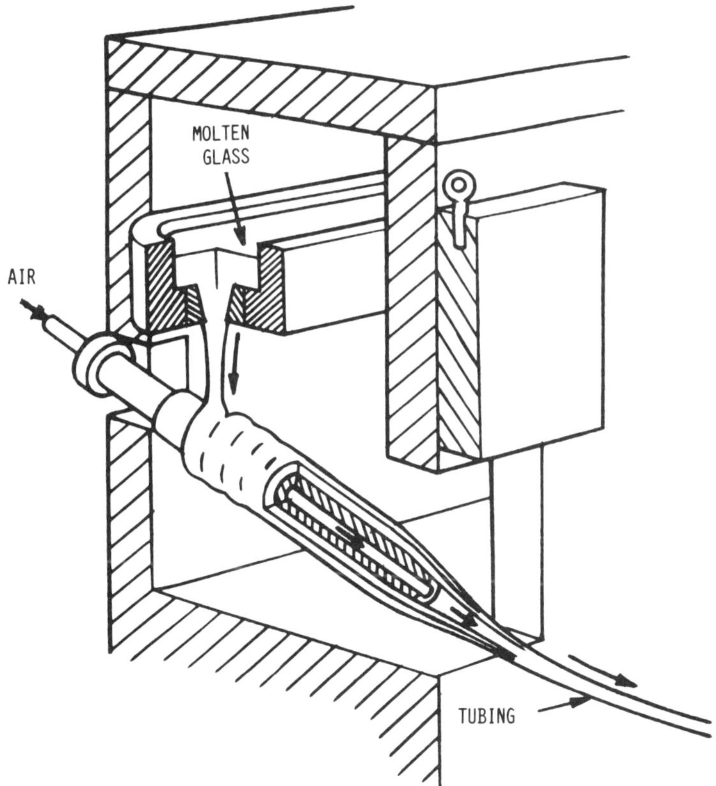

Figure 5 Continuous production of borosilicate glass tubing on a Danner machine.

on the cooled tubing many feet away from the Danner chamber. The tubing is uniform in thickness, and this uniformity is retained in the sidewalls of the containers into which it is converted. Because of this uniformity, these containers can be made relatively lightweight.

Figure 6 represents the steps by which tubing is converted to ampuls and vials on automatic lampworking machines. In the bottoming operation the tubing is heated in a narrow zone by intense flames until the glass softens, melts down, seals, and finally severs. A fume containing sodium, boron, oxygen, and perhaps other elements arises from the white-hot surface and deposits usually in a band about 2 mm above the bottom on the inside surface [7]. Most of this material is washed away when the container is rinsed before use. Although Type I ampuls and vials comply with the specification by virtue of their glass composition, some of them are sulfur-treated to neutralize the effect of this bloom and otherwise further enhance the chemical durability of the formed container [8]. This can be accomplished conveniently by spraying an ammonium sulfate solution into the containers, after which they are heated into the annealing range. The haze of sodium sulfate on treated Type I containers is usually less conspicuous than on Type II containers because there is less of it present.

Syringe bodies and cartridges are also formed from tubing. Of course, no bottoming operation is involved. The tubing is cut into appropriate lengths and both ends are tooled as needed. Several kinds are shown with other containers in Figure 7.

The chemical resistance of tubing-made Type I containers can also be improved severalfold by washing with dilute fluoride solution, e.g., 0.5–5% NH_4HF_2. The process also reduces the abundance of particulate matter adhering to the container surface more effectively than other common means [9]. It can best be carried out as an adjunct to the rinsing process just before filling. The solution is flushed over the internal surface of the container for about a second. The surface remains wet with the fluoride solutions for perhaps 60 sec. During this period the glass surface is attacked. Then thorough flushing with water removes the fluoride and products of attack along with any adherent particulate matter.

Ampuls are finished with either a plain tapered stem or one expanded to a funnel shape at the opening. After filling, the stem is heated and drawn down so that it welds shut. The excess stem material is discarded. Usually there is constriction between the stem and the body of the ampul, which is scored or coated with a narrow band of ceramic enamel of higher expansivity than the ampul glass to facilitate opening the sealed ampul. When the enamel band is applied and fired, a stress is generated at the interface between enamel and ampul glass as the ampul cools to room temperature. Later, after the ampul has been filled and sealed and the tip is flexed to open the ampul, the ring of stress aids in initiating and guiding the crack that severs the tip.

3. *Packaging and Shipping*

Large containers are generally packed in corrugated paperboard shipping cartons. For the packing of smaller containers, particularly vials, ampuls, and small Type I bottles, there is substantial use of plastic packaging materials to avoid contamination with paper fibers. Some vials and bottles are arranged in rectangular arrays, which are sealed as groups in heatshrinkable plastic film. Some syringe cartridges are washed and dried in equipment that delivers them into a clean room where they are sealed in plastic

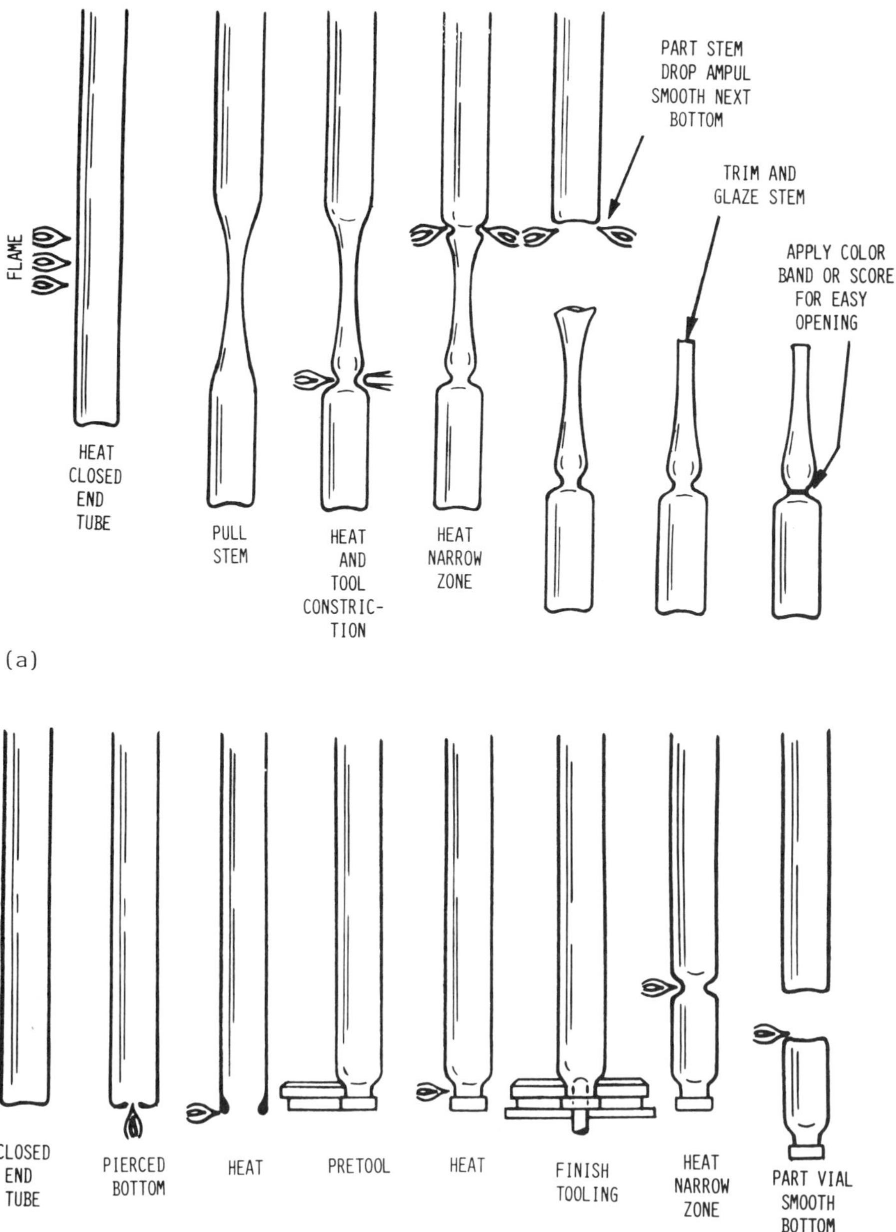

Figure 6 Principal steps in making containers from tubing. (a) Typical ampul forming. (b) Typical vial forming.

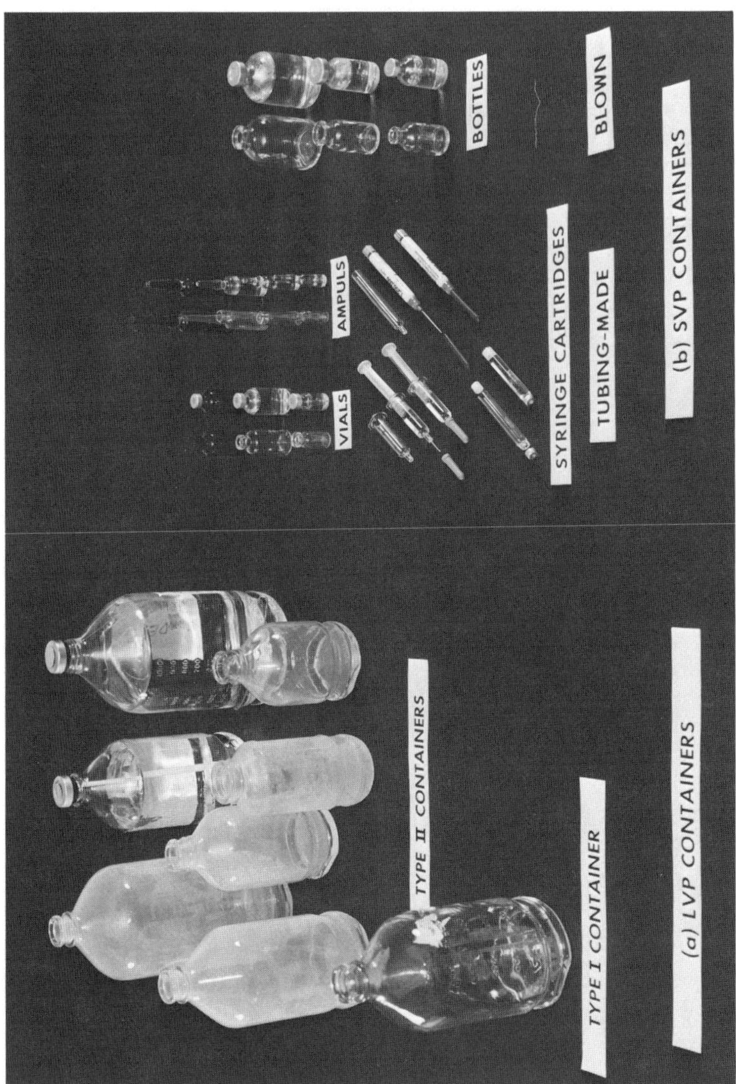

Figure 7 Typical glass containers for parenteral solutions. (a) LVP containers shown are all blown. They range in capacity from 150 to 1000 ml. Empty Type II containers are shown with haze of sodium sulfate present. (b) SVP containers shown are all made of Type I glass. Several kinds of disposable syringe cartridges are included. Vials are 2 and 10 ml capacity. Ampuls are 1, 2, 5, and 10 ml. Bottles are 6, 10, and 50 ml.

as just described. Many ampuls are packed in lightweight plastic boxes with well-fitting covers. Some of these packages are designed so that the containers can be introduced as a group in the pharmaceutical manufacturer's washing machine. The delivery of cleaner containers lessens dependence on the washer and helps to furnish the cleanest possible containers to the filling equipment.

4. General

The glassmaking raw materials are much more expensive for borosilicate glass than for soda-lime. The melting temperature required is substantially higher. The furnace size is generally less. These factors result in higher fuel and refractory costs. A measurable fraction of the B_2O_3 escapes as a fume. The glass produced is less homogeneous. Blow-molding operations must be carried out at a higher temperature. The extra cost of these factors is the price one must pay for the superior chemical durability and the higher resistance to thermal shock due to lower expansivity of borosilicate glassware.

Figure 7 shows typical containers of the various kinds discussed in this chapter.

V. CHEMICAL PERFORMANCE

Glass containers are inherently most resistant to dilute acidic products. The action that does occur is largely an exchange of hydrogen ions from the acidic solution for sodium ions from the glass. There are numerous sites within the glass structure than can accommodate a monovalent cation. Hydrogen ions diffuse inward and the sodium ions diffuse outward among these sites. The process is self-decelerating because additional sodium ions must come from greater depths within the glass body. Relatively minor amounts of calcium, magnesium, and silicon accompany sodium into solution. Lowering the Na_2O content of soda-lime and use of an optimum content of CaO or CaO plus MgO favor acid resistance [10, 11].

Products that are neutral react similarly at the outset but have some capacity to hydrolyze the skeletal glass structure, bringing all components into solution. As the solution becomes alkaline, this action is more rapid. The composition of extracted material resembles that of the glass from which it is extracted. Resistance to neutral solutions is favored by a high Al_2O_3 content, a low Na_2O content, and a suitable CaO or CaO plus MgO content in the glass [10, 11].

Substantially alkaline products attack glass most rapidly, yielding both soluble and insoluble decomposition products. Here, also, the soluble material is similar to the glass in composition. The insoluble material is a hydrous silicate, low in Na_2O and high in Al_2O_3, CaO, and MgO. A high Al_2O_3 content is favorable to alkali resistance [7, 10].

The only dilute acidic solution known to attack glass substantially is hydrofluoric acid. Its ability to break down the glass structure may be associated with formation of the soluble complex ion, SiF_6^{2-}. This reaction is used in chemical analysis as a step in decomposing glass and other silicates to obtain a solution of the ingredients [12].

Even though the materials extracted from glass by acidic and neutral solutions are slight and generally innocuous, it is desirable to keep parenteral solutions as free of extraneous matter as practical. The use of Type I or Type II glassware can usually reduce the extraction of ingredients from the glass by acidic or neutral products to one-tenth or less of that from untreated soda-lime glassware. For acidic and many neutral solutions, the effectiveness of dealkalization (Type II containers) preponderates the original glass composition in determining chemical performance. Most parenteral solutions are moderately acidic or neutral. Table 4 shows the amounts of several ingredients extracted from 4-oz blown containers in tests resembling the USP water attack at 121°C test [13]. Figure 8 shows the amounts of silica extracted from the same containers at 100°F by aqueous buffers of pH 7.5, 8.5, and 9.5 [10, 13]. This figure illustrates the reduced efficacy of dealkalized soda-lime glass containers as pH increases. The original glass composition becomes more important than the surface treatment. Hence, Type I containers are generally preferable for packaging alkaline parenterals.

The action of alkaline solutions includes the generation of a film of hydrous siliceous gel, an insoluble product of attack, on the exposed glass surface. Sometimes this breaks up, releasing flakes that become suspended in the product [10]. Adams [7] has identified crystalline material with the x-ray diffraction parameters of saponite, a hydrous magnesium silicate mineral, in such flakes. Borosilicate containers generally have the best resistance to flake formation. Dealkalization of soda-lime glass containers is effective in preventing flake formation in initially neutral products since it tends to prevent them from becoming alkaline.

An example of the relative behavior of ampuls is given by Hinson [14], who sealed water in 10-ml ampuls, autoclaved the sealed ampuls for 30 min, and then stored them for 2 years. Extreme precautions were taken to purify the water and prevent its contamination by CO_2 as the ampuls were sealed. The pH was measured by the isohydric indicator method in which

Table 4 Extraction by Water and Acid from 4-oz Blown Containers at 121°C for 1 hr

		0.0002 N H_2SO_4 (ppm)			Water (ppm)		
Bottle	Type	Na_2O	SiO_2	B_2O_3	Na_2O	SiO_2	B_2O_3
Untreated	III	2.4	0.50	—	6.6	30	—
		2.3	0.54	—	6.4	28	0.1
Treated	II	0.42	—	—	0.38	0.58	—
		0.40	0.06	—	0.40	0.56	0.1
Wheaton	I	1.14	0.28	—	0.56	4.8	0.9
		1.15	0.30	—	0.69	4.9	0.6
Kimble	I	0.54	0.19	0.3	0.26	0.78	0.4
		0.56	0.30	0.3	0.32	0.70	0.4
Pyrex[a] glass	I	0.87	0.20	1.6	0.58	0.40	1.2
		0.80	0.22	1.1	0.72	0.28	1.7

[a]Trademark of Corning Glass Works.
Source: Data from Ref. 13.

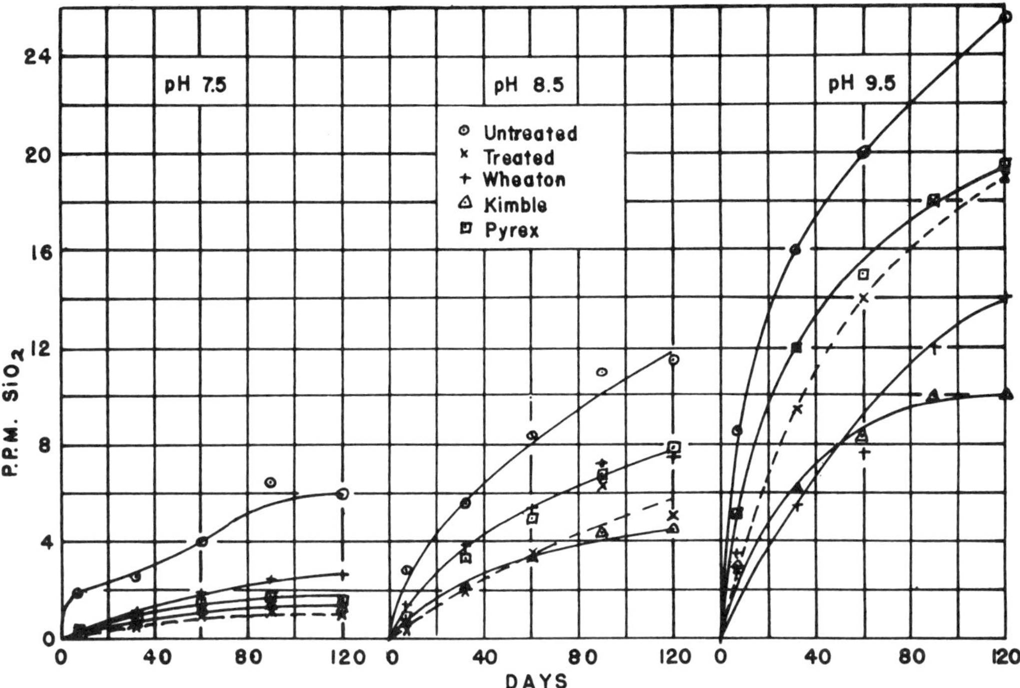

Figure 8 Extraction by borate buffers from 4-oz containers at 100°F. These buffers had the following compositions:

pH	B as H_3BO_3 (M)	Na as NaOH (N)
7.4–7.6	0.020	0.00053
8.4–8.5	0.020	0.045
9.4–9.5	0.020	0.0156

(After Ref. 13.)

any biasing of the pH of the unknown by the pH of the indicator solution is avoided. Total solids extracted were measured by evaporation to dryness with sulfuric acid and ignition at red heat. In soda-lime glass the pH rose from 6.8 to 10.3 and 100 ppm sulfated solids were found. In various high-resistance borosilicate glasses, the pH rose only to a range of 8–8.5, and from 5 to 12 ppm sulfated solids were found. Flakes formed during autoclaving in soda-lime ampuls and upon storage for a year or more in some of those made of borosilicate glass.

The action of neutral and alkaline solutions on glass is complex. Bacon and Raggon [15] found that the presence of certain anions, particularly citrate, causes neutral solutions to act similarly to alkaline solutions with substantial attack even on dealkalized glass containers. For example, when 200 ml of 4% sodium citrate or other salt solutions with approximately the same sodium content, all adjusted to a pH of 7.0, was added to ½-liter dealkalized containers and autoclaved at 121°C for 60 min, the SiO_2 dissolved was approximately 3 ppm for lactate, 6 for benzoate, 6 for acetate, 9 for succinate, 12 for ascorbate, 16 for malate, 28 for ethylenediaminetetraacetate, 30 for tartrate, 56 for oxalate, 64 for gluconate, 160 for fluoride, and 170 for citrate. Attack by the lactate solution was actually less than by plain water under the same experimental conditions. Strongly enhanced attack was interpreted as evidence of soluble complex formation by silica and the anion. For example, fluosilicic acid is quite soluble in water but silicic acid is not. The aggressive effect of citrate was eliminated by reducing the pH to about 5.5. At an initial pH of 7.0, borosilicate glass containers, particularly those with higher alumina content, were relatively resistant.

One practical consequence of these circumstances is that anticoagulant citrate dextrose solution with a pH of 4.5–5.5 can be packed in Type II containers with little interaction, but anticoagulant sodium citrate solution with a pH of 6.4–7.5 reacts extensively.

Degradation in the appearance of soda-lime glass containers on storage is called weathering. The reaction of the glass surface with atmospheric gases results in the formation of noticeable "weathering products" on the inside surface of ordinary soda-lime containers stored in unheated warehouses in all parts of the United States within 6 month's time. Continuous exposure to high humidity and temperature is somewhat detrimental. However, in areas where frequent, regular fluctuations in temperature and humidity occur, severe attack is sometimes encountered. The condensation of dew on the ware during cool periods and subsequent evaporation of the dew droplets during warm periods is a prominent factor in weathering [10]. The droplets of moisture extract sodium, becoming alkaline. As the solution becomes more concentrated during evaporation, further attack occurs.

In the early stages, the weathering product is mainly sodium carbonate, which does little damage if the containers are washed before filling. However, advanced weathering can increase the proneness of some glasses to release flakes after filling. Weathering can be avoided by the use of Type I borosilicate or Type II dealkalized glass containers. In the case of dealkalized containers the appearance may be changed by the solution of the byproduct, sodium sulfate, in condensed moisture and its subsequent recrystallization, but the underlying glass is virtually unaffected.

The concentration of material in a contained product migrating from a container wall increases with increase in container surface area per unit volume of contents [16]. If the shape and percentage fill of a container remain constant, the surface area per unit volume of contents is inversely proportional to the cube root of the volume. Thus it is increased 1.26 times when the capacity is cut to one-half and 2.15 times when it is cut to one-tenth. Hence, SVPs are exposed to potentially greater container influence than LVPs.

The total chemical performance of the parenteral container includes its stability in storage before use; the temperature and agent used in cleaning; its resistance to degradation during sterilization empty or to migration of ingredients into the contents if it is filled and sealed before sterilization; and its resistance to migration of constituents into the product during storage until the time of use.

As indicated above, it is desirable to sterilize Type III containers by dry heat prior to use. Type I and Type II containers may be sterilized by dry heat or by steam prior to use in aseptic filling operations or may be filled, sealed, and sterilized along with their contents by autoclaving. In terms of migration of container ingredients into the contents, sterilization of the sealed container at 121°C for 30 min is equivalent in severity to approximately 1 year at room temperature [10].

Of course, containers are not sterile and assuredly free of pyrogenic material when delivered to the pharmaceutical manufacturer. However, glass containers do have these attributes as they emerge from the high-temperature zone of the annealing lehr. Their surfaces are not capable of supporting the propagation of endotoxin-producing organisms that may be introduced during cooling, packing, storage, shipment, and handling prior to use by the pharmaceutical manufacturer. Further, the washing operation carried out by the user prior to filling is generally capable of removing pyrogenic matter that may be adventitiously present. The ability to withstand sterilization by heat without deformation or adverse effect on the contents is an important property of glass containers.

Container manufacturers can assist pharmaceutical manufacturers in the selection of containers that can be expected to meet the express requirements of individual parenteral preparations.

VI. MECHANICAL PERFORMANCE

The impermeability of glass to gases and liquids and the importance of fidelity in the finish dimensions to ensure effective mating and fastening of the closure have been mentioned above.

In view of the importance of glass wall thickness and surface condition to breakage resistance, the shape of the glass container must be well adapted to the bottle-forming process and the dimensions must be compatible with the bottle-handling elements of the washing and container-processing equipment used by the pharmaceutical manufacturer. Likewise this equipment must be designed to minimize the rubbing of bottle on bottle, the scraping of hard metal surfaces against the glass, and the impacting of bottles against one another or against conveyor elements to the extent compatible with efficient operation.

Thermal shock occurs when containers are heated or cooled rapidly during washing or sterilization. When one region of a container is hotter or colder than other regions, the region tends to expand or contract, generating temporary stresses in the rigid material. Thermal shock can be kept below levels that cause breakage by favorable container design, uniformity in heating or cooling, and moderation in heating and cooling rates. Type I glass containers have an advantage in their lower expansivity (see Table 1). In freeze-drying (lyophilizing) operations, Type I containers with thermal expansivity of about 32×10^{-7} per °C are less likely to crack than those with expansivity around 50×10^{-7}.

LVP containers usually have calibration marks and numerals embossed on the sidewall surface so that the approximate volume of contents can be seen with the bottle either upright or inverted. A depression is molded into the heel to serve as an index mark at the labeling machine. This enables the label to be placed in a proper position with respect to the calibration marks.

VII. QUALITY ASSURANCE

Throughout this chapter quality aspects of glass containers have been discussed in relation to official specifications, as affected by manufacturing

Table 5 Quality Aspects[a]

Chemical resistance
Powdered glass test (applicable to Types I and III)
Water attack at 121°C (applicable to Type II)
Dimensional conformity
Height
Diameter
Wall thickness variation
Perpendicularity
Concentricity of opening
Finish shape (except ampuls)
Internal neck diameter
Overflow capacity
Surface integrity
Absence of irregularities
Absence of checks
Absence of chipped edges
Glass quality
Freedom from cords
Freedom from stones
Freedom from seeds
Freedom from blisters
Whole container
State of annealing
Thermal shock resistance

[a]Definitions of trade terms that appear above. Finish: the part of a bottle holding the closure. Check: a tiny surface crack. Cord: an elongated region that differs in composition from the matrix glass. Stone: a crystalline inclusion. Seed: a tiny bubble. Blister: a relatively large flat bubble, usually near the surface.

parameters, and in relation to performance in the filling room on through use and disposal in the hospital or dispensary. Table 5 lists a number of these aspects which are susceptible to evaluation by examination or testing of the delivered container when warranted.

Normally, compliance with USP specifications and conformity of critical dimensions within defined tolerances are guaranteed by the supplier. The parenteral manufacturer may check these or rely on the guarantee. Numerous other aspects are considered or checked by the parenteral manufacturer. Generally these are a subject of private purchasing specifications that define the manner and extent of sampling and the frequency or extent of various defects that will be tolerated. They have the purpose of ensuring proper function and good appearance.

Those aspects that ensure the efficient filling, processing, storing, and delivery of contents sterile and without deterioration are vital. These include compliance with USP specifications, dimensional conformity to ensure compatibility with processing equipment and to ensure a hermetic seal, and the absence of abnormalities that would seriously undermine resistance to breakage—things such as finish shape, perfection of sealing surface, state of annealing, freedom from excessive checks, stones, or cords, and adequate thermal shock resistance.

Other aspects influence only appearance and are less critical. These include noncritical dimensions, abundance of seeds, and noncritical surface irregularities.

If purchaser and supplier work together starting with design of the container, including layout and maintenance of the purchasers' bottle-handling equipment and ending with review of the quality and performance of delivered ware, optimum performance of containers can be assured.

REFERENCES

1. SRM 622 and SRM 623 can be ordered from the Office of Standard Reference Materials, Room B311, Chemistry Building, National Bureau of Standards, Washington, D.C. 20234.
2. R. W. Douglass and J. O. Isard, The action of water and sulphur dioxide on glass surfaces. *J. Soc. Glass Technol.*, 33:289–335T (1949).
3. P. W. Anderson, F. R. Bacon, and B. W. Byrum, Effect of surface treatments on the chemical durability and surface composition of soda-lime glass bottles. *J. Non-Crystalline Solids*, 9:251–262 (1975).
4. ASTM Designation C729-75, Standard test method for density of glass by the sink-float comparator. In *1985 Annual Book of ASTM Standards*, Vol. 15.02, Philadelphia.
5. ASTM Designation C148-77, Standard methods of polariscopic examination of glass containers. In *1985 Annual Book of ASTM Standards*, Vol. 15.02, Philadelphia.
6. ASTM Designation C149-77, Standard method of thermal shock test on glass containers. In *1985 Annual Book of ASTM Standards*, Vol. 15.02, Philadelphia.
7. P. B. Adams, Surface properties of glass containers for parenteral solutions. *Bull. Parent. Drug Assoc.*, 31:213–226 (1977).
8. C. F. Stafficker, A comparison of blown bottles and tubing vials. *Bull. Parent. Drug Assoc.*, 17(5):31–40 (1963).

9. A. L. Hinson, Fluoride washing of glass containers. *Bull. Parent. Drug Assoc.*, 25:266–269 (1971).
10. F. R. Bacon, The chemical durability of silicate glass. *Glass Ind.*, 49:438, 439, 442–446, 494–499, 554–559 (1968).
11. F. R. Bacon, R. H. Russell, G. W. Baumgartner, and W. P. Close, Composition of material extracted from soda-lime glass containers by aqueous contents. *Am. Ceram. Soc. Bull.*, 53:641–645, 649 (1974).
12. ASTM Designation C169–80, Standard methods for chemical analysis of soda-lime and borosilicate glass. In *1985 Annual Book of ASTM Standards*, Vol. 15.02, Philadelphia.
13. F. R. Bacon and S. W. Barber, The chemical durability of sulfur-treated glass containers. Technical Bulletin, Owens-Illinois, Toledo, Ohio, 1948.
14. A. L. Hinson, D. C. Smith, and J. F. Greene, Changes in distilled water stored in glass ampuls. *J. Am. Ceram. Soc.*, 30:211–214 (1947).
15. F. R. Bacon and F. C. Raggon, Promotion of attack on glass and silica by citrate and other anions in neutral solutions. *J. Am. Ceram. Soc.*, 42:199–205 (1959).
16. J. F. Greene and A. L. Hinson, Glass durability tests—effect of shape and size of containers for injections. *Bull. Natl. Formulary Committee*, 17:61–66 (1949).

4

Plastic Containers for Parenterals

Donald D. Solomon,* Raymond W. Jurgens, Jr.,† and K. Lim Wong‡

American McGaw, American Hospital Supply Corporation, Irvine, California

I. INTRODUCTION

Subcutaneous, intramuscular, intrasternal, and intravenous injections have been routes used for parenteral medications since the late nineteenth century. The medications and vehicles were almost exclusively dispensed in glass containers due to the clarity, inertness, impermeability, and thermal resistance of these containers. Fragility, weight, and the necessity for a rubber closure represent the major inherent disadvantages of glass parenteral containers. With the development of polymer technology over the last 30 years, plastics have become logical alternatives for large volume parenteral (LVP) packaging. Although plastic containers have become well established as containers for LVP products, plastics are being used on a very limited scale for small volume parenterals (SVP). However, more interest has been shown recently in polyolefins for plastic SVP containers, especially those in the 100 ml and less volume range. Plastic containers for parenterals have a number of demonstrated advantages. They are relatively unbreakable and extremely light, less than one-tenth the weight of their glass counterparts. They are easily fabricated into any shape for ease of handling and effective packaging. Cost is also an important factor. Not only are plastic containers cheaper than glass but, in some cases, can be recycled as a fuel source.

The polymers used in plastic LVP containers must be carefully chosen or they can present several negative characteristics to the LVP manufacturer. The clarity of plastic LVP containers, in most cases, is inferior to that of

Current affiliation: Deseret Polymer Research, Warner-Lambert, Dayton, Ohio

†*Current affiliation*: Mallinckrodt, Inc., St. Louis, Missouri

‡*Current affiliation*: Rockwell International Corporation, Newport Beach, California

glass, although translucency and even transparency can be attained. Plastic containers cannot match the barrier properties of glass to moisture and oxygen, but adequate properties are achievable. Special attention must also be given to the additives present in the plastic due to the potential leachability of the additives into the parenteral medication.

Plastic parenteral packages have become commercially available only in the last decade. With the proliferation of new polymers and new polymer process technology, most of the less desirable characteristics of the plastic container have been overcome. This chapter will present an overview of the plastic parenteral containers used in the United States.

II. FUNDAMENTAL CONCEPTS

There is a wide variety of polymers on the market from which the parenteral product manufacturer may choose a packaging material. The selection of an appropriate plastic packaging material should be based upon a knowledge of the important properties and the unique processing and stability requirements of the material. The following subsections will serve as a foundation for later discussions and will provide the reader with an understanding of the basic terminology of polymers.

A. What Is a Plastic?

The American Society for Testing and Materials (ASTM) defines glass an an inorganic product of fusion that will cool to a rigid condition without crystallizing. Unlike glass, plastic is organic and polymeric in nature. A polymer is simply a large molecule built up by the repetitious joining of small molecules or monomers. These monomers are joined together by the process of polymerization. The monomers commonly consist of atoms of carbon, hydrogen, oxygen, nitrogen, and halogens (fluorine, chlorine, and bromine).

After the monomers have undergone polymerization, a repeat structure or unit becomes apparent and is usually equivalent or nearly equivalent to the monomer. The structural relationship between the monomer and repeat unit of three common polymers is shown in Table 1.

Table 1 Monomers and Repeat Units of Several Common Polymers[a]

Polymer	Monomer	Repeat unit
Polyethylene	$CH_2{=}CH_2$	$\leftarrow(CH_2CH_2\rightarrow$
Polyvinyl chloride	$CH_2{=}CHCl$	$\leftarrow(CH_2CHCl\rightarrow_n$
Polystyrene	$CH_2{=}CH$ (with phenyl ring on CH)	$\leftarrow(CH_2CH\rightarrow_n$ (with phenyl ring on CH)

[a]n signifies the finite number of repeat units that constitutes a single polymer chain.

The monomers shown in Table 1 closely resemble the structure of the polymer repeat unit. However, the repeat units of such polymers as polyesters are not as easily related to the monomers used in the polymerization. Polyesters are synthesized by reactions between bifunctional monomers, with the elimination of water:

$$\mathrm{HO{-}R{-}OH + HOCO{-}R'{-}COOH} \longrightarrow$$

$$\mathrm{HO{\left(R{-}OCO{-}R'{-}COO\right)}_n H + H_2O}$$

The portion within parentheses represents the repeat unit of the polyester.

There are basically two classes of plastics: thermoplastics and thermosets. Thermoplastics are polymers that soften upon heating at high temperature and solidfy again upon cooling. Thermosets are polymers that are only softened during the fabrication of an article and will harden permanently; therefore, they cannot be softened again upon heating. For parenteral packaging, thermoplastic polymers are preferred over the thermoset polymers due to their availability, reusability, and processibility.

B. Polymer Properties

The chemical structure of the polymer molecule, its molecular weight distribution, crystallinity, and additive content are the primary determinants of a plastic's physical, chemical, and mechanical properties.

Polymers that are formed into long linear chains will have different performance characteristics than those that are branched or interconnected to form a three-dimensional structure. The arrangements of the repeating structural units in a linear and branched polymer are illustrated in Figure 1.

Multi- or copolymer systems are those that have more than one type of repeating unit, and this often results in more favorable properties, such as toughness or flexibility, than are present in the individual homopolymers. The resulting properties are also influenced by the "manner" in which the repeating units appear in the polymer chain. The specific properties will be discussed in a later section. By employing different synthesis techniques, copolymers can be made with alternating, random, block, or grafted repeating units within the polymer chain. Each type of copolymer structure is illustrated in Figure 2.

Unlike small organic molecules, polymers contain molecules with different chain lengths. The chain length distribution of a polymer can be calculated statistically. This is generally referred to as the molecular weight distribution (MWD) of the polymer. This information can be used to predict or evaluate polymer processing parameters and performance characteristics. When two polymers have identical chemical structures but have different MWD, the processing parameters and performance characteristics of the two polymers may be considerably different.

The degree of order in a polymer system is directly related to the degree of crystallinity. By definition, a crystalline polymer system is one in which a high degree of order prevails. Conversely, an amorphous (noncrystalline) system is devoid of order. Generally speaking, most polymers have both amorphous and crystalline regions, the degree of each varying with the individual polymer system. Crystallinity is largely determined by the type and size of the repeating unit and how well the polymer chains

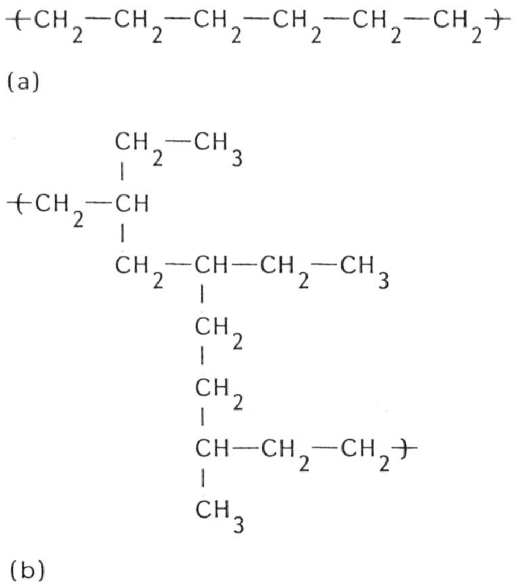

$+CH_2-CH_2-CH_2-CH_2-CH_2-CH_2+$

(a)

```
     CH2—CH3
     |
+CH2—CH
     |
     CH2—CH—CH2—CH3
         |
         CH2
         |
         CH2
         |
         CH—CH2—CH2+
         |
         CH3
```

(b)

Figure 1 The structure in parentheses represents arbitrary sections of polymer: (a) linear polyethylene, (b) branched polyethylene.

are arranged in a lattice array. Crystallinity is an important parameter in determining many of the plastic's physicochemical properties. In general, the higher the degree of crystallinity a polymer has the more brittle and rigid it will be. Such a polymer will also exhibit less permeability and transparency.

Since polymers are not generally as inert as glass, they may be subject to degradation and oxidation during the useful life of the product. Furthermore, degradation and process difficulties may be encountered during the fabrication of the product. These problems can be reduced or eliminated by the use of additives to protect the basic polymer.

C. Additives

Each polymer type has its own unique characteristics and end-use limitations. By the addition of other molecules, which are referred to as additives, it is often possible to improve a particular polymer's performance characteristics. The additives most commonly found in plastics used for LVP packages are antioxidants, heat stabilizers, lubricants, plasticizers, fillers, and colorants. These additives can be in liquid, solid, or fine particle form. The amount of additive combined with the base polymer varies from as little as 0.01% to as much as 60%, depending upon the type of polymer and additive. The following general discussion will introduce and define those additives that are used in plastics commonly used as parenteral plastic containers. Additives for each specific type of plastic used for LVP containers will be discussed in detail in Section IV.

Alternating

-A-B-A-B-A-B-A-B-A-B-A-B-A-B-

Random

-A-B-A-A-B-A-B-B-A-A-A-B-A-B-

Block

-A-A-A-A-B-B-B-B-B-A-A-A-A-A-

Graft

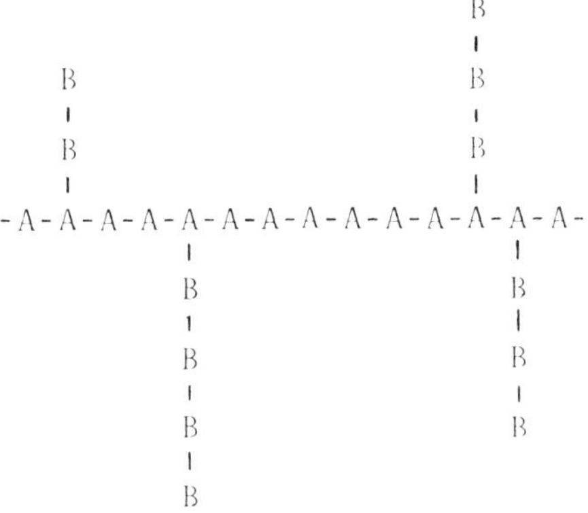

Figure 2 Four types of multicomponent polymer systems where A and B represent two different repeating units.

1. *Antioxidants*

Polymers are often exposed to heat, light, ozone, and mechanical stress in the presence of oxygen during processing and end use. The resulting oxidative effects will cause the formation of free radicals, which contribute, in turn, to the degradation of the polymer with a gradual loss of important physical and mechanical properties of the plastic. The presence of antioxidants in the plastic formulation will significantly reduce the degree of degradation and, therefore, help to preserve the lifetime of the plastic container.

There are two types of antioxidants:

Primary antioxidants: These are free radical chain terminators. They are basically a hydrogen donor that can terminate the free radical propagation reaction. Secondary arylamines and hindered phenols fall into this class.

Secondary antioxidants: These antioxidants destroy peroxide and thus eliminate the formation of free radicals. Phosphites and thioesters fall into this classification.

Very often, more than one antioxidant will be used in the polymer as a system to take advantage of the synergistic effects of the combined antioxidants.

2. *Heat Stabilizers*

During the manufacturing process of certain polymers, degradation byproducts will catalyze degradation reactions or cause discoloration of the polymer. Addition of a heat stabilizer will reduce these undesirable reactions. Heat stabilizers are generally required in the manufacture of polyvinyl chloride polymers (PVC). Metallic stearates and epoxidized plasticizers are the most commonly used heat stabilizers.

3. *Lubricants*

Lubricants are used to modify the surface characteristics of the molded polymer and facilitate processing. Addition of a lubricant to a polymer generally reduces the melt flow viscosity of the polymer, i.e., causes the polymer to be more free flowing during processing. Lubricants also modify the surface of the fabricated product to prevent polymers from sticking to the hot metal processing machinery. The most commonly used lubricants are fatty acids, fatty alcohols, fatty esters, fatty amides, metallic stearates, paraffin wax, and silicones.

4. *Plasticizers*

Plasticizers are used to improve the base polymer's workability, flexibility, extensibility, impact strength, and resilience. Addition of a plasticizer, on the other hand, will reduce the tensile strength of the polymer. The most commonly used plasticizers in parenteral plastics are dialkyl phthalates and low-molecular-weight polymers.

5. *Fillers*

Addition of fillers to the base polymer may result in improved flexibility, impact resistance, dimensional heat stability, and reduced material cost. In the parenteral plastic containers made from such plastics as PVC, small amounts of submicrometer fillers are used as brighteners and co-colorants. The addition of these fillers usually does not impair the transparency of the plastic container.

6. *Colorants*

Certain plastics have an inherent color that is not aesthetically desirable, and upon aging, the color becomes more intensified. To rectify this problem, parenteral manufacturers may add a colorant to hide the undesirable color of the polymer. Both dye and pigment colorants are available for use in plastics. Experience has shown that dye molecules have a tendency to bleed out of the polymer matrix upon aging, but pigments have been shown to be nonbleeding. Ultramarine blue is one of the most commonly used colorants for parenteral plastics.

From the foregoing discussion the reader is now equipped with a basic "plastics" vocabulary, making it possible to examine in detail the important polymers for the parenteral industry. In the following section polymer types will be described in a systematic manner to facilitate comparison. They will be discussed with consideration for the physical, chemical, and mechanical properties of the plastic, the additives necessary for processing and stability, and the potential problems which they (polymer and additives) might present to the parenteral manufacturer.

III. IMPORTANT PLASTICS FOR LVP PACKAGES

A. Polyolefins

Polyolefins represent one of the most widely used thermoplastic materials for packaging LVP. This section will deal with the three major polyolefin plastics of importance to the LVP industry: polypropylene, polyethylene, and copolymers of ethylene and propylene.

Polyolefins are formed by polymerization of unsaturated hydrocarbon monomers; the resulting polymer has a saturated structure composed of only carbon and hydrogen.

1. *Polypropylene*

Polypropylene is the most widely used polyolefin in the world. It has a number of attractive inherent properties for use as an LVP package material. It has excellent availability and is among the least costly plastics available. Polypropylene is the lightest major plastic and lends itself to a number of different packaging configurations.

Properties

Polypropylene is a linear, highly crystalline polymer. Its chemical structure is made up completely of carbon and hydrogen in a very orderly fashion.

$$\left(CH_2-\underset{\displaystyle CH_3}{\overset{|}{CH}}-CH_2-\underset{\displaystyle CH_3}{\overset{|}{CH}} \right)_n$$

The regularity of its structure imparts the high degree of crystallinity found in most commercially available polypropylenes. The crystalline nature of the polymer gives it a number of important properties. In the crystalline array, the $-CH_3$ groups add stiffness to the polymer. Polypropylene exhibits a high tensile strength, which is the ability to withstand forces tending to pull apart or distort. The high tensile strength, in conjunction with the high melting point of 165°C, is particularly important to the LVP manufacturer because containers made from polypropylene have the ability to withstand the high temperatures of steam sterilization without distortion.

Polypropylene is very resistant to chemical attack from organic solvents at room temperature, as well as strong acids and bases.

Polypropylene provides a good barrier to both gases and water vapor due to inherently high crystallinity. It also is very abrasion resistant and is capable of retaining a high surface gloss. LVP packages require a level of clarity that can be satisfied by polypropylene. Although there are a number of factors affecting the clarity of the material, such as processing and thickness of the final container, the containers vary from translucent to semiclear.

Additives

Polypropylene degrades when subjected to heat, ultraviolet (UV) light, and oxygen; it therefore must be stabilized by antioxidants. If polypropylene is not stabilized by the inclusion of appropriate antioxidants, degradation results in a material with low molecular weight, the generation of such compounds as butyric acid, poor processing characteristics, and a destruction of many of the plastic's useful properties.

There are a number of commercially available antioxidants that, either alone or in a synergistic system of two or more other antioxidants, can stabilize polypropylene against degradation. Hindered phenols, phosphites, and thioesters are the most common types of antioxidants used in polypropylene. Table 2 illustrates some of the more common variations of the three important classes of antioxidants used in polypropylene and other polyolefins.

Choosing the proper additives and concentration levels in a polymer system is extremely important. The volatility and mobility of the additives must be examined in light of current literature as well as specific end-use testing.

Conversely, choosing an improper antioxidant(s) or designating an insufficient antioxidant concentration level can result in premature yellowing of the plastic container, a higher degree of leachability due to degradation, and a higher potential for particulate matter formation. If the antioxidant is extremely mobile and/or the concentration is too high, the LVP manufacturer is faced with potentially high levels of antioxidants leaching into the parenteral solution, resulting in undesirable reactions with parenteral solutions.

Table 2 Antioxidants for Polypropylene and Other Polyolefins[a]

Chemical name	Type
Distearyl pentaerythritol diphosphite	Organo-phosphite
Tris nonylphenyl phosphite (TNPP)	Organo-phosphite
1,1,3-Tris-(2-methyl-4-hydroxy-5-*t*-butyl phenyl) butane	Hindered phenol
1,3,4-Trimethyl-2,4,6-tris [3,5,-di-*tert*-butyl-4-hydroxybenzyl] benzene	Hindered phenol
2,6-Di-*t*-butyl-*p*-cresol (butylated hydroxy toluene, BHT)	Hindered phenol
Octadecyl-3,5-di-*tert*-butyl-4-hydroxy-hydrocinnamate	Hindered phenol
Tetrakis[methylene-(3,5-di-*tert*-butyl-4-hydroxyhydrocinnamate)]methane	Hindered phenol
Dilauryl-3,3'-thiodipropionate (DLTDP)	Thioester

[a]Antioxidants in polypropylene and other polyolefins are usually found in levels of 0.01–0.25% for medical grade polymers.

Besides antioxidants, lubricants are the only other additives used in any significant amounts in polypropylene. Calcium stearate can be used to reduce frictional forces during the processing of polyolefins. Such lubricants as calcium stearate are commonly used in concentrations of 0.05–0.3% in polypropylene or polyolefin formulations.

Polymer Formulation Summary

The variety and concentration level of antioxidants are kept to a minimum in polypropylene containers. This is normally true also for other plastics used in the manufacture of LVP containers. The LVP container made from polypropylene is typically formulated with antioxidants and occasionally a lubricant. Table 3 illustrates the generally accepted components and concentration of each found in a polypropylene formulation.

Table 3 refers specifically to the parts of polypropylene LVP containers in direct contact with the intravenous (IV) or irrigation solutions. Other components, e.g., outer caps, retainers, and rings, can be manufactured from other polyolefins, such as high-density polyethylene and copolymers of ethylene-propylene. In general, Table 3 applies to the latter materials; however, components not in direct contact with solutions may be colored. In this case, the colorants are usually added in amounts ranging from 0.01 to 5%.

2. *Polyethylene*

Low-density or branched polyethylene was the first commercial branched ethylene polymer. This type of polyethylene is commonly referred to as LDPE. In many commercial applications LDPE is being replaced by linear-low-density polyethylene (LLDPE), which is less expensive to produce and has more desirable physical properties. Because of their low softening points, LDPE and LLDPE have virtually no application as container resins in the LVP industry. The vast majority of the LVP containers are subject to steam sterilization, which utilizes temperatures above their softening points.

High-density polyethylene (HDPE) is typically a highly crystalline linear polymer. HDPE, as its name suggests, is higher in density, 0.95–0.97 g/cm^3, compared with the 0.91–0.94 g/cm^3 found in LDPE. Crystallinity is the main contributor to the overall changes in properties. HDPE have greater tensile strength, are stiffer, and have a higher melting point (128–137°C) than the LPDE polymers. In Europe, sterilization cycles are

Table 3 Typical Formulation for a Polypropylene LVP Container

Component	Concentration range (%w/w)
Polypropylene resin	99.45–99.99
Antioxidant	0.01–0.25
Lubricant	0.05–0.3

being used where lower temperatures and longer cycle times are being used. Consequently, it is now possible to use some of the higher molecular weight HDPE having high melting points as LVP container resin. The latter is not, as yet, a common practice in the United States.

A final type of polyethylene needs to be at least mentioned. Ultrahigh-molecular-weight polyethylene (UHMPE) is commercially available. This type of polyethylene is defined as those linear polymers with a relative viscosity of at least 2.3 when dissolved (0.05%) in decahydronaphthalene at 135°C. Processing is much different than that of HDPE due to the high molecular weight of the polymers, typically 3–6 million. Powder processing is utilized for many applications. Although this type of polymer does not have any application as a LVP container resin, it is used for surgical implants, which require high abrasion resistance.

It is commonly known in the plastics industry that few additives are compatible with polyethylene in levels greater than 1%. Typically, antioxidants similar to those found in Table 2 are used.

3. *Copolymers*

Copolymers of ethylene and propylene are being successfully used in the LVP marketplace as LVP containers. In fact, polypropylene and copolymers of ethylene-propylene are the most commonly used polyolefins for LVP containers.

By combining a small fraction of ethylene as a block or random copolymer with propylene, a number of desirable properties can be attained (Fig. 3). The incorporation of ethylene decreases the stiffness of propylene, improves processability, and only slightly decreases the melting point of polypropylene. Typical melt temperatures are between 145 and 150°C. This makes ethylene-propylene (EP) copolymers appropriate for use under steam sterilization conditions. The clarity of most EP copolymers is quite sufficient to allow routine inspection for particulates and to observe the fluid level in the LVP container.

The EP copolymers, as with other polyolefins, require minimal levels of additives for processing and long-term stability. Generally, less than 0.2% of a hindered phenol antioxidant (see Table 2) is sufficient to prevent degradation during processing. Antioxidants at such low levels usually do not present a leachability problem with the common LVP products. EP copolymer containers provide an adequate moisture-vapor barrier to give a shelf life for products of a year or more. Therefore, LVP containers fabricated from EP copolymers do not require an outer wrap to prevent moisture loss.

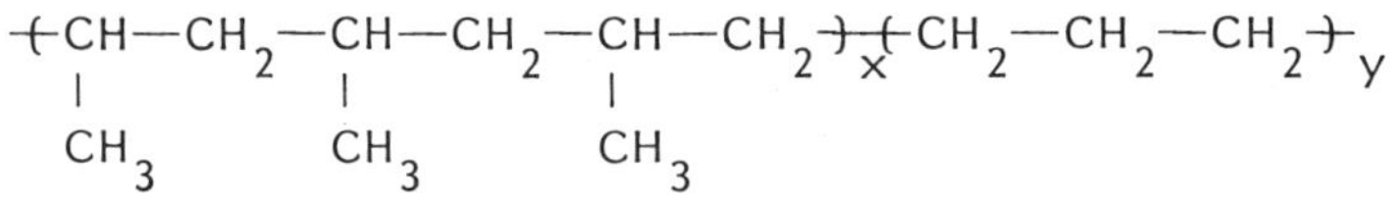

$$\left(\underset{\substack{|\\CH_3}}{CH}-CH_2-\underset{\substack{|\\CH_3}}{CH}-CH_2-\underset{\substack{|\\CH_3}}{CH}-CH_2\right)_x\left(CH_2-CH_2-CH_2\right)_y$$

Figure 3 An example of an ethylene-propylene block copolymer system where x and y represent the size of the blocks of ethylene and propylene, respectively.

B. Poly(vinyl Chloride)

Poly(vinyl chloride), or PVC as it is commonly known, is the dominant polymer resin in the vinyl family. PVC is used in the United States alone at the rate of more than 6 billion lb/year. Although PVC is the major polymer utilized in the medical industry, medical use of PVC represents only a very small fraction of the yearly PVC production.

PVC is one of the oldest polymers. As World War II approached, PVC became commercially significant, the primary interest being to find synthetic replacements for rubber. The medical use of flexible polyvinyl chloride resins encompasses IV tubing and drip chambers, catheters, blood bags, mixing bags, and LVP containers. PVC was the first polymeric material to replace glass for blood storage and LVP applications.

Poly(vinyl chloride), as the name implies, is based on the vinyl monomer of monochloroethene. PVC is produced by polymerizing vinyl chloride gas (CH_2=CHCl) in the presence of an initiator, such as an organic peroxide or an inorganic persulfate. The initiator acts to generate free radicals to propagate the polymerization reaction. It can be simply illustrated:

$$R_1OOR_2 \rightarrow R_1O\cdot + R_2O\cdot$$

where R_1OOR_2 represents an organic peroxide. After the peroxide free radical (an unpaired electron) is formed, reaction with the vinyl monomer takes place and then is propagated. This is shown in a general sense as

```
    H  Cl                         H  Cl  H  H
    |  |                          |  |   |  |
R—C—C• + CH2=CHCl → R—C—C—C—C•
    |  |                          |  |   |  |
    H  H                          H  H   H  Cl
```

which continues until the reaction is terminated.

Of all products made from PVC, 45% are flexible. In the LVP industry flexible PVC is used primarily for containers and rigid PVC as injection molded parts for IV administration sets.

In September 1975, the FDA proposed regulations to restrict the use of vinyl chloride (VC) in contact with food products. The principal concern was the potential migration of the VC monomer into food products. Since that time, great effort has been put forth by the PVC industry to reduce the residual levels of VC monomer to a level less than 1 ppm.

1. *Properties*

Plasticized PVC has found extensive application in the LVP and medical industry because of its unique physical properties, versatile fabrication properties, and relatively low cost. In general, PVC is a very tough and chemically resistant plastic. Poly(vinyl chloride) polymers are resistant to alcohols, aliphatic hydrocarbons, oils, weak acids, and alkalies. Articles made from plasticized PVC are mark and dent resistant. The density of PVC (1.16–1.35 g/cm^3) is significantly higher than that of other polymers, such as polyethylene (0.92–0.96 g/cm^3) and polypropylene ($\sim$0.90 g/cm^3). The moisture vapor transmission rate (MVTR) for PVC is higher than that of polyolefins (Table 4). Because of the high-moisture transmission rate

Table 4 Moisture and Oxygen Transmission Rates of Common Polymers

Polymer	Moisture (water)[a]	Oxygen[a]
High-density polyethylene	140	11
Polypropylene	672	23
Ethylene-propylene copolymer	609	20
Poly(vinyl chloride)	1550	1.2
Poly(vinylidene chloride)	13.5	0.05

[a]Permeation $\times 10^{10}$ ($cc/cm^2\ mm^{-1}/sec^{-1}/cm\ Hg^{-1}$) at 90% RH and 25°C.

of PVC polymers, most LVP are packaged with an outer wrap to reduce the water loss with the consequential concentration of the LVP product.

Unstabilized PVC is very susceptible to degradation and discoloration by heat and ultraviolet light. Degradation proceeds as a chain reaction initiated and propagated by a chlorine radical ($Cl^{\bullet}$). This is illustrated below.

$$Cl^{\bullet} + \sim CH_2-\underset{\displaystyle Cl}{\underset{|}{CH}}-CH_2-\underset{\displaystyle Cl}{\underset{|}{CH}}\sim \rightarrow \qquad (1)$$

$$\sim CH_2-\underset{\displaystyle Cl}{\underset{|}{CH}}-\dot{C}H-\underset{\displaystyle Cl}{\underset{|}{CH}}\sim + HCl \qquad (2)$$

$$\sim CH_2-\underset{\displaystyle Cl}{\underset{|}{CH}}-\dot{C}H-\underset{\displaystyle Cl}{\underset{|}{CH}}\sim \rightarrow \sim CH_2-\underset{\displaystyle Cl}{\underset{|}{CH}}-CH = CH\sim + Cl^{\bullet} \qquad (3)$$

The chlorine radical abstracts a hydrogen from the polymer chain (1) which then activates the polymer chain by forming a new chain radical (2) and hydrogen chloride. The polymer chain then deactivates to form a double bond and another chlorine radical (3). So proceeds the polymer decomposition until total decomposition has occurred. Color, due to decomposition, usually begins to develop when five to seven conjugated double bonds have been formed.

The degradation of PVC can generally be reduced sufficiently by the addition of stabilizers. It is important that sufficient levels of stabilizer be added to protect against degradation during the manufacturing process and stabilize the container for the life of the intended product. The HCl generated during decomposition can adversely lower the pH of many LVP solutions due to their relatively low buffering capacity. A certain amount of decomposition occurs during processing of PVC film or containers; therefore, it is essential to set stringent specifications for processing. Some of the important properties of PVC are summarized in Table 5.

Table 5 Properties of Poly(vinyl Chloride)

Property	Plasticized calendered PVC
Density (g/cm^2)	1.16–1.35
Tensile strength (psi)	1400–9000
Elongation (%)	100–500
Water absorption, 24 hr (%)	Negligible
Resistance to	
Strong bases	Good
Strong acids	Good
Alcohol	Good
Aliphatic hydrocarbons	Good
Sunlight	Fair
Heat sealing range (°C)	175–232

2. *Additives*

Flexible PVC is compounded by combining poly(vinyl chloride) homopolymer or copolymer, stabilizers, lubricants, and other additives necessary for a given final product. There is no single "standard" composition. Each flexible PVC formulation is designed for a specific product, and most are proprietary. However, some general well-known guidelines can be discussed. A summary of additives and levels present in typical flexible PVC formulations is shown in Table 6.

Heat stabilizers have been reviewed extensively [1]. The principal properties of an ideal stabilizer could be summarized as an ability to absorb HCl, displace chlorine radicals, disrupt double bonds, provide antioxidant protection, and provide UV screening. As with any additive, it should be nonmigratory, nontoxic, and odorless. In addition, it should not affect the physical properties of the compound, such as clarity or color. There are

Table 6 Components in Poly(vinyl Chloride) Formulations

Component	Level (phr)[a]
PVC resin	100
Plasticizer	30–40
Stabilizers	0.25–7

[a]phr = parts per hundred parts of resin by weight.

also processing considerations that must be reviewed before a stabilizer is chosen; however, these are not within the scope of this chapter.

Stabilizers fall into five main groups based on their composition:

Organo-tin compounds
Lead salts or soaps
Other metal salts or soaps
Synergistic mixed stabilizers
Organic and miscellaneous stabilizers

Of these only a very few can be used in medical applications due to their toxicity level.

Among those stabilizers that are FDA sanctioned are the calcium-zinc (Ca-Zn) types. In this same category there are other metal soaps, such as aluminum, magnesium, sodium, and tin, which are also FDA sanctioned.

Epoxides are commonly used as costabilizers. Among the most commonly used epoxides are epoxidized mono- and polyesters and ethers and epoxidized soybean oil. The epoxides also contribute secondarily to the plasticization of flexible PVC.

Lubricants rank as one of the most important components added to a PVC formulation. They facilitate the melt flow of the plastic during processing and prevent adhesion to metal surfaces. The addition of the proper lubricant can also result in much better appearance of the final product. The most common lubricants are fatty acid esters, fatty acids and alcohols, fatty acid amides, metallic soaps, e.g., zinc stearate, paraffins, and polyethylene waxes.

Plasticizers are responsible for modifying a normally rigid PVC into a flexible plastic. As the amount of plasticization in the formulation increases, the degree of "limpness" and "softness" of the material increases.

Plasticization dramatically improves the low-temperature properties of the material. Film is routinely manufactured showing excellent gloss and transparency. Plasticizer leachability is a primary concern when PVC is used as the material for LVP containers. There is an ongoing controversy surrounding the use of certain plasticizers. At the heart of the controversy is di-2-ethylhexylphthalate, commonly referred to as DEHP or DOP. The National Toxicity Program recently addressed the DEHP issue [2]. There has been no consensus reached about whether DEHP is a mutagenic hazard to humans.

Because of the wide use, economic considerations, and history behind DEHP, this plasticizer will no doubt continue to be used unless conclusive evidence of human hazard is established. The hint of potential human mutagenicity has caused some PVC, medical device, and parenteral manufacturers to investigate alternatives to DEHP. Some of the alternatives are listed in Table 7. Two of the key factors considered in designing alternative plasticizers were molecular weight and polymer miscibility. A higher molecular weight plasticizer, in general, is less likely to migrate or leach out of the plastic and into the parenteral solution. Trioctyltrimellitate (TOTM; see Table 7) is an example of a higher molecular weight plasticizer that is gaining wider acceptance. TOTM has been shown to be less leachable than DEHP [3]. There are some disadvantages in the use of TOTM; it is more expensive, and PVC compounds formulated with TOTM are slightly more difficult to process.

Polymeric plasticizers provide a large variety and a wide molecular weight range of plasticizers from which to choose. It must be remembered that

Table 7 Common High-Molecular-Weight Plasticizers

Plasticizer	Type	Molecular weight
Trioctyl trimellitate (TOTM)	Nonpolymeric	567
Polyester adipate	Polymeric	2000–3500
Polyester glutarate	Polymeric	2500

polymeric plasticizers, although high in molecular weight, are not monodisperse. The polymeric plasticizers, like all polymers, are composed of varied molecular chain lengths that translate into a range of molecular weights. It cannot be assumed that the leachability of polymeric plasticizers is inherently low. It is possible that a significant fraction of a given polymeric plasticizer is of sufficiently low molecular weight to be subject to a high level of leachability. Polymeric plasticizers are not as economically attractive as many of the other conventional plasticizers. Additionally, they also present a great challenge to the PVC formulator to achieve adequate processability.

The leachability of plasticizers is virtually impossible to predict a priori [4]. The safest approach is to evaluate the plasticizer under consideration in an appropriate PVC formulation. The PVC material should then be placed in contact with the LVP solution(s) that would be normally used. By choosing test conditions greater than the norm (e.g., 40 or 60°C) and comparing to a control, a logical choice can then be made.

IV. EVALUATION AND TESTING OF PLASTICS FOR LVP USE

The Pharmaceutical Manufacturers Association (PMA) recognized the need to develop standards for plastic materials as early as 1961. A committee was formed [5, 6] to establish procedures for testing and compile a data base for a number of plastic materials. Over a 2-year period, 20,000 tests were performed on 22 plastic materials [7]. The developmental work accomplished in that early study was eventually, with slight modifications, adopted by the U.S. Pharmacopeia (USP) and National Formulary (NF) [8, 9]. Since that time other revisions, modifications, and additions have been adopted and now appear in the current USP XXI-NF XVI [10]. Although the work culminated in today's biological and physiochemical test procedures, there are still no established positive standards of use analogous to FDA regulations for plastic packaging materials used in the food industry.

The FDA has given some limited direction concerning the evaluation and testing of polymeric materials. In presenting a plastic for use as the material for an LVP container, the following would probably be considered the basic framework for testing.

a. Determine, via USP XXI-NF XVI [10] procedures for biological and physiochemical testing, the amount and type of potentially leachable substances in any given plastic LVP container.

b. Determine integrity or stability by testing for the effects of storage conditions, i.e., time, temperature, light, and humidity, and the effect of a sterilization cycle on the physical, chemical, and biological properties of the container.
c. Perform any other tests, and generate an appropriate data base to assure the safety of the container.

In contrast to plastic materials, glass has enjoyed a traditional acceptance for use in LVP containers by virtue of early and long-time use. It should not be construed that glass materials should be used in LVP application without a reasonable battery of tests. However, an advantage of glass over plastics is that its use is aided by an existing USP XXI-NF XVI specification. In general, any container or component that comes in direct contact with an LVP solution should be evaluated with considerable care. Even glass has been shown to contain harmful extractables [11], and in some cases, glass has been shown to yield more extractables than comparable plastic containers [12].

With the increasing use of plastic for LVP containers, it is critical to become familiar with and establish appropriate up-to-date protocols for testing. The quality of testing is important. There are so many testing procedures available, it is important not to fall prey to testing for testing's sake. The following section deals with *some* of the more important methods and techniques used to test polymers. It must be stressed that these tests are generally regarded as appropriate but every test may not be necessary for each polymeric material. What is important is that a number of well-proven methods can increase the safety and efficacy of the plastic LVP container and, therefore, the product as a whole.

A. Qualifying New Plastics

1. Raw Materials Screening and Qualification

The first step after choosing a class of polymer in LVP containers is to screen several polymer resin manufacturers. This can be done easily by requesting samples from the plastics manufacturers of interest. Normally, product sheets, handling, and toxicity data can also be obtained.

The most basic tests are referenced in the USP XXI-NF XVI [10]. These tests include both biological and physicochemical tests. The biological tests are primarily toxicity screening tests, and all of the candidate raw polymer resins should be subjected to USP class VI biological testing (see Table 8). Current official biological procedures are primarily designed to determine the suitability of plastic materials intended for use in containers for parenteral preparations. These tests are performed using injected extracts prepared in a manner similar to the condition under which it is meant to be used. If the plastic is to be exposed to any cleansing or sterilization process prior to its end use, then the tests are to be conducted from a sample preconditioned by the same processing. To determine the reaction of living tissue, the injectable preparations are made by extracting the sample in either sodium chloride injection, a 1:20 solution of alcohol in sodium chloride, polyethylene glycol 400, or cottonseed oil at 50°C for 72 hr. After preparation of the extracts, specified doses are injected intravenously, subcutaneously, or intraperitoneally into mice or rabbits to observe for evidence of systemic toxicity or local tissue reaction. In these tests none of the animals injected with an extract of the sample should show a significantly greater reaction than that observed in animals injected with a blank.

Table 8 USP Class VI Biological Testing

Test material	Animal	Dose	Procedure
Extract of sample in sodium chloride injection	Mouse	50 ml/kg	Intravenous systematic injection
	Rabbit	0.2 ml/animal at each of 10 sites	Intracutaneous
Extract of sample in 1:20 solution of alcohol in sodium chloride injection	Mouse	50 ml/kg	Intravenous systematic injection
	Rabbit	0.2 ml/animal at each of 10 sites	Intracutaneous
Extract of sample in polyethylene glycol 400	Mouse	10 g/kg	Intraperitoneal systematic injection
	Rabbit	0.2 ml/animal at each of 10 sites	Intracutaneous
Extract of sample in vegetable oil	Mouse	50 ml/kg	Intraperitoneal systematic injection
	Rabbit	0.2 ml/animal at each of 10 sites	Intracutaneous
Implant strips of sample	Rabbit	4 strips/animal	Intramuscular implantation

Various biological testing of LVP plastics using these extracts are outlined in Tables 8 and 9. Biotesting from a quality assurance viewpoint, once the product is released, is held to a minimum by most pharmaceutical manufacturers due to the expense and time typically involved. If there is no animal facility in-house, there are a number of reputable laboratories available to do such testing on a contract basis.

A great deal of time and resources can be saved by obtaining an additives description from the polymer resin manufacturer. In many cases, the manufacturer will require a confidential disclosure agreement to be signed before information relating to the additive package is disclosed. The latter is a relatively common practice and will save many labor-hours in trying to discover the nature of the resin's additive package.

Once the preliminary information and resin samples have been obtained, a physicochemical test protocol can be written. The tests should include methods that characterize and challenge the plastic in relation to its final end use.

The physicochemical screening tests required by the USP XXI-NF XVI are very minimal. In the section relating to plastic containers found in

Table 9 Some Biological Testing of Polymers Used with Parenteral Products and Parameters Tested[a]

Tests	Injection site	Tested parameters or result(s)
Subacute testing (≤30 days)	Rabbit, ear Mice, tail	Hematology, blood chemistry, growth, organ weight, lethality
Chronic testing (≥45 days)	Mice, tail Rabbit, ear	Hematology, blood chemistry, growth, organ weight, lethality
Acute toxicity	Rabbit, ear Mice, tail	Behavior, and mortality and/or biopsy
Isolated muscle tests		Response versus a histamine standard (%)
Erythrocyte aggregation		Clumping of cells when neutralized indicates positive
Clotting time		Clotting time effects
Antigenicity		IP anaphylactic shock
Hemolysis		Comparison of positive and negative controls (15% used as a guideline for positive)
Dye extravasation	Subcutaneous infiltrating injection	Comparison of positive and negative controls

[a]These tests merely represent examples of biotesting that may be employed. Many other tests also exist and vary from company to company. In addition, many USP tests may be used for product testing, depending on the plastic container and the enclosed solutions. Also, due to cost, contaminants, and certain scientific rationales, not all tests are performed at each time interval in stability programs or QC laboratories. Although all tests listed may be employed, usually acute toxicity and/or subacute testing are the only ones employed.

USP XXI-NF, XVI [10], there are only three tests outlined: (a) nonvolatile residue, (b) heavy metals, and (c) buffering capacity.

The test samples are usually prepared by hot pressing a homogeneous plastic specimen. Enough samples should be prepared to be equivalent to 120 cm^2 when the thickness is less than 500 μm, or 60 cm^2 when the thickness is greater than 500 μm. This amount of surface area is required for every 20 ml of extraction medium. The pressed sample is then cut into strips approximately 3 mm in width and as near 5 cm in length as is practical. The test sample is then transferred to a glass-stoppered, 250-ml graduated cylinder of type I glass, and 150 ml of distilled water is added. Agitate briefly, drain, and discard the rinse liquid. Repeat with a second rinse.

Transfer the sample to a suitable flask, and add the required amount of extraction medium based on surface area. The flask should then be placed in an oven that has been equilibrated at 70 ± 1°C. After 24 hr, remove the sample from the oven and cool (not below 22°C). Decant the liquid extract into a well-cleansed flask, and seal. The extract is then subjected to physicochemical testing.

Blank and sample fused silica crucibles are tared in preparation for the *nonvolatile residue test*. Aliquots of 50 ml of sample extract and extraction medium (distilled water) are transferred to the individual crucibles. Both sample and blank are evaporated on a steam bath. The test samples are dried at 105°C for 1 hr and weighed. The difference between sample and blank should not exceed 15 mg.

With the nonvolatile residue obtained from the previous test, the residue is then charred, cooled, and moistened with sulfuric acid. It is then heated until white fumes are no longer being evolved. The crucible is then placed in a muffle furnace and heated to 800 ± 25°C until the carbon is consumed. The sample is cooled in a desiccator and weighed, and the percentage of residue is calculated. A distilled water blank is treated similarly. The difference between the amount obtained from the sample and the blank should not exceed 15 mg.

For the *heavy metals* test, 20 ml of water extract are pipeted into one of two matched 50-ml color-comparison tubes. The sample pH should be adjusted with 1 N acetic acid or 6 N ammonium hydroxide to yield a final reading between 3.0 and 4.0. Dilute with water to about 35 ml.

The second test color-comparison tube serves as the standard. Into the second tube are pipeted 2 ml of standard lead solution (0.01 mg/ml) and 20 ml of blank (distilled water). The pH is adjusted as with the sample tube and diluted to 35 ml.

Freshly prepared hydrogen sulfide TS (10 ml) is added to each tube and the contents diluted to 50 ml. Both standard and sample tubes are viewed downward over a white surface. If any brown color develops and does not exceed that of the standard tube, the sample passes this test (1 ppm or less in the extract).

Buffering capacity is measured by placing a 20-ml aliquot of extract into a suitable container. The sample is then potentiometrically titrated to a pH of 7.0, using either 0.010 N hydrochloric acid or 0.010 N sodium hydroxide, as needed. A blank sample is similarly treated. If the same titrant was used for both sample and blank, the difference between the two volumes should not exceed 10.0 ml. However, if acid was required for either blank or sample and base for the other, the total of the two volumes should not be greater than 10.0 ml.

With the heavy liability on the LVP manufacturer, these tests are clearly insufficient to base a judgment of a plastic materials physicochemical properties. It is important to establish a screening test regime (described below) to include the requirements of USP XXI-NF XVI and other tests to more completely characterize a given material.

A number of appropriate tests can be tailored to the plastic under consideration. The following sections will describe some of these tests and provide examples of their applicability and use.

Infrared Spectroscopy

One of the most basic tests that can be performed on a plastic material or one of its components is an infrared (IR) spectrum. An IR spectrum provides a fingerprint of the material being tested. This fingerprint is a means to detect any gross changes (5–10%) in the material formulation or additives.

The method is extremely versatile in terms of the sample requirements. For most cases, a hot-pressed thin film or solution cast film is sufficient for a good test sample. Extraction residues are also easily examined by combining the residue with dry potassium bromide powder and pressing the sample into a pellet. For samples with a high content of an inorganic filler, which thus are opaque, a technique called attenuated total reflectance (ATR) can be used. In this technique, test samples in the form of thin films are placed in contact with KRS-5 crystals (Fig. 4). The infrared radiation is internally reflected, and the result is a spectrum very similar to a transmission IR spectrum. Figure 5 shows a comparison between an ATR and transmission IR spectrum.

Reference spectra for the primary plastic materials are included in Figures 6 through 9. Some of the most common additive spectra can be found in Section VIII.A. As quick references, Table 10 and 11 are included to provide the characteristic IR absorption bands. The IR spectra for other materials, both polymer and additive, can be easily obtained in a number of good reference texts [13–18].

Ultraviolet Spectroscopy

Ultraviolet (UV) spectroscopy is a very useful tool in identifying and in some cases quantifying extracted additives containing conjugated double bonds or aromatic ring structures. Some of the additive components that can be examined by UV spectroscopy are found in Table 12. Normally, plastics are extracted by autoclaving or, at the very least, boiling the sample in distilled water. Soxhlet extraction is used in cases in which information concerning the additive package is needed. In this extraction method, a given quantity of polymer is placed in the extraction apparatus and then refluxed for up to 24 hr using a solvent, such as methylene chloride, chloroform, or diethyl ether. The extract is then evaporated, quantified, and prepared for spectroscopic examination using UV and IR techniques.

Atomic Absorption Spectroscopy

This is a rapid technique [19] used to analyze for the presence of elements such as lead and calcium. Sample preparation is relatively simple, usually involving autoclaving a sample with a high surface-to-volume ratio of polymer to distilled water. Sensitivity in the parts per billion range can be routinely obtained.

Chromatography

High-Performance Liquid Chromatography. HPLC has become an increasingly important tool in the last 10 years. Its versatility, ability to provide quantifiable data, and overall applicability have permanently etched HPLC as a key analysis technique. The versatility of the technique lies in the wide range of organic samples that can be analyzed. This is made possible by the numerous types of solvents, columns, and detectors that can be utilized. For example, there are currently available fluorescence, UV, refractive index, IR, conductivity, and several other types of detectors. A typical modern HPLC system can also be programmed to analyze and compare the data to internal standards. As can be seen in Figure 10, a state-of-the-art HPLC system is commonly a multicomponent instrument consisting of a data interpreting device-plotter, a microprocessor controlled programmer and pump control, pumps, detectors, columns, and a microprocessor-based autosampler.

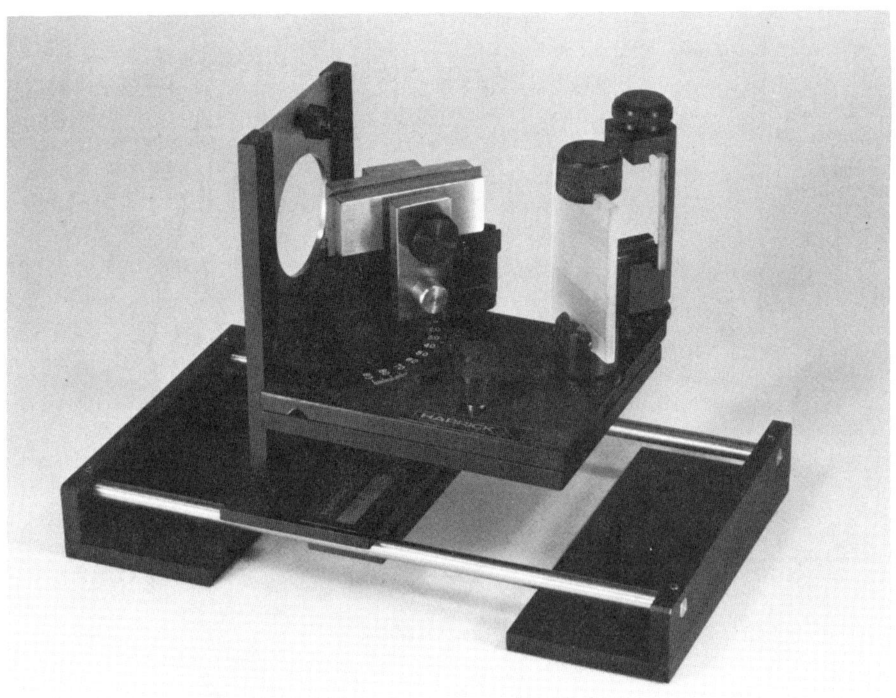

(a)

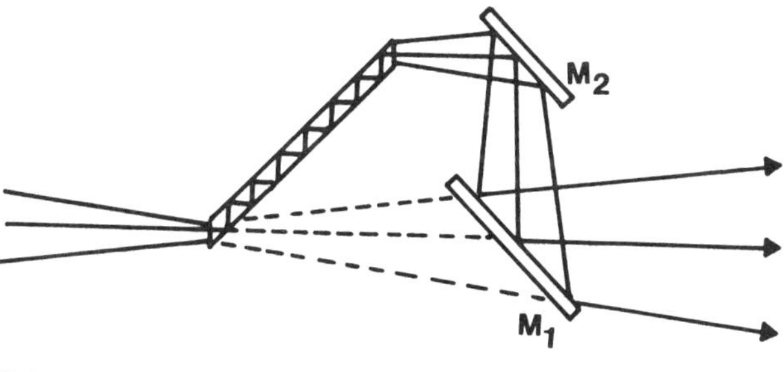

(b)

Figure 4 (a) An attenuated total reflectance (ATR) unit. (Courtesy of Harrick Scientific Corporation.) (b) The IR beam path through the crystal and the reflections on the surface of the sample. The IR beam is then focused into the detector by mirrors (M_1 and M_2).

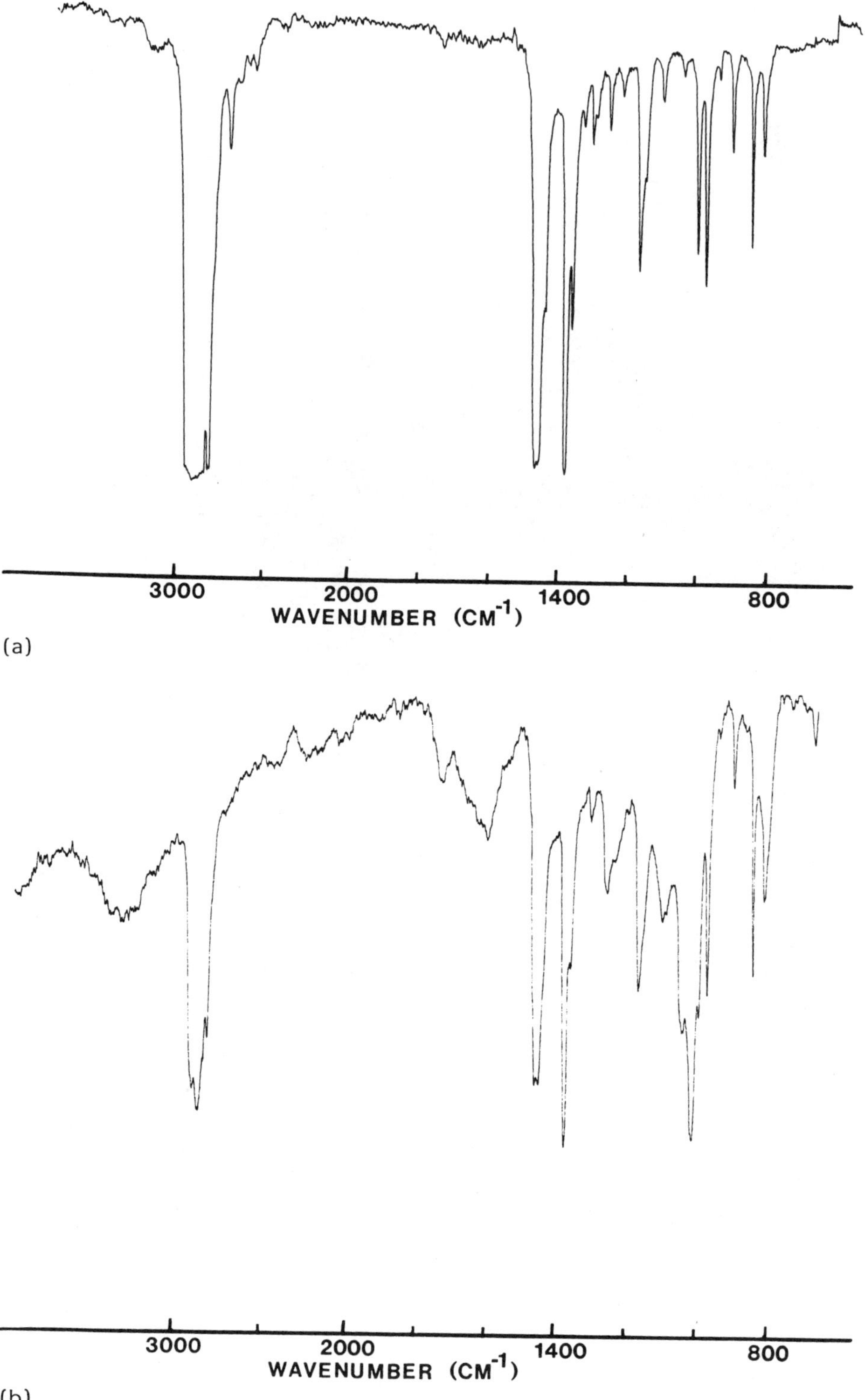

Figure 5 A comparison of transmission infrared (IR) spectroscopy to an attenuated total reflectance (ATR) spectrum. (a) Transmission IR spectrum of polypropylene. (b) ATR spectrum of polypropylene.

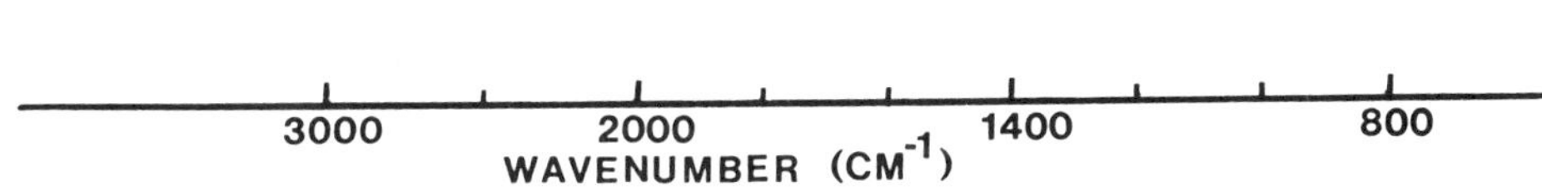

Figure 6 Infrared spectrum of high-density polyethylene.

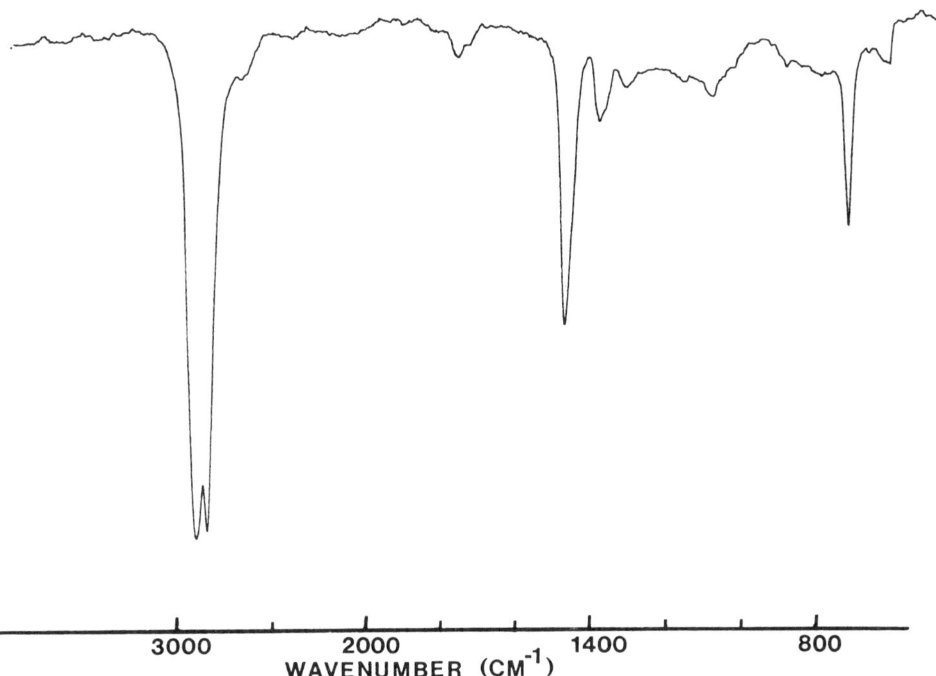

Figure 7 Infrared spectrum of low-density polyethylene.

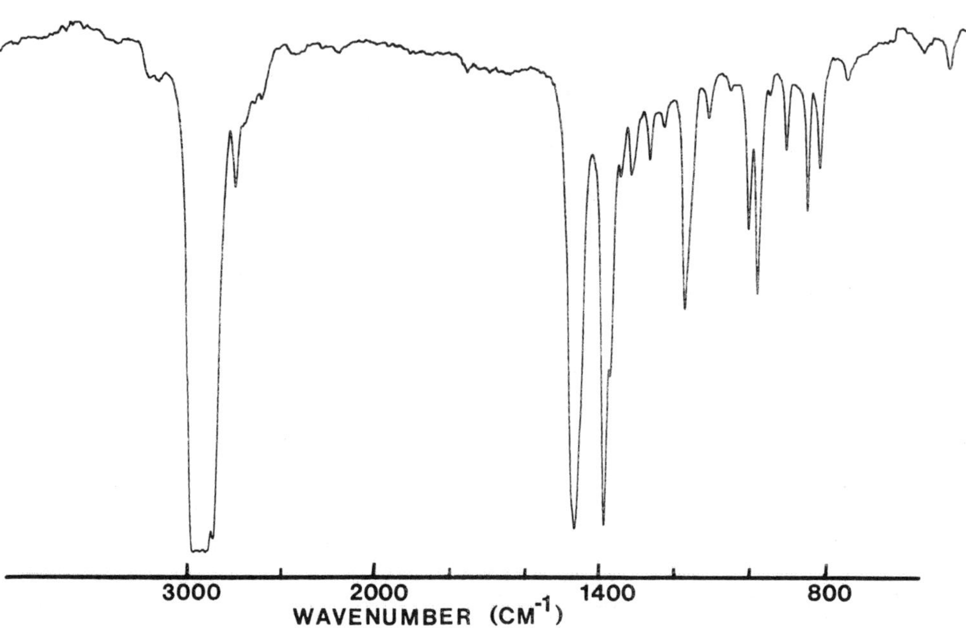

Figure 8 Infrared spectrum of an ethylene-propylene copolymer.

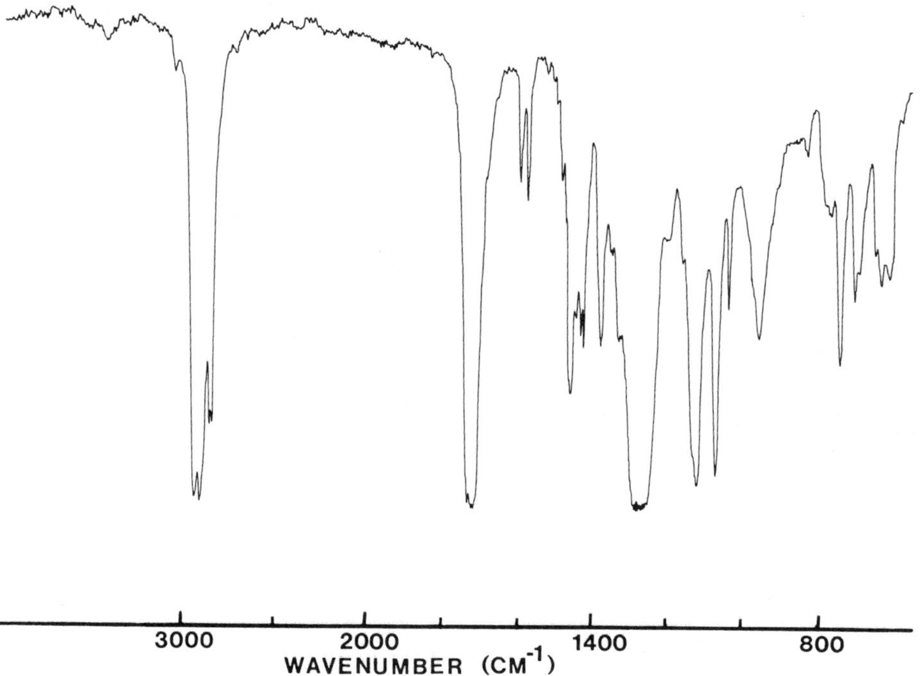

Figure 9 Infrared spectrum of plasticized PVC film.

Table 10 Characterization of Polyolefin IR Spectra

Wavelength (cm^{-1})	Polyolefin
Polypropylene	
2857	CH stretch due to polymer
1739	Ester carbonyl, DLTDP antioxidant
1471	CH deformation
1385	CH deformation, methyl groups
1366	CH deformation, methylene groups
1325	Crystalline-sensitive polypropylene absorption
1302	Crystalline-sensitive polypropylene absorption
1295	Crystalline-sensitive polypropylene absorption
1250	Crystalline-sensitive polypropylene absorption
1212	Crystalline-sensitive polypropylene absorption
1163	Crystalline-sensitive polypropylene absorption
1153	Shoulder-skeletal vibration, isopropyl groups
1099	Crystalline-sensitive polypropylene absorption
1042	Crystalline-sensitive polypropylene absorption
997	Crystalline-sensitive polypropylene absorption
974	Crystalline-insensitive polypropylene absorption
939	Crystalline-sensitive polypropylene absorption
898	Crystalline-sensitive polypropylene absorption
840	Crystalline-sensitive polypropylene absorption
810	Crystalline-sensitive polypropylene absorption
Polyethylene	
2857	CH stretch due to polymer
1460	CH deformation
1361	CH deformation, methylene groups
909	Vinyl unsaturation
730	Crystalline-sensitive polyethylene absorption
719	Skeletal vibration (linear methylene groups, $N \geqslant 4$)
Ethylene-propylene copolymers (see polypropylene + the bands listed below)	
730	Crystalline-sensitive polyethylene absorption
719	Skeletal vibration (linear methylene groups, $N \geqslant 4$)

Table 11 Characterization of Plasticized PVC Spectra

Wavelength (cm^{-1})	Plasticized poly(vinyl chloride)
2960	Aliphatic CH stretching
2900	Aliphatic CH stretching
1430	CH_2 bending
1420	CH_2 bending
1330	CH in CHCl
1255	CH in CHCl
1095	C-C stretching
960	CH_2 rocking
690	C-Cl stretching
640	C-Cl stretching
610	C-Cl stretching
1600 and 1580	Doublet, characteristic of DEHP plasticizer

Table 12 Common Additives That Can Be Examined by Ultraviolet Spectroscopy

Additive	Application	Wavelength (nm)
1,1,3-Tris-(2-methyl-4-hydroxy-5-*t*-butyl phenyl) butane	Antioxidant for polyolefins	280
1,3,5-Trimethyl-2,4,6-tris-3,5-di-*tert*-butyl-4-hydroxybenzylbenzene	Antioxidant for polyolefins	280
2,6-Di-*t*-butyl-*p*-cresol (butylated hydroxy toluene, BHT)	Antioxidant for polyolefins	280
Octadecyl-3,5-di-*tert*-butyl-4-hydroxy-hydrocinnamate	Antioxidant for polyolefins	280
Tetrakis methylene-(3,5-di-*tert*-butyl-4-hydroxyhydrocinnamate) methane	Antioxidant for polyolefins	280
Di-2-ethyhexyl phthalate (DEHP)	Plasticizer in PVC	280
Trictyl trimellitate (TOTM)	Plasticizer in PVC	280
Calcium stearate	Lubricant in polyolefins	240
Dilaurylthiodipropionate (DLTDP)	Antioxidant in polyolefins	230

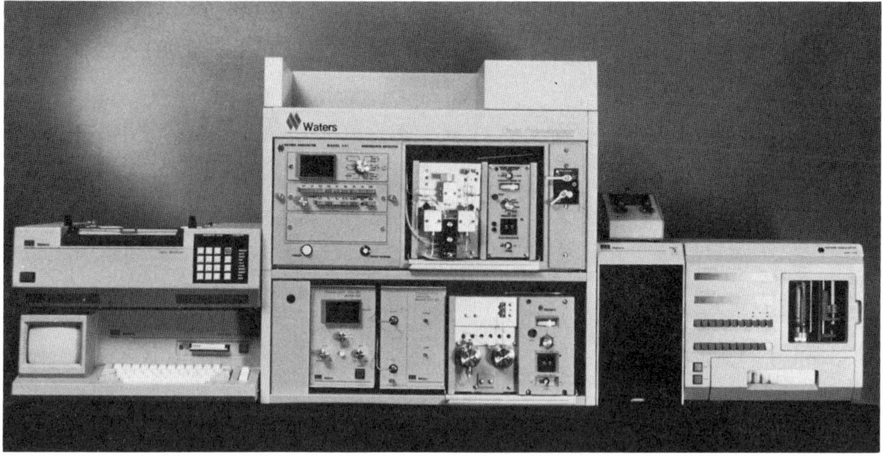

Figure 10 A modern microprocessor-controlled high-performance liquid chromatograph (HPLC). (Courtesy of Waters Associates, Inc.)

This powerful array allows the user rapid automated analysis of plastic extracts for degradation products, antioxidants and other additives, and contaminants.

The greatest use for HPLC in the analysis of plastics is the identification and quantification of additives. Soxhlet extraction of the plastic is commonly used to obtain the sample. The sample can then be diluted (or concentrated) appropriately and analyzed. Extensive references in the literature [20–26] detail excellent methods for using HPLC to analyze plastic additive packages. The containers should always be tested to determine whether they are leaching any of the additives into the solution from the container. Attention should be given to appropriate bracketing of all types of solutions that could be potentially placed in the LVP container. HPLC can then be used to test for the level of additive leachability of the plastic in each of the solutions. A common application for HPLC is the quantification of di-2-ethylhexylphthalate (DEHP). Details of the DEHP method are shown in Figure 12.

Gas Chromatography. GC can be used in much the same way as HPLC. It has the advantage of user-packed columns (less expensive than HPLC columns) and in some cases higher sensitivity. However, with one of the most common sensitive detectors, the high temperatures involved may degrade the sample before it is analyzed [21]. GC instrumentation has made great strides in recent years. A typical GC is shown in Figure 11. The automation and automatic sampling have freed the investigator from error due to hand sample injection techniques and also from the associated labor-intensive work injecting large numbers of samples. GC has been used extensively for the analysis of polymer additives, and the literature provides a number of appropriate methods [27–30].

Gel Permeation or Size Exclusion Chromatography. GPC, or SEC as it is more appropriately termed, is very similar in instrumentation to that used in HPLC. In fact, in most applications for which high temperature is not

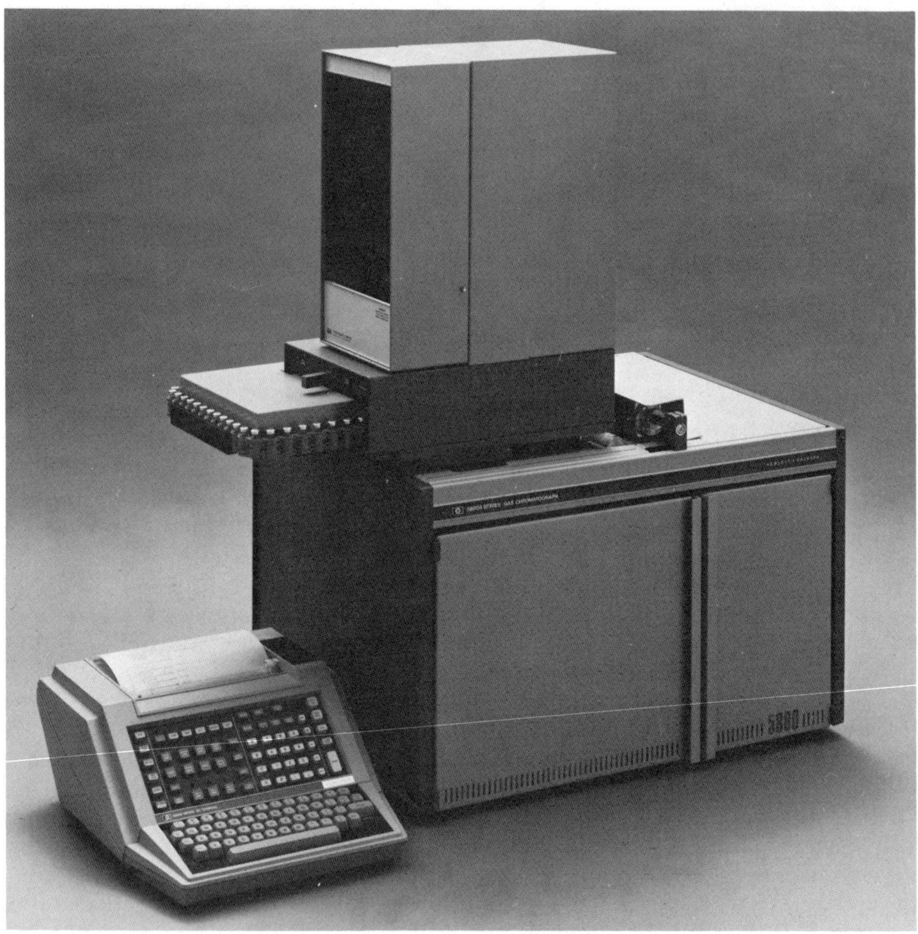

Figure 11 A state-of-the-art gas chromatograph (GC). (Courtesy of Hewlett-Packard.)

required, HPLC instrumentation can be used for SEC simply by connecting SEC columns. SEC, as the name implies, provides a separation of compounds based on the size of the molecule or hydrodynamic volume [31]. Molecular weight and distribution information can be easily obtained. This technique allows the comparison of lot-to-lot or manufacturer-to-manufacturer variations in the molecular weight properties of polymers. Such information is valuable in establishing raw material specifications and, at a later stage, solving processing problems. A typical GPC chromatogram is shown in Figure 13.

Thermal Analysis Methods

Differential Scanning Calorimetry. DSC [32] measures some very important thermal characteristics of plastics. Melting point thermograms and glass transition (T_g) thermograms are useful in comparing materials. These data can be used to grossly predict the processability of the polymer.

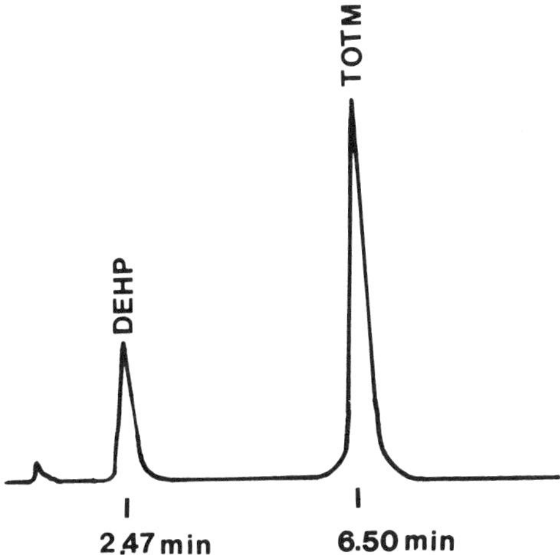

Figure 12 A reversed-phase HPLC method used to quantitate DEHP and/or TOTM leachables for plasticized PVC [3].

Thermal data are also very useful when comparing final product to resin. Thermal degradation due to processing can be followed using such techniques.

Among the most basic tests that can be applied to LVP containers are wet chemical methods [33]. Many of the previous testing methods require a considerable capital expense for the instrumentation. Wet methods require minimal equipment and are capable of resolving a number of key questions when investigating potential plastic materials. The most basic of the common tests include the following:

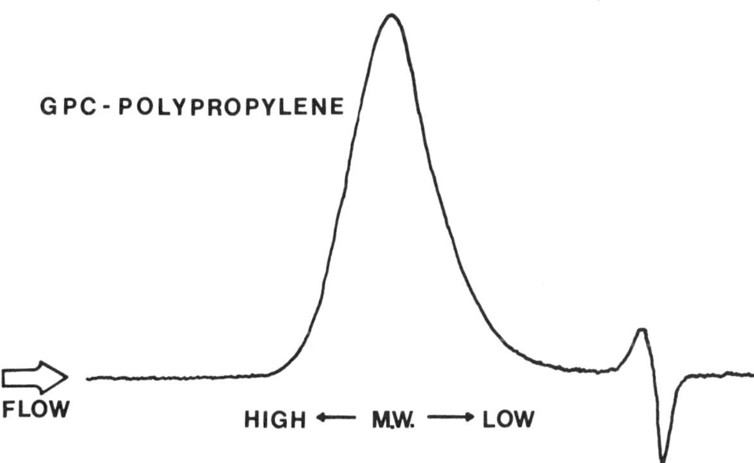

Figure 13 Polypropylene and other polyolefins are not soluble in organic solvents at room temperature. Temperatures of 145°C must be reached in solvents such as trichlorobenzene or *O*-dichlorobenzene to achieve polymer dissolution. A typical GPC chromatogram of polypropylene is illustrated.

pH
Buffering capacity
Heavy metals
Total solids
Oxidizable substances
Specific conductivity

B. Final Product Testing

After a raw material has been chosen, the prototype LVP container is manufactured. It is critical at this stage to retest the final product and each of its components, e.g., the closure system. The testing at this stage should be directed at

a. The effect of processing and sterilization on the end product
b. Determination of product specific leachability
c. Physical and functional tests of the final product
d. Long-term stability testing of the intended product(s)

The above concerns are most logically addressed in a final product protocol. Some of the essential points that should be included in such a test protocol are found in Section VIII.B.

It is a common practice in the LVP industry to bracket products in a stability test protocol. Bracketing simply means to take a critical look at all of the LVP formulations being tested and choose two or more formulations that cover the range of potential products. For example, if there are five LVP products to be tested with two major ingredients, X and Y, where percentage of X in the five solutions is 0.5, 1.0, 2.0, 3.0, and 5.0% and ingredient Y is a constant 0.25%, bracketing can be utilized to reduce cost and required labor to complete acceptable testing. In this case, the 0.5%X/0.25%Y product and the 5.0%X/0.25%Y product can be used to evaluate the entire range of formulations.

Most LVP test protocols run at least for 1 year, and many extend to 3 years with a more limited test schedule. It is important to glean as much information as possible in the shortest amount of time. Accelerated testing procedures, such as elevated temperatures (40, 60, or 70°C), are used to help predict a product's performance. The data accumulated are then used for internal product assurance and ultimately for submission to the Food and Drug Administration.

V. PROCESSING PLASTICS FOR FINAL PRODUCTS

Once the type of plastic is determined for use in large volume parenteral packaging, the next step is processing the raw material to final products. In the LVP industry, some manufacturing is vertically integrated, i.e., purchase the resin or raw material from the vendor and manufacture the final product in-house; other manufacturers rely on outside companies to produce either film or bottles and fabricate the finished products in-house. The sequence of events in making the final product generally involves

a. Film or bottle making
b. Bags or bottle prefabrication

c. Bag or bottle washing
d. Filling with IV solutions
e. Bag or bottle sealing
f. Sterilization
g. Labeling, final inspection, and packaging

A. Qualifying Raw Material Vendors

Raw materials play an important role in the quality of the final products. It is therefore very important to assure the cleanliness of the raw materials. The raw material to a LVP manufacturer can be resin, precompounded components, films, or bottles. In order to assure that the raw materials received from a vendor are free of contamination, the raw material vendor should have a manufacturing facility that has temperature and humidity control, good water and air quality, and minimum environmental particulate matter. This is possible by having a clean room or by enshrouding the processing area with polyethylene film and purging with filtered and dehumidified air. The machinery used to produce the raw material should be free of foreign materials, such as oil, water, dust, and dirt. Personnel who work in the area should be gowned and gloved and their hair and shoes covered. In order to eliminate in-line contamination with the material previously processed in the machinery, purging the equipment with the raw material to be used is very essential. Antistatic equipment, in the case of film production, is also needed to eliminate charge generation on raw material, which can attract airborne particles and cause a fire hazard. During the manufacture of the raw materials, the vendor should record all the manufacturing steps, such as weighing, mixing time, processing throughput, and observations. These data will provide a base for troubleshooting in case a product does not meet specifications. Ideally, the vendor should also have the capability to perform quality control (QC) release tests, such as melt index, extractables, pH, haze, tensile strength, creep modulus, and IR spectrum.

B. Techniques for Processing to Fabricate Containers

All the plastic LVP containers in the market are in either bag or bottle configuration. Most of the LVP bags are fabricated from film of lay-flat tubing. The films are generally made by calendering, extrusion, casting, or tubular blow molding; the lay-flat tubing can only be made by tubular blow molding. The bottles are made by blow molding, injection blow molding, or biaxially oriented blow molding. The preferred technique for processing often depends on the melt-flow properties of the resin and the end-use requirements of the container. Bag fabrication is generally accomplished by heating, radiofrequency (RF) welding, or induction heating. During the process, a functional injection molded part, such as a medication port or spike port, is often included in the fabrication process. Economic considerations also play an important role in the selection of a manufacturing process.

C. Washing, Filling, and Sealing

Most LVP containers require washing prior to filling and sealing. However, a process developed in Europe consists in the bottle making, filling, and sealing being done consecutively by one machine. This process is known as a blow-fill-seal process where the washing procedure is eliminated. Bag or bottle washing is sometimes done with detergent washing followed by distilled water rinsing or only distilled water rinsing. Bags made from lay-flat tubing, however, are not rinsed prior to filling to achieve minimal environmental exposure of the inner surface of the tube. Filling is normally accomplished by using conventional dispensing filling machines. After the container is filled, the container will be closed by insertion of an injection molded part followed by heat sealing. Once the product is sealed, it is ready for sterilization.

D. Sterilization

The most common method of sterilizing parenteral solutions in plastic containers is pressurized steam sterilization (121°C). Some European countries are using lower temperatures and longer times to attain the same degree of microbial destruction. The lower temperature sterilization permits the use of plastics, such as HDPE and PE, which generally cannot survive 121°C. A sterilization vessel usually contains several thermocouple temperature probes located at various sites within the vessel. These probes are used to monitor the temperature profile in the vessel as a function of time. The amount of sterilization time required for an LVP product also can be established by using biological indicators. In some cases, several strains of spores and bacteria are used to map out the optimized sterilization cycle. Once the sterilization cycle is established, the vessel temperature profile will be used to guarantee sufficient heat delivery to the LVP products to effect microbial kill. Sterilized products will then be ready for labeling, pressure testing for leakage, inspection for particulate matter, and packaging. For more details on sterilization, the reader is referred to Chapter 1.

VI. QUALITY CONTROL

Because the injectable contents of an LVP bypass all the body's natural defense mechanisms in IV therapy, the quality control of the parenteral container is extremely important. Numerous testing procedures must be followed to ensure the safety of any plastic being used. The quality control groups will test for compliance to the biological, physical, and chemical test specifications.

A. Sterility and Pyrogen Testing

The sterility and pyrogen testing of LVP plastic containers is a prominent topic of discussion in the health care industry. For plastic packaging materials, a number of sterilizing agents have been used but the most common are steam autoclaving and sterile filling of ethylene oxide-sterilized empty containers. However, steam can be used only on a few polymers due to their inability to withstand heat without distortion. The following commonly used plastic types can generally be steam sterilized at temperatures of 121°C: polypropylene, some high-density polyethylenes, and ethylene-propylene copolymers. After sterilization, pyrogen and sterility testing of the product becomes an essential part of the quality control check. Pyrogen testing is designed to limit the risk of a febrile reaction in the patient from an injection of the product. The rise in temperature above normal of rabbits from IV injections in a dose not to exceed 10 ml/kg over a 10-min period is measured. Pyrogen testing is incorporated as a release criterion for the product, but unlike sterility, it is rarely used as a test criterion after release of the product. Further discussion of these tests can be found in Chapter 9.

Sterility testing is designed to reveal the presence of any viable bacteria, fungi, and/or yeasts present in the LVP system (sterilized solution and container). Specific procedures to determine product sterility are provided in the official compendium. For certain LVP solutions in plastics, a sterility check is incorporated into the stability protocol to verify the integrity of the container at specified intervals. This procedure will detect susceptible areas of the container, potential problem sites, such as loosening of latex plugs at the medication site, air-inlet site, or improperly sealed rubber closures. The specific test intervals, when the test procedures are employed, depend on the LVP plastic container configuration and potential for microbiological efficacy. The more parts of the LVP container having potential areas of contamination, the more checkpoints for sterility should be placed onto quality control. Once adequate microbial kill has been established by sterilization cycle validation, QC would rely on less expensive physical testing, such as pressure leak tests or high-voltage leak tests, to ensure product integrity where potential lack of a seal or leaking part would possibly sacrifice the sterility or closed character of the container.

B. Physical Testing Procedures

Physical tests are applied to the plastic LVP containers to verify dimensional specifications, enclosure integrity, and suitability of the container design. Physical property testing will vary from company to company depending on whether the company is using blow molding or calendering its own container in-house or ordering the container from an external source and merely filling and sterilizing.

Resin testing. Upon receipt of the raw resin, the pharmaceutical manufacturer documents the raw resin lot number and relies to an extent on the release specifications established with the resin manufacturer. Incoming raw material specification checks usually are minimal. The physical tests employed would probably consist of a melt index measurement and measurement of specific gravity. Such physical checks may prove useful and important in the absence of better approaches as long as its empirical character is clearly realized.

Package testing. Physical testing of the completed filled container is the most common technique employed. Testing usually consists of many visual tests, such as clarity, film buildup, drop tests, and leak testing. Physical integrity tests employed would include those designed for body leakage, closure leakage and integrity, dimensional testing, and label damage.

Visual inspection for clarity and film buildup. A standard for container clarity will be established by the pharmaceutical manufacturer. This clarity should enable inspection of the container prior to dispensing to ascertain whether any particulate matter or "floaters" are present in the LVP. Particulates in finished products can be related to many sources. Obvious sources of particulate matter are "bad" resin lots, improperly cleaned equipment, bloom or migration of additive components to the surface of the polymer, or improper sterilization.

Container cracking and/or paneling. The container may become brittle due to improper sterilization or the manufacturing process. Visual inspection is done at the same time as clarity of the product. Paneling is a phenomenon in which the container exhibits a flattening of one side of the bottle. Besides user lack of acceptance, this makes for poor label adhesion if the container has an adhesive label as opposed to a hot stamp label.

Body leakage. This integrity test, after the product is filled into the LVP, may be done manually or through electronic instrumentation, which is designed to measure lesser resistance across a voltage bridge. The procedure detects any aqueous medium coming through defective areas in the container. LVP are discarded if any body leaks are present.

Closure leakage and integrity. Ports are usually sealed with latex plugs designed to handle air-inlet spikes or needles for medication addition. These plugs must assure the integrity of the container. Upon validation of the sterilization cycle of the specific LVP, these sites are of particular concern because if leaks exist, sterility could be affected.

Dimensional testing. Size and weight dimensions of the container must be verified before release. The fill volume also will be examined, as well as integrity of any overwraps.

Labeling. The label will be checked to verify the attachment of the label to the container, the inclusion of any expiration date, and the proper description of ingredients. If a hot stamp label is imprinted on the bag or bottle instead of a label, then leakage and integrity tests must be employed to confirm no damage to the container after this type of processing.

If quality control can select good physical tests that indicate container integrity, it may be possible to reduce some of the more expensive biological, microbiological, and chemical testing without sacrificing patient safety.

C. Chemical Testing Procedures

Chemical testing of the LVP container and the raw polymer material itself varies depending on the polymer used and the properties desired in the final container. Most commonly, the chemical description of the polymer used in the LVP container is provided by the polymer supplier. These descriptions usually contain an approximate molecular weight analysis, residue on ignition, percentage of heavy metals, solubility parameters, and an IR spectrum. Pharmaceutical companies usually run an IR scan, a test for heavy metals, and some testing for any additive systems, such as stearates or antioxidants. Typical QC testing will include the following:

IR spectra. An identification of the polymer using infrared spectroscopy is commonly done. Samples are prepared in potassium bromide pellets or hot pressed into thin film. Such groups as —OH, C=O, and —CH can be identified with reasonable certainty from the occurrence of a typical absorption band. This identification test is commonly done on incoming materials and bottles.

Heavy metal testing. Calcium and zinc are the most frequent metals tested, usually employing atomic absorption (AA) instrumentation. These heavy metals may be in the LVP polymer formulation as a stabilizer (metal oxides), mold-releasing agent (zinc stearate), or a pigment, such as calcium carbonate.

Additive fillers. These are low-cost particulate materials whose major functions are to extend the polymer and reduce the cost of the plastic. They have some mechanical reinforcing effect and reduce mold shrinkage and the thermal expansion coefficient. Calcium carbonate and talc are frequently used. Atomic absorption can be used to detect the calcium in calcium carbonate, and thermogravimetric analysis can be used to evaluate the amount of talc (inorganic) in filled polymers.

Plasticizers. Plasticizers, such as phthalate compounds (DEHP, di-2-ethylhexylphthalate commonly used in PVC bags), have been carefully scrutinized for potential leaching from the parenteral containers into the solutions with subsequent accumulation in the tissues and organs of patients.

Antioxidants. The polyolefin products contain certain antioxidants, such as BHT (butylated hydroxytoluene) and DLTDP (dilauryl thiodipropionate). For the extraction of these antioxidants, chloroform can be used as the extraction fluid. Currently, when a plastic material is used for the LVP container, QC testing will quantitate the antioxidants leached from the container into various LVP solutions to verify that the quantity leached is substantially below any toxic levels. Concerns over the risk of exposure to various additives, plasticizers, and antioxidants is appropriate, but a proper perspective must be maintained since these containers and many plastic biomedical devices provide therapeutic benefits, often lifesaving.

D. Biological Testing

Generally, once a new plastic material has been qualified and released, the material itself is not subjected to further biological testing. However, the LVP product, i.e., the solution within the container, is subjected to a battery of tests. The type and number of biological tests applied to the LVP product is largely dependent upon each company. Normally, QC testing for LVP products will include acute toxicity and pyrogen testing. Other more extensive tests can be done and may be done on a spot-check basis, however, the very high expense of biotesting is prohibitive for extensive routine testing.

In addition to assuring specifications and standards, the quality control unit also must be concerned with any lot-to-lot variation of the raw materials. Lot-to-lot variation problems occur primarily because of raw material manufacturer variation and processing differences. Raw material variation also occurs due to wide ranges on specifications from vendors and various merchandisers where the material is purchased. Heat sealing of bags is usually done by the company involved with selling the product and is another process that is subject to variation. If too much or too little heat, pressure, or time is employed for sealing, the container may not pass stability testing, may leak or crack, or be physically undesirable from a cosmetic viewpoint. Once all raw materials are assured to have correct specifications, the LVP container is filled with solution. The filled container then is tested to ensure that all specifications are met. In addition to the tests described in this section for the LVP container, testing of the filled solution to ensure efficacy and accuracy of its ingredients must also be accomplished. After QC releases the product with the proper labeling, it is then stored in the quarantine area for a prescribed period of time before being shipped. After the product leaves the plant, any problems arising are handled by the quality assurance (QA) group.

VII. THE FUTURE OF LVP PACKAGING

The future of new and innovative parenteral medications is inseparably tied to the development of plastic LVP packaging technology. As parenteral product researchers are challenged to provide new and improved forms of products for LVP therapy, the polymer chemists and plastic manufacturers must meet the needs. By providing new polymers and processes to improve such properties as clarity, lower moisture vapor transmission rates, flexibility, and inertness, new products will evolve.

Polymer processing techniques provide an important ingredient in developing new LVP containers. One of those processing methods is coextrusion. Coextrusion is the process by which two or more layers of plastic can be joined in the molten phase. Each layer retains its own unique properties, and the collective layers contribute to the overall properties of the coextruded film. The utility of such a product lies in the ability to join polymer films that would ordinarily be inadequate alone. Such properties as low moisture vapor transmission rate, low oxygen transmission rates, sealability, tear resistance, and low-temperature physical properties are but a few that are currently being addressed.

In those cases in which two polymers are not compatible at the hot melt interface, multilaminate construction is being investigated. Multilaminate plastics are thin films typically 0.5–2.0 mils in thickness bonded together with adhesives. Structures of this type can be made to include such layers of film as

Biaxially oriented polypropylene (BOPP) for strength and low MVTR properties
Linear low-density polyethylene (LLDPE) for tear resistence and flexibility
Nylon for low oxygen transmission properties
A low additive level ethylene-propylene copolymer for LVP fluid contact

Multilaminate packaging forms will gain wider acceptance as high-molecular-weight nonmigrating adhesives are developed.

The need for reduced labor-intensive LVP therapy products is now being voiced. These convenience products are and will provide a means to decrease the work load on hospital pharmacists. Products are emerging for which no admixing of drugs with LVP is necessary. Commonly used drugs, such as lidocaine, are becoming available in an appropriate LVP medium.

Economic considerations are also a driving force in the development of new parenteral packages. Such factors as freight savings derived from lighter and smaller cubage of plastic containers and savings associated with in-house manufacture of plastic LVP are but a few of the motivating factors for more plastic LVP containers.

Successful development of innovative LVP packaging depends to a great extent upon the interdisciplinary efforts of pharmaceutical researchers, polymer scientists, and the packaging industry. The plastic LVP containers development is still in its infancy. Many parenteral solutions have not been studied in relation to the wide variety of new polymer and copolymers currently available. Technology is leading the plastic LVP container to a dominant position among parenteral containers in the medical marketplace.

VIII. APPENDIX

A. Infrared Spectra of Common Polymer Additives

IRGANOX 1010

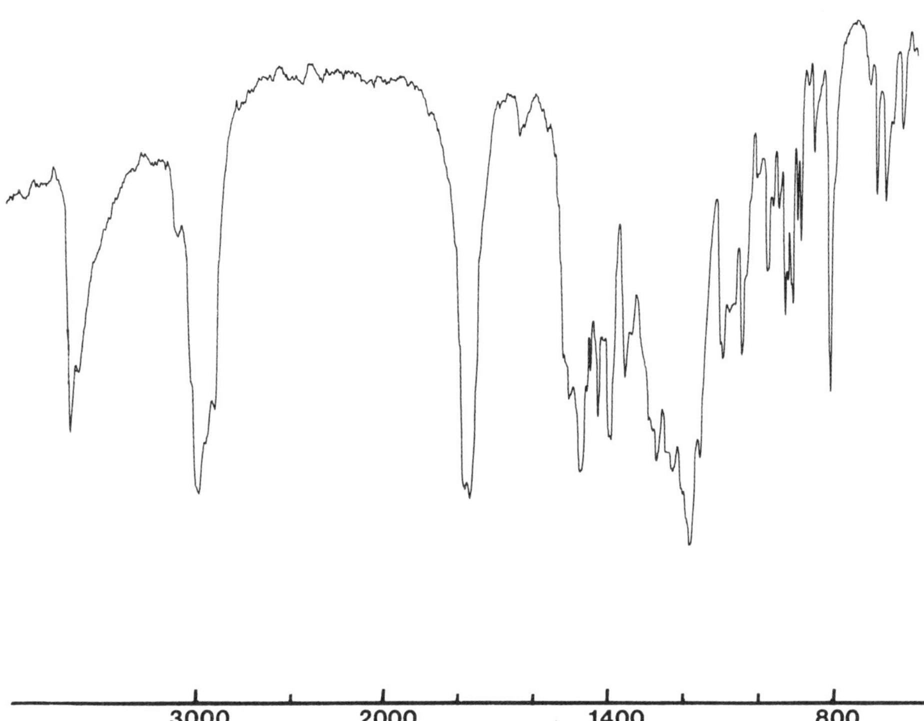

IRGANOX 1076

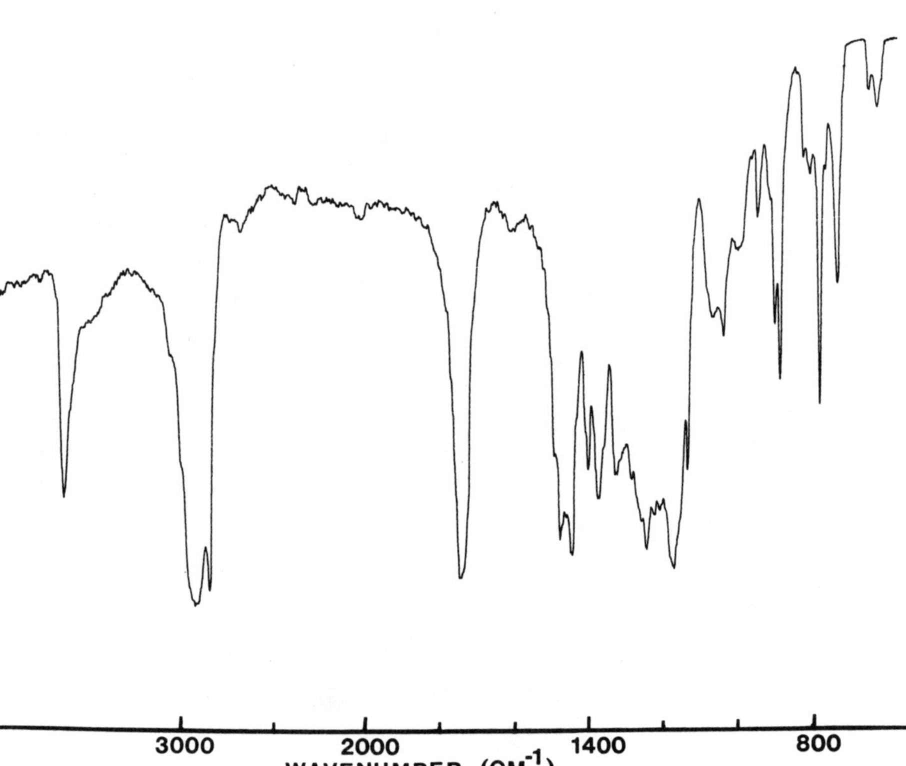

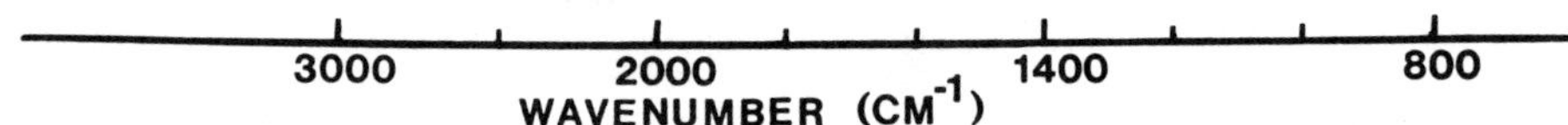

SANTANOX R

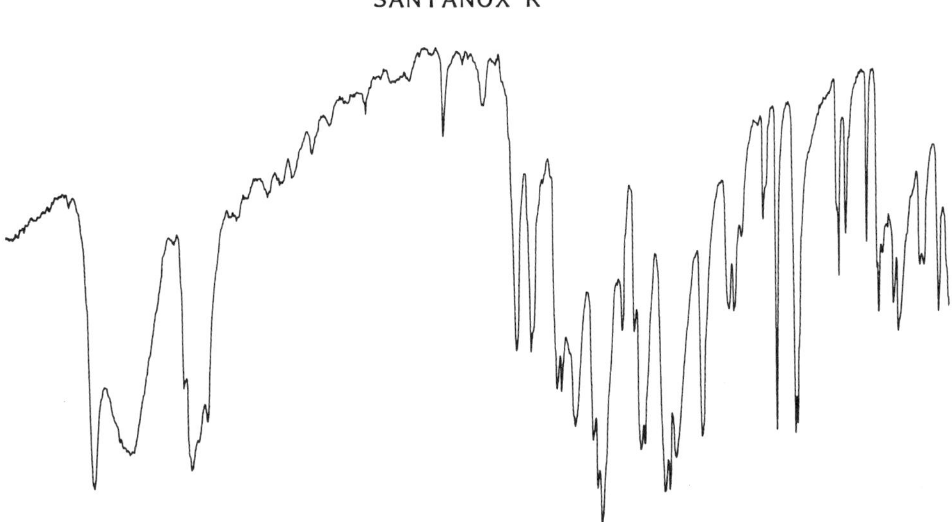

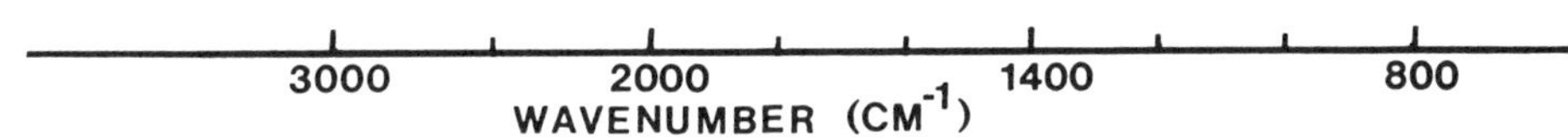

DEHP

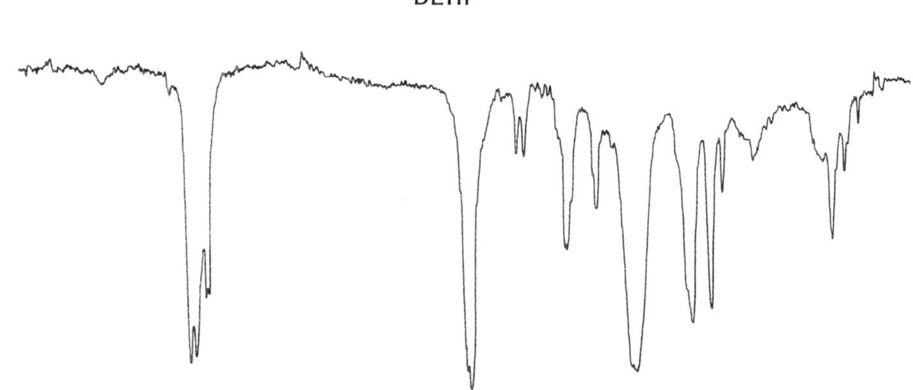

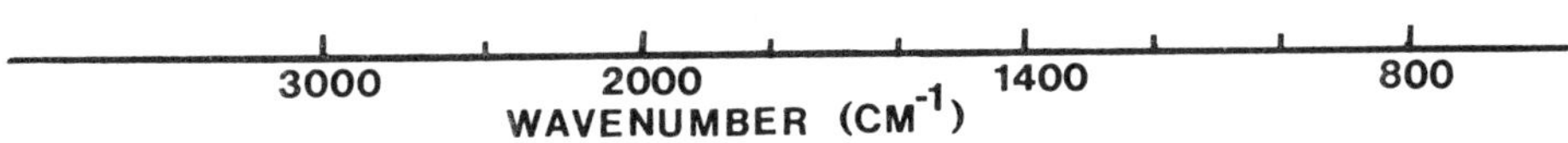

B. Long-Term Stability Testing Protocols

Final product testing protocols are generally long-term stability testing protocols, i.e., up to 3 years of testing. The purpose of these long-term tests is to establish the stability of the plastic container and its components in contact with specific parenteral formulations. The data gathered throughout the testing interval will be used to apply to the FDA for approval to use the new LVP container with specific parenteral formulations. In the following text a generalized long-term stability protocol for a new LVP container will be outlined.

As with any protocol, it is important to write a short *introduction* to the protocol. Background relating to the LVP container development, advantages of the new container, objectives, salient features (in brief) of the testing protocol, such as length of the testing intervals and general conditions, can be included. This section provides a basis for anyone at any time during the test to quickly grasp the intent of protocol design.

The *formulation* section might include a description of all container components with lot numbers and a listing of the formulation of each parenteral solution to be tested.

Preparation of stability samples should be described. Each component of the container should be prepared according to a standard operating procedure. Preparation includes how they will be washed, assembled, filled, sealed, and sterilized. The "fill volume" should also be documented. For example, if a new 500-ml LVP container were being tested it might be appropriate to test it at fill volumes of 100 and 500 ml. The purpose behind testing at a 100-ml fill volume (even though it will only be a 500-ml product) is to provide the greater challenge to the container. By using a smaller volume of parenteral solution, leachable substances will be greatly exaggerated and thus provide information that will help predict the success of the product.

Storage conditions for the stability test should be outlined, for example, temperature: ambient warehouse temperature, 4, 40, 60°C, and so on. The interval at each storage condition should be described and when testing will be conducted. For example, a potential product would be commonly tested at

Ambient warehouse temperature
At a given fill volume
Tested at 0 time, 1, 3, 6, 12, 24, and 36 months

The *testing regime* should use previously documented and validated test methods. The individual tests should be specifically outlined for each parenteral solution along with the interval storage condition. Each test should be evaluated as to its applicability to each solution under test. At the appropriate scheduled test interval, enough LVP containers are removed from storage to complete the required testing. Generally, the testing is divided in physicochemical, biological, and physical integrity categories. Some of the possible tests are as follows.

Physicochemical (tests how the plastic LVP containers affects the parenteral solution): APHA color (American Public Health Association), Hunter color, pH, oxidizable substances, UV spectroscopy, nonvolatile residue, heavy metals, specific conductivity, analysis of formulation ingredients,

HPLC or GC analysis for plasticizers or other specific leached additives, particulate matter (USP XXI-NF XVI) or HIAC particulate matter testing, moisture or water vapor transmission rate.

Biological: Subacute toxicity, sterility, pyrogen

Physical testing (testing directly on the container): drop impact, body leaks, seal and injection port integrity, spike insertion and retention, other tests specific to the design of the LVP container

A sample testing schedule for one product at one storage condition is given:

Sample Schedule,
"Parenteral Solution X,"
100-ml Partial Fill Volume,
250-ml LVP Container Z

	No. of units required for testing[a]					
	Testing interval (months)					
Tests	0	3	6	12	24	36
Physicochemical	40	40	—	40	40	40
Biological	20	20	—	20	20	20
Physical testing	100	—	100	100	100	100

[a]Storage condition, 40°C.

From the example, the great amount of labor, expense, and time involved in a long-term stability program is easily seen. Realizing that for a complete program the number of units must be multiplied by each parenteral solution and by each storage conditions, which would normally include 4°C, ambient warehouse, 40°C, and an accelerated storage condition, such as 60 or 70°C. In most cases, the accelerated storage condition rarely runs longer than 12 months due to the effects of high temperature on the parenteral solution as well as the container. The accelerated test conditions are normally conducted at 0 time and 1-, 3-, and 6-month intervals. They provide an early alert to potential problems that may appear at other less harsh storage conditions. They are also useful in predicting shelf life of a given container-solution combination.

It must be emphasized that *every* long-term storage program should be designed with as complete an understanding of the plastic material and its additive system as possible. This means extensive qualification and characterization work on the resin and final container configuration *before* the stability program begins. The storage stability testing regime of the filled LVP containers should include tests that truly challenge the potential product. Each program should be designed *specifically* for the parenteral solutions and container under test.

REFERENCES

1. *Encyclopedia of PVC*, Volumes 1–3, Leonard I. Nass, ed. Marcel Dekker, New York, 1976, 1977.

2. *Food Chemical News*, June 15, 1981, pp. 55–56.
3. C. E. Kurachi, K. L. Wong, S. Saxena, and D. D. Solomon, Abstr., The 1982 Pacific Conference on Chemistry and Spectroscopy, San Francisco, Oct. 27–29, 1982.
4. T. W. Downes, *Pharm. Tech.*, 5:45 (1981).
5. O. M. Netzer, Report on plastics, Prepared by the Committee on Plastics of the Quality Control Section and Biological Section of PMMA, *PMMA Year Book*, 6:234 (1964–1965).
6. E. L. Meyer, The Food and Drug Administration's Role in the Use of Plastic Materials, *AAAS Interdisciplinary Symposium in the Medical Sciences*, Berkeley, California, December 19, 1965.
7. J. H. Brewer, Toxicity standards for plastics. *Bull. Parent. Drug. Assoc.*, 19:22 (1965).
8. *U.S. Pharmacopeia*, 18th Revision. Mack Publishing, Easton, Pennsylvania, 1970, p. 926.
9. *National Formulary*, 13th Revision. Mack Publishing, Easton Pennsylvania, 1970, p. 840.
10. *The United States Pharmacopeia*, 21st Revision. National Formulary, 16th Revision, Mack Publishing, Easton, Pennsylvania, 1985, pp. 1235–1238.
11. J. P. Majeske, *Bull. Parent. Drug Assoc.*, 16:1 (1962).
12. A. Rodeyns, *Trans. J. Plastics Inst.*, April 1967, p. 453.
13. *Polymer Characterization, Spectroscopic, Chromatographic, and Physical Instrument Methods*, Ed. C. D. Craver. Advances in Chemistry Series 203, ACS, Washington, D.C., 1983.
14. J. Urbanski, W. Czerwinski, K. Janicka, F. Majewska, and H. Zowall, *Handbook of Analysis of Synthetic Polymers and Plastics*. Halsted Press, New York, 1977.
15. J. Hasham, H. A. Willis, and D. C. M. Squirrell, *Identification and Analysis of Plastics*. Butterworth Group, Woburn, Massachusetts, 1972.
16. D. O. Hummel, *Atlas of Polymer and Plastics Analysis*, Vol. 1, *Polymers: Structures and Spectra*. Carl Hansen Verlag, Munich, 1978.
17. F. Scholl, *Atlas of Polymer and Plastics Analysis*, Vol. 3, *Additives and Processing Aids*. Carl Hanser Verlag, Munich, 1980.
18. S. J. Borchert, G. A. Kelly, and E. A. Hardwidge, *Pharm. Tech.*, 7:72 (1983).
19. W. T. Elwell and J. A. F. Gidley, *Atomic-Absorption Spectrophotometry*. Pergamon Press, New York, 1966.
20. M. A. Haney and W. A. Dark, *J. Chromatogr. Sci.*, 18:665–659 (1980).
21. S. Hyden, *Anal. Chem.*, 35:113 (1963).
22. J. F. Schabron and L. E. Fenska, *Anal. Chem.*, 52:114–115 (1980).
23. J. F. Schabron, V. J. Smith, and J. L. Ware, *J. Liq. Chromatogr.*, 5:613–624 (1982).
24. R. G. Lichtenhaler and F. Ranfelt, *J. Chromatogr.*, 149:553–560 (1978).
25. J. M. Howard, III, *J. Chromatogr.*, 55:15–24 (1971).
26. A. W. Wims and S. J. Swarin, *J. Appl. Polym. Sci.*, 19:1243 (1975).
27. J. A. Denning and J. A. Marshall, *Analyst*, 97:710–712 (1972).
28. T. R. Compton, *Eur. Polym. J.*, 4:473–496 (1968).
29. D. A. Wheeler, *Talanta*, 15:1315–1334 (1968).
30. K. T. Hartman and L. C. Rose, *J. Am. Oil Chemists Soc.*, 47:7 (1970).

31. W. W. Yau, J. J. Kirkland, and D. D. Bly, *Modern Size-Exclusion Liquid Chromatography*. John Wiley & Sons, New York, 1979.
32. *Thermal Characterization of Polymeric Materials*, (E. A. Turi, ed.). Academic Press, New York, 1981.
33. D. A. Skoog and D. M. West, *Fundamentals of Analytical Chemistry*, 2nd Ed. Holt, Rinehart, and Winston, New York, 1969.

5

Elastomeric Closures for Parenterals

Edward J. Smith and Robert J. Nash

The West Company, Phoenixville, Pennsylvania

I. ELASTOMERIC PARENTERAL PACKAGING COMPONENTS—A PHYSICAL DESCRIPTION

Elastomers have been in commerical use as materials for parenteral packaging components since the early part of the twentieth century because they possess unique physical properties that are important to the functions of the total parenteral package system. Elastomers, sometimes known simply as "rubbers," are moldable into an almost limitless variety of permanent shapes and forms to meet specific package design requirements. Examples of the desirable properties of elastomers are compressibility and resealability. Properly formulated elastomeric closures seal small fissures or voids in mating surfaces, such as the inside necks of parenteral vials or the inner surface of hypodermic syringes. Other types of materials, such as glass, metal, or conventional thermoplastic, do not possess this ability. Elastomers are easily penetrated by a hypodermic syringe needle and reseal rapidly after needle withdrawal. Hopkins [1] presents a lengthy list of pharmaceutical uses of elastomeric materials. Representative elastomeric packaging components are shown in Figure 1.

A. Vial Closures

Elastomeric vial stoppers, used as primary closures for parenteral vials, are one of the most commonly used forms of pharmaceutical closures. Rubber has been molded into all types and sizes of vial closures, from unit-dose to closures for containers with volumes of several liters. A flange stopper, shown in Figure 2, consists of a hollow plug and disk designed as one unit. Both the cylindrical surface on the inside of the vial neck and the circular surface at the top of the neck finish are sealed with a properly placed flange stopper. Table 1 lists the nominal dimensions of the most

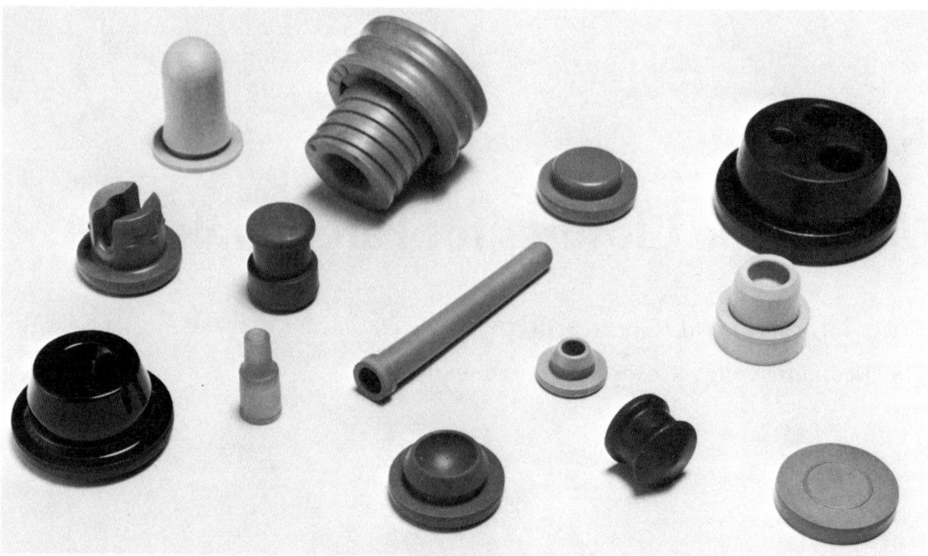

Figure 1 Elastomeric pharmaceutical packaging components. Top row: Dropper bulb, specialty syringe plunger stopper, coated flange stopper, large volume parenteral stopper. Middle row: Lyophilizing stopper, specialty two-compartment vial closure, cannula cover, diagnostic tube stopper. Bottom row: Large volume parenteral stopper, sleeve stopper, flange stopper, molded disk. (Courtesy of the West Company, Phoenixville, PA.)

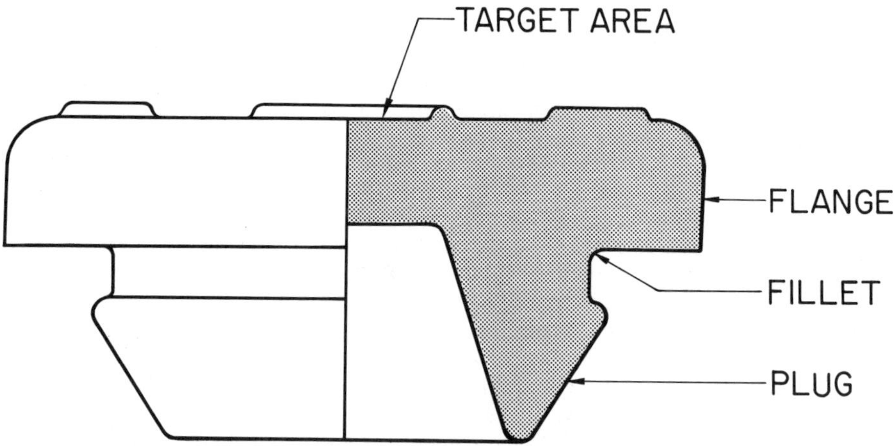

Figure 2 Typical flange stopper.

Table 1 Nominal Dimensions of Representative Flange Stoppers

Stopper	Flange diameter (in.)	Plug diameter (in.)	Diaphragm thickness (in.)
West V-24	0.400	0.226	0.088
West V-35	0.500	0.305	0.082
West S-127	0.750	0.524	0.110
West S-51	1.103	0.623	0.157

commonly used sizes of vial stoppers. The flange stopper is held in place by a metal seal applied over it and crimped around the bottom ledge of the glass finish. This is shown in Figure 3. A special design of flange stopper, a lyophilizing stopper, permits evacuation of the liquid vial contents prior to final stoppering. These closures are used for freeze-dried products intended for reconstitution at point of use. A schematic use of a lyophilizing stopper in freeze drying is shown in Figure 4.

Sleeve stoppers (Fig. 5) are occasionally used as vial closures, particularly for extemporaneous preparations. Sleeve stoppers, however, are most often used as injection sites for intravenous fluid therapy systems. In use, the plug end of the sleeve stopper is inserted into the bottle hole or injection port and the sleeve is folded back to form a seal over the bottle lip and mouth or injection site opening. Usually, a band of shrink wrap material is placed around the retracted sleeve to hold it in place.

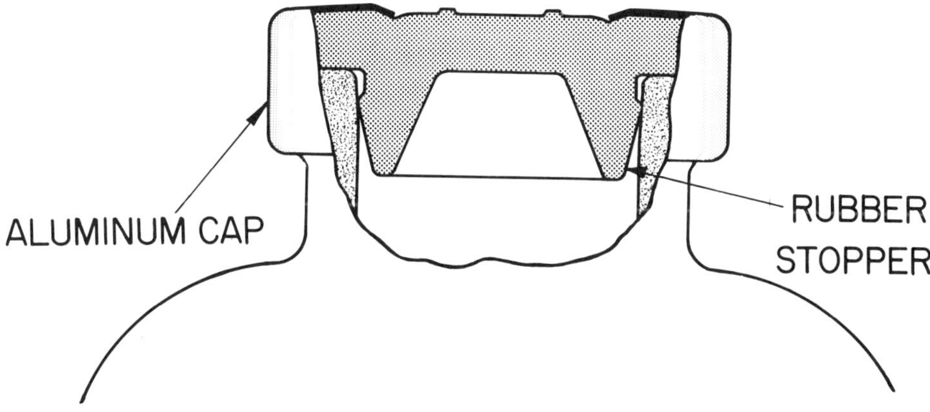

Figure 3 Sealed parenteral closure system.

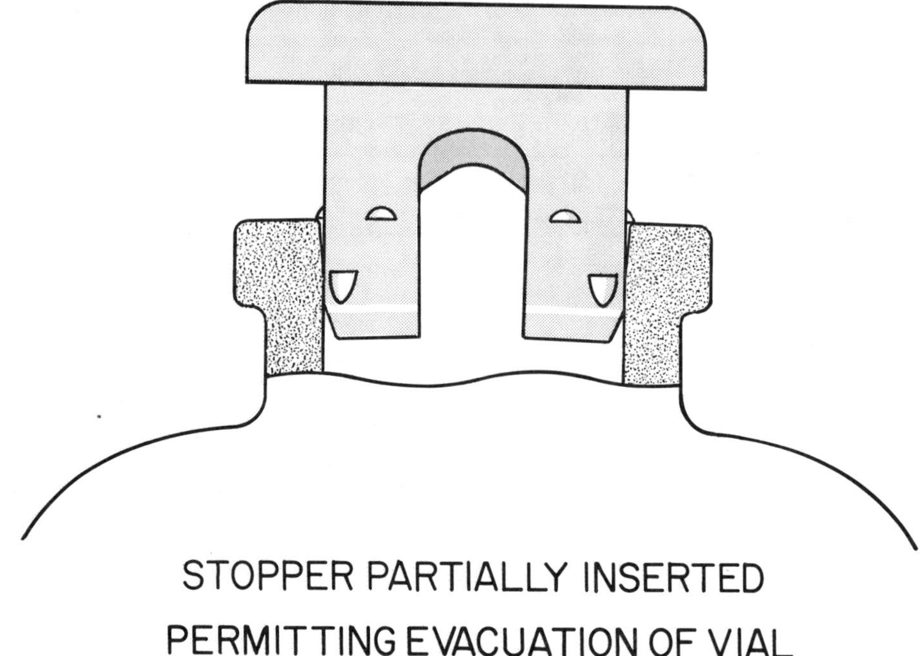

Figure 4 Use of a lyophilizing stopper in freeze drying.

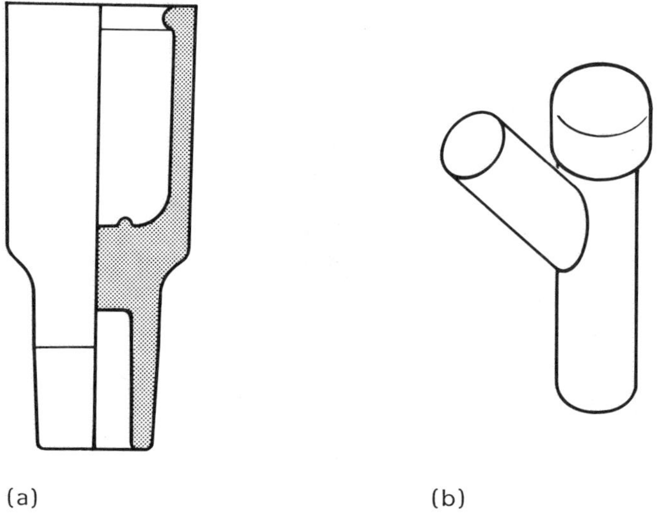

Figure 5 (a) Sleeve stopper. (b) Sleeve stopper assembled with Y-site connector.

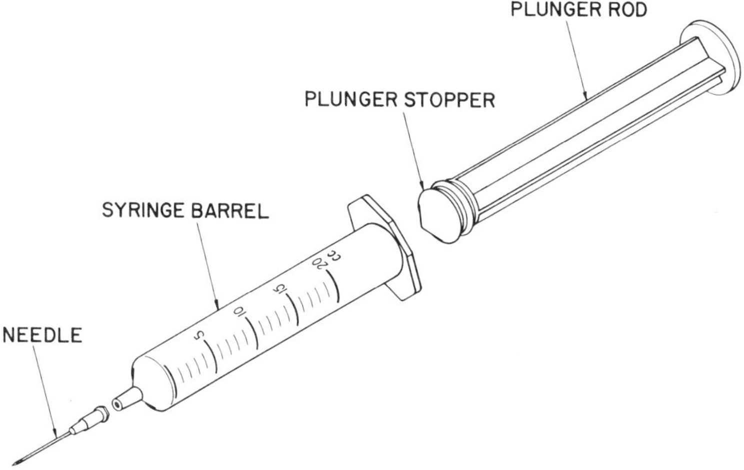

Figure 6 Disposable syringe assembly.

Laboratory stoppers are simple cork-shaped sealing devices that are removed when the drug is withdrawn. It is impractical to withdraw parenteral solutions through a laboratory stopper with a hypodermic needle and syringe because of the thickness of the cork itself.

Disks are used as primary closures in conjunction with aluminum sealing caps. Disks can be either molded or punched from a flat sheet of material, depending on the thickness of the disk. Thick disks are difficult to punch cleanly during manufacture and must be molded. Molded disks permit the feature of a target ring, which is a raised circle enclosing the area of the closure designed for needle penetration.

B. Syringe Plungers

Syringe plungers were one of the early uses of rubber as a pharmaceutical packaging component [2,3]. A typical application of a syringe plunger is shown in Figure 6. Disposable hypodermic syringes contain a rubber piston, usually with two ribs. The piston is attached by an interference friction fit to a plastic plunger rod, which serves to aspirate the fluid into

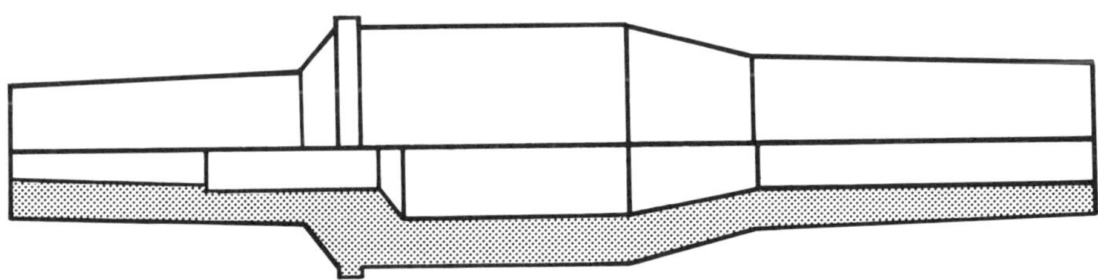

Figure 7 Intravenous fluid line connector.

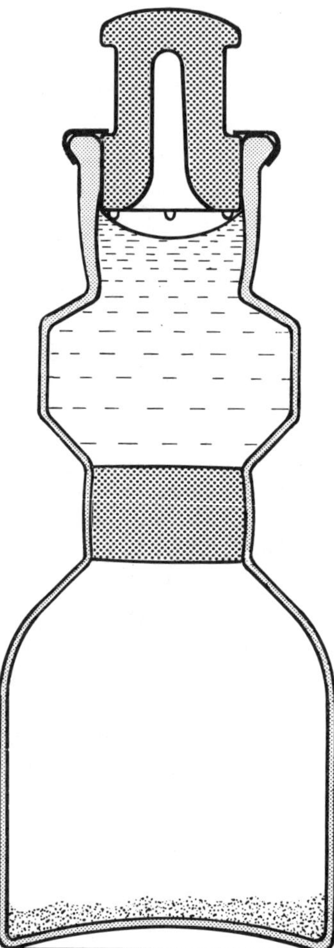

Figure 8 Univial parenteral package. Pushing on the top plunger causes hydrostatic pressure to dislodge the center seal, permitting mixing and dissolution of the powder in the lower compartment.

the syringe and to push the fluid through the cannula during injection. The design of the plunger tip and a mating plastic rod must be such as to prevent the plastic rod from pulling out during use. The front edge of the plunger tip (the distal end) must be molded to a suitable sharpness to permit easy reading of the syringe scale. Dental anesthetic cartridges are another major use of pharmaceutical closures. This packaging form actually contains two rubber components, a plunger to close the back end of the cartridge and a plug to close the front end. The syringe plunger for prefilled cartridges generally consists of a three-ribbed plunger tip, which is pushed by a rod to expel the enclosed drug.

C. Intravenous Therapy Drug Delivery Components

Intravenous drug delivery systems often contain sites for the additional introduction of drugs to the fluid stream. Turco and King [3] describe intravenous fluid (IV) systems in current use. Several styles of rubber components are available permitting direct injection into the fluid stream. The rubber connector for intravenous systems is shown in Figure 7. In addition to the rubber connectors, which are placed in the main flow of intravenous fluid, a Y site is often attached to the point of injection to permit auxiliary delivery of medication. These plastic Y sites are closed with the sleeve stopper style described previously.

D. Specialty Components

Medication fluid delivery systems have been developed in many forms utilizing a wide variety of rubber shapes. Drugs that are unstable in solution are maintained in a dry condition until they are reconstituted at the time of use. A convenient method of reconstituting on a unit-dose basis is the Univial system (Fig. 8). The powdered drug is contained in the lower half of an hourglass vial and the sterile diluent is contained in the upper half. The two vial halves are separated by a rubber barrel, which is displaced with hydrostatic pressure from pressure applied to the Univial plunger.

II. PHYSICAL DESCRIPTION OF RUBBER

Polymers exhibit characteristic stress and strain properties (Fig. 9). Stress is the applied force per unit area which causes a deformation. Strain is the deformation per unit length in tensile tests or deformation per unit distance between the contacting surfaces in shear tests [4].

A brittle plastic undergoes very little deformation before breakage occurs (Fig. 10, curve A). A yielding plastic deforms to a yield point, then deforms with low applied stress for a period of time before resuming a positive stress-strain ratio (Fig. 10, curve B). This phenomenon can be seen during testing as a sudden "necking" of the test specimen. Elastomers undergo considerable deformation with a long linear stress-strain region (Fig. 10, curve C).

The American Society for Testing Materials (ASTM) definition of rubber (D1566) is "a material that is capable of recovering from large deformations quickly and forcibly, and can be, or already is modified to a state in which it is essentially insoluble (but can swell) in boiling solvent. . . ."

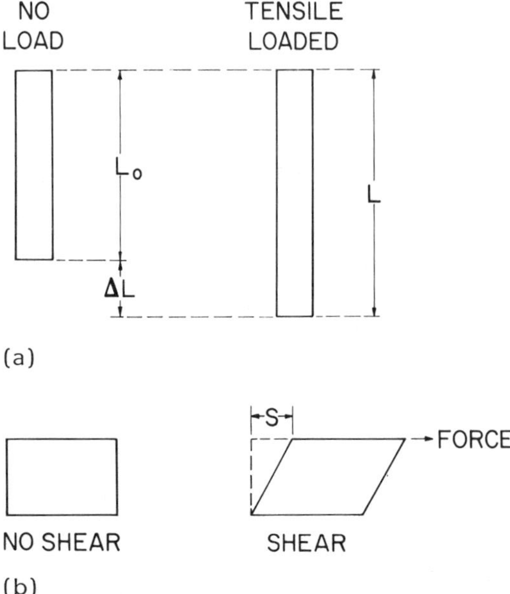

Figure 9 (a) Tensile stretching of a bar. (b) Shear of a rectangular block.

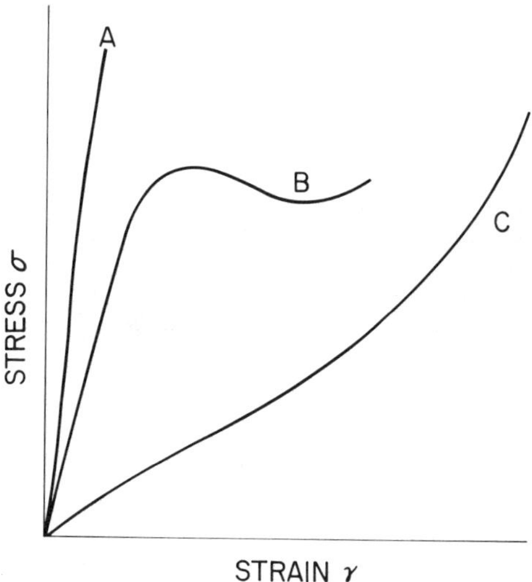

Figure 10 Stress-strain properties of polymers.

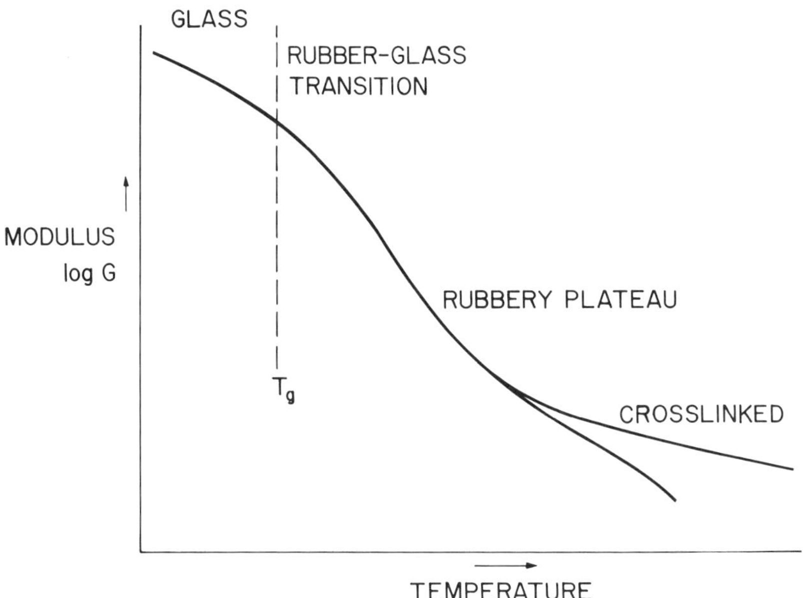

Figure 11 Phase diagram of an elastomeric material.

The ratio of stress to strain is called the *modulus* and is a measure of the rubber stiffness. Young's modulus is the stress-strain ratio applied to elongation; shear modulus is the same ratio applied to shear. The regions of viscoelastic behavior are defined in terms of the temperature dependence of the modulus (Fig. 11).

Ultimate tensile strength is the force per unit area required to break a specimen of specified geometry when it is subjected to a stress applied at a constant rate. Elongation is the percentage increase in linear dimension that the test specimen has experienced up to a point that it breaks. The use of these properties for the characterization of specific rubber formulations is discussed in Section VI.

III. TYPES OF RUBBER USED IN PARENTERAL PACKAGING

A. Historical Development

In the broadest sense, *rubber* is a polymeric material that at room temperature can be stretched to at least twice its length and then on release will return quickly to its original length [5]. Although simple by definition, rubber is a complex material commonly composed of two to ten or more raw materials. The chief polymeric component of rubber is the elastomer. Other components and their role in a rubber formulation will be described later. When a rubber is referred to as "butyl" it is understood that the elastomer used in that rubber formulation is a butyl elastomer. Thus, the terms "elastomer" and "rubber" are commonly used interchangeably.

The historical development of rubber parallels the development of unique elastomers. Some selected important events are listed in Table 2. An

Table 2 Important Events in the History of Rubber

1496	Columbus reports natives of Haiti using balls which bounced in games
1770	Joseph Priestly names the elastic, bouncy material rubber since it could be used to rub off pencil marks
1839	Hancock and Goodyear discover vulcanization of natural rubber
1855	Use of rubber in medicine, such as bandages, gloves, and syringes, noted in book by Goodyear
1878	Thomas Foster patents the fabrication of rubber surgical gloves
1914–1918	Methyl rubber (dimethylbutadiene polymers) produced in Germany
1930	Thiokol, an oil-resistant polysulfide rubber, introduced into the United States
1930s	Commercially available intravenous administration sets
1931	Neoprene (DuPont) production started
1933	Buna S, a butadiene-styrene copolymer, made in Germany
1936	Buna N, a butadiene-acrylonitrile copolymer, made in Germany
1940	Butyl rubber, used in tires and inner tubes, made in United States
1942	Butadiene-styrene copolymers made in United States
1944	Silicone elastomers introduced
1946	Polyurethanes made in Germany
1954	First fluorocarbon elastomers available
1955	"Synthetic natural" rubber, polyisoprene, made
1960	Commercial production of cis-polybutadiene
1960	Chlorobutyl rubber produced in United States
1963	EPDM elastomers commercially available
1963	Ziegler and Natta awarded the Nobel prize for chemistry for work on catalysis of ethylene-propylene rubber

extensive history can be found in the book by Stern [6], and a recent paper by Wright reviews the history of rubber in medicine [7].

B. Classification of Elastomers

Elastomers are usually classified as unsaturated or saturated, based on the fraction of reactive double bonds in the main chain or side chain of the elastomer. The higher the unsaturation, the greater is the fraction of reactive carbon-carbon double bonds.

Commonly used saturated and unsaturated elastomers and their ASTM abbreviation (D1418) are listed in Table 3 [8].

The degree of unsaturation determines both the physical and chemical properties of the elastomer, which in turn very strongly influences the properties of a rubber formulation. In a general sense this can be summarized as follows.

Polymer type	Physical properties	Chemical properties
Highly unsaturated	Excellent	Poor
Slightly unsaturated	Good	Good
Saturated	Poor	Excellent

For example, an injection flashball on an IV set is usually made from natural rubber (unsaturated) because the physical properties, such as resilience and ability to reseal after injection, are of primary importance. On the other hand, implantable devices are usually made from silicone rubber (saturated) because its chief chemical property, inertness, is of paramount importance [9].

Table 3 Saturated and Unsaturated Elastomers

Saturated	Unsaturated
Butyl (IIR)	Natural (NR)
Halogenated butyls, chloro and bromo (CIIR & BIIR)	Styrene butadiene (SBR)
Ethylene-propylene rubber (EPM)	Polyisoprene (IR)
Ethylene-propylene-diene rubber (EPDM)	Nitrile (NBR)
Silicone (Q)	Neoprene (CR)
Urethane (U)	Polybutadiene (BR)
Fluoroelastomers (FKM)	

Source: From Ref. 8.

Table 4 Selected Physical and Chemical Properties of Elastomers[a]

Type elastomer	Butyl/ halobutyl	Natural	Neoprene	NBR
Chemical name	Isobutylene-isoprene copolymer	Cis-1.4-polyisoprene	Polychloro-prene	Butadiene-acrylonitrile copolymer
Moisture vapor resistance	Excellent	Good	Fair	Fair
Gas transmission resistance	Excellent	Good	Fair	Good
Coring	Fair	Excellent	Good	Fair
Compression recovery	Poor	Excellent	Good	Good
Shelf life	Good	Fair	Good	Fair
Automatic handling ease	Poor	Good	Fair	Good
Heat resistance	Excellent	Good	Good	Good
Resistance to				
Water	Excellent	Good	Fair	Good
Animal oil	Excellent	Poor	Good	Excellent
Vegetable oil	Excellent	Poor	Good	Excellent
Mineral oil	Poor	Poor	Good	Excellent
Aliphatic solvents	Poor	Poor	Good	Poor
Aromatic solvents	Good	Good	Poor	Good
Chlorinated solvents	Poor	Poor	Poor	Poor
Acid dilute	Good	Good	Good	Fair
Alkali dilute	Good	Good	Good	Fair
Abrasion resistance	Fair	Good	Fair	Good
Resilience	Poor	Excellent	Good	Good
Ozone resistance	Excellent	Poor	Good	Poor
Radiation resistance	Fair to Poor	Good	Good	Good

[a]Ratings expressed in this guide are average values for typical rubber formulations using these base elastomers. Ratings can vary significantly with specific rubber formulations.

Silicone	Fluoro-elastomers	Urethane	EPDM	Polybutadiene
Polydimethyl siloxane	Fluoro-rubber	Polyester isocyanate	Ethylene propylene diene monomer	Cis-polybutadiene
Poor	Good	Poor	Fair	Fair
Poor	Good	Poor	Fair	Fair
Poor	N.D.	Excellent	Fair	Fair
Poor	Good	Excellent	Good	Good
Excellent	Excellent	Excellent	Excellent	Fair
Fair	N.D.	Fair	Fair	Good
Excellent	Excellent	Poor	Very good	Good
Excellent	Good	Poor	Good	Good
Good	Excellent	Excellent	Fair	Fair to poor
Excellent	Excellent	Excellent	Fair	Fair to poor
Fair	Excellent	Excellent	Poor	Poor
Poor	Excellent	Excellent	Good	Poor
Poor	Excellent	Poor	Fair	Poor
Poor	Excellent	Good	Poor	Poor
Fair	Fair	Poor	Good	Fair
Good	Good	Poor	Good	Fair
Fair	Good	Excellent	Good	Fair
Good	Fair	Good	Good	Good
Excellent	Excellent	Good	Good	Fair
Fair to good	Fair to good	Fair	Fair	Poor

C. Typical Physical and Chemical Properties of Elastomers

Table 4 lists some selected physical and chemical properties of nine common elastomers used in the pharmaceutical packaging industry. The ratings assigned are typical indications since properties can vary significantly with the type of other ingredients in the rubber formulations, their quantity, and degree of cure. The degree of cure is the extent of cross-linking between the elastomer chains. It is influenced by time and temperature of cure.

A rubber rated excellent for moisture vapor or gas transmission resistance will be relatively impermeable to water vapor or gases, such as O_2, N_2, and CO_2. It would be a good choice for vial closures used to package lyophilyzed or other powdered drugs. Butyl rubber has excellent gas resistance [10–12].

Coring resistance is the ability to resist fragmentation during puncture. A multidose vial, requiring many seal punctures during its use, would be better sealed with a natural rubber stopper than with a silicone.

Compression recovery is a measure of the resiliency of the rubber. It is the ability to recover to its original dimensions after being compressed for a given time at a given temperature. A natural rubber would be a better choice than a butyl for a syringe piston, which must remain resilient and not leak during storage or use.

Shelf life is related to the chemical properties of the rubber compound. It is the ability to maintain its properties after exposure to oxygen, ozone, heat, light, and moisture. The silicones and fluoroelastomers (saturated) are more long-lived than unsaturated natural rubber. Heat resistance runs parallel to shelf life in most pharmaceutical applications [13].

Resistance to solvents is an important property for pharmaceutical rubber items since they are frequently in contact with liquids. The ability of a rubber to resist solvent transmission, swelling, extraction, and degradation is an important packaging parameter. Vegetable oil is compatible with butyl rubber but not mineral oil.

Abrasion resistance is not as important a property with pharmaceutical items as it is in more mechanical items, such as tires or wire coatings. However, pharmaceutical items are in intimate contact with one another during manufacture, shipping, washing-processing, and assembly. The ability to resist surface disruption and the generation of particles is important in all parenteral applications [14].

Resilience is related to compression recovery. It is a measure of the elasticity of the rubber. A natural rubber ball will bounce; a butyl ball will not. An item, such as a blood valve commonly used with evacuated blood collection tubes, must be able to spring back and forth many times along the length of a needle to open and reseal the blood path. Natural rubber is the elastomer of choice.

Ozone is a common rubber degradant. It is present in the atmosphere, especially near ultraviolet lamps and electrical equipment. Ozone (O_3) resistance is poor for natural rubber; it hardens and cracks the rubber; ethylene propylene diene rubbers (EPDM) are quite resistant.

Radiation resistance, the ability to resist a change in properties after exposure to gamma rays or an electron beam, is more important now since radiation sterilization of many pharmaceutical items is common. Natural rubber syringe pistons, used in disposable plastic syringes, are commonly sterilized in this manner.

Table 5 Common Elastomers and Chemical Structure

Common name	Chemical name	Structure
Butyl rubber	Poly(isobutylene-isoprene)	$[-(CH_2-C(CH_3)_2)_{50}-(CH_2-C(CH_3)=CH-CH_2)-]_n$
Halobutyl rubber	Halogenated poly(isobutylene-isoprene)	$[-CH_2-C(CH_3)_2-)_{65}(CH-C(CH_3)-CH(X)-CH_2)-]_n$ X = Cl or Br
Ethylene-propylene rubber	Poly(ethylene-propylene)	$[(CH_2-CH_2)_3(CH_2-CH(CH_3))]_n$
Ethylene propylene-diene rubber	Poly(ethylene-propylene-diene)	$[(CH_2-CH_2)_{15}(CH_2-CH(CH_3))_5(\text{diene})-]$
Silicone rubber	Polydimethylsiloxane	$[-Si(CH_3)_2-O-]_n$

Table 5 (continued)

Common name	Chemical name	Structure
Urethane rubber	Adipic acid-ethylene glycol polyester	$HO(CH_2)_2[O-\overset{O}{\overset{\Vert}{C}}-(CH_2)_4-\overset{O}{\overset{\Vert}{C}}-O(CH_2)_2-]_nOH$
Fluoroelastomers	Poly(tetrafluoroethylene)	$[-CF_2-CF_2-]_n$
Natural rubber	Cis-1,4-polyisoprene	$[-CH_2-C(CH_3)=CH-CH_2-]_n$
Polyisoprene rubber	Cis-1,4-polyisoprene	$[-CH_2-C(CH_3)=CH-CH_2-]_n$
Neoprene rubber	Polychloroprene	$[-CH_2-C(Cl)=CH-CH_2-]_n$
Styrene butadiene rubber	Poly(butadiene-styrene)	$[(CH_2-CH=CH-CH_2)_4(CH_2-CH(C_6H_5))]_n$
Nitrile rubber	Poly(butadiene-acrylonitrile)	$[(CH_2-CH=CH-CH_2)_5(CH_2-CH(CN))_2]_n$
Polybutadiene	Polybutadiene	$[-CH_2-CH=CH-CH_2-]_n$

D. Chemical Structure of Elastomers

The properties of a rubber formulation are dependent on the chemical structure of the base elastomer used in its formulation. The structures of common elastomers are given in Table 5. Simple low-molecular-weight monomers, such as butadiene, isoprene, ethylene, propylene, and isobutylene, are used either exclusively (polybutadiene) or in combination (butyl rubber) to form high-molecular-weight polymers.

E. Manufacture of Elastomers

Rubber manufacturers combine the elastomer with other chemicals to produce a vulcanized product having specific physical and chemical properties that meet unique needs. Previously elastomers were divided into saturated and unsaturated types. Elastomers may also be classified as either natural or synthetic. The principal source of natural rubber is the tree *Hevea brasiliensis*, which is grown principally in Malaysia, Indonesia, Thailand, Celon, Africa, and other locations with similar tropical climates. Guayule rubber, obtained from a shrub that grows in arid environments, may become an alternate source [15]. Pharmaceutical rubber manufacturers usually use a grade that is virtually free of mold, specks, resinous matter, sand, bark, and blemishes [16].

Synthetic elastomers are those produced by humans, principally from petroleum products, using a highly automated continuous process that is well controlled. As a result, the shipment-to-shipment consistency of synthetic elastomers is better than that found in natural elastomers, where natural phenomena have a strong influence on the final product. A description of the production of synthetic elastomers can be found in the book by Morton [4].

IV. CLOSURE DESIGN

Standard rubber closure designs are offered by pharmaceutical closure manufacturers in a large number of configurations that mate with other packaging components [17–24]. The Glass Container Manufacturers Institute (GCMI) standard for biological glass finish, Number 2710, specifies the dimensions and tolerances for the finish of glass vials that have been adopted by the pharmaceutical industry. Information on the dimensions and tolerances for aluminum seals packaging can be obtained from the aluminum seal manufacturers (e.g., The West Company, Phoenixville, PA [25]). Available as standard rubber molded items are flange stoppers, sleeve stoppers, laboratory stoppers, syringe plunger tips, and dropper bulbs. The design details of these components are available from rubber closure manufacturers. For specialty applications, specialty closures must be designed. This section presents some design considerations that are presented as guidelines for closure design. Close cooperation between the package designer and the closure manufacturer throughout the development stages of a rubber closure design is needed to assure a satisfactory design.

Closures are designed to possess a slight "interference fit" with their mating parts. An interference fit is one in which the closure diameter is slightly larger than the inside diameter of the mating part, usually by approximately 2–10%. The amount of interference required for proper function varies greatly with the hardness of the rubber. The required interference is also influenced by the performance requirements of the closure system, such as the breakloose and extrusion specifications for syringe pistons, removal forces required for laboratory stoppers, and the pull-off strength of a needle shield-cannula hub connection.

The package designer must also consider the processability of the intended closure design in its intended assembly operation. If the closures are to be mechanically transported in the drug-packaging operation, the transport stability of the closure should be assured through proper design. The center of gravity of the molded part must be placed such that the part is not excessively top-heavy, causing wobbling or tipping during transport. The tracking system itself should be designed to avoid sharp bends or constricted areas that could cause line jams, requiring operator intervention and the increased potential for contamination of the packaged product. Pairing (sticking together) of flat surfaces of rubber closures, which occurs frequently in washing and autoclaving operations, can often be prevented by the addition of raised dots, approximately 0.005–0.010 in. high, added to the surface of the part. Nesting, another problem in handling certain styles of stoppers, especially sleeve stoppers, should be anticipated and corrected in the stopper design stage; when possible, parts should not be designed so that one portion of a part can interlock or nest with a portion of another part.

To improve stopper moldability, a radius is used to break all sharp corners of molded parts. The greater the radius, the easier it is to fill the mold, avoiding molding nonfills and feathered edges. Sharp corners are usually broken with a mild radius of 0.005 in. When possible, a fillet is designed as a part of the closure (see Fig. 2). The fillet is placed in the section of the vial closure between the intersection of the bottom flange and the plug. This fillet serves to break the sharp corner at that intersection, permitting the stock to flow efficiently in that area of the mold, thus minimizing the tendency to create molding splits in that section. With a vial closure, this fillet takes advantage of the rounded radius of the GCMI finish.

The tolerances for closures molded in the compression molding process are generally ±0.005 in. for tooling-controlled dimensions, such as molded diameters. This tolerance is generally applicable for diameters up to 0.500 in. A tolerance of ±0.008 in. is normally required for nominal diameters between 0.500 and 1.000 in. Above 1.000 in., a tolerance of ±0.010 in. is needed.

Very thin sections are very difficult to fill uniformly and should be avoided. Diaphragms should be at least 0.050 in. thick at their thinnest cross section.

Diaphragm designs have been introduced that minimize stopper coring. One of the more effective designs is the V diaphragm in which a V section of the diaphragm acts as the needle target area. Two problems associated with the V design are the accumulation of debris in the recess of the top of the stopper and the extreme difficulty in filling the diaphragm during molding. This design, while effective in minimizing coring, is susceptible to diaphragm imperfections, such as holes or tears, as a result of the molding process and should be adopted only when absolutely necessary.

The eccentricity, or relationship of the diameters of the flange and the plug, should be taken into consideration when designing closures. For large compression molds, a tolerance of 0.020% maximum total indicator readout (TIR) is required. The TIR requirement can be lowered for products produced by transfer molding or injection molding.

Barrier coatings are available to reduce extractable substances from rubber closures. The most common barrier coating is a cured epoxy resin, which reduces but does not completely eliminate extractable substances. Hopkins [1] describes application of epoxy-type coatings to pharmaceutical closures and their barrier properties. Recently, Teflon coatings have been applied to molded rubber closures. Teflon coatings have been shown to be highly effective as barriers [26,27].

V. RUBBER COMPOUNDING

A. Rubber Formulation Ingredients

As stated previously, a rubber formulation is a complex combination of two to ten or more ingredients. Ingredients are classified according to their function in the formulation. Ingredients used in pharmaceutical rubber are

a. Elastomer or polymer
b. Curing or vulcanizing agent
c. Accelerator
d. Activator
e. Antioxidant-antiozonant
f. Plasticizer-lubricant
g. Filler
h. Pigment

Other types of materials are used in rubber but not usually in pharmaceutical rubber. These include blowing agents that produce gas to make sponge rubber and odorants that mask the natural odor of rubber.

B. Function of Rubber Ingredients

1. Elastomers

This is the basic component of any rubber formulation. The properties of the rubber formulations are largely dependent on the properties of the elastomer. Types of elastomers and their properties were discussed previously.

2. Curing or Vulcanizing Agents

Chemicals used to cross-link elastomer chains into the three-dimensional network required to give a rubber formulation the desired physical and chemical properties are called curing or vulcanizing agents. The term "vulcanization" is used to indicate that heat is employed in the curing process. Cross-linking with gamma radiation or an electron beam is still loosely referred to as vulcanization, even though no heat is used. Common curing agents and elastomers cross-linked by them are shown in Table 6.

A desirable property of pharmaceutical rubber formulations is that they be "clean," that is, that they contain materials that neither extract nor volatilize into the headspace of a packaged pharmaceutical. Sulfur-cured rubber, because it requires the use of other chemicals to effect an efficient cure, are not as clean as resin-, metal oxide-, or peroxide-cured formulations.

Table 6 Typical Curing Agents and Elastomers Crosslinked

Elastomer type	Curing agent
Natural rubber and polyisoprene	1. Sulfur 2. Sulfur-containing chemicals, e.g., tetramethylthiuram disulfide 3. Peroxides
Styrene butadiene rubber	1. Sulfur
Nitrile rubber	1. Sulfur 2. Peroxides 3. Cadmium and magnesium oxides
Neoprene	1. Sulfur 2. Sulfur-containing chemicals 3. Zinc and magnesium oxides
Polybutadiene	1. Sulfur 2. Sulfur-containing chemicals 3. Peroxides
Butyl and halobutyl	1. Sulfur 2. Resins 3. Zinc oxide (halo only)
Ethylene propylene	Peroxides
Ethylene propylene diene rubber	1. Peroxides 2. Sulfur-containing chemicals
Silicone	Peroxides
Urethane	
Polyesters	1. Peroxide 2. Sulfur
Polyethers	Sulfur
Fluoroelastomers	Amines

The demands of the pharmaceutical industry and regulatory agencies are such that these relatively clean cure systems are becoming more common.

3. *Accelerators*

Accelerators reduce the cure time by increasing the vulcanization rate. These materials are not catalysts since they are chemically altered and in many cases also act as cross-linking agents. Sulfur cures always require an accelerator to produce an effective degree of cross-linking. Common sulfur cure accelerators are listed in Table 7. Some accelerators, because of their reactivity, may form toxic extractables, such as 2-(2-hydroxyethylmercapto)benzothiazole from mercaptobenzothiazole [28,29]. Such accelerators as tetramethylthiuram disulfide can form toxic nitrosamines [30,31].

Table 7 Sulfur Cure Accelerators

Amine	Hexamethylene tetramine
Dithiocarbamate	Zinc dibutyldithiocarbamate
Sulfenamide	*N*-*t*-butyl-2-benzothiazole Sulfenamide
Thiazole	2-Mercaptobenzothiazole
Thiuram	Tetraethylthiuram disulfide

4. *Activators*

Activators increase the rate of cross-linking by reacting with accelerators to form materials that are more efficient. Zinc oxide is a common activator, as is stearic acid. In conventional sulfur cure systems, zinc oxide and stearic acid are routinely used as coactivators. Zinc stearate is formed as a by-product of the vulcanization reaction. Zinc salts may be extractable from rubber closures containing zinc oxide. This may not have any effect on the drug packaged, but a zinc-sensitive drug may lose potency.

5. *Antioxidants-Antiozonants*

Antioxidants and antiozonants are classified as antidegradants or age resistors. An antioxidant is a chemical that protects against oxygen attack; an antiozonant is specifically designed to protect against the more reactive ozone. These chemicals are commonly used to improve the age resistance of unsaturated elastomers. (See Table 5.) Saturated elastomers, such as silicones or fluoroelastomers, need no antidegradants. Antidegradants are of the chemical or physical types. Chemical antidegradants, such as hindered phenols and amines, protect the rubber by preferentially oxidizing in place of the polymer. Physical antidegradants are waxes that "bloom" or migrate to the surface of the rubber to form a protective shield. These waxes may also act as lubricants that allow the smooth movement of such items as syringe pistons.

6. *Plasticizers-Lubricants*

These ingredients are used in a rubber formulation to assist in the mixing or molding of the rubber, to soften the final vulcanized rubber, or to add lubricity to the closure. Included in this group of materials are paraffinic wax, silicone oil, paraffinic and naphthenic oils, phthalates, and organic phosphates. Paraffinic wax and silicone oil are commonly used in syringe pistons that must slide freely within a glass or plastic barrel. Silicone oil decreases the coring tendency of vial stoppers. Organic phosphates, such as tributoxyethyl phosphate (TBEP), are used rather than paraffinic oils in acrylonitrile rubber (NBR). TBEP can interfere with certain clinical tests if it is used in evacuated blood tube stoppers [32,33].

7. *Fillers*

Rubber may be formulated without a filler. If so, the resultant product is called "gum rubber." Gum rubber is usually translucent. Baby nipples, flashballs, and sleeve stoppers (for IV sets) are common items utilizing gum rubber. In most rubber applications, however, it is desirable to modify the hardness of a formulation, improve its physical characteristics, increase its abrasion resistance or density, or reduce its cost. Fillers do all of the above. A number of fillers are utilized by the rubber industry [4,6,34]. Those most frequently used in pharmaceutical applications are carbon black, hydrated or calcined aluminum silicates (clay), barium sulfate, magnesium silicate (talc), zinc oxide, and hydrated or anhydrous silica [35].

Modification of the physical properties of a rubber formulation is dependent on the amount of interaction between the polymer and the filler [36]. The amount of filler used, the surface activity of the filler, its particle size, and its shape are the four most important factors. Carbon blacks are the most effective materials and are considered reinforcing fillers. Barium sulfate and talc are considered nonreinforcing fillers, and their primary use is to increase the density of a formulation or add lubricity. The other fillers, such as clays and silica, are semireinforcing materials. A reinforcing filler is one that interacts with the polymer system and adds structure and strength to the rubber formulation. The particle size of most fillers range from 15 to 500 nm. Fillers add or enhance specific rubber properties when used judiciously. Coring and gas transmission can be reduced by the use of talc. Swelling (solvent resistance) is reduced by clays and carbon blacks. Pharmaceutical rubber manufacturers are limited in the grades of fillers they can use. Certain carbon blacks have high concentrations of polynuclear aromatic hydrocarbons (PNA), which can be extracted into the packaged drug. Clays may contain extractable metals, such as aluminum, that may not be compatible with certain drug formulations [37,38].

8. *Pigments*

Pigments are either inorganic salts and oxides, carbon black, or organic dyes that are used for aesthetic or functional purposes. Aesthetically, a pharmaceutical supplier may want the rubber closure to match the aluminum seal or label to enhance the look of the package. More importantly, color may also identify a drug or designate a dosage. Carbon black is used to produce gray or black rubber; titanium dioxide is used for white. Iron and chromium oxides are used for shades of yellow, red, and green. Organic dyes, such as phthalocyanines and ultramarine blue for blues and greens, are also used, but the color fastness of these organics is not as good as the inorganic oxides.

The eight ingredients discussed here do not represent all the possible materials available to the pharmaceutical rubber formulator. An exhaustive list of "allowable" materials can be found in the Code of Federal Regulations Sec. 177.2600 or in Technical Methods Bulletin No. 1 of the PDA [39].

C. Typical Rubber Formulations

To paraphrase a recent paper on the validation of elastomeric closures, "The perfect closure probably does not exist" [40]. Therefore, the need for further research to improve polymers, especially natural rubber, is obvious [41]. No one rubber formulation will meet all the requirements of the pharmaceutical packaging industry since the items and the drugs to be packaged are too diverse. There is a need for good communications both within and between the closure supplier and the drug packager to define the precise requirements of the closure system [42]. Table 8 lists

Table 8 Factors Affecting the Selection of Rubber Closures

Drug-medicament
Solvent-vehicle
Preservative
pH of packaged product
Buffer system
Metallic sensitivities
Moisture vapor-gas protection required
Configuration of closure
Color

nine factors that influence the selection of a rubber formulation. In a later section, tests that may be used in the selection of rubber formulations will be discussed.

Tables 9 through 12 show typical pharmaceutical formulations based on natural, halobutyl, ethylenepropylenediene (EPDM), and silicone elastomers. In these formulations the amount of each ingredient is expressed in parts per hundred polymer (php) or weight of ingredient relative to the elastomer, which is arbitrarily set equal to 100. The function of each ingredient is also given.

A formulation may be optimized to meet specific requirements, such as coring and reseal. But for each gain in one parameter, there may be concurrent losses in others [43]. For example, when coring and resealing parameters are enhanced, resistance to gas transmission may be reduced.

Table 9 Red Natural Rubber Pharmaceutical Closure Formulation

Ingredient	php	Function
Natural rubber	100	Elastomer
Calcined aluminum silicate	50	Filler
Paraffinic oil	5	Plasticizer-lubricant
Iron oxide	2.5	Pigment
Zinc oxide	3	Activator
Stearic acid	1	Activator
Thiuram accelerator	0.5	Accelerator
Thiazole accelerator	0.25	Accelerator
Butylated hydroxytoluene (BHT)	1	Antidegradant
Sulfur	2	Curing agent

Table 10 Gray Halobutyl Rubber Pharmaceutical Closure Formulation

Ingredient	php	Function
Halobutyl rubber	100	Elastomer
Calcined aluminum silicate	75	Filler
Naphthenic oil	8	Plasticizer-lubricant
Titanium dioxide	2	Pigment
Carbon black (furnace type)	0.25	Pigment
Butylated hydroxytoluene (BHT)	1	Antidegradant
Zinc oxide	3	Curing agent
Thiuram accelerator	0.35	Accelerator

Table 11 Black EPDM Rubber Pharmaceutical Closure Formulation

Ingredient	php	Function
EPDM	100	Elastomer
Carbon black (furnace)	100	Filler
Naphthenic oil	40	Plasticizer-lubricant
Zinc oxide	5	Activator
Stearic acid	1	Activator
Thiuram accelerator	1.5	Accelerator
Zinc dithiocarbamate	1.5	Accelerator
Sulfur	0.5	Curing agent

Table 12 Gray Silicone Rubber Pharmaceutical Closure Formulation

Ingredient	php	Function
Dimethylpolysiloxane polymer	100	Elastomer
SiO_2	25	Filler
Carbon black	0.25	Pigment
2,4-Dichlorobenzoyl peroxide	0.75	Curing agent

D. Raw Materials and Vendor Selection by Pharmaceutical Rubber Manufacturers

In previous sections the function of the various raw materials used in a formulation of rubber was explained. Material specifications must be rigidly controlled from batch to batch so that the final rubber formulation is maintained within desired limits. A small change in the purity or activity of even one raw material may affect the final rubber product. The key word in raw materials for the pharmaceutical rubber manufacturer is consistency. Pharmaceutical rubber manufacturers commonly have drug master files (DMF) for both raw materials and finished goods. A DMF filed with the FDA is a reference source providing detailed information about the composition, specifications, and testing procedures of materials [44].

Once a rubber formulation is filed, its composition must be maintained within specified narrow limits. If the activity of a given lot of accelerator does not allow a rubber formulation to cure properly, there is no allowance for substitution with another accelerator or even a change in the amount of accelerator. A manufacturer of rubber bands or floor mats can probably do either or both. Before a new material is even evaluated for routine use in pharmaceutical products it must meet three criteria:

a. It must be readily available from the supplier in sufficient quantity to meet anticipated needs.
b. It must either be listed as GRAS (generally regarded as safe) in the appropriate sections of the Code of the Federal Regulations or at least the material must not specifically be prohibited.
c. The suppliers published specifications must meet or exceed any generally applicable specifications of the user.

The approval of a new raw material is a two-phase process. First, it is evaluated in the laboratory, then in a manufacturing environment. In the laboratory, tests for identity, purity, and functionality are developed. The material is then evaluated for toxicity. Only after it meets all laboratory specifications is it evaluated in a plant. After both approvals the material may be filed with the FDA in a drug master file that will describe the material and list specifications and test methods that will be used to control the quality of the material on an ongoing basis. The approval of a new vendor-manufacturer of an existing raw material follows the same general procedure. The use of different antioxidants or plasticizers in a raw material may not make materials from two vendors-manufacturers functionally different, but they are chemically different and therefore would not be approved as equivalent by a pharmaceutical rubber manufacturer.

Specific raw materials and tests are too numerous to discuss here, but at least one test for purity, identity, and functionality is desirable on each sample of raw material. Of course, good analytic practices in the quality control of raw materials like those outlines by Bernard et al. must be observed [45]. This means qualified people, standard materials, and validated and audited test procedures. Retained samples are often kept for 5 years to allow retesting if required. Pharmaceutical rubber manufacturers purchase their raw materials from the same sources as do the manufacturers of tires or other mechanical goods. Since there are often different standards of quality and specifications, the pharmaceutical rubber manufacturer must work with suppliers to obtain required materials. Using increased and/or specific manufacturing controls and increased testing by both the suppliers and users, better quality raw material may be obtained for use in pharmaceutical rubber items. Carbon black with a low PNA content and calcined clay with low soluble aluminum are two good examples of the result of supplier-user cooperation.

VI. VULCANIZATION PROCESS

A. Definition and Properties

Vulcanization is to rubber manufacturing as baking is to the culinary arts. Vulcanization is discussed briefly in the section on curing or vulcanizing agents. Once the elastomer and other formulation ingredients are mixed to form a homogenous mass, the unvulcanized rubber is usually processed either into sheets of uniform dimensions or into small pellets. At this point the material is plastic; that is, it will flow easily under pressure into molds that will shape and hold the rubber in the desired configuration during vulcanization. During vulcanization or curing the material changes from a plastic nonelastic material to an elastic resilient material.

The changes that take place during vulcanization can be divided into microscopic (or molecular) and macroscopic (or observable) changes.

1. *Microscopic Changes*

Before vulcanization, the elastomer chains are twisted, coiled, and randomly oriented in the homogenous mass of rubber ingredients much like spaghetti and sauce on a plate [46]. There are no links (chemical bonds) between the elastomer chains; they are essentially free to move about independently of each other. During vulcanization the individual elastomer chains are linked (cross-linked) together to form a three-dimensional network in which freedom of motion is now restricted. The rubber is no longer plastic because elastomer chains are not free to slide by one another. In sulfur-cured systems, the link between chains, known as cross-links, are single sulfur atoms or short chains of sulfur atoms. In peroxide-cured silicone rubber, carbon atoms in the elastomer chains are linked directly together by a single chemical bond via a free radical mechanism. These are illustrated in Figures 12 and 13.

Physical properties of the vulcanized rubber are dependent on the number and type of cross-links [47]. Cross-link density or tightness of cure increases as the number of cross-links increases. Compression set, the amount of permanent deformation a rubber sample will retain after it has been compressed or deformed for a given period of time at a specified

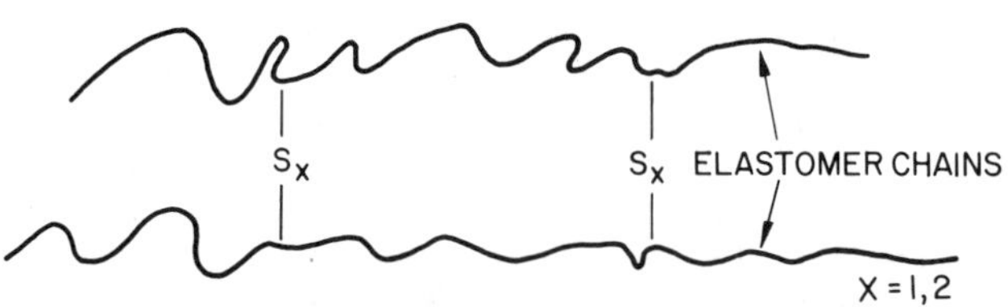

Figure 12 Sulfur cross-linking of polymer chains.

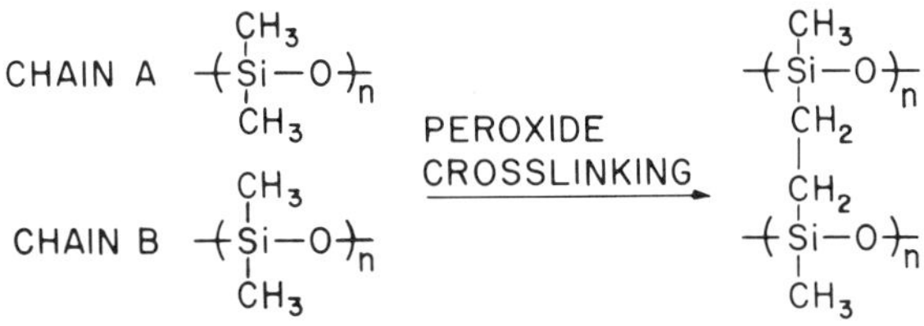

CHAIN A $\left(\begin{matrix} CH_3 \\ | \\ Si - O \\ | \\ CH_3 \end{matrix}\right)_n$

CHAIN B $\left(\begin{matrix} CH_3 \\ | \\ Si - O \\ | \\ CH_3 \end{matrix}\right)_n$

PEROXIDE CROSSLINKING →

$\left(\begin{matrix} CH_3 \\ | \\ Si - O \\ | \\ CH_2 \end{matrix}\right)_n$
$\begin{matrix} | \\ CH_2 \end{matrix}$
$\left(\begin{matrix} | \\ Si - O \\ | \\ CH_3 \end{matrix}\right)_n$

Figure 13 Peroxide cure of silicone rubber.

temperature, is decreased (improved) by monosulfide (-S-) cross-links; the X in Figure 12 is equal to one. On the other hand, tensile strength, or the force required to stretch a sample to the breaking point, is increased (improved) by polysulfide cross-links ($-S-S_X-S-$). Thus the formulation and cure can be adjusted to give the specific rubber properties required for the application. Low compression set, or monosulfide cross-linkage, is required for vial stopper applications; high tensile strength, or polysulfide cross-linkage, for rubber bands.

2. *Macroscopic Changes*

Observable differences in the properties of uncured and cured rubber are listed in Table 13. These are observable more than measurable parameters; quantifiable parameters on uncured and cured rubber will be discussed later. The change from uncured rubber to cured rubber is a continuum and therefore so are its properties. Also, the state of being cured is not an absolute. Rubber cured to a given degree to optimize one property might be under- or overcured for another. The "optimum" cure state is that which gives the required collective physical and chemical properties for satisfactory performance.

The properties listed in Table 13 are only general indicators of cure. For example, natural rubber will be tacky before being cured. The tack

Table 13 Comparative Macroscopic Properties of Uncured and Cured Rubber

Interaction	Uncured	Cured
Inorganic solvent	Dissolves	Swells
Under pressure	Flows (plastic)	Elastic
On touch	Very tacky	Slightly tacky to slippery
When stretched	Breaks easily	Springs back
In aqueous alkali-acid	Ingredients easily extractable	Slight or no ingredients extractable
When dropped	No bounce	Slight bounce to complete rebound
On weathering, (heat, light, O_3, O_2, time)	Deteriorates rapidly	Weathers well

will disappear over a range of cures, then reappear if the rubber is overcured or reverted. By reversion is meant that some of the cross-links formed during vulcanization are broken, and as a result, the rubber is reverting or returning to its un-cross-linked state. Excessively tacky parts mean that the rubber is either over- or undercured. On the other hand, butyl rubber is inherently tacky, and therefore, tack may not be an indicator of poor cure.

B. Measure of Vulcanization

The vulcanization process can be measured on a sample of uncured rubber. This is commonly done as an in-process control test to assure the rubber compounder that all batches cure within a specified range of time and temperatures. Uniformity of the batch of rubber leads to a more consistent molded item from the press.

The purchaser of pharmaceutical items receives and utilizes only vulcanized parts. The manufacturers of rubber may do testing on three kinds of samples: (a) uncured rubber, (b) cured items of special geometry, such as dumbbell-shaped slabs or cylindrical plugs, to facilitate physical testing and, (c) the molded pharmaceutical rubber items that will be sold. The pharmaceutical rubber customer only tests one type of sample—molded parts that are purchased.

1. *In-Process Testing of Uncured Rubber*

Only one type of curemeter, the oscillating disk rheometer, will be described here since it is the most commonly used device. Details can be found in ASTM Method D2084 [8]. Other methods are described adequately in the text by Morton [4].

In the oscillating disk cure meter, such as a Monsanto Rheometer, a grooved biconical disk is embedded in an 8- to 12-g sample of uncured rubber and oscillated. While the temperature is held constant, the force or torque required to oscillate the disk is recorded as a function of time. A typical cure or rheometer curve is shown in Figure 14. The torque initially decreases as the sample begins to soften, then rises as the rubber begins to cure. The torque continues to rise as the cross-link density increases and finally may reach a maximum value as equilibrium is reached.

There are four important pieces of information obtained from the rheometer curve (Fig. 14):

Minimum torque M_L is a measure of the viscosity of the unvulcanized rubber. Viscosity is a measure of the deformability or flow characteristics of the rubber. The lower the viscosity, the easier it is to fill complex mold cavities.

Scorch time t_s2, essentially is the time the molder has to get the stock in place in the mold cavities before vulcanization begins. Scorch is normally taken as the time on the rheometer curve necessary for the torque to rise two units above the minimum (M_L). The longer the scorch time, the longer the rubber can be moved within the mold.

The time necessary for the torque to reach 90% of the increase from M_L to M_H (torque maximum) is t(90). Stated another way, t(90) is the time to reach $0.9(M_H - M_L) + M_L$ torque units and is commonly referred to as the cure time. The t(90) is inversely proportional to cure rate; the smaller the value of t(90), the faster the cure.

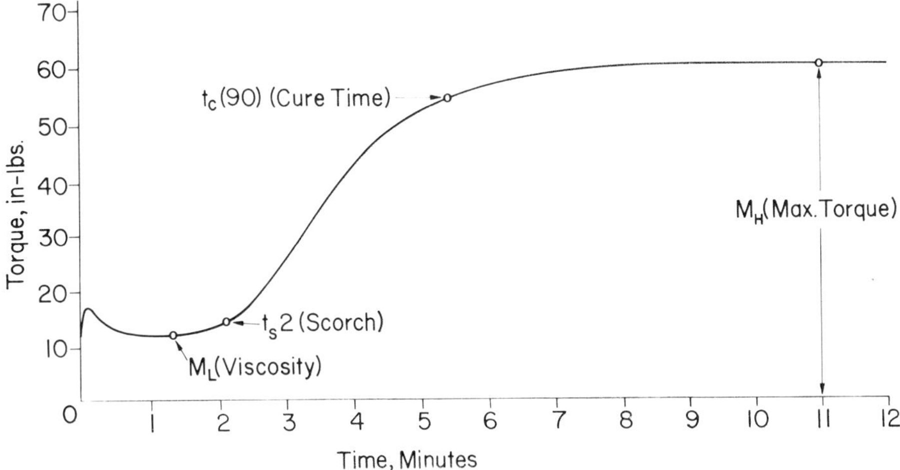

Figure 14 Rheometer curve.

The maximum torque is M_H and is a measure of the stiffness of the cured rubber. The M_H has a strong influence on the tensile strength or force required to rupture a sample of rubber.

In Figure 15a the torque reaches an equilibrium value and is constant. In Figure 15b the torque reaches a maximum but then decreases since the rubber sample is reverting (cross-link density decreases). This type of curve is common for sulfur-cured natural rubber formulations. In Figure 15c the torque and therefore cross-link density continues to rise with time. Both a and c are typical of synthetic rubbers, such as butyl or EPDM.

Although cure meters give the rubber manufacturer valuable information about the cure process, they do not predict the degree of curve on finished vulcanized parts nor do they accurately mimic the cure process in the press. The use of cure meters is limited to the quality control of unvulcanized stock [48]. Often cure windows, maximum and minimum values for M_L, t_s2, t(90), and M_H are established and used by manufacturing plants to control the consistency of mixed stock.

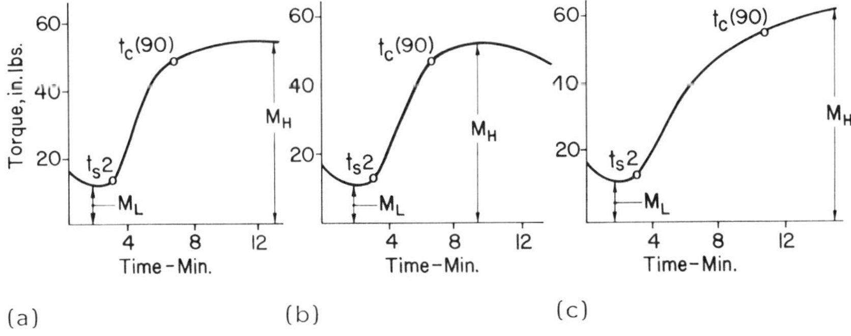

Figure 15 Types of cure curves.

2. *Physical Cure Tests on Items of Specific Geometry*

Various physical tests are often useful for indicating the degree of cure of rubber, provided parts of specific geometry are available.

Tensile and Modulus

Usually a dumbbell-shaped specimen is used in these tests. The specimen must be flat and have a thickness between 1.5 and 3 mm [8]. Several standard lengths and widths may be used. Dumbbells are cut with a die from square test plates molded under selected standard conditions of time and temperature. ASTM-recommended procedures are found in D3184 [8]. In the modulus and tensile tests, the specimen is stretched at a constant rate and the force (in psi) required to either stretch the specimen to a 300% increase in length (four times original length) or until the breaking point is measured. The former number is known as 300% modulus, or modulus at 300% elongation, and the latter as tensile strength.

ASTM Method D412 contains the standard procedure for these tests [8] which are normally performed on an instrument such as the Monsanto Tensometer (Monsanto Co., Akron, OH). Tensile strength and 300% modulus increase with cross-link density and will reach a maximum value then decrease if the rubber reverts [1,46].

Hardness

The hardness of rubber may be measured on a device such as the Shore Conveloader (The Shore Instrument & Mfg. Co., Jamaica, NY) using a type A durometer. The method is based on the penetration of a standard indentor forced into the rubber under specified conditions (ASTM Method 2240) [8]. The A scale extends from zero for liquids to 100 for a hard surface, such as glass. Typical pharmaceutical rubber formulations may range from 25 for a soft nipple formulation to 60 for a hard plunger formulation. The durometer test requires a test specimen that is at least 6 mm in thickness and 24 mm in diameter and therefore usually cannot be done on molded pharmaceutical items. A special test plate mold that gives a sheet of rubber for tensile and modulus tests and a cylindrical plug for the durometer test is commonly used. Hardness increases as cross-link density increases and may be used as an indicator of degree of cure, but the relationship must be empirically demonstrated in each case before it can be used for control purposes.

Compression Set

Compression set is the amount of permanent deformation a sample retains after it has been compressed for a given time at a specified temperature. ASTM D395 (method B) is most commonly used in the pharmaceutical rubber industry [8]. The test specimen is usually a cylinder 6–12.5 mm in thickness and 13–30 mm in diameter, which is compressed to 75% of its initial thickness for 22 hr at 70°C. After the specimen is removed from the compression device and allowed to cool for 30 min, thickness measurements are made and compression set calculated. Compression set (expressed as a percentage) decreases as cross-link density increases [6]. A good plunger rubber formulation will have compression set of 10–30%.

Tear Tests

ASTM D624 describes standard methods for measuring the tear resistance (in psi) of three types of rubber specimens. Tear resistance is quite sensitive to the degree of cure in some formulations [4]. Tear resistance is highest at low cross-link density.

Friction Tests

Since tack may be an indicator of cure, the friction between the surface of rubber and a flat stainless steel plane may be used to measure tack and therefore cure. In one device, four small rubber plugs are placed in individual cavities of a heavy stainless steel block. The plugs fit snugly and protrude several millimeters above the surface. This block with samples is placed face down on a flat stainless steel plane, and the angle of incline is increased until the block begins to move. The angle of first movement is a function of tack [49].

Other Methods

Table 14 lists other standard ASTM methods that may be used to determine cure when all other variables in a formulation are constant. The applicability and sensitivity of these methods will depend on the specific rubber formulation and must be empirically determined.

3. *Chemical and Physical Cure Tests on Molded End-Use Items*

Ideally, cure tests should not depend on the dimensions of the item or on the surface condition of the item. Many physical and chemical properties are cure related but are also strongly related to other parameters. Tests that the pharmaceutical industry may utilize can be classified as (a) cure specific, (b) cure related, or (c) independent of cure. Such tests as percentage ash and specific gravity [50,51] are independent of cure. Compression set and the coring tendency of a closure [52] may be affected by the degree of cure depending on the formulation type and the cure characteristics of the formulation.

The two cure-specific tests commonly used are free sulfur [53] and swelling [54]. Free sulfur can be measured only on sulfur-cured formulations that are extractable. These include natural, isoprene, butadiene,

Table 14 Miscellaneous Physical Cure-Related Test Methods

Test description	ASTM method	Type of specimen
Adhesion	D429	Cylinder
Dynamic fatigue	D430	Dumbbell strips
Crack growth	D813	Molded or cut strip
Vibration test	D945	Cylinder
Cut growth flexing	D1052	Cut strips
Resilience (rebound)	D1054	Rectangular blocks
Abrasion resistance	D2228	Cylinder
Forced vibration	D2231	Cylinder
Resilience (vertical rebound)	D2632	Slabs

chloroprene, SBR, and NBR rubbers. Sulfur-cured butyl rubber is notably absent from this list. The most common procedure is that found in ASTM D297 [8]. It involves the reaction of sodium sulfite with elemental or free sulfur to form thiosulfate, which is then titrated with a standard iodine solution. The amount of free sulfur found is a function of the amount used in the formulation and the amount consumed during vulcanization; both elemental sulfur and sulfur-containing accelerators will contribute to the free sulfur value [53]. Free sulfur, expressed as a percentage of total sample weight, will decrease as cure is increased. Typical free sulfur values of pharmaceutical rubber are less than 0.50%.

Swelling in an appropriate solvent may be useful as means to monitor and control the cure of rubber. Typically a 0.5-g sample of rubber (one or more small rubber parts or a section of a large part) is immersed in a solvent, such as trichloroethylene, for 24 hr at 45°C. The sample is cooled, patted dry, and then weighed. The percentage weight gain is taken as the percentage swell by weight [55]. Other solvents, such as iso-octane, *n*-heptane, and toluene, may also be used [56]. Percentage swell is a function of cure and the fraction of filler in a given formulation. A gum, nonfilled rubber will swell more than a clay-filled rubber having the same degree of cure. To correct for filler content, the percentage swell by volume may also be determined if the volume of filler, the specific gravity of the solvent imbibed, and specific gravity of the rubber sample are also known. Volume swell and weight swell will have different absolute values, but plots of these values versus cure time (at constant temperatures) will parallel one another. Swelling data may be used to calculate the cross-link density of rubber, cross-links per gram of rubber, but percentage swell is usually all that is needed for control purposes [54,57,58].

VII. CLOSURE MANUFACTURE AND CONTROL

A. Technology of Closure Manufacture

The manufacturing steps for the production of pharmaceutical closures are similar to those in general use in the rubber industry. Morton [4] describes rubber manufacturing in general. The quality requirements of pharmaceutical closure manufacture necessitate rigid raw material specifications and control, strict material traceability, absence of contamination, and tight dimensional tolerances.

The first step in the manufacturing process is the measuring of the individual batch ingredients. The tolerance for the weight of an individual batch ingredient is generally less than 1% of its absolute amount. When an ingredient is required in a relatively small amount (approximately 4 oz or less), it is preblended with a portion of the elastomer to minimize the relative weighing error. This preblending (or master batching) also facilitates the dispersal of the small amount of ingredient throughout the entire batch during mixing.

The mixing of rubber for pharmaceutical closures is a batch process using open mills and internal mixers. In the two-roll mixing mill, the two rolls rotate toward each other at different speeds, creating a shearing action in the open space between them. The rolls are equipped for chilling in order to control the temperature of the batch. The elastomer is introduced first while the rolls are in motion. The elastomer softens and becomes plastic. The powdered fillers are next added, and the shearing action of the roll breaks up the filler agglomerates and disperses the particles throughout the plasticized elastomeric matrix. After this dispersion is complete, the plasticizers, if any, and coloring agents are added and dispersed. The curing system is generally added as the last step because of the sensitivity of many rubber formulas to premature vulcanization. After mixing, the batch is calendered or extruded into the form required for molding.

Internal mixing, an alternative to open mill mixing, offers greater flexibility in the order of addition of ingredients. The usual sequence is to masticate the elastomer, then add the fillers, cure accelerators, and coloring agents, and blend for a prescribed time. In most cases, the cure ingredients are held out entirely and added on a finishing mill. The completed batch is then usually taken off the mill and calendered or extruded into a form suitable for molding.

Most rubber closures are formed by molding. Three types of molding are in general use: compression molding, transfer molding, and injection molding. The majority of pharmaceutical closures are manufactured by compression molding. Compression molding offers an economy of scale and satisfactory dimensional control for almost all applications (Fig. 16). With the mold open, the compounded stock is placed on the mold surface. Most compounds require treatment of the mold surfaces with a release agent, such as a silicone emulsion or a water-soluble or dispersible surfactant. The mold is closed, and the combination of heat and pressure momentarily softens the rubber, forcing it into the mold cavities. Continued application of heat cross-links the rubber compound, resulting in a sheet of cured stoppers. The molding press can be controlled to automatically open at a prescribed cure time. While the sheets of molded stoppers are cooling from the press operation, the selvage edges are trimmed and the molded sheet is inspected.

Trimming the molded stoppers from the molded sheets is the next operation. Using a mechanical punch press, the individual stoppers are trimmed from the molded sheet. A lubricant is applied to the sheet in order to make the die cut as clean as possible and to extend the die life. The last operation routinely performed is stopper washing.

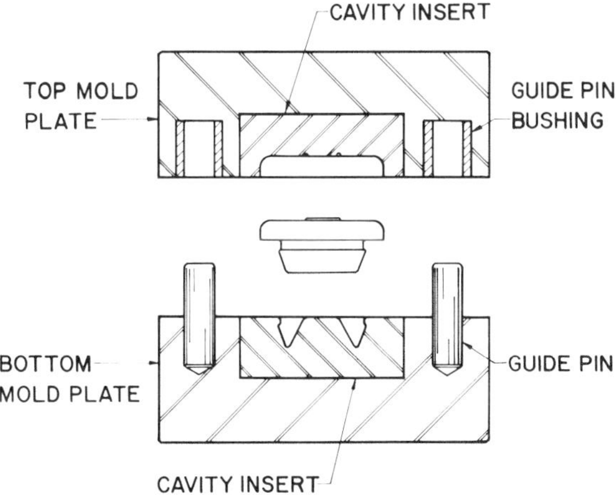

Figure 16 Compression molding process.

Several auxiliary finishing operations are occasionally performed by the closure manufacturer for special purposes. Surface chlorination (oxiglazing) is a process in which the surface of the rubber is oxidized in a controlled manner, causing a marked decrease in the coefficient of friction of the rubber surface. The major reason for surface chlorination is to aid in the movement of rubber components during high-speed automatic assembly. Another auxiliary operation sometimes required by pharmaceutical packagers is siliconization of the rubber closures. The silicone film acts as a lubricant, aiding in stopper transport during high-speed filling operations. The pharmaceutical packager should siliconize the stoppers in the facility at the time of use because of the absorption of the silicone fluid into the rubber over time. The siliconization process is achieved by tumbling a quantity of closures with a measured amount of silicone fluid in order to uniformly coat the surfaces of the stoppers.

With some closure formulations, an objectionable amount of extractable materials may remain in a molded closure regardless of the amount of press cure that can be achieved. In those cases, the closure manufacturer or the pharmaceutical manufacturer performs an auxiliary extraction procedure. One of the most common extraction procedures is an extended autoclave cycle, sometimes cycling with vacuum, to reduce the residual extractable substances. Care should be taken to avoid excessive heat input to the closures to prevent deterioration of physical properties through reversion of the rubber.

B. Inspection

Inspection, the checking or testing of an individual product against established standards, is conducted throughout the manufacturing process at all stages. The inspection procedures are formalized where possible, although much informal and unreported inspection occurs naturally as a result of employee concern for manufacturing product of high quality in conformity to user requirements. All formal inspection procedures, written in concise detail sufficient to guide trained inspectors (and operators when an inspection step is one of their operations) and approved by appropriate quality department management, must be fully documented, reviewed, retained as required, and used as indicators for both remedial and corrective action. All standards—attribute, variable; sensory, quantifiable—should relate either to product specifications directly or to processability requirements.

Raw materials and purchased components are inspected immediately upon receipt for container damage, container seal integrity, ingredient labeling agreement with purchase order, label legibility, and proper package coding if relevant. Normally this inspection can be performed as the carrier unloads the material; this inspection must occur before acceptance of the shipment. Any claims against the carrier for transit damage should be made at this time. Because the shipment acceptance protocol requires chemical tests for raw materials that are highly sensitive to contaminants and visual sample inspection for purchased components for which particulate matter judgment is critical, each container chosen for sampling must be cleansed prior to being opened. A portable vacuum cleaner is well suited for removal of dust from container surfaces. During sampling, the raw material should be inspected for foreign matter, variations in color or consistency, and stratification. Likewise, purchased components should be inspected at this time for the presence of foreign parts; acceptance inspection of the samples is usually performed in an area specially equipped for inspection.

In the compounding of rubber batches, testing is needed for those characteristics that are related to the further processability of the material; no dimensional or visual aspects of the molded part—except color—are directly related to the dimensions or appearance of the unvulcanized compound. If the mixing procedures have been adequately qualified and validated and are performed under controlled conditions, no formal inspection by quality control personnel should be necessary: operator observation of thoroughness of mixing as each batch is completed should be sufficient, given proper process control. Setup verification of the batch finishing equipment, i.e., the calender or extruder, must be performed and checked to assure that in-tolerance stock will be produced to supply the molding operation. This verification must include heater temperatures, machine speeds, calender opening thicknesses, calender collar placements, lubricant application rates, and finished stock take-up rates. For batches that are calendered, the sheet thickness must be measured with a suitable indicator gauge either automatically or manually, to assure the correct amount of material per mold charge, and the sheet must be continuously inspected for holes or voids that could cause poorly formed molded sheets. Extruded stock must likewise be controlled dimensionally and visually, and if the extruded stock is pelletized as a part of the stock preparation process, the pellets must be checked for size. Color is routinely checked as a batch control test, but the *uniformity* of the batch's color needs to be inspected in-process.

Inspection at the molding process is performed against standards directly related to the product end-item specification, dimensionally and visually. In addition, the overall molded sheets from compression molding are examined at this point for excessive warpage or distortion, which could lead to poor seating in their trimming dies, causing trim lips and cutoffs. Molded sheets of stoppers are inspected more easily than trimmed stoppers for operator-controlled dimensions and molding defects because the stoppers are geometrically oriented on the sheet, permitting rapid row-by-row visual inspection and facilitating dimensional gauging. Dimensional gauging of the "overflow" or web that connects the stoppers in the sheet is performed with a low-force dial indicator with a relatively broad foot and anvil (to minimize inaccuracy caused by rubber deflection); the overflow thickness and the associated dimensions that incorporate the overflow are the only dimensions of the end-item controlled by the operator. The remaining dimensions, e.g., diameters and some of the internal part lengths, are not under operator control and must be controlled through a tooling control program and confirmed by measuring samples either at the molding station or at final inspection. The inspector uses special fixtures to visualize hidden or not readily visable defects, such as splits, tears, holes, sponginess, and foreign matter. The design of these fixtures ranges from pliers and pincer devices to specially lighted probes that stretch and challenge vulnerable sections of the subject part, permitting defects to be seen. Backlighted inspection tables are especially useful for inspection of membrane integrity of thin sections, and lighted magnification, usually three to five power, is required for the inspection of very small molded parts less than 1/8 in. largest dimension.

In certain circumstances, mechanized inspection, which is more reliable and faster than human inspection for some applications, is preferred for detecting and culling defective finished parts. Certain types of gross part malformations, such as large trim lips (untrimmed molded web) and trim chopped parts, can be easily sorted mechanically with vibrating gravity-fed drop-through plates containing holes or slots cut to the correct size. These simple sorting machines are used instead of human operator inspection because they are faster and not subject to inspector fatigue and distraction. Some types of critical defects may occur at very low levels during manufacture, for example, a pinhole in the diaphragm of an intravenous bottle stopper. These critical defects, which occur very infrequently in the molding process, nevertheless must be detected and removed with a very high degree of confidence. Here mechanized sorting is required. One effective defect-sensing technique is fluidic inspection, in which the differential air pressure is measured across the tested membrane. Information on fluidic inspection technology is available from Corning Glass Works (Corning, NY).

C. Statistical Sampling for Attributes

Statistical sampling and sample inspection at the manufacturing stage of packaging are performed to confirm the acceptable quality of finished product; final sample inspection is *not* for the purpose of controlling quality: this must be done in process. Any attempt to rely solely on final sample inspection for total quality control is doomed to failure and will lead to great mounds of scrap and excessive reinspection and rework of manufactured product. With proper process quality control, resulting in a controlled process, the amount of final sampling required is minimized and sampling schemes can be designed for maximum final inspection efficiency.

A controlled process permits final sampling for defect attributes, leading to great simplicity of the inspection process and easy to understand and apply sampling decision rules. For inspection purposes, an attribute can be defined as any characteristic of the subject that can be classified as either conforming or nonconforming to an established standard without reference to any degree of conformance or measurement of magnitude. Measurements of variable quantities, such as dimensions, can be reduced to attribute measures by classifying them as either conforming or nonconforming to a specification range without regard to how close or far the measured quantity is to the specification limit. In recognition of the differences in seriousness of nonconforming conditions that range further from the specification limits than those that are close to specification, nonconformances are often graded into multiple categories with tighter AQL (acceptable quality levels) assigned to the further-out conditions. Of course, specification values should be established on a rational basis consistent with actual end-item usage requirements. AQL is a statistical term applied to acceptance sampling of a continuing supply of material. The AQL is the poorest level of quality or maximum fraction defective for the supplier's process that the consumer would consider to be acceptable as a process average for the purposes of acceptance sampling [59]. MIL-STD-105D [60] or other sampling plans with substantially equivalent sampling risks are generally used for acceptance sampling; these risks are tabulated and shown graphically in MIL-STD-105D.

Attribute inspection plans offer several advantages. Because actual measurements are not recorded, attribute gauging of dimensions is performed very rapidly. Results of attribute inspection plans are eaisly interpreted: X nonconforming items in a sample of N items. Decision making is straightforward; for single sampling plans, if the number of nonconforming items in a sample exceeds the acceptance number, the sample fails. There are disadvantages, also, to attribute plans. The lack of numeric measurements prevents the estimation of the process average fraction nonconforming and the process variability from attribute inspection alone. However, this use of final sampling data is not required if the proper process quality control plan is in effect. Attribute sampling requires larger sample sizes than variable plans, but this is almost always compensated by the far greater ease of making attribute measurements. Finally, strict attribute classification does not permit defects to be "scored" by degree of seriousness, but careful inspection to clearly established categorical standards can overcome this drawback.

In the U.S. pharmaceutical industry, acceptance specifications for packaging components, including closures, are written categories of nonconforming attributes; each category is indexed by an AQL.

Although widely used for acceptance sampling of incoming shipments, AQL sampling plans are inapproapriate for outgoing final inspection sampling. The AQL plans offer far too little protection against the approval and shipment of product of less-than-specified quality, and the risk of approving a defective sublot under an AQL plan increases as the number of sublots in a shipment lot increases [61]. To overcome this deficiency with AQL plans, sometimes a sampling scheme indexed on an average outgoing quality limit (AOQL) is employed. AOQL plans are based on the following practical assumptions:

Sublots that pass the plan are approved for shipment as is.
Sublots that fail the plan are sorted. Defective items in these sublots are replaced with nondefective items.

An efficient family of AOQL sampling plans for final inspection is presented in Table 15. The performance curve of a typical plan is shown in Figure 17.

Table 15 Average Outgoing Quality Limit Double-Sampling Plans for Final Inspection

AOQL (%)	Sample size	Acceptance number	Rejection number	Sample size	Acceptance number	Rejection number
0.10	400	0	2	400	1	2
0.25	180	0	2	180	1	2
0.40	110	0	2	140	1	2
0.65	110	0	2	140	3	4
1.0	110	1	3	140	4	5
1.5	110	2	5	140	6	7
2.5	110	3	6	140	10	11
4.0	110	6	10	140	14	15

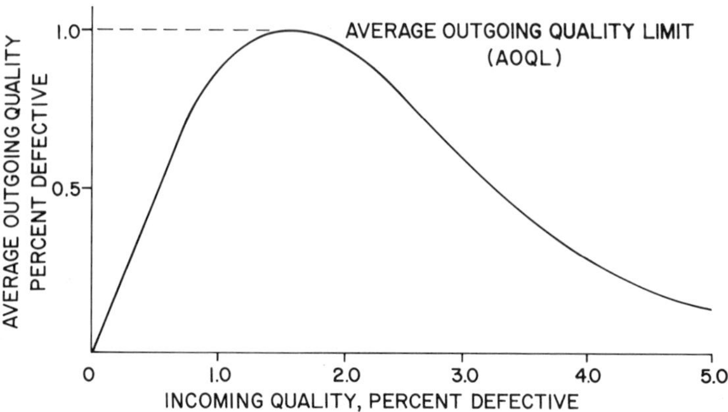

Figure 17 Performance characteristics of a typical AOQL scheme.

The inspection criteria used at final inspection must be identical to that required by the product specification. The specification should be written in a clear and unambiguous style to avoid differences in interpretation between vendor and customer. Defects must be described in precise detail, and methods of measurement and test must be straightforward. When possible, defect classifications that require inspector judgment for their correct interpretation should be confirmable with a functional test, such as a leakage test for the correct AQL assignment of a rubber void defect. After sufficient correlation experience of defectiveness level with functionality, limit conditions should be documented in the form of matched samples, photographs, or sketches, each approved by both vendor and customer. The size of defects of rubber closures can be estimated easily with the aid of size charts available from the Technical Association of the Pulp and Paper Industries (TAPPI) (Atlanta, GA). Reference overlays for optical comparator measurement for attribute dimensional gauging are readily drawn from approved product drawings and are often used in final inspection. Simple dimensions are easily confirmed with carefully machined go—no go gauges, although inspection skill is required to avoid error due to the deflection (compression) of the rubber surfaces under measurement.

D. Testing and Control

1. *Raw Materials*

The eight classes of raw materials used in pharmaceutical rubber formulations were discussed in the section on rubber formulation ingredients. These classes are elastomer, curing or vulcanizing agents, accelerator, activator, antioxidant-antiozonant, plasticizer-lubricant, filler, and pigment. A more exhaustive directory of commercially available raw materials listed by class can be found in the rubber *Blue Book*, published annually [16]. This book lists the trade name, composition, supplier, physical properties, and function of more than 10,000 materials. Another good source of general information is the handbook published by the R. T. Vanderbilt Company [62].

Since rubber, like all other materials, is not absolutely inert, the composition of rubber formulations used to package or deliver drugs is restricted to the safest raw materials available. There are no direct FDA regulations regarding the use of rubber and rubber ingredients for drug packaging, but those regulations that apply to foods are generally used [39]. Applicable segments of the code of Federal Register [63] are

CFR 175: Indirect food additives, adhesive coatings, and components
CFR 177: Indirect food additives, and polymers
CFR 178: Indirect food additives, adjuvants, production aids, and sanitizers
CFR 182: Substances generally recognized as safe (GRAS)
CFR 184: GRAS direct food additives
CFR 185: GRAS indirect food additives

Tests on raw materials are usually performed to identify the material, to measure the purity of the material, and to evaluate the functional ability of the material. Both chemical and physical tests are used, and more than one test may be required to meet each of the three testing objectives. Tests for the eight classes of raw materials are discussed below.

Elastomers

Specific gravity is a commonly listed physical property of elastomers. Specific gravity values of elastomers are listed in Table 16. Elastomer type and grades of elastomer within a type may be distinguishable by specific gravity. Thus specific gravity is an identity test and may be measured either by using a pycnometer or by hydrostatic weighing using water for

Table 16 Specific Gravities of Elastomers

Elastomers	Specific gravity[a]
Urethane	0.80–1.23
Ethylene-proplylene	0.86–0.87
Ethylene propylene diene (EPDM)	0.87–0.90
Polybutadiene	0.90–0.93
Polyisoprene	0.91–0.95
Natural	0.92
Butyl	0.92
Halobutyl	0.92–0.95
Styrene butadiene rubber (SBR)	0.94–1.00
Nitrile butadiene rubber (NBR)	0.98–1.18
Silicone	0.98–1.70
Neoprene	1.23
Fluoroelastomer	1.72–2.02

[a]Relative to water at 25°C.

those elastomers with gravities greater than 1 and isopropanol for elastomers with gravities less than 1. The specimen must be free of dirt and air bubbles or erroneous results will be obtained. ASTM Method D297, Section 15, outlines the procedure [8].

The percentage ash can be used as a measure of purity of elastomers. ASTM Methods D1278 and D1416 give procedures for natural and synthetic elastomers, respectively [8]. Samples weighing 3–6 g are heated in a porcelain crucible at 550°C for several hours. Silicone elastomers are difficult to analyze precisely because of the loss of ash. The grade of natural rubber may be identified using the ash test since the better grades have lower ash contents than the others; e.g., SMR 5 is 0.6% and SMR 50 is 1.5%.

The control of both specific gravity and percentage ash in elastomers is important since these tests are frequently used by end users to identify compounded vulcanized rubber formulations [34,50,51,64].

An infrared spectrum of an elastomer is the most frequently used identity method. ASTM Method D3677 outlines procedures for preparing both thin films and pyrolyzates [8]. Tables of diagnostic wavelengths and actual spectra are presented, but working reference standards should be prepared by each laboratory using their own spectrophotometers. Fourier transform methods (FT IR) have increased the speed and accuracy of elastomer identification [65].

Analysis of extracts is a test for identity and purity. Acetone is commonly used since it does not dissolve the elastomer. Acetone extracts acids, resins, sterols, and proteins from natural rubber; emulsifiers, antioxidants, and uncombined chain terminators are extracted from synthetic elastomers [53]. The acetone may be evaporated off and the extract weighed as in ASTM Method D297 [8], or the extract may be analyzed by spectroscopic or chromatographic methods as in ASTM Method D3156 [8]. The better grades of natural rubber will not contain more than 5% by weight of extractable materials.

The viscosity of an elastomer is one measure of its functionality. The Mooney viscometer, commonly used to measure viscosity, is an instrument very similar to the rheometer described elsewhere in this chapter. It consists of a motor-driven rotating disk within a die cavity containing a sample of elastomer. The effect of temperature and time on the viscosity of elastomers is measured using the procedures described in ASTM Method D1646 [8]. The Mooney viscosity is a standard specification for most elastomers, and its value will have a great effect on the mixing and molding characteristics of a rubber formulation [16].

Last but not least are visual and olfactory tests. Elastomers look and smell differently; they range from light amber, odorless bales to gray extruded chips with a mild pleasant odor. These simple tests are easily performed yet sensitive enough to be used as tests for identity and sometimes purity.

Curing Agents, Accelerators, Activators, Antidegradants, and Plasticizers

The tests given these rubber chemicals include infrared spectroscopy (D2702), ultraviolet spectroscopy (D2703), density (D1817), melting point (D1519), thin-layer chromatography (D3156), and other specialized ASTM tests [8]. Often standard test formulations are developed to evaluate the functionality of active rubber chemicals, such as accelerators. ASTM Methods

D3184 through D3192 list formulations and mixing procedures for many kinds of materials [8].

Fillers

The weight loss on ignition at 1000°C is used as a measure of purity on most fillers except carbon black, which is heated to 550°C (ASTM Method D1506) [8,34,62].

A test for moisture content is also conducted along with the loss on ignition. This test, done at 105°C, measures not only some water of hydration but also water picked up from the environment during transportation and storage of the filler (ASTM Method D1208) [66].

The pH of fillers is usually measured by making a 5–10% slurry in water containing a small amount of potassium chloride to increase ionic strength and conductivity. ASTM Method D1512 outlines the method for carbon black, which may be adopted for other fillers [8]. The pH of the filler is important since cure rate of the rubber formulation is affected by the acidity or alkalinity of ingredients [4]. The pH range of calcined clays is normally in the range 5.0–8.5. As the pH decreases, the rate of cure of clay-filled formulations will increase.

Particle size is an important physical property of a filler; size determines the surface area per unit weight of the filler [4]. Wire cloth sieves are commonly used to determine the size distribution of fillers. ASTM Method D1514 for carbon black is typical [8]. Vanderbilt methods T-14 and T-14-C measure the "fineness" of fillers [62]. Both pH and particle size are part of the supplier's specifications.

An infrared spectrum is the primary identification technique. A mull or pellet is usually prepared for analysis. One source of reference spectra is the handbook by Sadtler [67].

The concentration of such metals as lead, zinc, and aluminum is an important purity test since extractable metals may interfere with the successful packaging of certain drugs [37,38]. Total metals may be determined by ashing followed by dissolution of soluble metals then analysis by atomic absorption [68]. Soluble metals are determined in appropriate solvents under defined test conditions [37,69]. No "official" limits exist for extractable metals, but a limit such as 10 ppm total lead is commonly used.

Pigments

Pigments may be purchased and used either as loose powders or as masterbatches. Masterbatches (also referred to as color concentrates) are dispersions of the loose powders in an elastomer matrix; small amounts of a filler, such as calcium carbonate or titanium dioxide, and an antioxidant may also be present in the masterbatch. Masterbatches obviate the handling of loose materials that are easily carried about the manufacturing area and may contaminate other materials. Pigment concentrations of 50% are typical.

Dry pigments may be analyzed using standard procedures found in ASTM Method D1208 [66] or other appropriate tests [68]. The composition of most pigments may be found in the handbook by Patton [70].

Pigment masterbatches are given the following tests. The percentage ash is used for purity and identification purposes as found in ASTM Methods D1278 and D1416. Specific gravity, like percentage ash, is an identity and purity test (ASTM Method D297) [8]. An infrared spectrum of a pyrolyzate is commonly used to identify the polymer in the masterbatch (ASTM Method D3677) [8]. Color evaluation is usually done by using the color masterbatch in a test batch of rubber and then comparing the color of a test plate of rubber to a standard. Tristimulus color values may be obtained on an appropriate reflecting colorimeter. Dispersion of the pigment may be done by milling a piece of masterbatch into a very thin sheet and inspecting this sheet under intense light. Color and dispersion are functional tests to assure proper pigmenting of the rubber formulation. The antioxidant and filler may be identified using ASTM Methods D3156 and D297, respectively [8].

The testing of all raw materials for identity, purity, and functionality is important in rubber compounding in general but is especially important with pharmaceutical rubber formulations since adjustments in the quantity or type of raw materials from batch to batch is not permitted. Extensive raw material testing reduces processing costs by allowing the use of established validated manufacturing conditions. This in turn leads to a better quality, more consistent, molded product. The establishment of user's specifications and a validated testing program also leads to better quality raw materials from vendors.

2. *In-Process Batch Testing*

Once raw materials are tested and approved for use they are mixed to form a homogeneous mass using either a roll mill or an internal mixer. A roll mill consists of two steel cylinders mounted side by side and rolling in opposite directions. Mixing is caused by the shear between the rolls, which is a function of the space (nip) between rolls and the roll ratio or difference in speed. Mill rolls range in size from 6 × 13 in. to 28 × 84 in. and will mix 1.25–300 lb, respectively [4,62]. In an internal mixer, rubber is forced down between rotating blades in a mixing chamber. These blades knead the raw materials until they are dispersed uniformly. Production batch sizes may vary from 100 to 370 lb [71].

The mixed rubber formulation must be tested and approved before it is molded into final end-use items.

Cure Tests

Rheometer testing using "cure windows" for scorch, minimum torque, maximum torque, and t(90) is common practice. The use of the oscillating disk rheometer is described in Section VI.B. Batches that meet rheometer specifications will cure under previously established molding conditions, and parts produced will have predictable chemical and physical properties. The rheometer test is a measure of batch-to-batch consistency regarding the amounts and activity of ingredients.

Identity Tests

A test plate, a small thin slab of rubber, is molded for physical and chemical testing.

Specific gravity is measured on a test specimen to identify the formulation. Gravity is a function of the type and amount of each raw material used in the formulation [50,64].

Durometer, or hardness, is a function of formulation composition and is sensitive to cure. ASTM Method D2240 is described in another section [8].

Color of the test plate is matched against a standard as identity test.

To identify that the correct antioxidants and accelerators were incorporated into the formulation, these substances may be extracted using dilute 0.01 M sodium hydroxide and analyzed via ultraviolet spectroscopy [72].

3. *Chemical and Physical Testing of Finished Goods*

In 1968, Hopkins proposed four basic tests that manufacturers could use as outgoing quality control tests on pharmaceutical closures [53,64]. These are identity tests that, taken together, will distinguish one formulation from another and will assure the pharmaceutical customer that a product that is received is consistent from shipment to shipment. These tests are simple, reliable, and accurate and have become industry standards. Complete test methods have been published in Parenteral Drug Association (PDA) Technical Bulletin No. 2 [72]. A short description of these four tests follows.

Percentage Ash

A 1–2 g sample is weighed accurately in a porcelain crucible. The sample is ashed in a muffle furnace for 4–8 hr at 550°C. If calcium carbonate or other materials that decompose at this temperature are part of the formulation, a lower temperature may be used, i.e., 450°C. Chlorine-containing polymers, such as neoprene and chlorobutyl, and zinc compounds cannot be ashed reproducibly since volatile halides are lost during the ashing [8]. Silicone rubber is also not easily ashed with precision since the ash is easily lost.

The percentage ash of a rubber formulation is a function of the weight W and percentage ash A (at the temperature selected) of each of the ingredients.

$$\% \text{ Ash} = \frac{A_1W_1 + A_2W_2 + \cdots + A_iW_i}{W_1 + W_2 + \cdots + W_i}$$

Ash specifications are determined from the weight and ash variability of each of the ingredients. Typical specifications are

Ash (%)	Allowable tolerance
0–4.9	+1 to −0.5
5–9.9	±1
>10	±2

Specific Gravity

A 1–2 g sample is weighed in air, then in a fluid such as water or isopropanol. Care must be taken to avoid both trapped air in the cavities of the item and adsorbed air bubbles on the surface. Cutting the item to a suitable shape and dipping it in alcohol before weighing in water will obviate both problems. The specific gravity of the part relative to water at 4°C is calculated by the equation

$$\text{Specific gravity} = \frac{\text{weight in air}}{(\text{wt in air} - \text{wt in liquid})} \times (\text{sp. gr. of liquid})$$

If the liquid is at 25°C (77°F), use 0.997 for the specific gravity of water and 0.785 for isopropanol. Isopropanol is recommended since many rubber formulations will float in water. Specific gravity like ash is a function of the weight W and specific gravity G of each of the formulation ingredients. The usual specification tolerance limits for the specific gravity of a rubber formulation is ±0.04 units. Specific gravity can be calculated using the following relationship, where W1 is the weight of ingredient number one, G1 the specific gravity of ingredient one, and so on.

$$\text{Specific gravity} = \frac{W1 + W2 + \cdots + Wi}{(W1/G1) + (W2/G2) + \cdots + (Wi/Gi)}$$

Both percentage ash and specific gravity are primarily functions of the filler type and content since elastomers and other organic ingredients have low ash contents and similar gravities (see Table 12).

Infrared Spectrum of Pyrolyzate

A small sample in a Pyrex test tube is heated slowly over a Meker burner flame. Holding the test tube at 15° from the horizontal, first water vapor then liquid pyrolyzate will form at the top of the tube. Using KBr crystals, a transmission spectrum of the pyrolyzate is obtained from 2.5 to 15 μm (4000–667 cm^{-1}). ASTM Method D3677 contains spectra of typical elastomers [8].

The IR spectrum obtained in this method is used as a qualitative tool to identify the elastomer(s) only. If two or more elastomers are present in the formulation, only those present at 20% or more by weight of the total elastomer content will be detected.

Ultraviolet Spectrum of Extracts

A small sample of rubber is extracted in 0.1 M NaOH at 100°C for 15 min. Accelerators and antidegradants are extracted, and a spectrum from 220 to 380 nm is characteristic of the cure and antidegradant system used in the formulation. Characteristic absorption bands for several accelerators are shown in Table 17. These absorptions are characteristic of accelerators in the rubber after the rubber has been vulcanized. Extent of accelerator

Table 17 Characteristic Absorption Wavelengths for Common Accelerator Types in 0.1 M NaOH

Cure system	Wavelength of absorption (nm)
Thiuram	276 (peak)
Dithiocarbamate	258 (peak)
	282 (peak)
Thiazole	232 (peak)
	252 (shoulder)
	310 (peak)
Aldehyde-amine reaction products	280 (shoulder)
	306 (weak shoulder)
	320 (weak shoulder)

reaction and post treatments of rubber [64], such as washing or autoclaving, will affect the relative intensity of absorption. Comparison with an approved reference is recommended.

When each of these four basic tests are performed, the resultant data will allow the analyst to make a reliable decision regarding the identity and consistency of a closure formulation. When two or more formulations have matching percentages of ash, specific gravity, IR, and UV specifications, other distinguishing tests must be utilized in place of or in addition to these four.

Frequently used supplementary and complimentary control tests to aid in the identity or to assess the consistency of outgoing finished goods are described below.

Free Sulfur

This test determines the amount of uncombined or free sulfur and is a measure of the degree of cure or cross-linking in some sulfur-cured formulations. However, if the amount of free sulfur is plotted versus cure (time at constant temperature), the value will decrease and asymptotically approach zero even if the rubber later reverts or cross-links are broken by excess heat. A low free sulfur value, compared with the value on an unvulcanized sample, therefore may not indicate optimum cure; it may mean either optimum or overcure. This test is discussed in detail in Section VI.B.3, and the complete procedure can be found in ASTM Method D297 [8].

Percentage Swelling

Swelling, like free sulfur, is an indicator of cure. Once an acceptable degree of cure and its relationship to swelling is established, swelling may be a useful control test. Variations of ±10% in the weight percentage swell are generally acceptable. Depending on the temperature, time, elastomer, the percentage filler, the solvent used, and the degree of cure, values typically range from 200 to 1200%. Swelling may be calculated as

$$\%\ \text{Swelling} = \frac{\text{wt after swelling} - \text{wt of original sample}}{\text{wt of original sample}} \times 100$$

Swelling is discussed in detail in Section VI.B.3 [54–58].

Durometer Hardness

Hardness may be used as both a cure and identity test provided the specimen has appropriate geometry and dimensions. A large IV stopper would be suitable because of its thickness and large flat surface; a small vial stopper or syringe piston would not. Since durometer hardness is a function of temperature and time of storage after vulcanization and the temperature and relative humidity at the time of measurement, care must be taken to assure precise measurements. Hardness is discussed in more detail in Section VI.B.2.

Other Physical and Chemical Tests

Hopkins noted that such tests as nephelos or turbidity and concentration of heavy metals could also serve as control tests for consistency and/or identity [50]. Most commonly used are the physicochemical test procedures recommended by the United States Pharmacopoeia [73]. These tests are performed on the extracts of closures. Solvents recommended include purified water, drug product vehicle, and isopropanol. Other solvents, such as saline, and dilute acid or base may be used as long as the solvents are applicable for the purpose intended. No specifications are recommended by the USP; these must be established by the user. A brief description of each USP test follows.

Turbidity. The clarity of the closure extract is measured using a nephelometer with appropriate standards. The standards available from one supplier, Coleman Instruments [74], range from 0 to 100 Coleman Nephelos units; those available from Hach [75] range from 0 to 200 nephelometric turbidity units. Turbidity is a measure of the insoluble extractables from a closure and is affected by the type and amounts of ingredients in a formulation, such pretreatments as washes, extractions, or sterilizations [76], and cure.

Reducing agents. Organic extractables that are oxidizable by iodine are determined in this procedure. It is affected by the same variables as turbidity.

Heavy metals. Extractable lead as well as other metals, such as zinc and cadmium, may be determined either colorimetrically or by atomic absorption. Lead and cadmium would be regarded as contaminants in a pharmaceutical rubber formulation, but zinc is a common element added as the oxide or as a salt to promote cure.

pH Change. The pH of the extract is a measure of the acidic and alkaline water soluble extractables from a formulation. Since pH may affect drug stability or efficacy, it is an important parameter [77].

Total extractables. The sum of the inorganic, organic (nonvolatile), soluble, and insoluble extractables is measured in this test. The weight of total extractables is an indication of the cleanliness of a formulation. Although no specifications exist, Table 18 lists value ratings for test results obtained using these USP-NF methods. Other groups, such as the British Standards Institution [78], the German DIN [79], and the Japanese Pharmacopoeia [80], have published test procedures similar to those of the USP and have recommended specifications.

Table 18 Value Ratings of USP-NF Test Results

	Value ratings		
Test (units)	Excellent	Good	Poor
Turbidity (Coleman turbidity units)	<20	30–40	>80
Reducing agents (ml of 0.1 N I_2)	<0.25	0.5–1.0	>1.5
Heavy metals (ppm Pb)	<0.1	0.1–0.5	>1.0
pH Change (pH units)	<0.5	0.5–1.0	>1.5
Total extractables (mg per 100 ml)	<2	3–6	>10

Other specialized test procedures have been developed to identify or measure the consistency of closures. A manufacturer may measure the amounts of paraffinic wax, silicone oil, or plasticizer in each sample of closures. If such coatings as lacquers, Teflon (DuPont), or polypropylene are placed on closure surfaces, tests to verify the identity and uniformity of these coatings would usually be part of the manufacturer's release test program.

A syringeless gas chromatographic method was developed by Mattson et al. to fingerprint pharmaceutical rubber formulations [81]. In this modified headspace technique, small samples of rubber are heated in an aluminum capsule in the injection ports of a gas chromatograph and the volatiles are chromatographed under programmed column temperature conditions.

Pyrolysis gas chromatography was used by Krishen and Tucker [82] to identify polyisoprene, styrene-butadiene rubber, ethylene-propylene-diene rubber, polybutadiene, and chlorobutyl elastomers in rubber formulations. Mixtures of elastomers, when the minor component was only 10% of the total elastomer content, were analyzed successfully. Reviews of the application of pyrolysis gas chromatography to polymer analysis proves the future viability of this method as a quality control tool [83,84].

A technique called chromatopyrography by Hu [85] is a combination of headspace and pyrolysis gas chromatography. In this technique, first volatile components in a rubber are vaporized at 270°C and identified then the polymer is identified by pyrolysis at 1000°C. Ethylene-propylene, butyl, and neoprene rubbers were characterized by this technique in less than 40 min.

The combination of gas chromatography and mass spectrometry (GC-MS) is used to separate then identify the components in a rubber formulation. Kiang [86] reported the utility of this technique in the analysis of pharmaceutical packaging materials. Pyrolysis GC-MS is also used to characterize silicone polymers [87].

Both thin-layer and liquid chromatography (LC) may be used to identify antioxidants, antiozonants, plasticizers, and accelerators from vulcanized rubber. Protivova et al. separated and identified more than 15 antidegradants and 22 accelerators and other rubber additives by liquid chromatography [88]. LC conditions for the extraction and separation of curing agents, antioxidants, accelerators and plasticizers are also given in the paper by Majors and Johnson [89].

The review article by Krishen discusses chromatographic, spectroscopic, and thermal methods of rubber characterization [90].

4. *Incoming Quality Control Tests: Identity and Consistency*

Formulation-Specific Properties

The Code of Federal Regulations Section 211.84 of Current Good Manufacturing Practices requires the testing of closures and components [63]. Some generic tests for the identification and measurement of the chemical properties of a rubber formulation were discussed in detail in the previous section.

PDA Technical Methods Bulletin No. 2 outlines the procedures for four identity tests—percentage ash, specific gravity, infrared analysis, and ultraviolet analysis [51]. In addition, the physicochemical test procedures outlined by the USP measure the extraction characteristics of elastomers [73].

These extraction tests should yield results that are consistent for incoming lots of a particular item in a given elastomeric formulation. Once typical values for each of the five tests (turbidity, reducing agents, heavy metals, pH change, and total extractables) are established, these tests may be utilized for incoming control. The paper by Mattson et al. outlines a gas chromatographic method for the identity of closures [81]. Chromatograms of several plunger formulations indicate that the method is sensitive enough to differentiate formulations in approximately 22 min.

Each end user of pharmaceutical closures must choose formulation-specific tests that unequivocally identify each of the formulations purchased. Since there are many similar formulations available from each supplier, consultation with the supplier to select effective tests is imperative.

Design-Specific Properties

The current Good Manufacturing Practices embodied in the Code of Federal Regulations, Section 211.84, require that closures be tested "for conformance with all appropriate written procedures" [63]. These procedures are those on which the vendor and customer have mutually agreed and have included in the purchase specification. They may include functional tests as described in PDA Technical Methods Bulletin No. 2 [72] or specific functional tests that relate directly to the drug package or device. The test methods should be worked out between the vendor and the customer so that there is complete understanding of closure acceptance criteria between them. If the vendor cannot agree with certain functional tests that are critical to the customer's final package integrity because the manufacturer does not supply the mating components or control the assembly operation, for example, these tests should be performed by the pharmaceutical or device manufacturer nevertheless for information purposes. Preferably, however, the packaging engineer should identify which physical or dimensional characteristics of the closure components are critical to the proper functioning of the finished assembly and specify tests for those characteristics.

A healthy vendor-customer relationship depends on a steady diet of performance dialogue between them, especially information about perceived quality trends and changing quality requirements. A formal method of achieving this is through communication of periodic vendor ratings from the drug packager to the closure vendor. These should be accompanied by periodic meetings between responsible individuals from both companies to share inspection results and review actual product samples and defects found during acceptance sampling.

VIII. CLOSURE DESIGN QUALIFICATION

Effective quality assurance of a drug-packaging system begins with the assurance of the adequacy of the package design, including the closure system. The design must be tested and proved to be adequate for all intended purposes, including the fulfillment of regulatory requirements, the assurance of drug-closure chemical and physical compatibility, assurance of the biosafety of the closures, assurance of mechanical and dimensional compatibility with mating packaging components, adequacy of processability of the closures, and assurance of the mechanical performance of the closure in the intended application. The manufacturing process of the closure itself must be qualified and adequately controlled by the manufacturer. Proper specifications and test methods are necessary to assure fitness for use as defined by the above design qualification criteria. A suggested procedure for the validation of elastomeric closure systems has recently been proposed by Wood [40]. There must be close cooperation of the closure manufacturer and drug packager in qualifying and validating closure formulations and designs. A necessary first step in qualifying an elastomeric formulation should be prescreening compatibility tests conducted by the closure vendor. An outline of a prescreening protocol has been described [91].

Regulatory requirements for design considerations are found in the provisions for submitting a new drug application (NDA) for market approval for new drugs as well as in the Current Good Manufacturing Practices (CGMP) pomulgated by the Food and Drug Administration (FDA). The submission of a new drug application must include evidence of the stability of the drug in its marketed package. This requirement is specific to the primary container and closure system. Any change in the composition of the elastomeric closure requires the notification and approval of FDA. CGMP requires that the closures demonstrate lack of reactivity, additivity, or absorptivity to the drug system such as will alter the safety, identity, strength, quality, or purity of the drug beyond the official or established requirements. Also, the design of the container-closure system must provide adequate protection against foreseeable factors in storage and use that can cause deterioration or contamination of the drug product. The assurance of drug-closure chemical compatibility is the first consideration in choosing a closure design.

A. Chemical Compatibility

A generalized procedure for prescreening may be briefly described as follows [91]. After consultation with a drug manufacturer regarding anticipated processing and stability requirements, the closure manufacturer selects a number of candidate rubber formulations for prescreening. Teflon-lined closures are used as controls because of the relative inertness of Teflon. The closure manufacturer molds the candidate elastomeric formulations into closures. The sample closures and vials are rinsed with filtered distilled water and dried under laminar flow conditions. The test drug solution, which is obtained from the drug manufacturer, is filtered through a 0.45-μm membrane filter and then used to fill the cleaned vials. A volume of solution is chosen to purposely exaggerate the ratio of exposed elastomer surface to drug solution. The vials are sealed with aluminum caps using a standard capping apparatus. For drugs known to be oxygen sensitive, the vial headspace is flushed with nitrogen prior to sealing. The samples and controls are autoclaved in an inverted position for 30 min at 250°F to ensure sterility. (Solutions known to be heat sensitive are not heat sterilized.) The test vials are stored at room temperature and at an elevated temperature of 45°C in an inverted position. A storage time of at least 8 weeks is used for preliminary screening. The vials are examined periodically for signs of precipitate or discoloration of the solution. At the completion of the storage time, the closures are removed from the vials and examined for signs of discoloration or swelling. For aqueous materials, pH and ultraviolet absorption spectra are recorded.

As a result of these prescreening studies, the closure manufacturer recommends a choice of several candidate closure formulations to the drug manufacturer. This prescreening service has been estimated to save considerable amounts of time and expense for the drug manufacturer's stability testing program. Close cooperation between the drug manufacturer and the closure supplier must be maintained throughout the closure development planning stages in order to derive the maximum amount of information from these studies.

As a result of the prescreening studies, pilot quantities of closures are offered to the drug manufacturer for chemical and mechanical testing. The importance of thorough testing cannot be overlooked at this point. The chemical literature contains numerous reports of chemical and physical degradation of products in which the closure system is implicated. FDA cites inadequacy of one stability testing program where the product on stability test was not stored with the drug product in contact with the closure [92]. Gas transmission has been implicated in the loss of stannous ion in radiopharmaceutical test kits [93]. High levels of extractable aluminum have been found in a parenteral solution using a chlorobutyl rubber closure [37], rubber closures have been investigated as a source of haze in freeze-dried parenterals [94], and several other reports of closure-implicated drug stability problems have been found in the literature [26, 95–107].

B. Mechanical Testing

The important performance tests for the qualification of closure designs are suggested by the Parenteral Drug Association (PDA) [63]. It should be emphasized that these tests are designed to be qualification tests for design approval only, not routine incoming quality control tests.

1. *Vial Closures*

Needle penetration and resealability testing is an important aspect to consider in the qualification of an elastomeric closure. This test measures the force required to penetrate the diaphragm of the stopper with a hypodermic needle and the ability of the closure to reseal when the needle is withdrawn. In the test procedure, ten closures of each formulation or design are used. Half the closures are used to measure penetrability and the other half resealability. After thorough cleaning, five containers are sealed with one each of the clean closures. The containers are placed on a constant-speed mechanical testing machine set at an appropriate sensitivity range (usually 0–5 lb) and punctured with a needle pushed at the rate of 10 in./min. The maximum force required for penetration is recorded as the penetrability force. A new needle is used for each puncture. To test resealability, deionized water equal to one-half the designated capacity of the container is placed in the test vial. The prepared closure is sealed and a 10-ml syringe fitted with a 20/21 gauge needle is used to inject a volume of air equal to the normal dose to be withdrawn. The needle is rapidly withdrawn while the container is inverted, and a visual observation is recorded of any spraying, leaking, or drop formation occuring at the puncture site.

Moisture vapor transmission (MVT) is described in the USP-NF [73]. In this test, ten test bottles and two controls are tested for moisture gain when stored for 28 days at 75% relative humidity at 22°C. Carefully dried calcium chloride desiccant is measured into ten of the bottles and the remaining two bottles (the control bottles) are filled with an equivalent weight of glass beads. At the end of the 28-day storage time, the weight of the individual bottles is determined and the rate of moisture permeability, in units of weight per day per unit volume, is calculated.

Coring is defined as the cutting of rubber from a closure during insertion of a hypodermic needle, resulting in the production of elastomeric particles or fragments. A testing apparatus to measure coring is shown in Figure 18. The preparation and application of the test closures must be carefully controlled in order to obtain reproducible coring results. After a prescribed washing and drying procedure, the stoppers are inserted into empty vials and aluminum seals are applied under simulated or actual production conditions. The surface of the test closure is swabbed with alcohol to simulate actual use. A supply of hypodermic needles of a selected type and gauge, all from a single lot of manufacture, must be available. The needles should be checked under a microscope for evidence of burrs before and after use. The PDA recommended coring procedure [72]

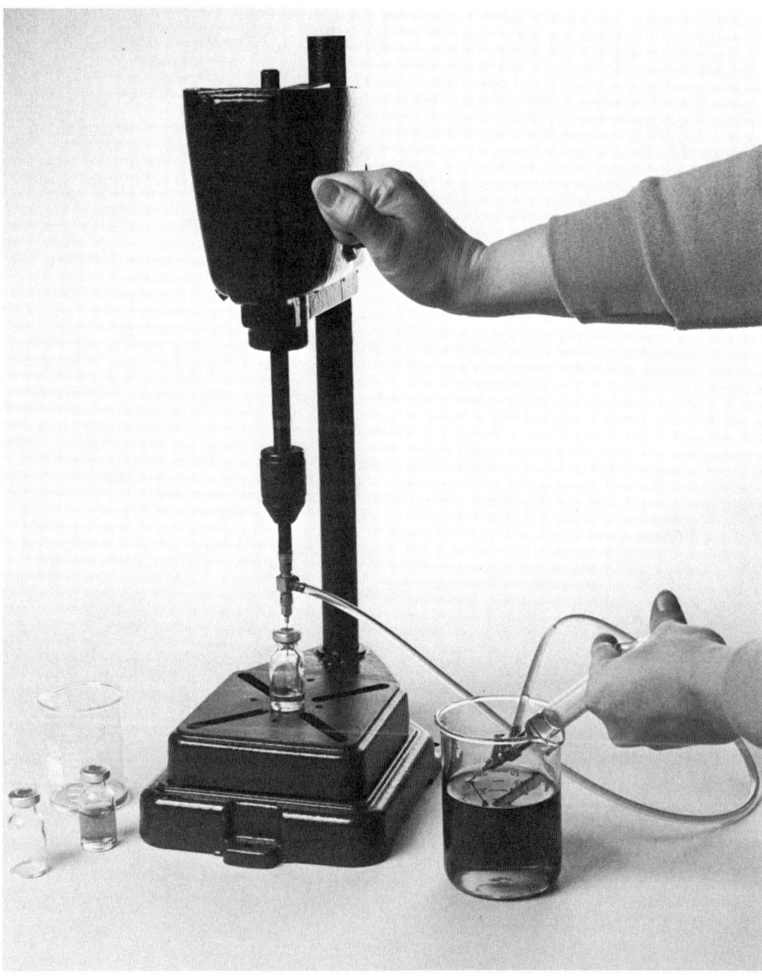

Figure 18 Coring testing apparatus.

specifies the number of punctures permitted for different needle classifications. The test vials are assembled in an order specified by the PDA procedure, and the first vial is inserted using the drill press. While the needle is inserted, 1–1.5 ml of filtered water is expelled from the syringe through the needle to dislodge any cores that may have been lodged in the lumen of the needle. The needle is withdrawn, and the test closure is rotated and punctured repeatedly for a total of ten punctures. After all the punctures have been completed, each vial is shaken vigorously to dislodge any cores and the aluminum seal and closure are removed. The contents of the vials are filtered through filter paper and examined under magnification for cores or fragments. The results are tabulated and reported as cores per 100 punctures for each formulation or configuration.

2. *Syringe Plungers*

Breakloose and extrusion forces are defined in PDA Technical Bulletin No. 2 [72]. Breakloose is the term applied to the force required to initiate plunger movement. After movement begins, the maximum force recorded as the plunger travels to the end of its path is called the plunger's extrusion force. These forces are measured using a crosshead tension-testing machine equipped with a load cell. The test results can be significantly affected by sample preparation methods, and exact conditions of sample preparation must be recorded and maintained. Using a compression cell sensitivity of approximately 0–10 or 0–20 lb, 20 syringes each are tested at a crosshead speed of 10 in./min and 20 in./min. The breakloose force and extrusion force are recorded as shown in Figure 19.

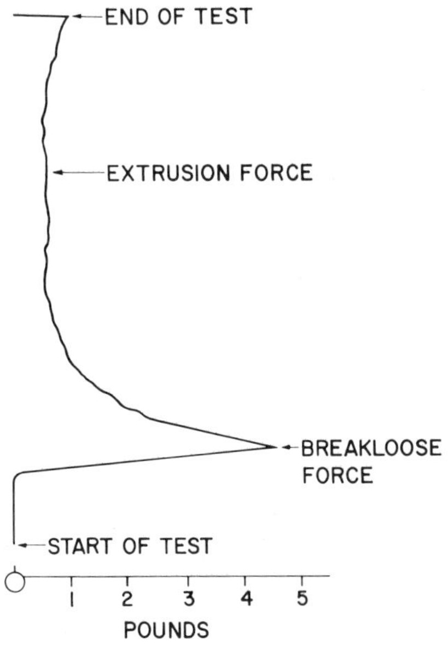

Figure 19 Breakloose and extrusion force chart.

C. Vendor Qualification

A good vendor-vendee relationship built on mutual trust and respect is a business treasure to be nourished and built upon. From the customer's point of view, the establishment of a continuing business relationship with a vendor begins with the qualification of the vendor in the eye of the customer to possess the ability to supply consistently the required quantity and quality of material.

The potential vendor of raw materials for pharmaceutical closures must thoroughly understand the requirements of the closure manufacturer with respect to delivery quantity, schedule, and quality. These are preferably contained in a purchasing manual provided to potential vendors. Communication of detailed specifications for raw materials and purchased components is especially important. The bulk of raw material production for the rubber industry is used in the tire and mechanical goods segments, whose quality requirements take on a different emphasis from those of the pharmaceutical closure manufacturer. Specifications of physical properties dominate the former; the latter requires very tight control of chemical properties. Raw material vendors are responsive to the special needs of closure manufacturers when these needs are clearly expressed and communicated. This is the first step in vendor qualification; the communication of the special requirements of the pharmaceutical closure manufacturer and the commitment by the potential vendor to fulfill those requirements. Two avenues of communicating these special requirements are successfully followed. First, rubber closure manufacturers have actively addressed industry trade groups through presentation of technical papers explaining their requirements and through publication of relevant information in the trade press and journals. Second, closure manufacturers have established technical exchange sessions with major vendors for the purpose of fostering better understanding of the needs and capabilities of each party.

The closure manufacturers must thoroughly test a potential source of a new or substitute raw material or purchased component. Qualification samples are not only subjected to the tests that have been written into the specification for the commodity, but also need to be as completely characterized as possible for biosafety, chemical, physical, and processability properties. The chemical tests should include sensitive qualitative and quantitative methods for the determination of trace impurities that need to be assessed for their biosafety and processability effects. Depending on the chemical nature of the candidate material, x-ray, spectroscopic, chromatographic, mass spectroscopic, and electrochemical methods, such as those described elsewhere [29,34,39,53,86], are applicable to the initial sample qualification phase. Likewise, biosafety and physical properties need to be determined. Finally, production trials are carried out on candidate material that passes laboratory screening.

Initial purchases of a new brand of a raw material are monitored closely for physical and chemical properties. In-depth sampling of the initial shipments yields valuable information on the material's intralot homogeneity, and lot-to-lot comparison with previously used material should be performed. It is important that the closure manufacturer must communicate the results with the vendor at this point as a check on the mutual understanding of the material's requirements, specifications, test methods, and test results.

The closure manufacturer should perform an audit of the vendor's production facility. The audit should address the vendor's technical capability to produce the quantity, quality, and consistency of material required. Business policies should be probed and confirmed in the audit. The quality control system should be analyzed—recognizing company-to-company differences in procedures—for its ability to maintain control. The actual observation of the production and quality control systems will help to confirm the qualifications of the subject vendor.

D. Closure Specification

The specification document serves several purposes in the relationship between the closure manufacturer and the closure user. By direct statement or by reference, the specification serves as a description of the closure, details the characteristics and requirements expected of the closure, describes the sampling, evaluation, and test methods for incoming shipments, and outlines a decision scheme for shipment acceptance.

In order to fully describe a rubber pharmaceutical closure, several characteristics must be defined. The geometry and dimensional tolerances are usually described by reference to an engineering drawing. The engineering drawing is very complete and describes all dimensions and tolerances of the closure. For incoming inspection purposes, however, very few of the dimensions need to be measured on a routine basis because of their interdependent relationship and because most of them are controlled by the closure manufacturer's tooling control program. The important dimensions should be separately specified in the closure specification for lot-by-lot measurement. The rubber formulation is specified by reference to a formulation number. Usually these numbers are codes assigned by the closure manufacturer. Finally, a description of any auxiliary treatments such as barrier coatings or surface treatments, should be specified in the description section of the specification. The specification should reference any applicable compendial or otherwise published rubber standards or test methods such as those found in the USP-NF or ASTM.

Packaging and labeling instructions are recommended as a part of the purchase specification. The packaging instructions should include the description of the primary and outer packaging as well as complete labeling requirements.

The method of sampling for chemical and physical attribute testing should be defined. For chemical tests, a given weight of stoppers per lot is required. Physical and dimensional sampling, however, requires a variable number of samples depending on the number of items in the lot. The most used acceptance sampling plan for attributes is ABC-105-D (MIL-STD-105-D).

The list of defect attributes is usually the lengthiest section of the closure specification. Generally the defects are classified according to seriousness into several categories, and each category is assigned an acceptable quality level (AQL). The AQL is defined as the maximum percentage defective permitted as a process average as long as certain conditions, such as continuity of production, are met. Acceptance sampling is described by Grant and Leavenworth [61].

The specification should contain directions for lot disposition depending on the outcome of the acceptance testing. A material review board should be invoked for questionable or marginal inspection results and also to keep interpretation of the product specification current with actual requirements.

IX. REGULATORY CONSIDERATIONS

Pharmaceutical closure manufacturers are not subjected to the requirements of the Food and Drug Acts or FDA CGMP regulations per se. However, they adopt those features of the regulations that fit their control purposes and adapt others where required. A closure manufacturer will maintain a drug master file. A convenient way to maintain such a file for a large number of different products manufactured from a common list of raw materials using similar processes is to write the file in two sections, a raw materials processing section and a formulation section. The first section lists the properties of all raw materials, their specification values, and their test methods. Important process parameters should be described here also. The second section lists the percentage composition of each formulation number. A model formula filed in this manner is shown in Table 19.

These files are used by FDA personnel in reviewing new drug applications and field problems involving a particular closure. Although the closure manufacturer is not directly regulated by the FDA, the closure supplier does cooperate with the FDA at the request of its customer, the drug manufacturer, in the investigation of field complaints and questions relating to drug-closure interaction.

Table 19 Typical Formulation as Listed in a Drug Master File

File Number DMF XXXX, January 18, 1985
Formulation 1111/45 red

Ingredient	Description	Amount (%)
1	Polymer	61.3
2	Filler	18.4
3	Masterbatch	1.1
4	Plasticizer	9.2
5	Activator	6.1
6	Vulcanizer	5.0 max.
7	Accelerator	3.0 max.

For information relating to raw material specifications, laboratory test methods, and manufacturing procedures, see Reference File Number DMF ZZZZ.

We request that all information in this file be treated as confidential, within the meaning of Regulation 314.11, and that no information from the file be submitted to an applicant without our written consent to an authorized member of your department.

Confidential and trade secret information
Exempt from the Freedom of Information Act
under 5 U.S.C. Section 552(b)(3) and (4)
and subject to 18 U.S.C. Section 1905.

X. INTERACTION OF DRUG FORMULATIONS WITH RUBBER CLOSURES

The primary requirements of a closure system are to protect and preserve the drug formulation until it is delivered to its recepient and to facilitate the delivery itself. The ideal closure should be chemically inert; that is, it should neither adsorb nor absorb any components of the drug formulations. Neither should any of the components of the closure chemically react with any of the components of the drug formulation. The ideal closure should also be selectively permeable. It must be penetrable by a hypodermic needle when used as a vial closure, yet must be a barrier to gases, such as oxygen or water vapor. The ideal closure will be flexible, resilient, and elastic. The physical qualities required by closures, such as vial stoppers, needle shields, syringe plungers, and IV delivery components, are diverse.

Rubber is a unique packaging material. In its diversity, it is closer to ideal than any other material available to date. But as ideal as it is, rubber reacts with drug formulations in several ways.

Adsorption is the phenomenon of concentration of a substance on the surface of the closure.

Absorption may follow adsorption. It is the process whereby a substance passes through the closure surface and is distributed throughout its mass.

Permeation occurs when sorption (adsorption and Absorption) is followed by the transmission of a substance through the closure.

Leaching is the phenomenon of a substance migrating from the closure into the drug formulation.

The extent (equilibrium state) and rate (kinetics) of these processes is affected by the specific drug formulation and rubber closure system and by such variables as temperature, surface area, volume, pH, concentration, pressure, and external environment. An excellent review of examples from the literature as well as a mathematical description of these processes may be found in PDA Technical Report 5 by Wang and Chien [108].

It is often difficult to distinguish if the adsorption process alone or if the processes of adsorption and absorption are active in a particular experimental system. However, adsorption alone takes up a smaller quantity of material and requires less energy than the combined process.

Lachman et al. studied the absorption of preservatives, such as benzyl alcohol, chlorobutanol, and methylparaben, by natural, neoprene, and butyl rubber [109]. The natural rubber closures exerted the least deleterious effect on preservative content. Loss of preservative increased with time and temperature. Wang and Chien [108] list the partition coefficients (closure-water) for several preservative-rubber systems. Those preservatives with the lowest partition coefficients (e.g., benzyl alcohol, phenol, and cresol) are sorbed less than those (e.g., phenylmercuric chloride) with higher coefficients. The tendency for sorption is, in descending order, neoprene, natural, butyl, and silicone rubber.

Permeation is a consideration from both the aspects of keeping undesirable materials out of the pharmaceutical package and of keeping critical components of the drug package contained at acceptable concentrations.

Lyophilization stoppers are formulated from rubber that has a low water vapor transmission rate; usually a butyl or halobutyl-natural blend is used.

Materials that are sensitive to oxidative degradation may also require a closure with a low gas transmission rate to keep oxygen out and, perhaps, keep a nitrogen blanket in. Table 4 lists the moisture and gas transmission resistance of most common elastomers. Natural rubber is 18 times as permeable to oxygen as butyl; silicone rubber is 400 times that of butyl. For water vapor the relative permeation is butyl = 1, natural = 92, and silicone = 1400. For a given rubber, permeation of gases varies, in increasing order, nitrogen, oxygen, and carbon dioxide [108].

Volatile drug formulation components may permeate the closure system. Such solvents as ethanol and such preservatives as methylparaben are permeable to rubber closures [110]. Loss of a component may lead to an ineffective or perhaps unsafe drug formulation.

PDA Technical Bulletin No. 1 [39] lists closure formulation ingredients likely to be leached as (a) low-molecular-weight polymers, (b) fillers, (c) activators, (d) curing agents-accelerators, and (e) other ingredients, such as antioxidants, plasticizers, and lubricants. This bulletin also provides procedures to identify and quantitate extracts. The monograph by Wake et al. [53] is another good source of methodology.

The extractability of a common rubber accelerator, 2-mercaptobenzothiazole (2-MCBT), has recently been brought to the attention of drug manufacturers by the FDA. In 1965, Inchiosa found a material similar to 2-MCBT in two brands of disposable syringes [28]. In 1981, Peterson et al. identified 2-(2-hydroxyethylmercapto)benzothiazole (HMBT) as a contaminant in the extract from disposable syringes [29]. The HMBT is a product of the reaction between 2-MCBT and ethylene oxide, which was used to sterilize the syringes. Danielson et al. [111,112] reported 2-MCBT in 12 lots of large volume parenteral solutions. One consequence of extractables is the toxicity of resultant drug formulation. Guess and O'Leary found HMBT to be more toxic than 2-MCBT in single-dose studies. However, the 2-MCBT was more toxic in repeated-dose studies [113].

Another consequence of extractables is the interference with drug assays. 2-MCBT is a strong ultraviolet absorber (312–320 nm) and will interfere with the UV or liquid chromatographic UV analysis of many drug formulations. In clinical studies, 2-MCBT was found to be the cause of increased failures in amniocentesis tests [114].

Products of the cure reaction may also be extracted. The FDA has set an action level of 10 parts per billion of volatile *N*-nitrosamines in rubber baby bottle nipples [115]. Preston and Anderson recently studied the effect on the pH shift of solution in contact with resin-cured butyl rubbers [116].

Metal ions, such as zinc from cure activators and aluminum from fillers, have been found in parenteral solutions [37,38,69].

REFERENCES

1. G. H. Hopkins, *J. Pharm. Sci.*, 54:138–143 (1965).
2. The West Company, Phoenixville, Pennsylvania, *Herman O. West, A Man and His Company*. Livingston Publishing, 1968.
3. S. Turco and R. E. King, *Sterile Dosage Forms*, 2nd ed. Lea & Febiger, Philadelphia, 1979.

4. M. Morton (ed.), *Rubber Technology*, 2nd ed. Van Nostrand Reinhold, New York, 1973.
5. K. F. Heinisch, *Dictionary of Rubber*. John Wiley and Sons, New York, 1966.
6. H. J. Stern, *Rubber: Natural and Synthetic*. Palmerton Publishing, New York, 1967.
7. J. I. Wright, *Elastomerics*, 114(12):28–32 (1982).
8. Am. Soc. Test. Material, *1984 Annual Book of ASTM Standards*, Section 9, Volumes 09.01 and 09.02. ASTM, Philadelphia, 1984.
9. M. Szycher, V. L. Poirier, and D. Dempsey, *Elastomerics*, 115(3): 11–15 (1983).
10. G. H. Hopkins, West Company Technical Report No. 10. The West Company, Phoenixville, Pennsylvania, 1963.
11. G. H. Hopkins, West Company Technical Report No. 8. The West Company, Phoenixville, Pennsylvania, 1955.
12. J. J. Farley and J. N. Drummond, *Bull. Parent. Drug Assoc.*, 30: 187–194 (1976).
13. G. H. Hopkins, *Bull. Parent. Drug Assoc.*, 22:181–185 (1968).
14. G. H. Hopkins and R. W. Young, *Bull. Parent. Drug Assoc.*, 28: 15–25 (1974).
15. M. Moore, *Rubber Plastics News, XIV*, (Jan. 28):1 (1985).
16. D. R. Smith (ed.), *The Blue Book*. Lippincott & Peto, Akron, Ohio, 1984.
17. The West Company, West Bridge Street, Phoenixville, PA 19460.
18. Tompkins Rubber Company, P.O. Box 160, 550 Township Line Road, Blue Bell, PA 19422.
19. Plasticoid Company, 249 West High Street, Elkton, MD 21921.
20. Helvoet Pharma, 9012 Pennsauken Highway, Pennsauken, NJ 08110.
21. C. F. Ross, *Packaging of Pharmaceuticals*. Newnes-Buttersworths, London, 1975, pp. 76–79.
22. K. E. Avis, Sterile products. In *The Theory and Practice of Industrial Pharmacy*, 2nd ed. (L. Lackman, H. A. Lieberman, and J. L. Kanig, eds.). Lea & Febiger, Philadelphia, 1976, p. 597.
23. G. H. Hopkins, *J. Pharm. Sci.*, 54:138–143 (1965).
24. F. M. Keim, *Bull. Parent. Drug Assoc.*, 29:46–53 (1975).
25. The West Company, Phoenixville, Pennsylvania 19460, Bulletin A-3.
26. L. Lachman, W. Pauli, P. Sheth, and M. Pagliery, *J. Pharm. Sci.*, 55(9):962–966 (1967).
27. E. Adams, The West Company Technical Report, November 1978.
28. M. A. Inchiosa, *J. Pharm. Sci.*, 54:1397–1381 (1965).
29. M. C. Peterson, J. Vine, J. J. Ashley, and R. L. Nation, *J. Pharm. Sci.*, 70:1139–1143 (1981).
30. F. W. Yeager, N. N. Van Gulick, and B. A. Lasoski, *Am. Ind. Hyg. Assoc. J.*, 41:148–150 (1980).
31. C. B. Ireland, F. P. Hytrek, and B. A. Lasoski, *Am. Ind. Hyg. Assoc. J.*, 41:895–900 (1980).
32. D. C. Farshy, *Appl. Microbiol.*, 27:300–302 (1974).
33. K. M. Kessler, et al., *Clin. Chem.*, 28:1187–1190 (1982).
34. F. M. Keim, *Elastomeric Closure Formulations: Composition, Development, Evaluation and Control*. Presented at the 19th National Mtg. of the Academy of Pharmaceutical Sciences, Atlanta, Georgia, 1975.
35. L. Mullins, Effects of fillers in rubber. In *The Chemistry and Physics of Rubber-Like Substances* (L. Bateman, ed.). John Wiley and Sons, New York, 1963.

36. A. R. Plank, *Rubber World*, 186(May):35–36 (1982).
37. E. A. Milano, S. W. Waraszkiewicz, and R. Dirubio, *J. Parent. Sci. Technol.*, 36:117–120 (1982).
38. E. A. Milano, S. W. Waraszkiewicz, and R. Dirubio, *J. Parent. Sci. Technol.*, 36:232–236 (1982).
39. Extractables from Elastomeric Closures: Analytical Procedures for Functional Group Characterization/Identification, Technical Methods Bulletin No. 1, Parenteral Drug Association, Philadelphia, 1980.
40. R. T. Wood, *J. Parent. Drug Assoc.*, 34:286–294 (1980).
41. W. L. Fuess, *P&MC Ind.*, 2(2):30–31 (1983).
42. J. J. Farley, Parenteral Drug Association, Fall Meeting, Philadelphia, Nov., 1984.
43. R. Mastromatteo, et al., *Rubber World*, 187(5):24–32 (1983).
44. G. R. Personeus and P. Ascione, *J. Parent. Sci. Technol.*, 35:63–69 (1981).
45. A. J. Barnard, R. M. Mitchell, and G. E. Wolf, *Anal. Chem.*, 50: 1079A–1086A (1978).
46. A. M. Gessler, Compounding concepts and physical testing of elastomeric compositions. In *Elastomers Technology* (J. V. Fusco, ed.). Center for Professional Advancement, East Brunswick, New Jersey, 1980.
47. D. L. Hertz, Jr., *Elastomerics*, 116(11):17–21 (1984).
48. R. H. Norman, *Polymer Testing*, 1:247–257 (1980).
49. West Co. Method, CF-01, The West Co., Pharma Packaging Div., Phoenixville, Pennsylvania, 1982.
50. G. H. Hopkins, *Bull. Parent. Drug Assoc.*, 22:48–52 (1968).
51. Generic Test Procedures for Elastomeric Closures, Information Bulletin No. 2, Parenteral Drug Association, Philadelphia, 1979.
52. G. H. Hopkins, West Company Technical Report No. 9. The West Company, Phoenixville, Pennsylvania, 1958.
53. W. C. Wake, B. K. Tidd, and M. J. R. Loadman, *The Analysis of Rubber and Rubber-Like Polymers*, 3rd ed. Applied Science, New York, 1983.
54. L. Bateman, et al., Chemistry of vulcanization. In *The Chemistry of Physics of Rubber-Like Substances* (L. Bateman, ed.). John Wiley and Sons, New York, 1963.
55. West Company Method, Swelling-01, The West Company, Pharma. Packaging Division, Phoenixville, Pennsylvania, 1981.
56. S. Davison, *Rubber Age*, 100:76–80 (1968).
57. H. P. Schreiber, H. W. Holden, and G. Barana, *J. Polym. Sci. Part C*, 30:471–484 (1970).
58. N. Kawasaki and T. Hashimoto, *J. Polym. Sci.*, 11:671–673 (1973).
59. A. J. Duncan, *Quality Control and Industrial Statistics*, 4th ed. Richard D. Irwin, Inc., 1974.
60. United States Department of Defense, Military Standard, Sampling Procedures and Tables for Inspection by Attributes (MIL-STD-105D). U.S. Government Printing Office, Washington, D.C., 1963.
61. E. L. Grant and R. S. Leavenworth, *Statistical Quality Control*, 5th ed. McGraw Hill, New York, 1980.
62. R. O. Babbit (ed.), *The Vanderbilt Rubber Handbook*. R. T. Vanderbilt Co., East Norwalk, Connecticut, 1978.
63. Code of Federal Regulations, Title 21, U.S. Government Printing Office, Washington, D.C., April 1981.
64. G. H. Hopkins, *Bull. Parent. Drug Assoc.*, 23:105–113 (1969).

65. W. A. McAllister, F. D. Sancilio, and G. W. Martin, *Pharmaceut. Technol.*, 3(April):51–56 (1979).
66. ASTM, *1984 Annual Book of ASTM Standards*, Section 6, Volume 06.02. ASTM, Philadelphia, 1984.
67. J. R. Ferraro (ed.), *The Sadtler I.R. Spectra, Handbook of Minerals and Clays*. Sadtler Research Laboratories, Philadelphia, 1982.
68. F. J. Welcher (ed.), *Standard Methods of Chemical Analysis*, 6th ed., Vol. 2, Part B, Chapter 43. Van Nostrand Reinhold, New York, 1963.
69. D. Mondimore and C. Moore, *J. Parent. Sci. Technol.*, 37:79–81 (1983).
70. T. C. Patton (ed.), *Pigment Handbook*, Vol. I, II, and III. Wiley Interscience, New York, 1972.
71. F. R. Eirich (ed.), *Science and Technology of Rubber*. Academic Press, New York, 1978.
72. Elastomeric Closures: Evaluation of Significant Performance and Identity Characteristics, Technical Methods Bulletin No. 2, Parenteral Drug Association, Philadelphia, 1981.
73. USP XXI/NF XVI, General Chapter 381, United States Pharmacopoeia Convention, Rockville, Maryland, 1985.
74. Coleman Instruments, Inc., Magwood, IL.
75. Hach Co., Loveland, CO.
76. J. Kapoor and R. Murty, *Pharmaceut. Technol.*, 1(Nov.):53, 80, 83 (1977).
77. A. I. Kay, *Pharmaceut. Technol.*, 7(May):54–61 (1982).
78. *British Standards*, British Standards Institution, British Standards House, London, 1960.
79. *DIN Standards*, Deutsches Institut for Normung e.v., Berlin, W. Germany, 1982.
80. *The Pharmacopoeia of Japan*, 10th ed. Society of Japanese Pharmacopoeia, Yakuji Nippo, Ltd., Tokyo, Japan, 1982.
81. L. N. Mattson, et al., *J. Parent. Drug Assoc.*, 34:436–446 (1980).
82. A. Krishen and R. G. Tucker, *Anal. Chem.*, 46:29–33 (1974).
83. C. J. Wolf, M. A. Grayson, and D. L. Fanter, *Anal. Chem.*, 52: 348A–358A (1980).
84. N. Iglauer and F. F. Bentley, *J. Chromatog. Sci.*, 12:23–33 (1974).
85. J. C. Hu, *Anal. Chem.*, 49:537–540 (1977).
86. P. H. Kiang, *J. Parent. Sci. Technol.*, 35:152–161 (1981).
87. J. C. Kleinert and C. J. Weschler, *Anal. Chem.*, 52:1245–1248 (1980).
88. T. Protivova, J. Pospisil, and J. Holcik, *J. Chromatogr.*, 92:361–370 (1974).
89. R. E. Majors and E. L. Johnson, *J. Chromatogr.*, 167:16039 (1978).
90. A. Krishen, *Anal. Chem.*, 53:159R–162R (1981).
91. G. H. Hopkins, *Bull. Parent. Drug Assoc.*, 29:278–285 (1975).
92. GMP Trends, GMP Trends, Inc., Boulder, Colorado 80306, September 15, 1980.
93. N. Petry, S. Shaw, W. Kessler, G. Born, and P. Belcastro, *J. Parent. Drug Assoc.*, 33:283 (1979).
94. M. Pikal and J. Long, *J. Parent. Drug Assoc.*, 32(4):162–173 (1978).
95. G. Van Amerongen, *J. Polym. Sci.*, 5:307 (1950).
96. P. Van Damme, *Pharm. Acta Helv.*, 45(9):564–571 (1970) (*Chem. Abstracts* 73:9121u).
97. H. Gildmeister, *Deutsch. Gesundheitsw.*, 22(7):307–310 (1967) (*Chem. Abstracts*, 67:41582t).

98. J. Viska, *Cesk. Farm.*, 15(9):501–503 (1966) (*Chem. Abstracts*, 63:68904r).
99. B. Johnannsen, *Medd. Norsk. Farm. Selskap.*, 27(2):15–19 (1965) (*Chem. Abstracts*, 63:438f).
100. J. Birner and J. Garnet, *J. Pharm. Sci.*, 53(11):1424–1426 (1964).
101. L. Lachman and P. Sheth, *J. Pharm. Sci.*, 53(2):211–218 (1964).
102. I. Csato, J. Nuridsany, A. Bincze, and L. Lang, *Gyogyszereszet*, 6:380–384 (1962).
103. V. Bondar, F. Konev, I. Kovalev, and K. Kulesk, *Parm. Zk.*, 5:68–71 (1976) (*Chem. Abstracts*, 86:127169t).
104. J. Boyett and K. Avis, *Bull. Parent. Drug Assoc.*, 30(4):169–179 (1976).
105. M. Jetton, J. Sullivan, and R. Burch, *Arch. Intern. Med.*, 136(7): 782–784 (1976) (*Chem. Abstracts*, 85:68242r).
106. S. Dixon, A. Missen, and G. Down, *Forensic Sci.*, 4(2):155–159 (1974) (*Chem. Abstracts*, 82:81252b).
107. S. Motola and C. Clawns, *Bull. Parent. Drug Assoc.*, 26(4):163–171 (1972).
108. Y. J. Wang and Y. W. Chien, PDA Technical Report No. 5. Parenteral Drug Association, Philadelphia, 1984.
109. L. Lachman, S. Weinstein, G. Hopkins, S. Slack, P. Elsman, and J. Cooper, *J. Pharm. Sci.*, 51:224–232 (1962).
110. N. R. Anderson and J. J. Motzi, *Am. J. Hosp. Pharm.*, 36:161 (1982).
111. J. W. Danielson, G. S. Oxborrow, and A. M. Placencia, *J. Parent. Sci. Technol.*, 37:98–92 (1983).
112. J. W. Danielson, G. S. Oxborrow, and A. M. Placencia, *J. Parent. Sci. Technol.*, 38:90–93 (1984).
113. W. L. Guess and R. K. O'Leary, *Toxicol. Appl. Pharmacol.*, 14: 221–231 (1969).
114. J. V. Burles, M. P. Hexley, and T. S. Kennedy, *Lancet*, June 11: 1336–1337 (1983).
115. 49 Fed. Reg. 50789 (Dec. 31, 1984).
116. W. A. Preston and N. R. Anderson, *J. Parent. Sci. Technol.*, 38: 237–246 (1984).

6

Particulate Matter

Patrick P. DeLuca

College of Pharmacy
University of Kentucky
Lexington, Kentucky

Julius Z. Knapp

R&D Engineering Associates
Somerset, New Jersey

I. INTRODUCTION

The parenteral routes of administration have over the past few decades increased in usage due to the inherent advantages of reaching the systemic circulation quickly. That parenterals gain entry to internal body compartments by circumventing the body's most protective barriers, the skin and mucous membranes, makes these dosage forms vulnerable to strict specifications. Freedom from particulate contamination is one specification essential to ensure function and integrity of the product and safety for the consumer. The attribute of freedom from undesirable particulates must not only be built into the product and exist when the product is released by the manufacturer, it must be maintained during shipping and storage and upon administration to the patient.

Particulate matter in injectable solutions has been defined as foreign insoluble material (other than gas bubbles) inadvertently present in a given product [1]. The presence of foreign materials in solutions to be administered directly into the bloodstream is of deep concern to drug-safety regulators, manufacturers, clinicians, and consumers. Not only do particulates constitute potential adverse clinical consequences, but the quality of the product becomes suspect when undissolved material is observed. Although the clinical effects have not been thoroughly assessed, manufacturers have improved the quality specifications of component materials and processing techniques in order to provide a high-quality product. Additionally, the technology for manufacturing, monitoring, and administering parenterals has advanced so significantly in the last two decades that quality assurance personnel are often uncertain about what constitutes suitable standards.

An appreciation of the magnitude of the problem of particulates can be illustrated by an example of "purity" and "impurity" of a material. A product that is 99.99% pure contains only 0.01% impurity, or 100 parts per million. Although this generally is an acceptable amount of impurity, even

Table 1 Number of Spherical Particles in a Milligram[a] of Insoluble Material as a Function of Density

Diameter (μm)	Density		
	0.5	1.0	1.5
1	3.8×10^9	1.9×10^9	1.3×10^9
5	3.0×10^7	1.5×10^7	1.0×10^7
10	3.8×10^6	1.9×10^6	1.3×10^6
25	2.4×10^5	1.2×10^5	0.8×10^5
50	3.0×10^4	1.5×10^4	1.0×10^4

[a]The quantity 1 mg/liter represents 1 ppm.

on a 100-fold smaller scale of 1 ppm, i.e., 1 mg/liter, such a level of insoluble impurity or contamination is equivalent to 120,000 particles (assuming a density of 1), 25 μm in diameter. This level of particulate contamination is well above the USP allowable limit for intravenous infusion solutions [1]. The number of spherical particles per milligram of substance can be calculated from the formula

$$\text{Particles/mg} = \frac{1.91 \times 10^9}{dD^3} \tag{1}$$

where d is the density of the particle and D is the diameter in micrometers. Table 1 shows the number of spherical particles in a milligram of insoluble impurity or contaminant at various diameters and densities.

II. SOURCES OF PARTICULATE MATTER

The principal sources of particulate matter contamination encompass the product, the manufacturing process, and the administration system. Hospital practices as well as the hospital environment also constitute sources of contamination. Although considerable efforts are made to avoid or minimize particulate contamination by pharmaceutical manufacturers during the production of parenteral products, the administration of the solutions will inevitably lead to the inadvertent administration of small particles. Unfortunately, compendial standards and guidelines apply to levels of particles occurring during manufacturing and storage and do not take into account those that arise from the handling and manipulations during administration.

A. Product

Product-related particles are those that arise within the solution due to instability or interaction with the container components. Contaminants in distilled water and raw materials may be colloidal in nature and escape removal during filtration only to aggregate into subvisible and visible particles on storage. Such contamination has been reported in intravenous solutions [2] and dextran [3] and dextrose [4] solutions. The latter two were the result of polymerization. Particulate matter was reported in commercial antibiotics [5] and implicated in the manufacturing process. Subsequent studies utilizing scanning electron microscopy [6,7] revealed the residues isolated from the antibiotic products represented less than 0.1% of the drug substance and were most likely due to subtle degradation and the formation of insoluble degradation products.

B. Container

If it were possible to remove all particulates from the parenteral solution and eliminate degradation, the solution still would be in contact with the container, either glass or plastic, and possibly a rubber closure. Glass particles illustrated in Figure 1a are shed from glass containers or may be generated during processing or upon high-heat water attack during the sterilization and pyrogenation processes. Soluble materials can be leached from the glass containers and react with the drug or added substances, resulting in a precipitate (Chap. 3, Vol. 2). Type I glass often contains a small percentage of barium oxide, which has been shown to leach into the product as barium ions [8]:

$$BaO + H_2O \rightarrow Ba(OH)_2 \rightarrow Ba^{2+} + 2OH^- \qquad (2)$$

if the active ingredient is a sulfate salt, or the product is stabilized by bisulfite as an antioxidant, after some time $BaSO_4$ crystals will form and grow to a fine precipitate.

$$Ba^{2+} + SO_4^{2-} \rightarrow BaSO_4 \qquad (3)$$

Barium sulfate crystals, such as illustrated in Figure 1b, were isolated from six products: three were sulfate drugs and three contained a bisulfite or metabisulfite as an antioxidant. Additionally, flakes can form in acid, alkali, or alcoholic solutions and appear to be the result of interactions involving Mg, Ca, Al, CO_3, and PO_4 ions. The process of autoclaving and the addition of electrolytes often induce or accelerate the formation of such flakes.

C. Closure

The rubber closure is regarded as a major source of particulate contamination. Rubber is used for closures on multidose vials and large volume containers as well as plungers in disposable syringes. The closures are made of natural latex, synthetic butyl and neoprene polymers, and silicones and contain numerous fillers, antioxidants, activators, and vulcanizing agents (Chap. 5, Vol. 2). Leaching of organic and inorganic materials into the solution often occurs. A common extractable from rubber closures is zinc ion, originating from catalysts and lubricants used in the vulcanizing and molding process. A phosphate salt or a phosphate buffer system present in the product can result in the formation of insoluble zinc phosphates.

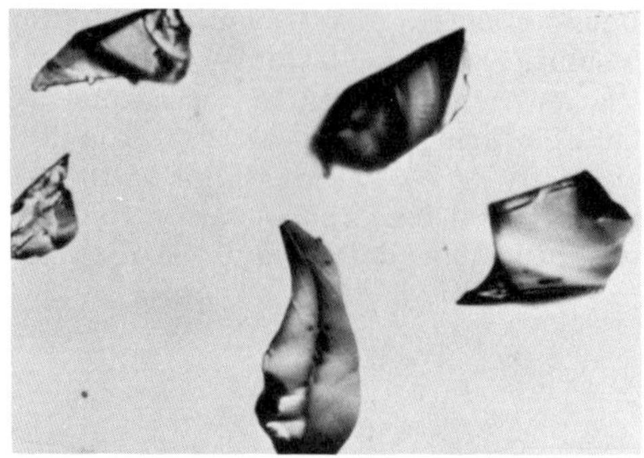

(a)

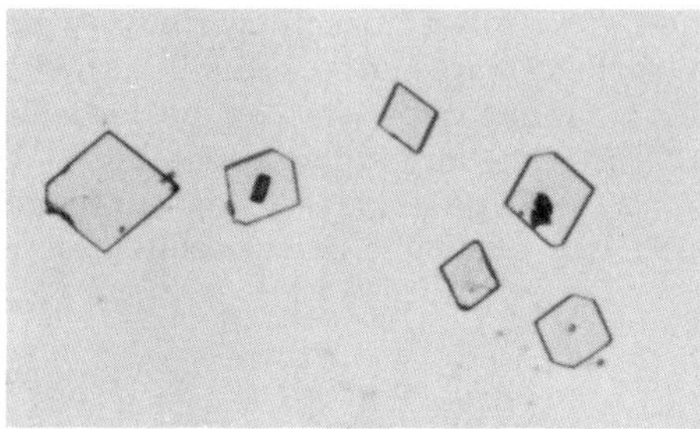

(b)

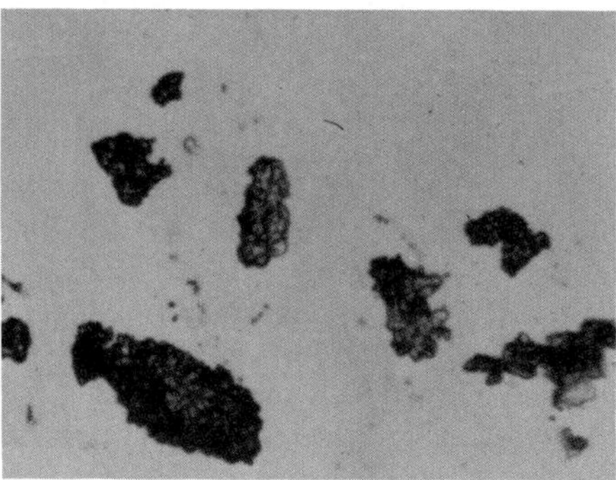

(c)

Figure 1 Optical micrographs of (a) glass, (b) barium sulfate, (c) coating from a rubber closure, (d) stainless steel, and (e) starch grains.

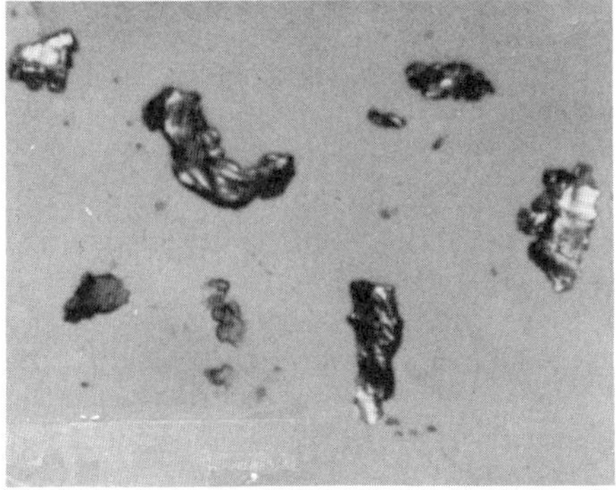

(d)

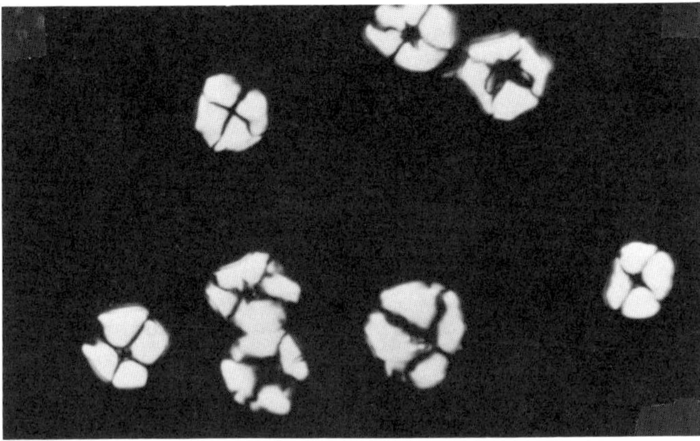

(e)

Figure 1 (continued)

Surface materials illustrated in Figure 1c can slough off rubber closures and are often visible as fragments exceeding 100 μm in size. Lacquered closures and Teflon coatings have been shown to reduce the particulates generated [9].

D. Manufacturing Process

The manufacturing process can contribute to particulates in the product. Significant technological advances have been made in facility design, processing techniques, and clean room garments to minimize contaminants from the environment, personnel, and materials. Nevertheless, nothing can be taken for granted when dealing with trace contaminants. For example, invariably water will be used not only as an ingredient but as a means of achieving the desired level of cleanliness of equipment, vials, and closures. No doubt the water is controlled to meet certain specifications, for instance, total dissolved solids. But once the water is evaporated, as it would be during dry heat sterilization of washed containers, a residue would remain. There is no guarantee that the minute amount of residue can be redissolved in the product. This is particularly true, for instance, in the case of soluble silica, which once "baked" is nearly impossible to redissolve. The problem becomes even more complex when detergents and their potential residues are involved.

Automatic processing equipment, i.e., feeder bowls for closures and syringe fillers and stoppering devices, can induce the generation of particles due to attrition or mechanical agitation. Stainless steel, as shown in Figure 1d, has been isolated from several products [10], as well as starch grains, shown in Figure 1e, which are often a component of the lubricant on clean room gloves.

The sources of particulate matter are many, and one must be alert to combinations of factors or interactions between individual sources. Although the active ingredient may be compatible with extractibles from filters, containers, and closures, a minute amount of degradation product of the drug, which may eventually form, may not be compatible. Compared with such potential interactions, contamination from the environment and processing steps are generally easier to diagnose and correct.

E. Administration System

Contamination of the product can occur during removal from the container by the clinician prior to administration. The breaking of ampuls results in the introduction of glass particles into the solution, and the piercing of the rubber closure with a hypodermic needle causes the generation of rubber fragments. Similarly, particles are generated during the spiking of

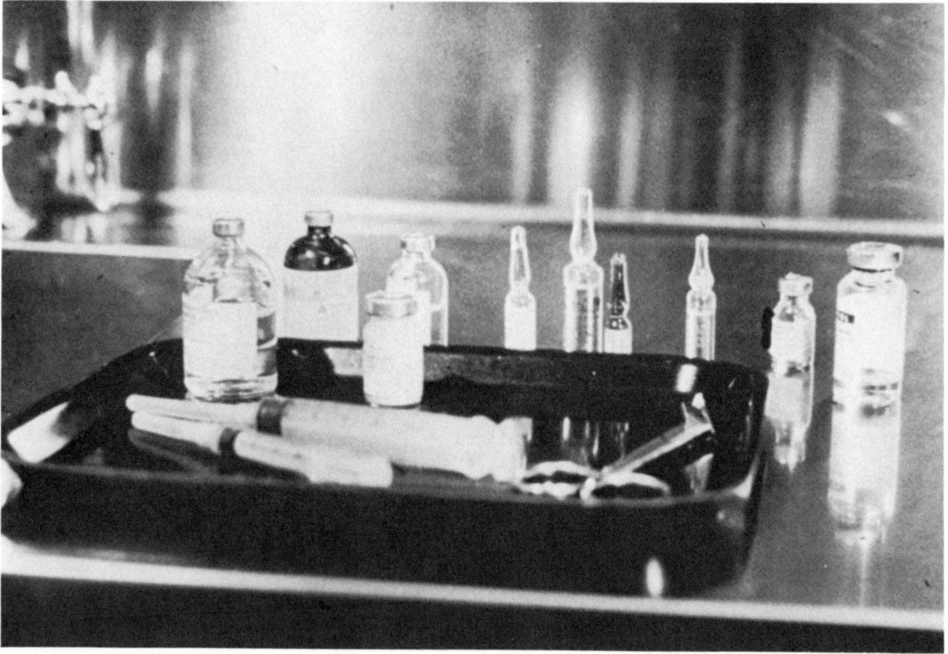

Figure 2 Parenteral products and administration devices.

large volume parenteral solutions with an administration set and when adding drugs, electrolytes, minerals, and vitamins to medication chambers and administration devices.

Parenteral solutions are administered to the patient through administration sets, cannulae, and filters, as well as syringes. Some of the many devices used are shown in Figure 2. These products are composed of plastic, glass, rubber, filters, and metal parts and are the potential sources of particulate contamination. The prevention of contamination therefore depends on the proper use of these devices, further emphasizing the importance of training (Chap. 10, Vol. 1).

III. BIOLOGICAL (CLINICAL) SIGNIFICANCE

Some of the more easily recognized problems associated with intravenous therapy include postinfusion phlebitis, fever, and septicemia. However, the consequences that could arise from occlusion of small blood vessels and other effects caused by foreign particulate matter present in injectables are still to be defined. Thus in addition to sterility, the current requirement for "absence" or minimization of foreign particulate matter in injectables is certainly a reasonable safeguard against suspected and observed consequences.

To better understand the potential problems arising from the injection of parenteral fluids contaminated with particles, a consideration of the circulatory system and the lines of defense against foreign matter is helpful. As shown in Figure 3 there are two main circulations, the high-pressure systemic system through the body and the low-pressure pulmonary circuit through the lungs.

The pump for the circulatory system is the heart, which supplies both circuits simultaneously. A particle injected into the systemic circulation via a radial vein will travel to the right side of the heart. The diameter of a vein increases as it approaches the heart so there is little chance of the particle becoming lodged. The particle then enters the right atrium of the heart, passes into the right ventrical via the tricuspid valve, and is pumped out into the pulmonary artery. The diameter of an artery decreases the farther it is from the heart. The pulmonary artery terminates in the massive capillary network of the lung. Since the diameter of the capillaries is between 8 and 12 μm particles above 8 μm can be expected to lodge in the lung following intravenous administration. Particles less than 8 μm localize in the liver, spleen, and bone marrow [11,12].

The principal defense mechanism against foreign materials is the reticuloendothelial system, which as shown in Figure 4, is comprised of fixed and mobile phagocytic cells. Phagocytosis is the ingestion and digestion of foreign matter, i.e., microorganisms and particles by cells, usually leukocytes.

When monographs for injectable solutions were first included in the National Formulary in 1926, there were no statements regarding foreign insoluble material in this "new" approach to therapy. This lack of concern was reflected in early studies of the fate of particulate matter injected intravenously [13,14]. Reports involving silica dust highlighted the chemical toxicity rather than the potential hazard of particulate matter.

The concern that particulate matter could represent a health hazard began to surface in the late 1940s. Although one study reported no adverse effects in rabbits injected with ground glass for extended periods of

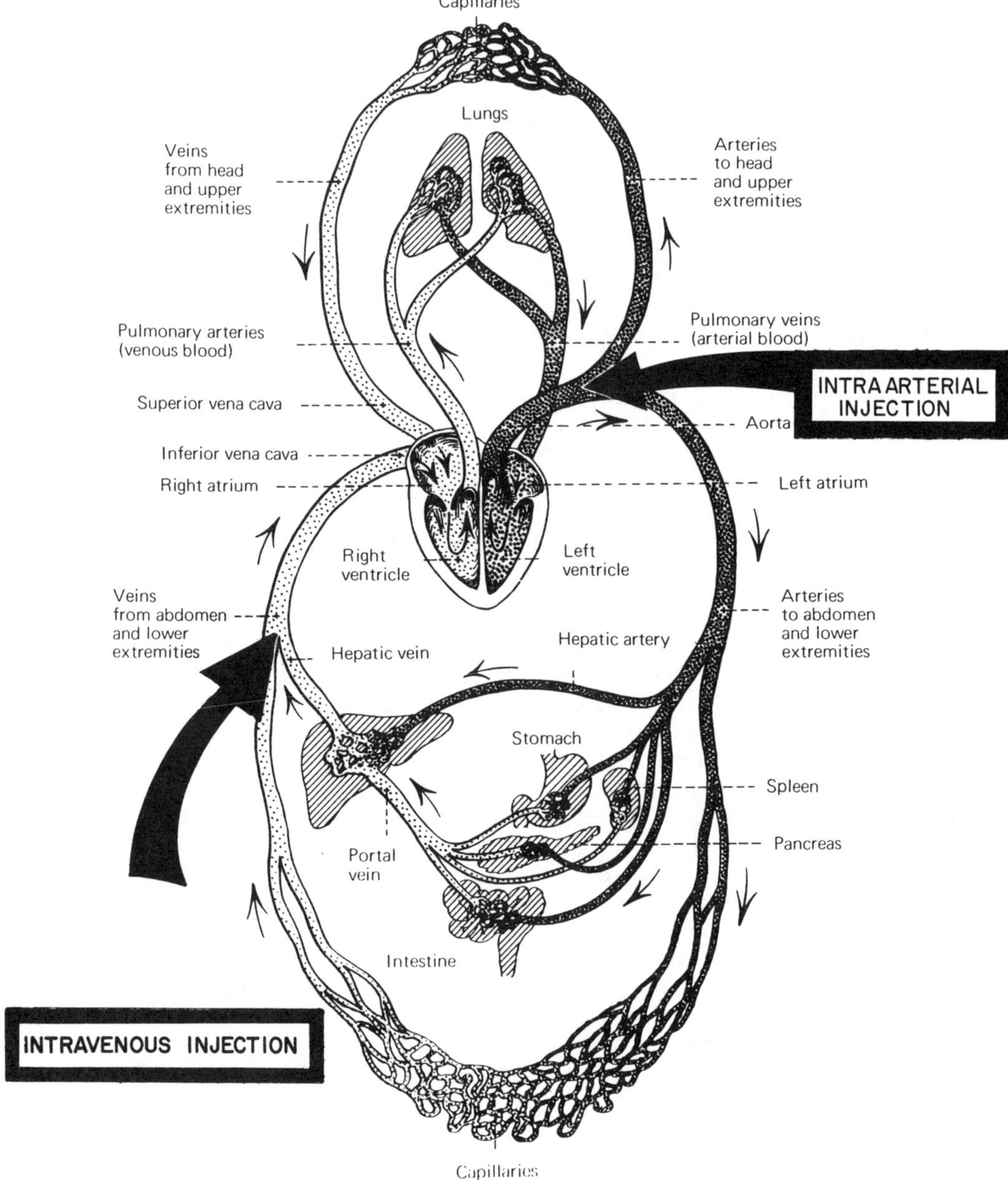

Figure 3 Diagrammatic representation of systemic and pulmonary vascular systems.

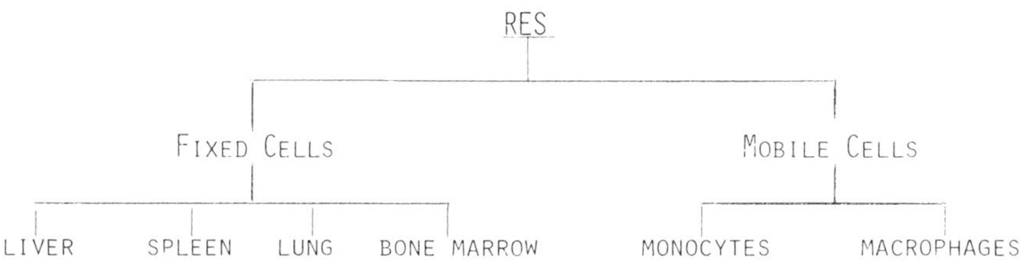

FUNCTION

REMOVE CONTAMINANTS IN INTRACELLULAR VASCULAR SYSTEM

ANTIGEN PROCESSING

METABOLIZE DENATURED PROTEINS

Figure 4 Components of the reticuloendothelial system (RES).

time and attached limited significance to the presence of emboli [15], there were several reports of pulmonary emboli caused by cotton fibers in necropsies and animal studies [16,17] and the autopsy results of lungs of 210 children revealed foreign materials in the lung tissue [18]. Of the 210 autopsies, 150 patients received intravenous injections before death. Thrombi observed were predominantly aggregated platelets to which leukocytes, erythrocytes, and foreign debris had adhered. Platelet aggregation was observed in several other studies involving particulate matter [19,20].

In 1960, Sarrut and Nezelof [21] autopsied premature infants that had received intravenous (IV) therapy and found a high number with pulmonary arterial lesions. The lesions were attributed to cotton fibers. Cotton fibers were also reported in the brains of five individuals in whom cerebral angiography had been performed [22], and in two of the cases the foreign particles were suspected of causing brain damage. Drews reported finding microscopic particles in the fluid of the anterior chamber of cataract surgery patients and traced the source of these particles to the saline and drug products used for irrigation [23]. Other opthalmologists soon confirmed Drews' findings with reports of particles in ophthalmic solutions and drugs [24]. Far from being benign, these particles were soon implicated in a number of conditions, including a partial occlusion of the central retinal artery. Drews found particle counts ranging from 453,000 to 958,000 per liter in his solutions. The size varied from 5 to 300 μm (particles larger than 50 μm are visible with the unaided eye). The classic investigations of Garvan and Gunner [25–27], which showed particles present in practically all the commercially available intravenous fluids, were most responsible for raising the concern of potential hazards of particulate matter in injectable preparations. Capillary and arterial granulomas were cited as the major histopathological changes in experimental animals as well as in lung tissue of patients who had received intravenous fluids. Each granuloma was found to contain fragments of cellulose fibers that came from the solution. Growing concern in this country about particulate matter was evidenced by the symposium, "The Safety of Large Volume Parenterals," convened by the Food and Drug Administration in 1966 [28].

The effect of deliberately injecting particulate matter has never been investigated in humans, but a review by Turco and Davis cited incidences of accidental administration of particulate matter by drug abusers and the inadvertent administration of particles and air in the hospital setting [29]. Capsules and tablets dissolved and injected by abusers contained such fillers as cornstarch and talc, and the insoluble particulates were injected along with the drug [30–32]. Other reports deal with the consequences of accidental administration of air that resulted in massive embolism [33,34] and accidental intravenous administration of suspensions not intended for such use [35,36]. The pharmacological observations associated with this type of mistake included dizziness, shortness of breath, cyanosis, tachycardia, increase in blood pressure, and death [37].

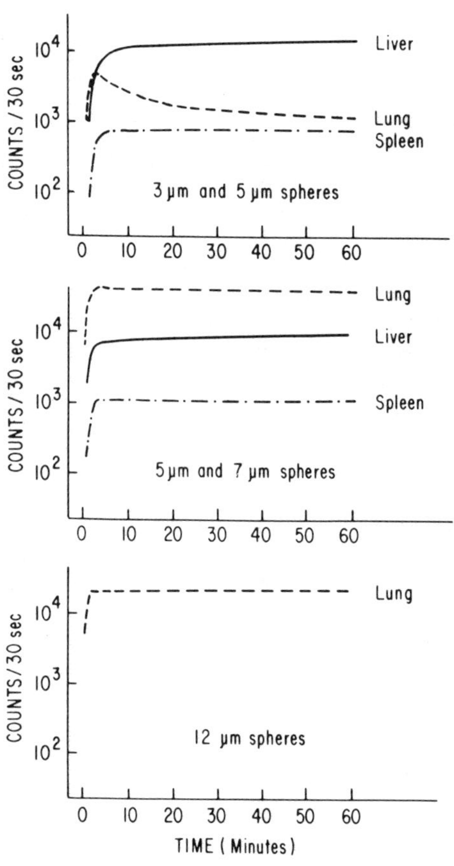

Figure 5 Distribution patterns of microspheres obtained by rapid frame sequential scanning. (From Ref. 12.)

The administration of radiolabeled polystyrene microspheres to beagle dogs [11,12,38,39] resulted in differences in distribution patterns according to size. As shown in Figures 5 and 6, 12-μm spheres as well as a good percentage of 7-μm spheres were retained in the lungs; smaller spheres, 3–5 μm, cleared the lungs and were trapped in the liver and spleen. The smaller spheres were found consistently in vascular channels, Kupffer cells, and the sinusoids of liver, spleen, and bone marrow within phagocytizing cells (Figs. 7 and 8); the 12-μm spheres were found predominantly in the capillaries of the alveolar walls, and occasionally free spheres were seen in the alveolar lumina of the lungs (Fig. 9). The presence of spheres in the lungs caused occasional vascular engorgement, but the integrity of the cellular organelles at the substructural level was not affected.

The rate of clearance of particles is believed to be a function of particle size, shape, chemical properties, charge, and the amount and rate of injection. Clearance of polystyrene spheres from the blood of beagle dogs was found to be size dependent and more rapid with larger spheres [11,12,39]. As shown in Figure 10, 12-μm spheres were eliminated rapidly from the circulation, with a half-life of 0.52 min. Although the smaller spheres cleared the circulation rapidly in the first 10–30 min, concentrations of 10^4 of 3-μm spheres and 10^2–10^3 of 5-μm spheres per gram of blood remained in the circulation for up to 2 hr. This prolonged residence in the blood suggested interaction with the circulating blood cells, and subsequent study [40] revealed 1- and 3-μm spheres in the lysosomes inside the cytoplasm of monocytes and granulocytes (Figs. 11 and 12). The residence time of the spheres in the white blood cells was up to at least 24 hr with 1-μm spheres and up to 4 hr with the 3-μm spheres. There was no evidence of damage

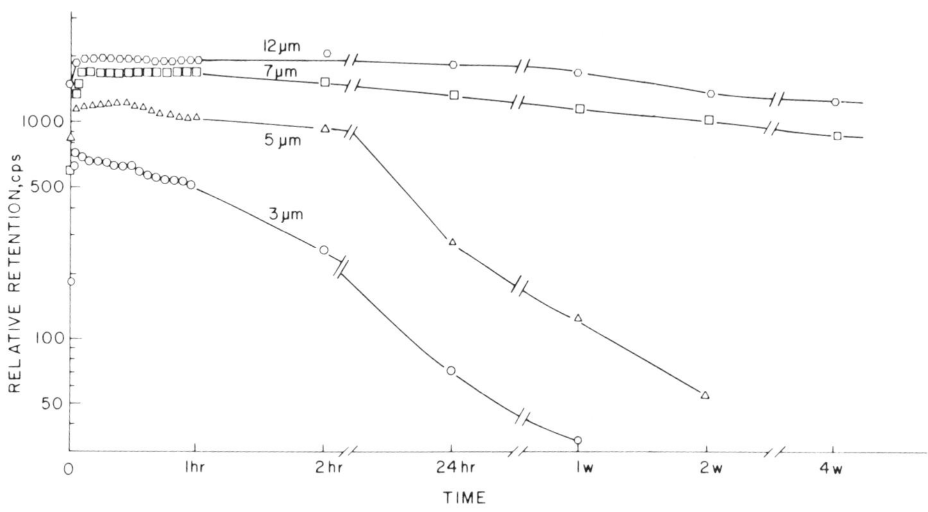

Figure 6 Relative retention of ^{141}Ce-labeled microspheres in beagle dog lungs; obtained by external scanning. (From Ref. 12.)

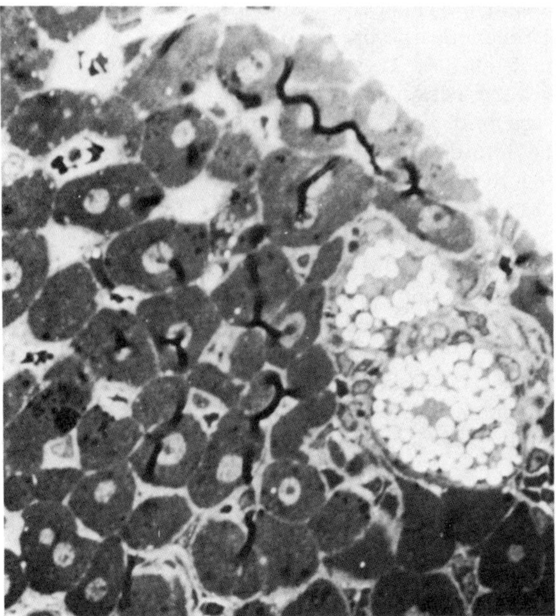

Figure 7 Optical photomicrograph of liver section of beagle dog showing localization of 3-μm spheres.

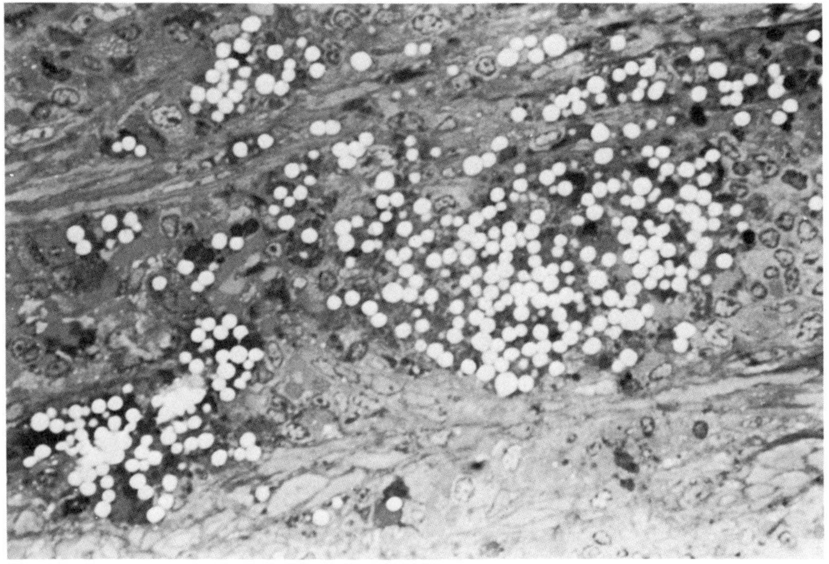

Figure 8 Optical photomicrograph of liver section of beagle dog showing localization of 5-μm spheres.

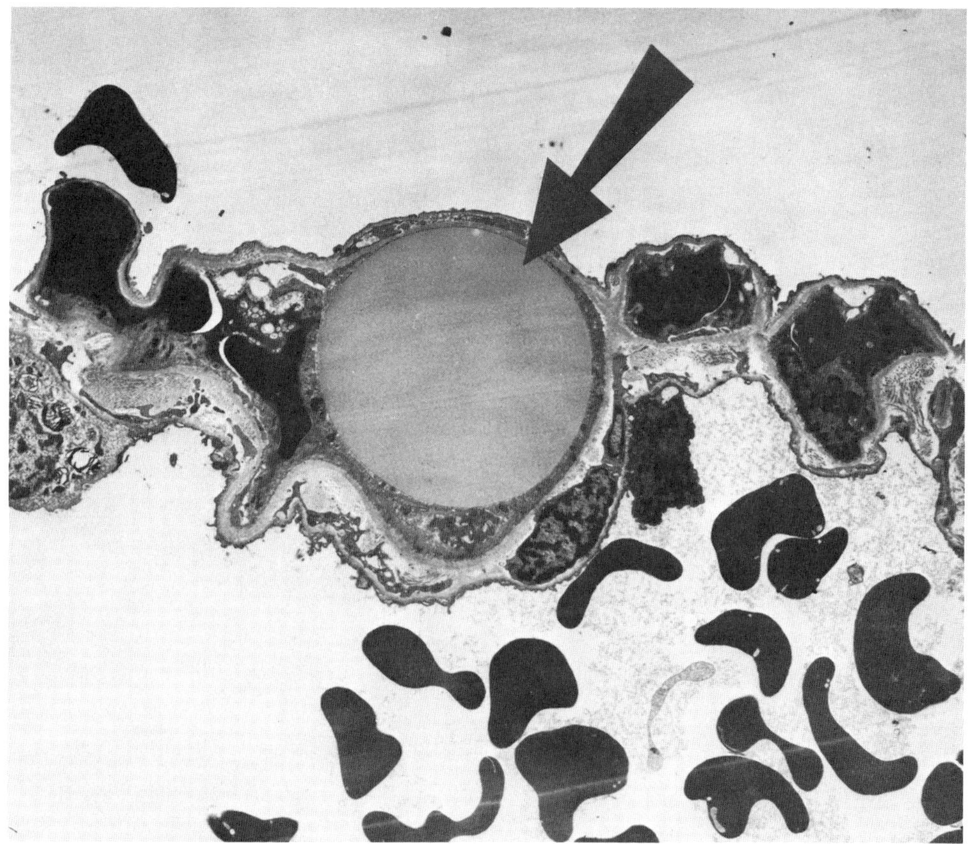

Figure 9 Scanning electron photomicrograph of lung section of beagle dog showing localization of a 12-μm sphere. (From Ref. 40.)

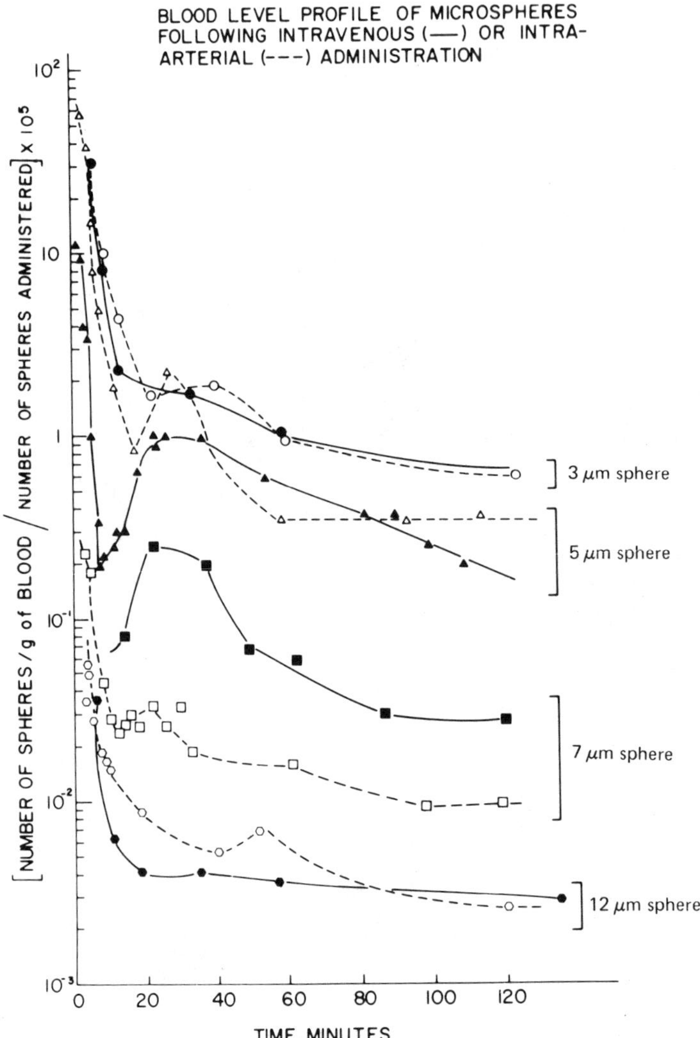

Figure 10 Clearance of polystyrene microspheres from the circulation. Closed figures and solid lines represent intravenous administration, and open figures and broken lines represent intra-arterial administration. (From Ref. 12.)

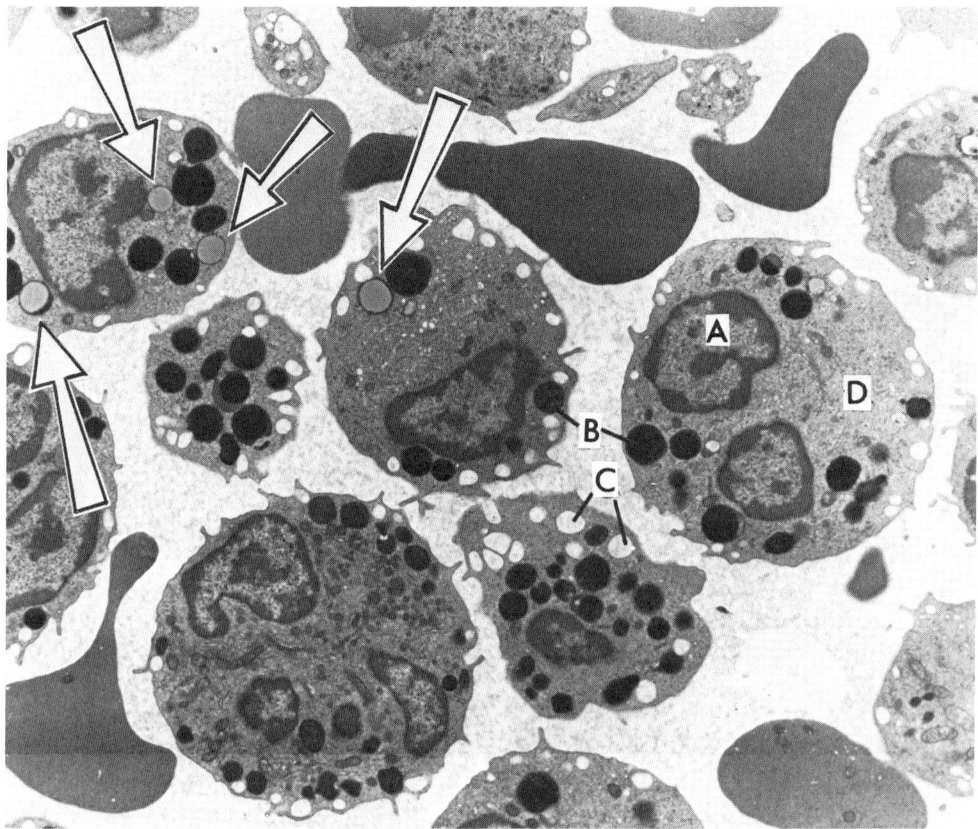

Figure 11 Electron micrograph with arrows showing 3-μm spheres in granulocytes 5 min after administration, 2830X magnification. (A), nucleus; (B) specific granules; (C) vacuole; (D) endoplasmic reticulum (smooth) with ribosomes. (From Ref. 40.)

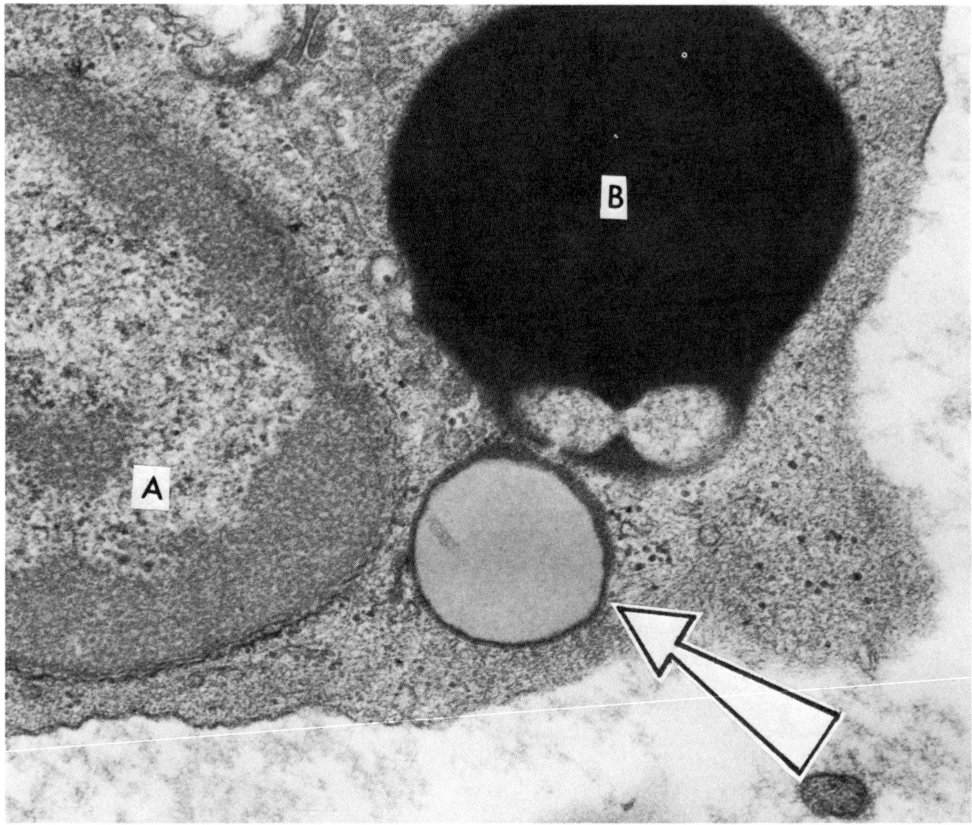

Figure 12 Electron micrograph showing a 1-μm sphere in the lysosome of a monocyte 24 hr after IV administration, 16,900X magnification. (A) nucleus; (B) specific granule. (From Ref. 40.)

to the lysosomes or other cellular organelles. Spheres smaller than 1 μm (nanoparticles, 80 nm to 1 μm) have been reported to localize in the liver within 7 days following IV administration in rats [41,42].

IV. REGULATIONS AND STANDARDS

Particulate matter in parenteral solutions has been a matter of concern to the FDA and USP for a number of years [43]. It was not until 1936, when 26 monographs for parenteral preparations were introduced in the NF VI, that a requirement for clarity was included. This was under the heading "Clearness:" "Aqueous ampul solutions are to be clear, i.e., when observed over a bright light, they shall be substantially free from precipitate, cloudiness or turbidity, specks or fibers, or cotton hairs, or any undissolved material."

For the three decades following the inclusion of a monograph for visible inspection in the official compendia, the definition for clarity changed repeatedly to permit a less subjective and more enforceable standard. Prior to 1965, there were no limit standards for particles in the subvisible (microscopic) range. Particulate matter observed in solution upon resting would often disappear upon shaking, not to reappear unless the container was allowed to rest for several days. The amount of particulate matter was too small to isolate and characterize by existing methods of analysis.

Concern and reports like those cited in the clinical section of this chapter highlighted the fact that the presence of foreign particulate matter in injectable products is undesirable and hence should be avoided if at all possible. Considering that the use of the IV route of administration was increasing, as was the number of products and administration devices intended for such use, the development of standards to regulate or control the amount of foreign material injected was a logical step in the sequence of events.

The first attempt at setting standards was made by Vessey and Kendall of the National Biological Standards Laboratory, Canberra, Australia, in 1965, when the following specifications were proposed for intravenous solutions [44]:

Not more than 25 particles per milliliter above 10 μm
Not more than 100 particles per milliliter above 5 μm
Not more than 250 particles per milliliter above 3.5 μm
Not more than 1000 particles per milliliter above 2 μm

This event was closely followed by an international conference on particulate matter convened by the FDA in July 1966. Industry, academia, and government participated and agreed that particulates were undesirable in parenteral solutions and limits should be established [45].

The pressures for limit standards in intravenous solutions in the United Sates increased because during the period that followed the conference there was a significant increase in (a) intravenously administered products, (b) devices for IV administration, and (c) literature on the existence of particulates and potential hazards in IV solutions. At the same time the technology for reducing particulates had been advanced.

Ideally, standards should be established on the basis of the clinical hazards since there would be little argument or controversy of establishing regulations on a sound moral basis considering the safety of the patient. The noble goal "zero particles" would therefore be ideal. However, in the absence of conclusive clinical evidence concerning the hazards of particulate matter, it was prudent to establish strict but attainable standards. As a result, the state of the art became an important factor in setting meaningful guidelines.

In 1973, an expert advisory panel of the USP-FDA sponsored National Coordinating Committee on Large Volume Parenterals reviewed the existing methodology for monitoring particulate matter and presented recommendations for standard methodology. After reviewing the various methods, including electric resistivity, light blockage, light scattering, and light microscopy, and assessing reports in which these methods were used to compare existing products [46–50], the microscopic method was selected. The technique of membrane filtration followed by microscopic viewing offers the advantage that identification of the contaminants can be performed. The limitations of a microscopic method based on incident light techniques in discerning particles less than 10 μm in size were cited, and it was suggested that if microscopic monitoring of particles less than 10 μm was desirable, new methods based on transmitted lighting would have to be developed.

As will be pointed out further in the section pertaining to monitoring methodology, it is not possible to separate the actual limit values from the monitoring methodology chosen. Due to the advantageous potential for particulate matter identification, the United States Pharmacopeia in 1975 [51] opted for a microscopic technique as the standard procedure. At that time the standard applied only to large volume parenterals (LVP), excluding multidose injections, single-dose small volume injections, and solutions reconstituted from sterile solids. The USP standard states that a LVP meets the requirements of the regulations if it contains no more than 50 particles per milliliter equal to or larger than 10 μm and not more than 5 particles per milliliter equal to or larger than 25 μm in effective linear dimension. Information available at the time indicated that the particle size distribution for most products parallels the line described by the two points plotted on a log-log scale, as shown in Figure 13, and that the state of the art in production technology was such that the particulate level in LVP could realistically be maintained below the proposed pass-fail line. The technology has advanced to such a degree that particulate matter levels encountered in current LVP products fall short of reaching the limit at 10 μm by almost one order of magnitude. Official standards for particulate matter in large volume parenteral solutions for other countries are shown in Table 2 and compared to the USP standard.

Limits for small volume parenterals (SVP) were included in USP XXI [52]. Unlike the LVP standard, which is on a per milliliter basis, the limit for SVP is on a per container basis. The small volume injection, regardless of type, meets the requirements of the test if it contains not more than 10,000 particles per container equal to or greater than 10 μm in effective spherical diameter and not more than 1000 particles per container equal to or greater than 25 μm in effective spherical diameter.

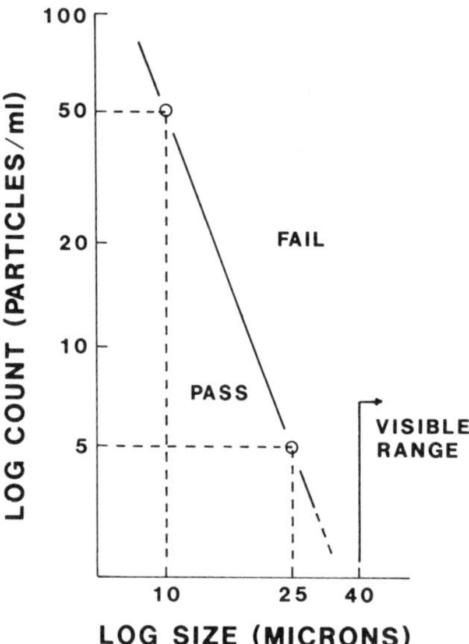

Figure 13 USP pass-fail standard for particulate matter in large volume parenterals.

Table 2 Comparison of Official Standards for Particulate Matter in Large Volume Parenterals

Australian (1974):
max 100 particles per ml > 2 μm, max 2 particles per ml > 20 μm.
The sum of the mean and twice the standard deviation should not exceed twice these values.

British Pharmacopeia (1980):
Coulter counter:
max 1000 particles per ml ⩾ 2 μm, max 100 particles per ml ⩾ 5 μm.

HIAC counter:
max 500 particles per ml ⩾ 2.0 μm, max 80 particles per ml ⩾ 5.0 μm.

USP XXI (1985):
max 50 particles per ml ⩾ 10 μm, max 5 particles per ml ⩾ 25 μm.

Considerable controversy surrounds both the rationale of the standard on a per container basis and that the standard does not differentiate the type of small volume injection, i.e., single or multidose, dry fill for reconstitution or prefilled disposable syringe. The rationale for the standard for SVPs is arbitrarily based on the number of additions to a large volume infusion solution. The 10,000 particles per container limit comes from an assumption that generally five SVPs are added to an LVP and it was thought that the amount of particles a patient might receive should not be more than double that allowed in the LVP as a result of adding five SVPs. Since the limit for the LVP is 50,000 particles not greater than 10 μm/liter, then five additives should not add more than 50,000 additional particles. It has been reported that, because of the container-closure surface area to the product-volume ratio factor in the small SVP units, a higher count on a per milliliter basis than that in the LVP can be expected. A recent study on 50 marketed products of various types revealed that the LVP limits per milliliter would not be suitable for use as a starting point for SVPs [10]. The data are listed in Table 3, and Figures 14 and 15 graphically show the population of particles found in the products. The much higher levels in dry products, ampuls, and multidose vials emphasize that the standards should take into account the type of product.

The methodology for LVPs is optical microscopy following membrane filtration. The particles are isolated on a contrast filter substrate and counted using incident illumination. For SVPs, an electronic liquid-borne particle counter system using a light blockage sensor or equivalent is recommended. Both the microscopic and electronic monitoring methods will be described under the monitoring section of this chapter, but the standard for SVPs on an effective spherical diameter basis is subject to criticism since the light blockage methods monitor particles by an equivalent diameter of a circle since it measures an area blocked.

Since the particle size distribution follows the log-log line, the count of larger particles will give a relative indication of the amount of smaller ones (⩽10 μm) present. Under ideal conditions, particles of the order of 50 μm in effective linear dimension can be detected by visual inspection. Thus the additional requirement for 100% visual inspection of final containers

Table 3 Microscopic Monitoring of Particles in Parenteral Products[a]

Product type	Number of particles per ml (median values reported)			
	≥5 μm	≥10 μm	≥25 μm	≥40 μm
LVP (7)[b]	10	3	1	<1
Single dose[c] (12)	343	36	11	4
Multiple dose (14)	311	106	19	4
Dry products[d] (10)	703	148	48	12
Prefilled syringes (6)	33	6	3	<1

[a]Two containers of each product were counted.
[b]Number of products in parentheses.
[c]Excludes one product that reportedly forms fibrous degradation upon exposure to air.
[d]Reconstituted according to manufacturer's directions.

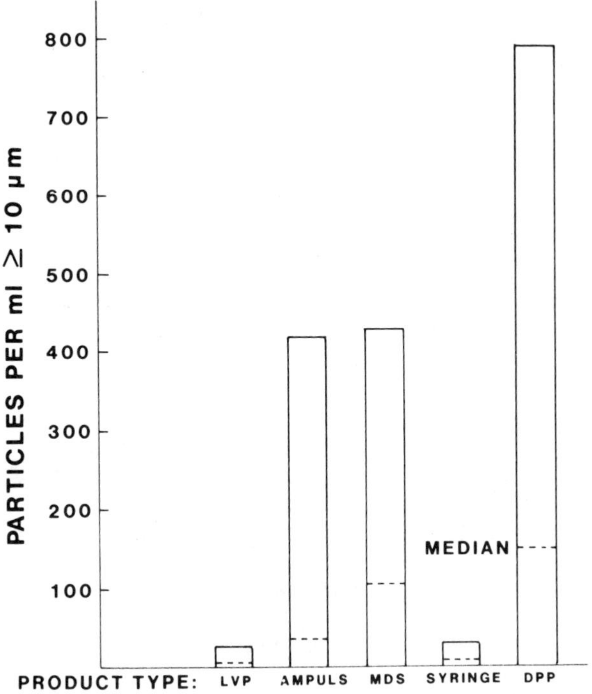

Figure 14 Particle populations in various product types for particles greater than 10 μm.

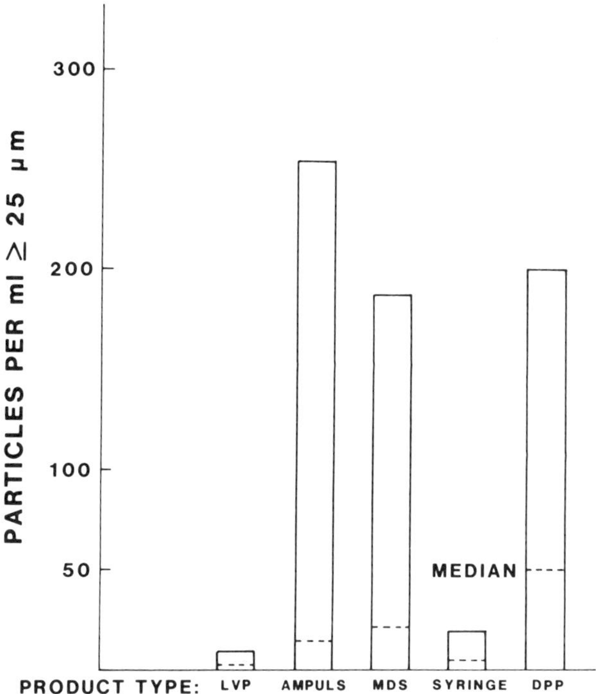

Figure 15 Particle population in various product types for particles greater than 25 μm.

of injectables adds some additional assurance against excessively large numbers of subvisible particles in containers not subjected to the destructive USP test. Visible inspection is not included in the reference section of the USP on particulate matter standards but in the General Information Section under General Tests and Assays and pertains to all parenterals. It states that "Good pharmaceutical practice requires that each final container of injection be subjected individually to a physical inspection, whenever the nature of the container permits, and that every container whose contents show evidence of contamination with visible foreign material be rejected."

V. METHODS OF DETECTION, COUNTING, AND SIZING PARTICLES

The particles found in injectables are commonly measured in units of micrometers, formerly referred to as microns because of their small size. There are 1000 μm to a millimeter or 1 million μm to a meter. Particulate matter data are reported as frequency according to size. For example, the data recorded in Table 4 can be represented by a frequency histogram shown in Figure 16, which displays the data in a differential mode. The same information could be expressed in size ranges as reported in Table 5 and plotted in a cumulative mode shown in Figure 17. Although both modes are interchangeable, the cumulative mode is generally used and the one upon which the USP standards for LVPs are stated.

Table 4 Particular Distribution in Various Size Ranges

Size range (μm)	Count
0–5	4
5–10	20
10–15	46
15–20	23
20–25	6
25–30	1
>30	0

A. Optical Microscopy

1. *Principle*

The particulate matter present in injectable solutions is not readily visible to the unaided eye. For this reason, the particulate matter is collected and fixed on a substrate suitable for microscopic analysis. The most common approach is to filter the solution through a membrane capable of retaining the particles and then viewing the membrane under magnification. The USP recommends a dark contrast membrane, to be viewed with a total 100-fold magnification under oblique incident light. "Blank" determinations

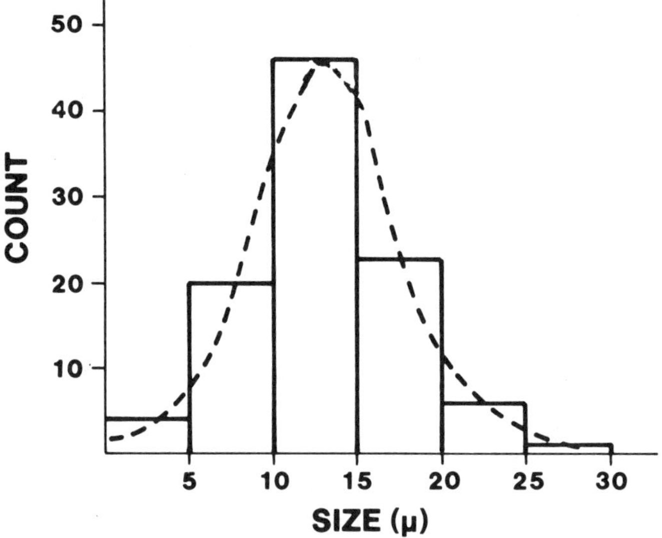

Figure 16 General distribution of particulates plotted in the differential mode.

Table 5 Particle Population Greater Than a Stated Size

Size range (μm)	Count
>0	100
>5	96
>10	76
>15	30
>20	7
>25	1
>30	0

are made by substituting an equivalent volume of filtered fluid for the sample. By performing a simple calculation on the total counts obtained to correct for sample size, the concentration of particulate matter can be derived. Training aids are available for those who must prepare and monitor filters. Nevertheless, data collected on supposedly identical sample vials often differ because of the choice of substrate membrane to collect the sample, the choice of lighting approach, and overall quality of the microscope used [53,54]. An inherent advantage of the microscopic method is that the filter membrane provides a permanent record of each sample. Validation of the various procedures involved in microscopic monitoring is important.

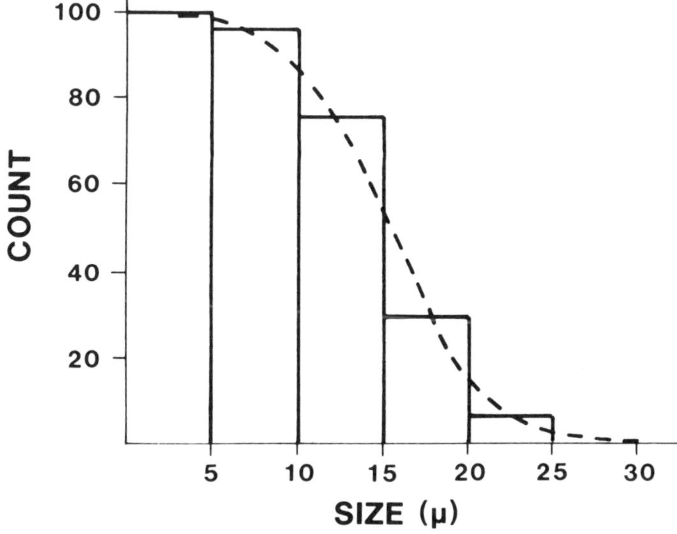

Figure 17 General distribution of particulates plotted in the cumulative mode.

These procedures include equipment precleaning and preparation, sampling and filtation of parenteral products, and preparation and counting of filters. For a detailed description of such procedures, the reader is referred to the literature [10].

2. *Sample Preparation*

Operators preparing samples for microscopic testing should wear head covers and flexible nonpowdered gloves. A clean, properly functioning laminar airflow hood should be used. Sufficiently thin membrane filters with 0.4- to 0.8-μm pore sizes are recommended. When assembling the filter and filtration apparatus, both sides of the filter should be rinsed with ultraclean water. Once the filter membrane is in place, the assembled filtration funnel and exposed membrane surface should be rinsed. Blanks should be counted as soon as possible before sample filtration to verify the efficiency of the cleaning and assembly procedures.

A good practice is to visually examine each intact container before sampling for the presence of particulate matter. Prior to removing the solution, the outer surface of the container should be cleaned thoroughly with a warm detergent and rinsed. For ampuls, score the ampul lightly with a file at the breaking point (Fig. 18a), rinse the surface with distilled water from a filter jet apparatus (Fig. 18b), and dry with a lint-free cloth. Then carefully break the ampul (Fig. 18c) and withdraw the solution with a rinsed syringe. For vials, remove the tear-off seal and clean the outer surface with a lint-free cloth moistened with isopropyl alcohol (Fig. 19a and b). Rinse the glass-closure junction (Fig. 19c), and carefully remove the closure with the aid of forceps (Fig. 19d). Pour the solution into the filter funnel. For dry-filled products, add the reconsitution vehicle to the material after removal of the closure and return the closure. Gently shake to dissolve, then remove the closure and filter the contents.

At least two filters should be prepared for each product using the contents of one container for each filter unless the particulate level is too high and produces a crowded filter. In this case, dilution of the contents of the container to obtain a fraction of the contents will be necessary. In the case of large volume parenterals, 250 ml of the solution should be used.

The solution should be added to the filter funnel along the sides of the funnel without applying vacuum. Once the solution is added and the turbulence dissipates, vacuum can be applied. After sufficient rinsing, the filter is removed with the aid of forceps, placed on a microscope slide, and transferred to a petri dish until ready for viewing.

3. *Description of the Microscope*

Basically, two types of microscopes are used in the laboratory. One, a wide-field steroscopic microscope, is a very simple instrument to use because lighting the stage is not difficult and the image is not reversed. However, magnification is limited to 5–100X. The second type of microscope, a compound microscope (sometimes called a biological or medical microscope), has a useful magnification of 20–1000X. Care has to be taken to obtain proper lighting, and the images are reversed. This causes difficulty in manipulation of the particles.

There are several modifications of the compound microscope. One is the polarizing microscope, which provides plane-polarized light and is usually used to discern optical characteristics. Several texts are available on microscopy if the reader is interested in a more detailed discussion.

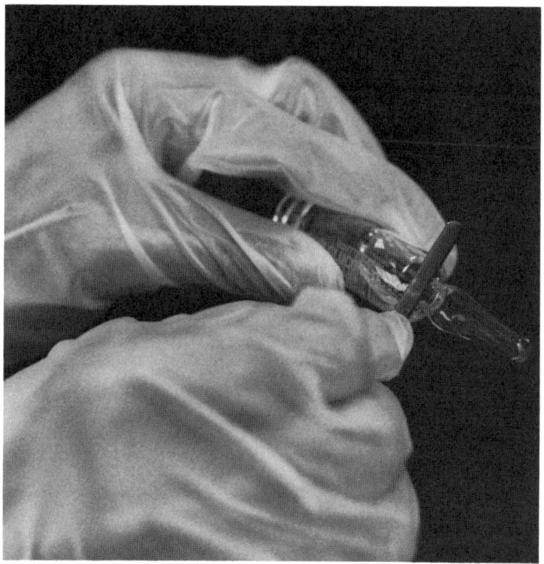

(a)

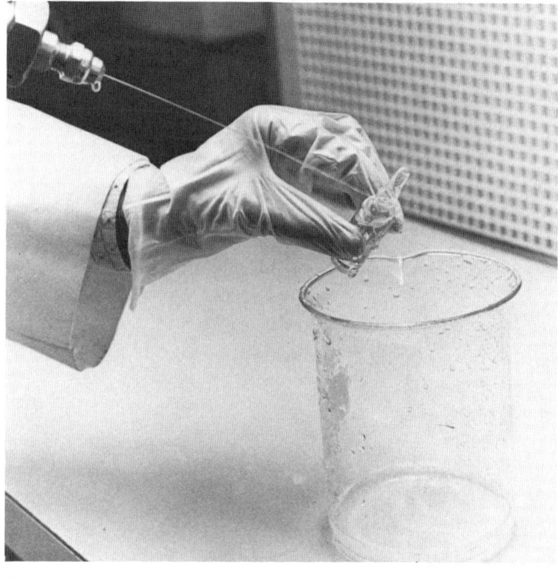

(b)

Figure 18 Procedure for removing solution from glass ampuls: (a) scoring of ampul at the breaking point, (b) rinsing with ultraclean water, (c) breaking of the ampul, and (d) withdrawal of solution.

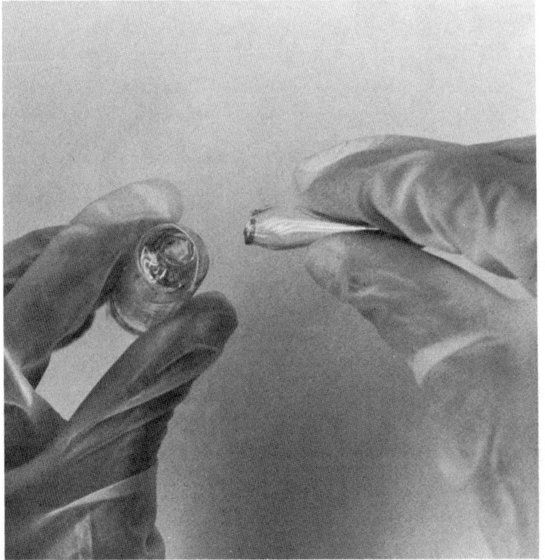

(c)

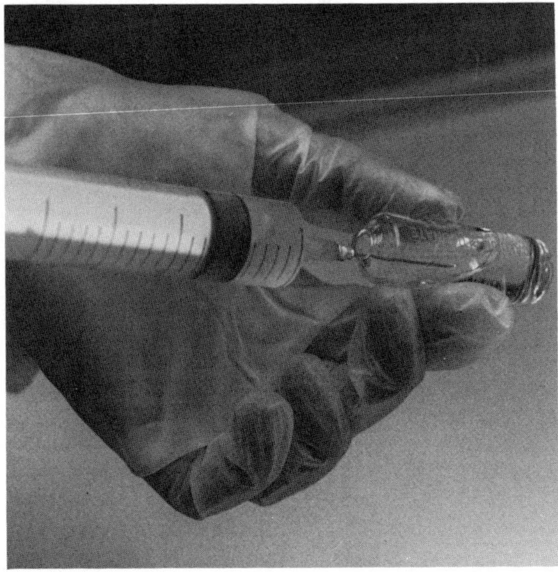

(d)

Figure 18 (continued)

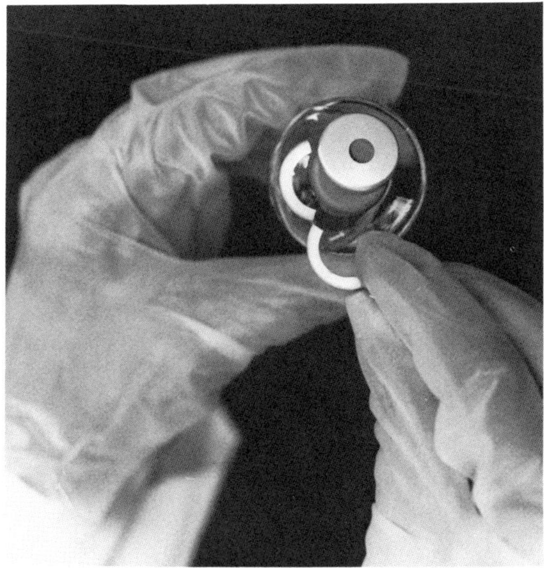

(a)

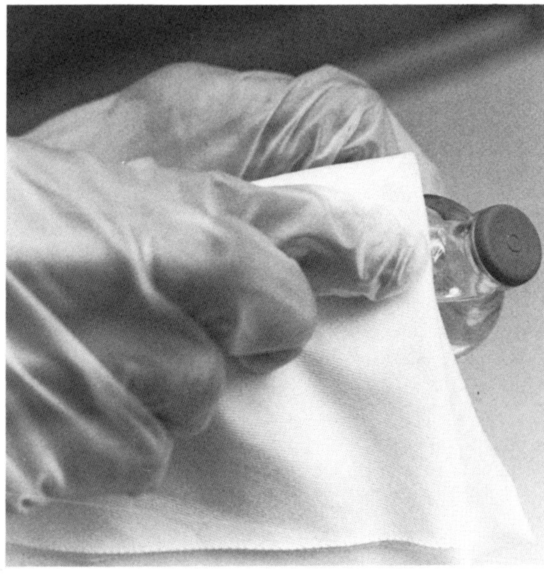

(b)

Figure 19 Procedure for removing solution from vials: (a) removal of tear-off seal and inner seal, (b) cleaning outer surface of vial with isopropyl alcohol, (c) rinsing of rubber closure and glass-closure junction with ultraclean water, and (d) removal of rubber closure with forceps.

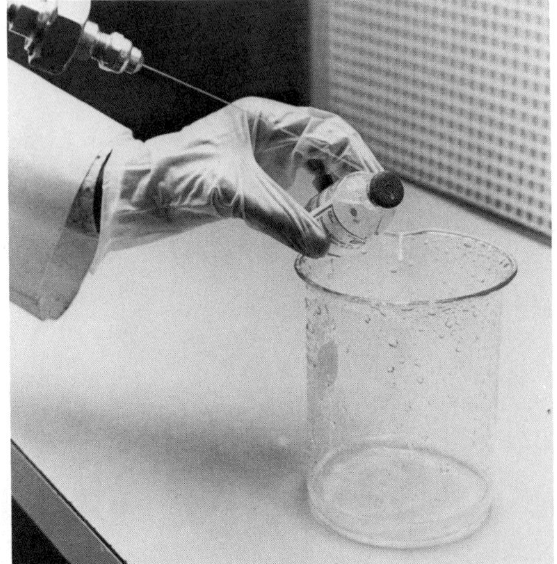

(c)

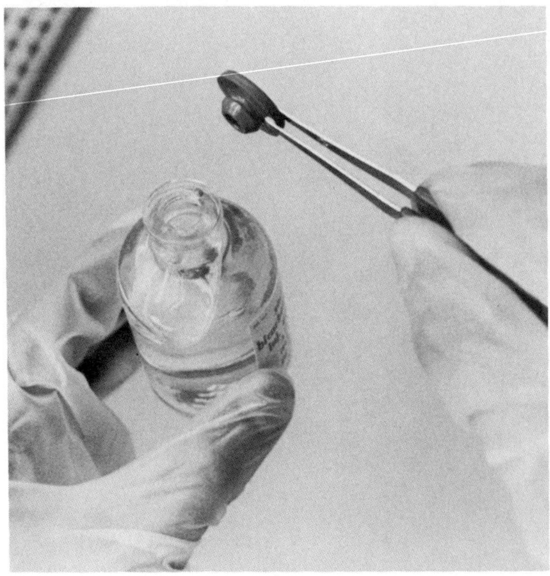

(d)

Figure 19 (continued)

4. *Calibration of the Ocular Micrometer*

Unilateral oblique illumination, depicted in Figure 20, is the official method for microscopic monitoring with a compound microscope, although vertical illumination with Epilum objectives has been shown to be more reliable with certain particle types [53]. To size the particles through the microscope, one must use an ocular micrometer scale that has been calibrated against the stage micrometer for each objective used. Once this is accomplished, it is possible to calculate the micrometer value, which indicates the number of micrometers corresponding to each graduation on the ocular scale. Each objective on the microscope should be calibrated.

5. *Method of Counting Particles*

As particles remain on the membrane in a stable position, they can be perceived in two dimensions and could be sized by several parameters, such as their cross-sectional area, perimeter, longest linear dimension, or a ratio of any of these parameters. As defined in the USP, the size of a particle is determined by its greatest projected dimension, which as illustrated in Figure 21 represents the longest effective linear dimension. The parameter could be visualized as the diameter of the circle circumscribing a given particle. The number of particles on the filter can be counted in two ways: (a) counting the particles of all size ranges in the entire effective area of the filter, and (b) statistical counting of particles of all size ranges in 20 or 40 fields of view.

Counting the entire effective filter area requires considerable training and skill. Beginning at a fixed location, the entire filter surface is scanned and total counts are recorded in all fields of view using a manual counter in various size ranges, such as 10–24, 25–40, and >40 μm. The time for counting and the tedium can be reduced by utilizing a statistical counting technique. In this method, a minimum of 20 fields is selected from predetermined areas and counted. The fields should be randomly selected from the upper, middle, and lower portions of the effective filtration area

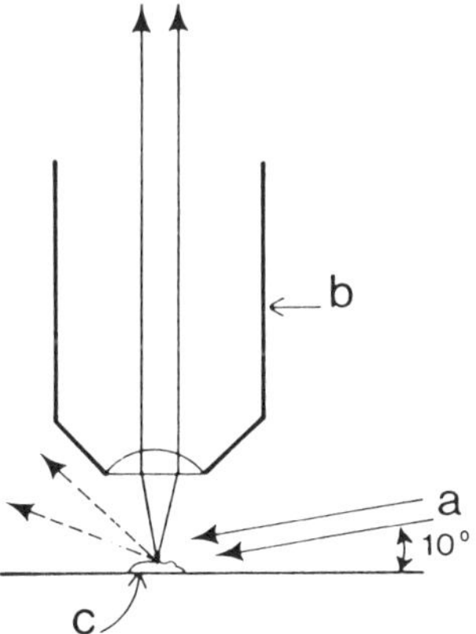

Figure 20 Unilateral (oblique) illumination. The light rays from the auxiliary illuminator (a) are directed downward to the specimen (c) at a 10–15% angle of incidence and are diffracted by the specimen to the microscope objective (b). (From Ref. 53.)

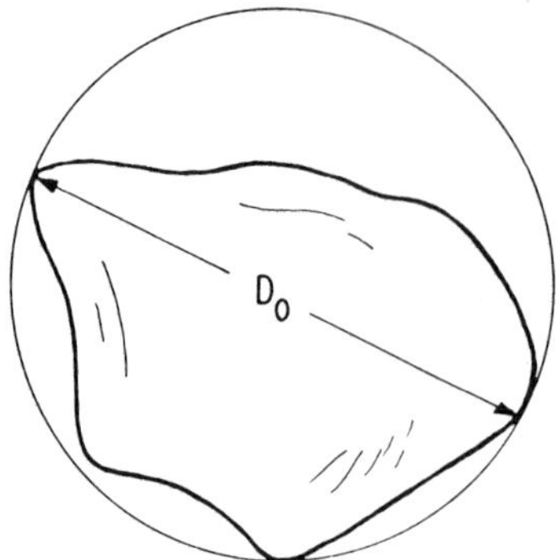

Figure 21 Size determination by the USP method. The longest effective linear dimension D_0 is measured independent of orientation.

(Fig. 22). The sum of the particles in each size range is divided by the total number of fields counted to give an average count per field of view. Using this average, the total number N of particles on the filter in each size range can be calculated using the formula

$$N = \frac{nD^2}{d^2} \tag{4}$$

where n = average count per field, D = the inside diameter of the funnel or the effective filtration area, and d = the diameter of a field of view. For statistical particle counting, the particle distribution should be uniform and the quality of particle distribution should be checked by scanning the entire filtration area before attempting to count the particles.

Microscopic techniques utilizing other forms of illumination have been explored. These include vertical illumination, in which the opaque illuminator of a universal polarizing microscope combined with Epilum objectives provides bright-field illumination; transmitted light illumination requiring a cleared membrane substrate; and incident dark-field illumination.

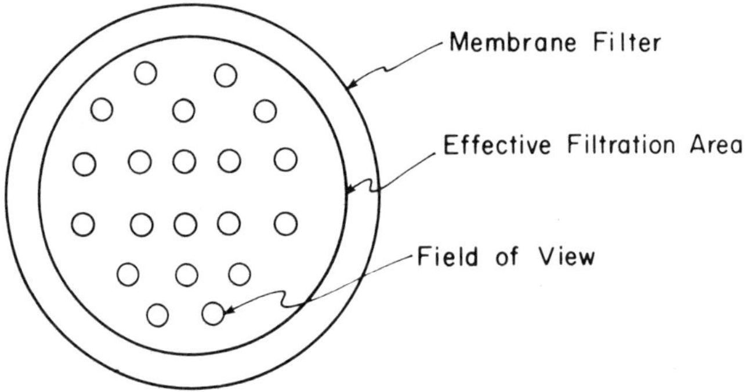

Figure 22 Random selection of fields for statistical counting of particles.

6. *Image Analysis*

Substantial time savings in counting the preparations can be achieved by an automated microscope approach referred to as image analysis. In essence, the microscope view is monitored by a TV camera, and the corresponding signals are analyzed by a computer. This type of equipment, illustrated in Figure 23, is capable of providing a great deal of information about the shape and size parameters of individual particles, including the USP parameter D_O. Although most image analysis equipment is capable of measuring the longest dimension of an individual particle, for convenience particles are often counted on an entire field basis, using the horizontal projection as a sizing parameter (Fig. 24). Since the size measurement will depend on the orientation of the particle, counts based on the horizontal projection D_H will generally be lower than USP counts based on D_O.

7. *Advantages and Disadvantages of Microscopic Approaches*

Microscopic monitoring has the advantage of fixing the particle on a substrate for subsequent viewing and reviewing. Several counts can be made on the same sample by different microscopists. That counting is tedious and time consuming can lead to inaccurate and irreproducible results. For this reason, training in the use of the microscope and microscopic counting is essential. Numerous practice samples should be counted under the guidance of an expert microscopist.

The microscopic approach also offers the advantage of retention of the particles for identification purposes. In many cases the contaminants can

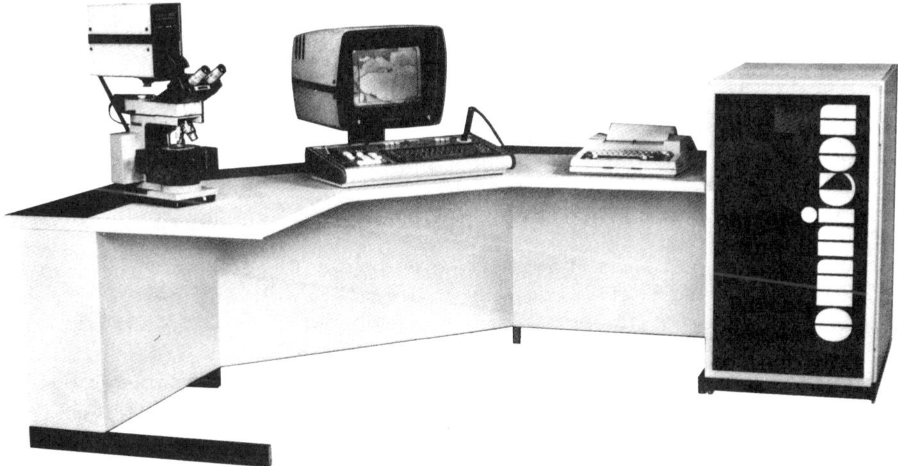

Figure 23 The Milton-Roy Corporation image and analysis system.

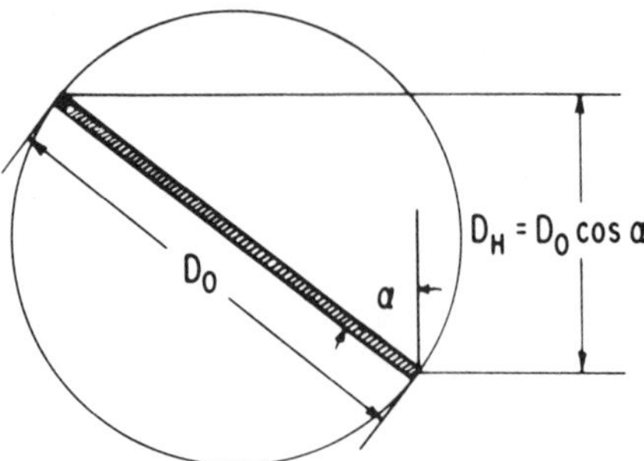

Figure 24 Size determination by horizontal projection. (From Ref. 54, reprinted with permission of the Parenteral Drug Association.)

be recognized on sight by experience, and if not, the particles can be retrieved and subjected to other types of identification analysis. By tracing the source of the contamination, some type of corrective action can be taken. Unlike most instrumental approaches, bubbles do not interfere with counting, but as is the case as well for most instrumental approaches, microscopic analysis is destructive in nature. Almost any sample volume can be adapted to be counted by the microscopic method, but most instruments have a requirement for a minimum volume necessitating dilution.

Most microscopes cost less than automatic counters. If versatility for research purposes or microphotographic equipment is desired for documentation of the contaminants, the cost of the microscope becomes comparable. Automatic image analyzers are much more expensive than elaborate research microscopes and fully automated electronic counters.

B. Automated Methods of Monitoring and Sizing

1. *Principle*

Electronic instruments basically consist of a sensing zone through which the particles pass and generate electrical signals or pulses proportional to the size of the particles. The design or approach to sensing determines the characteristic parameter measured. For most common instruments the pulse is treated in a similar fashion, independent of how the signal was generated. As illustrated in Figure 25, the signal is amplified, then electronically classified by magnitude of threshold setting and eventually displayed if it is of the appropriate magnitude. Figure 26 schematically represents an idealized set of response pulses for a multichannel instrument. Events 1, 4, and 5 would trigger the counter/display of channel 1, events 3 and 7 would be recorded in channel 2, events 2 and 8 in channel 3, and event 6 in channel 4 if the instrument were operated in a differential mode (Table 4 and Fig. 16). In the cumulative mode, channels 1, 2, 3, and 4 would display total counts of 8, 5, 3, and 1, respectively (Table 5 and Fig. 17). To obtain this distribution with a single-channel instrument, the sample would have to be counted four times at the four corresponding sensitivity levels.

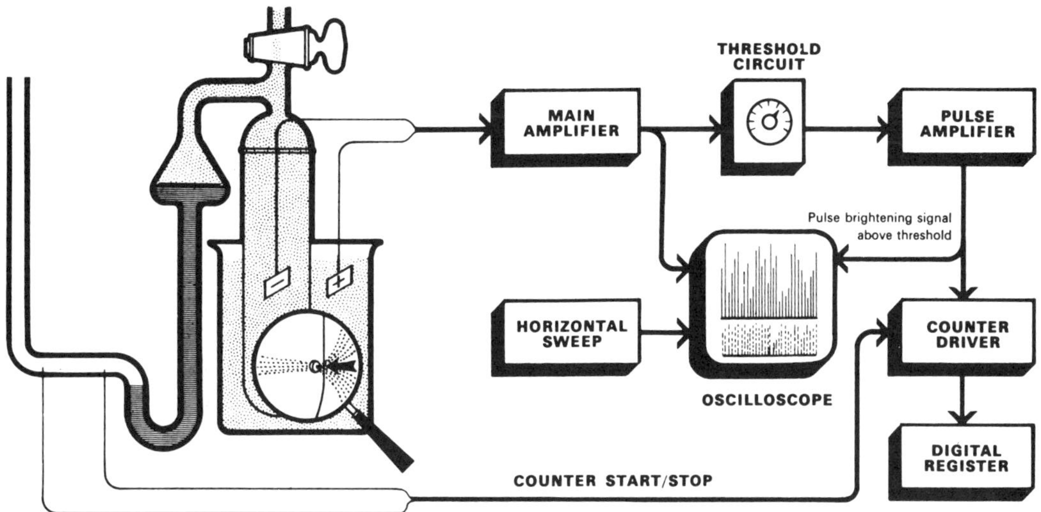

Figure 25 Illustration of the monitoring components of an electronic counter.

2. *Calibration of Electronic Instruments*

The thresholds discussed can be set for infinitely variable sensitivity, but for any of the settings to be meaningful, the response of the instrument has to be calibrated. There are two basic approaches to correlating the pulse magnitude to actual size. The first is theoretical. If the maximum response for a given instrument is known (for instance, total blockage of light for the light blockage approach to be discussed), a partial response can be expressed as a percentage of the maximum response; thus a corresponding percentage of the maximum size can in some cases be attributed

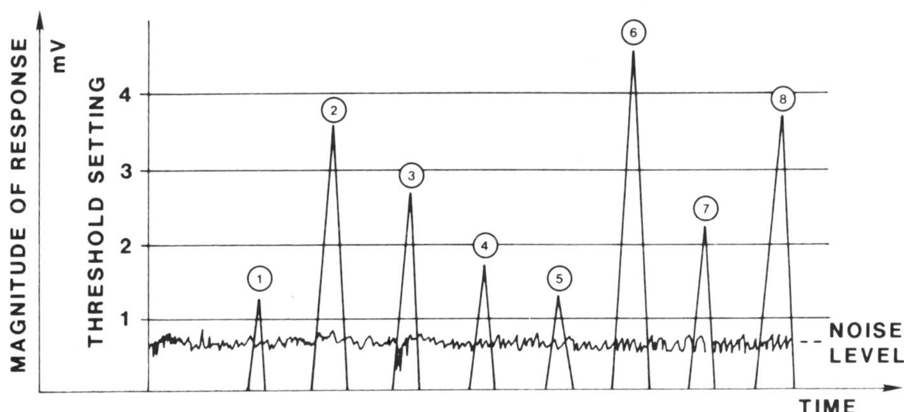

Figure 26 Schematic illustration of the monitoring channels of an electronic counter.

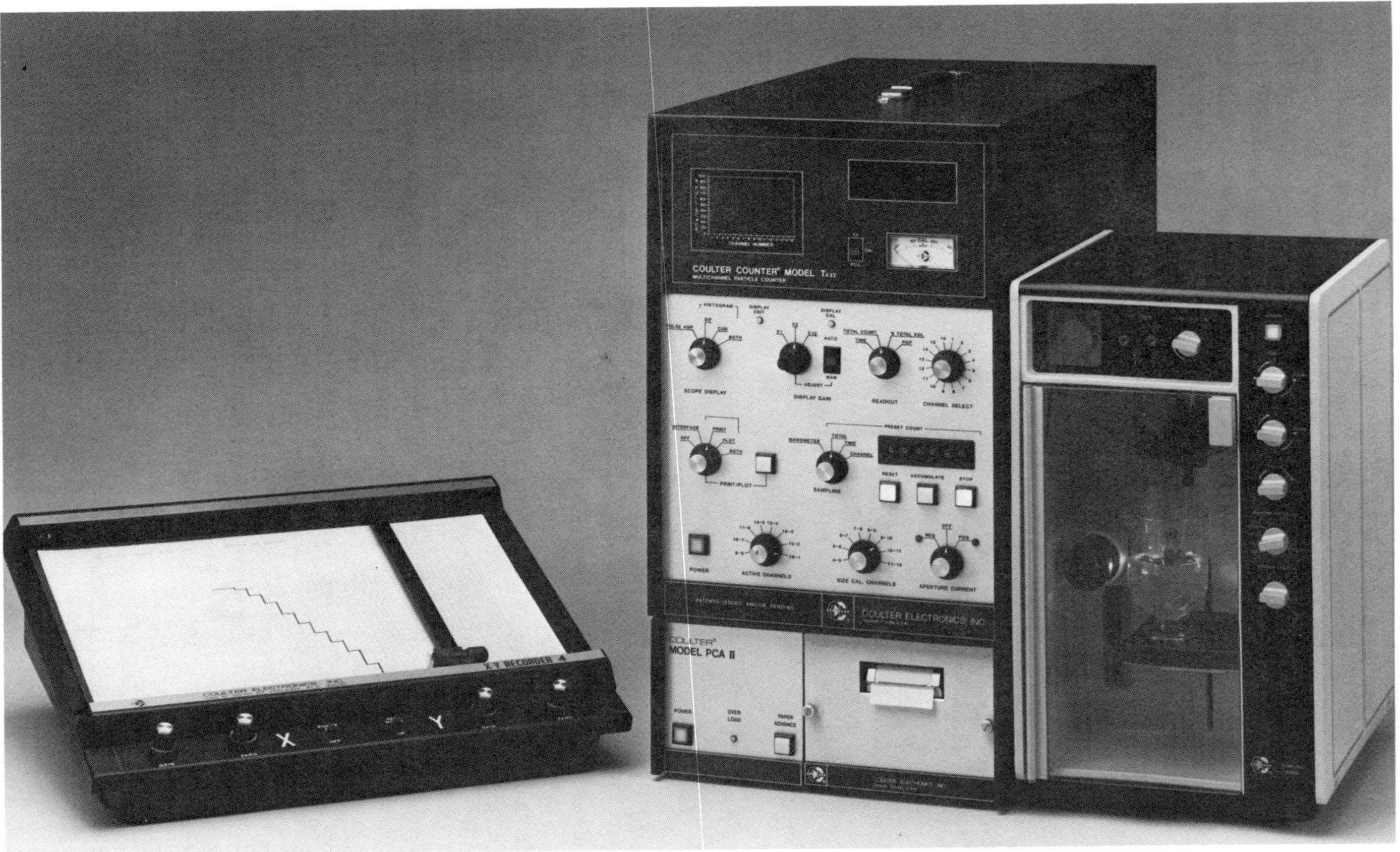

Figure 27 Coulter counter, Model TAII. (Courtesy of Coulter Electronics.)

to a given response. This approach requires the sensors from one instrument to another to be identical and that they will not change with time. This is not possible, and so the supplier adjusts the threshold settings initially and can readjust them periodically. The second is an empirical method, referred to as primary calibration. Particles of known size distribution and total number are exposed to the sensor, and the thresholds are adjusted until the "known" count and distribution are matched. Primary calibration suspensions are commercially available or can be freshly prepared prior to use. Two types of particles are widely used to prepare such suspensions: AC fine test dust and polystyrene or glass beads, also available from the National Bureau of Standards. Suspensions of AC fine test dust have the advantage that they resemble actual contaminants, and suspensions of known concentration (in milligrams per liter) have been shown to exhibit consistent particle counts. To obtain significant particle counts in the size range of 10 μm or larger, a large number of finer particles are invariably present, which could interfere with the proper performance of the instrument. For this reason the use of microspheres is recommended, as these are also easily counted and sized by microscopic methods. Microspheres can be obtained in narrow verifiable size distributions. The size calibration can be accomplished by following the instruction manual for various instruments.

3. *Particulate Matter Monitoring by Electrolytic Displacement*

A schematic of an electrolyte displacement sensor is shown in Figure 25. As the particle enters the sensing zone, it displaces a portion of the electrolyte in the carrier solution, causing a measurable change in the resistance between the two electrodes. This change in resistance is proportional to the volume of the particle. The instrument displays the counts as a function of volume directly or as an option; D_V, the diameter of a sphere of equal volume, can be cleared from the following equation and counts are reported as a function of D_V.

$$\text{Volume observed} = \frac{\pi D_V^3}{6} \tag{5}$$

Figure 27 shows the components of the Coulter Counter, an instrument that operates by electrolytic displacement.

4. *Particulate Matter Monitoring by Light Blockage*

A schematic of a light blockage sensor is shown in Figure 28. The basis for measurement is the reduction of light received by the photocell due to the presence of the particle in the sensing zone. This reduction of light and the consequent measurable drop in the photocell output is proportional to the area of the particle exposed to the light beam. The suspended particle is free to rotate and, due to turbulence, will rotate through all possible orientations. Ideally the instrument will size the particle based on the largest shadow. Rather than reporting counts based on the actual area

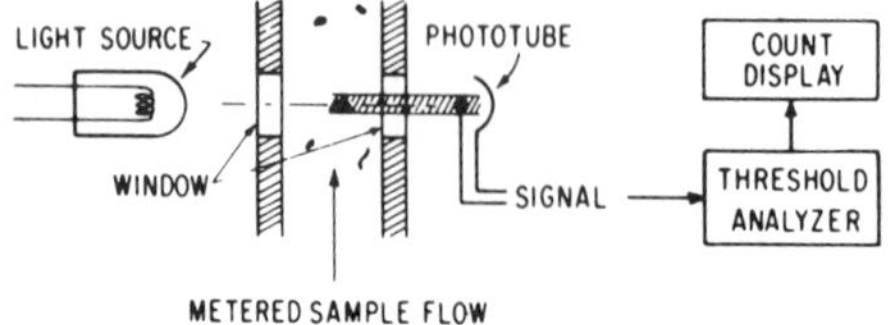

Figure 28 Schematic diagram of a light blockage sensor. (From Ref. 54.)

observed, the instrument clears D_A from the following equation and reports the counts as a function of the diameter of a circle of an area equal to the area observed for the particle in the sensor.

$$\text{Area observed} = \frac{\pi D_A^2}{4} \tag{6}$$

Figure 29 shows the HIAC-Royco Counter, an instrument that operates by light blockage.

5. *Particulate Matter Monitoring by Near Forward Light Scattering*

Light scattering methods are used to monitor airborne aerosols, for which this type of sensor is probably best suited. The approach has been adapted

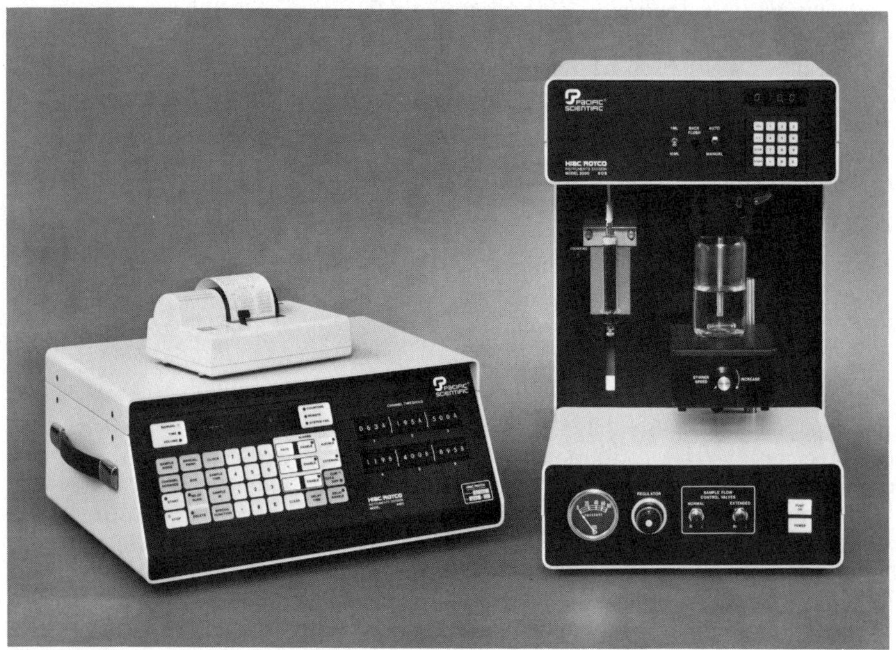

Figure 29 The HIAC-ROYCO counter, Model 3000. (Courtesy HIAC Royco, Inc.)

to solutions and is schematically depicted in Figure 30. This is a nondestructive method in which a laser beam is focused to a point within the sealed container. The contents of the container are agitated by shaking or rapid rotation prior to analysis. Particles in motion within the container will at some time enter the region exposed to the laser beam. The main portion of the beam itself will exit the container and impinge on an opaque absorptive target, but the light scattered by the particle in the near forward direction is collected by a lens focused on a photomultiplier tube. The near forward scattered light will elicit a response from the photomultiplier, and the intensity of this response is proportional mainly to the cross-sectional area of the particle. This approach has been shown to yield reasonable results when carefully selected containers are used, as surface irregularities of the container interfere with focusing and contribute to some degree to the total light scattering.

An innovative concept in the monitoring of particulate matter is the use of pulsed ultrasonic waves. This approach is applicable to in-line monitoring of large process streams, generally water systems. A sensing element imbedded in the wall of a pipe sends out a wave to the opposite wall of the pipe. The return or "echo" signal is detected by the same sensor. If the return wave encounters a particle, the particle echo is detected.

6. *General Advantages and Disadvantages of Instrumental Methods*

Instrumental methods generally provide greater reproducibility of results than microscopic methods. In addition, sample preparation and analysis for instrumental methods is less cumbersome and less time-consuming and the results obtained are not operator dependent. As most instruments monitor or control the sample flow, the results can generally be displayed directly as a concentration without performing additional calculations. Instruments also have shortcomings. First is the dependence on accurate

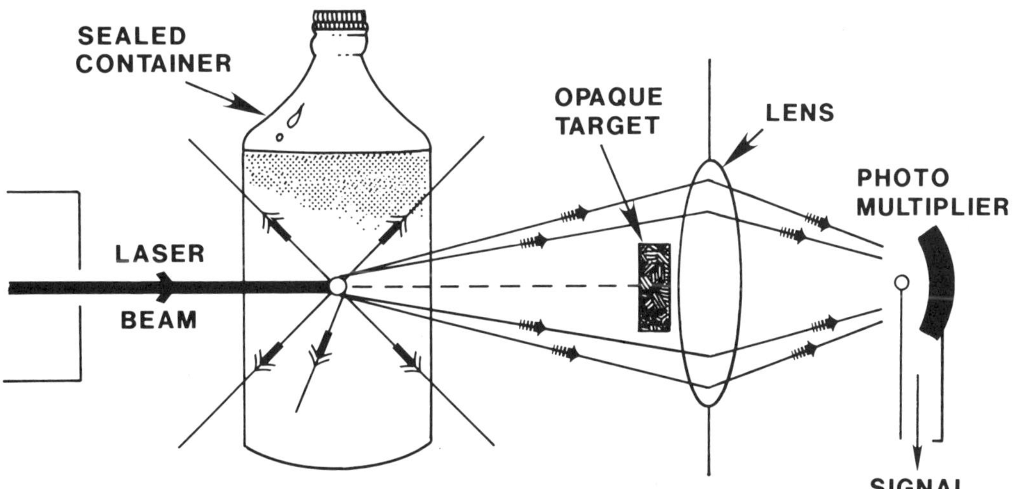

Figure 30 Illustration of a laser instrument using near forward light scattering.

calibration, which if done inaccurately can introduce large counting errors. Most instruments also count bubbles that would be excluded in microscopic evaluations. Generally, analysis is destructive, and instruments lack the identification capabilities of the microscope.

When the particle concentration of a given sample becomes too high, most instruments will give erroneously low results as a consequence of either "coincidence counting" (several smaller particles being recorded as one larger one) or "electronic saturation," the inability of the counter to "keep up" with the incidence rate. These phenomena generally occur at counts of several thousands of particles per milliliter, thus constituting no problem for fluids in which the count is not "allowed" to be over 50 particles per milliliter.

Another disadvantage of instruments is that none will measure D_o, the dimension tested using the USP method. This will result in differences between methods, since the shape of commonly found particles generally differs from the shape of the material used for calibration. The influence of shape of the particles on the sizing by instrumental methods has been treated [54]. Since the instrumental methods based on light blockage and electrolytic displacement converts the parameter measured to a diameter of a circle of equivalent area or of a sphere of equivalent volume, then for nonspherical particles the measurement will be less than that obtained microscopically. For example, a rod-shaped particle with a 10:1 length-width ratio will have a longest linear dimension equal to 10L. By light blockage, the particle will be sized as 3.57L, and by electrolytic displacement, 2.47L. On the basis of these geometric considerations, it is difficult to understand why the British Pharmacopeia allows for fewer particles when using light blockage compared with that when using electrolytic displacement (Table 2). Considering the example of a rod with a 10:1 length-width ratio, a particle sized as 10 μm by light blockage would be sized at 7 μm by electrolytic displacement.

VI. IDENTIFICATION OF PARTICULATE MATTER

Guidelines for the routine identification of particulates in parenterals have been developed. These have been published in detail elsewhere [10]. However, this chapter will cover the highlights of the guidelines and comment on their application.

In any type of particle identification work, it is important to stress that, although this area has emerged as both a science and an art, a great deal of information has been compiled in the *Particle Atlas* in six illustrative volumes, all of which should be used as reference sources (Fig. 31) [55]. Additionally, the facilities required for particulate identification should be sufficient to prevent extraneous particles from contaminating the samples under investigation, and appropriate validation procedures of the various steps of the identification process should be performed to verify the absence of extraneous contamination.

A. Facilities and Clean Room Equipment

A laminar-flow hood should be used for sample filtration and preparation and at least a class 10,000 clean room for optical microscopy. The clean room should be air-conditioned and of sufficient space to accommodate a

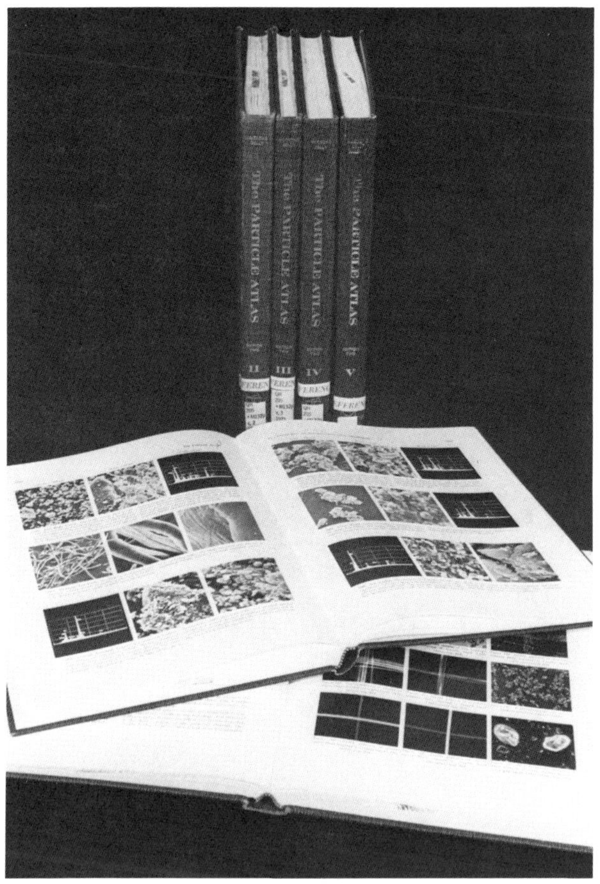

Figure 31 *Particle Atlas* as a reference source.

work station, two microscopes and other accessories (Fig. 32). A stereo-binocular microscope and a polarizing compound microscope equipped for transmitted and incident illumination, with photomicrography capabilities, are essential. A hot-stage, reference file of known particles, chemical reagents for performing microchemical tests, refractive index oils, universal illuminators, tungsten needles, and assorted devices for particle handling are also required in the clean room. Various filtration equipment and glassware are required for particle isolation and transfer, operations that should be carried out in a laminar-flow hood in close proximity to the clean room.

B. Validation Procedures

During the various steps of the identification process, extraneous particles could contaminate the particulate samples. It is therefore essential to validate procedures for filtration, sampling, and particle handling.

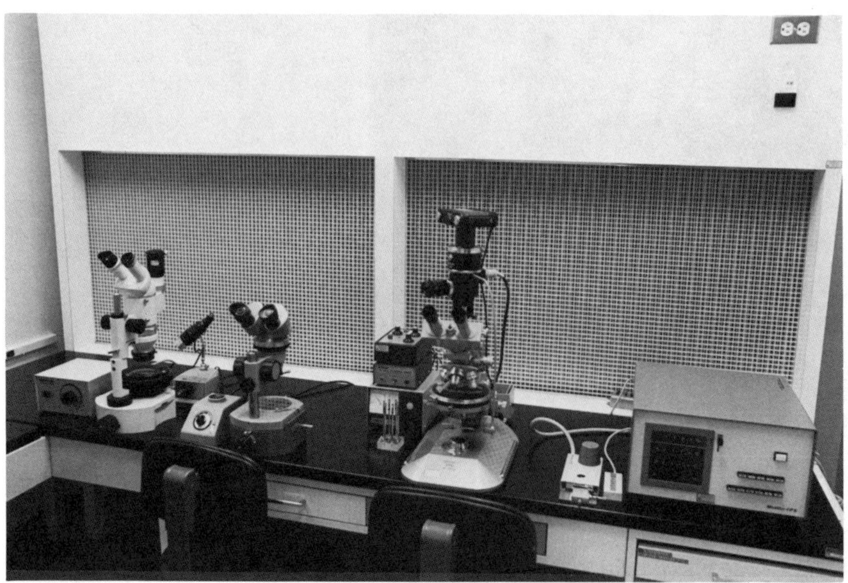

Figure 32 Work station for microscopes. (Courtesy University of Kentucky, College of Pharmacy, Lexington, Kentucky.)

C. Validation of Filtration

The cleaning procedures for filtration equipment and glassware can be validated along with the filtration procedure. At least three filtration blanks should be prepared using ultraclean water. (Ultraclean water refers to distilled water containing not more than 10 particles $\geq$ 10 μm per 10 ml.) The procedure for preparing the blanks should be the same as that for filtering samples, and the filter blanks when viewed microscopically should not contain more than 5 particles $\geq$ 25 μm.

A more stringent validation of the filtration procedure and setup would be to filter a suspension of known particles and then examine the filtrate for the absence of these particulates.

D. Validation of the Sampling Procedure

Often the outside of a parenteral container is contaminated with fibrous materials, environmental contaminants, skin flakes, and components of the label paste. These contaminants result from the repeated handling of the container following the aseptic operation. It has been found that the water rinse or an alcohol wipe does not guarantee removal of these contaminants, especially skin flakes. However, a wash with a warm detergent solution prior to water and alcohol rinses will effectively remove the skin flakes as well as the other contaminants. To validate the cleaning of the containers prior to sampling the contents, it is necessary to fill clean containers with ultraclean water and seal under laminar-flow conditions. Such containers are then subjected to routine nonaseptic handling and deliberately contaminated. Following contamination with known particles, the washing and sampling procedures are then performed and filtration blanks are prepared. The absence of particles used to contaminate the exterior of the containers validates the washing and sampling procedures.

E. Validating the Isolation of Particles

The procedure for selecting particles from a filter membrane and transferring the particles to a glass slide or a stub for scanning electron microscopy must also be validated. The glass slide or SEM stub should be prepared by the appropriate technique and at least 20 polystyrene microspheres or other known particles transferred from a membrane to the glass slide or SEM stub using a tungsten needle. The absence of foreign particles on the glass slide or the SEM stub validates the particle transfer process.

VII. PROCEDURES FOR PARTICLE SAMPLING

A. Equipment Precleaning and Preparation

All glassware should be washed in an ultraclean bath with warm detergent solution, rinsed, and allowed to dry in the laminar-flow hood. The membrane filter should be cleaned on both surfaces. The bottom side can be cleaned by letting it overfloat briefly on a layer of ultraclean water on the filter holder base (Fig. 33a). Then, rinse the upper side with ultraclean water while holding the membrane filter in place on the filter holder base with the aid of a forceps (Fig. 33b). Position the membrane filter on the base with the glossy side up. Apply the vacuum, and clamp the clean filtration funnel on the base (Fig. 33c). This should be done in such a manner as not to slide the funnel over the membrane surface. Once assembled, the filtration unit can be removed from the filtration flask for a final rinsing. Invert the funnel, and rinse the inside with ultraclean water (Fig. 33d). Then return the funnel to the collection flask.

B. Preparation and Counting Filtration Blanks

Blanks should be counted as soon as possible prior to sample filtration in order to verify the efficiency of the cleaning procedures. For each of two blanks, an appropriate volume of ultraclean water is filtered. Care should be exercised to avoid transferring the solution directly on the filter surface and to allow turbulence in the filter funnel to dissipate before the vacuum is applied. Following filtration, the filter is removed with forceps and transferred to a glass slide for observation and counting at about 150X magnification. If more than 5 particles ≥ 25 μm are found on either of the blank filters, the cleaning procedures must be repeated.

C. Sampling Various Product Types and Filtration

The procedures described in the monitoring section should be followed.

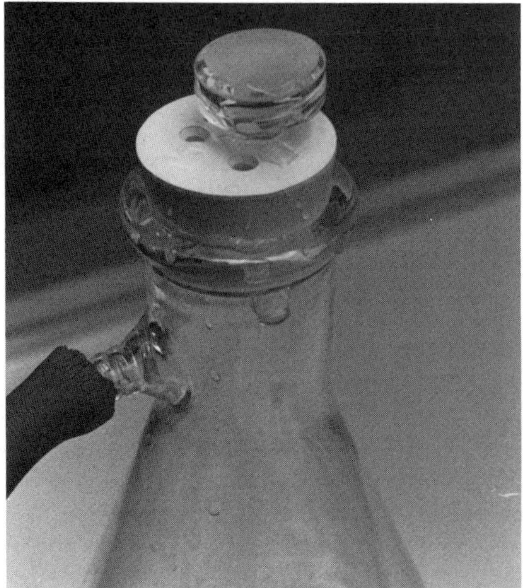

(a)

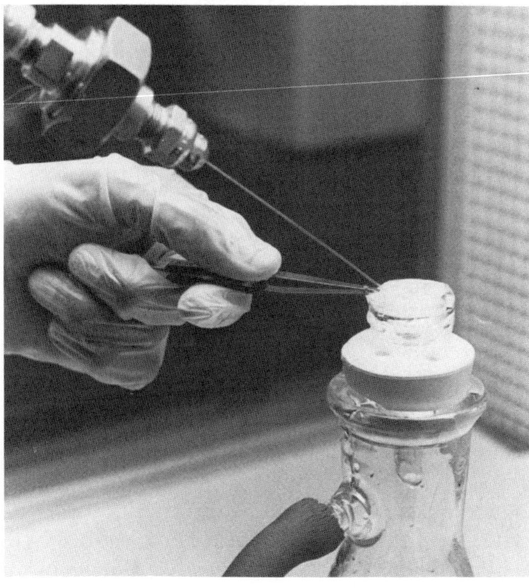

(b)

Figure 33 Cleaning of membrane filter and filtration assembly: (a) cleaning bottom side of the filter, (b) rinsing top side of the filter, (c) assembled unit, and (d) final rinsing of the funnel and filter.

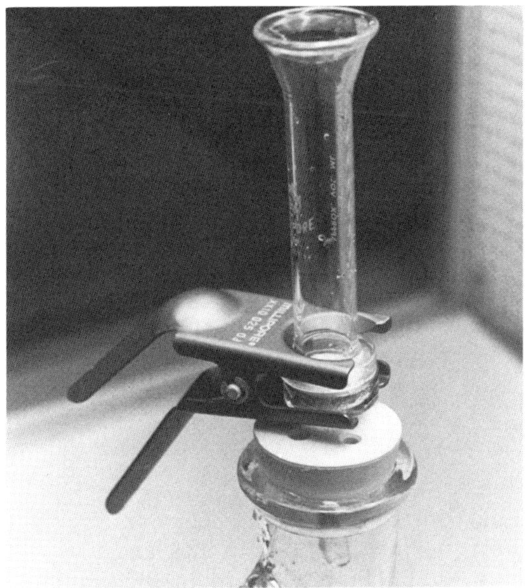

(c)

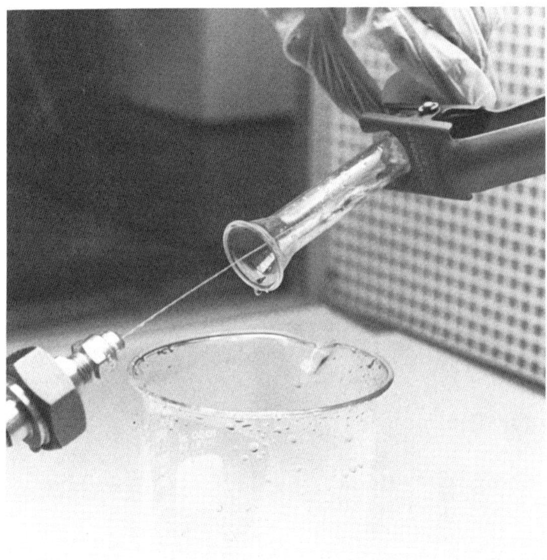

(d)

Figure 33 (continued)

VIII. PARTICULATE ISOLATION AND HANDLING

A. Mounting Media

Although particles can be examined microscopically without being immersed in a mounting medium because of the difference in refractive index between air and the particles, high-viscosity liquids are commonly used to disperse particles so that they can be microscopically examined individually and their refractive index determined. Such liquids are also employed for preparing permanent mounts for later reference. The mounting medium should not dissolve any portion of the particles being analyzed, and its refractive index must differ from that of the particles by at least 0.2 units so that the particles can exhibit distinctive refraction and reflection effects. The most common mounting media used in optical microscopy are listed in Table 6.

B. Tools for Particle Handling

Special fine tools and materials, such as tungsten needles, micropipets, glass flakes, and coverslips, refractive index oils, and solvents are required to manipulate small particles. Tungsten needles come in different sizes to facilitate transfer of subvisible particles from one location to another under the microscope, often from one microscope to another. Flexible polyethylene micropipets are used to deliver tiny droplets of liquid onto the surface of the microscope slide. For refractive index determination, glass flakes, small coverslips, and membrane filter triangles are custom-made materials used with calibrated mixed liquids whose refractive indices and temperature coefficients are known. Three solvents most often needed in the manipulation of particles are collodion, redistilled amyl acetate, and double-distilled water. Collodion is used to mount the particles in a film. Water is used to float the collodion film off a surface, and amyl acetate is required to dissolve such films in order to recover the particles.

Table 6 Common Mounting Media for Particulates

Compound	Refractive index (n_D^{25})
Viscous mounting media	
Glycerol	1.47
Mineral oil	1.47
Canada balsam	1.53
Aroclor 1260[a]	1.64
Permanent mounting media	
Collodion	1.52
Aroclor 5442[a]	1.66

[a]Available from McCrone Associates, Chicago, IL.

C. Isolation of Particles

Once the particles have been collected by filtration, isolation of single particles or groups of particles is necessary to study the particles microscopically. Those particles that appear to be similar upon initial microscopic examination are transferred in groups while viewing under the compound microscope to a glass slide positioned on the stage of the stereomicroscope. Once this is accomplished, the isolated particles can be viewed under the compound microscope or can be further separated. Additionally, they can be mounted in collodion and amyl acetate for further analysis. Single-particle isolation is shown in Figure 34. A drop of collodion in amyl acetate (about 0.5 mm in diameter) is transferred on the tip of a tungsten needle to the filter and spread over the particle. Once the collodion dries, the thin film containing the particles can be lifted with a tungsten needle and transferred to a clean glass slide. By placing a small drop of amyl acetate on the glass slide next to the collodion film containing the particle, the collodion can be softened with the tip of the tungsten needle, thereby thinning out the mixture. By this procedure, the particle is embedded in a clear collodion film, allowing its microscopic examination by transmitted polarized light.

D. Scanning Electron Microcopy/Energy Dispersive X-ray Analysis

Aluminum stubs coated with graphite are used for the SEM/EDXRA analysis. A thin membrane (0.8 μm polycarbonate), marked with two indentations, is fixed onto the stub (Fig. 35) and coated with a thin layer of 10% collodion solution in amyl acetate. The indentations facilitate the retrieval of the different types of particles which will be placed on the filter. The Type I particles represent a predominant type. Less numerous types are grouped as Types II and III. Type IV designates a random selection of particles. At least 5 particles of each type are transferred and approximately 10

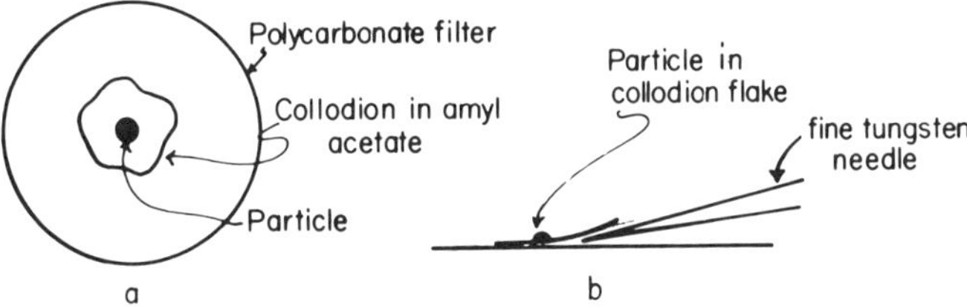

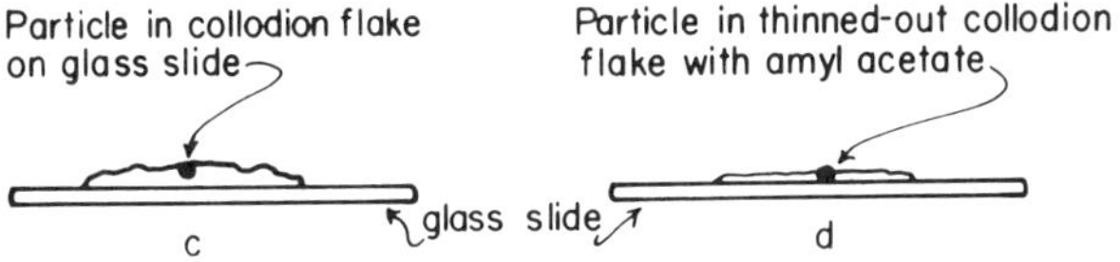

Figure 34 Isolation of a single particle.

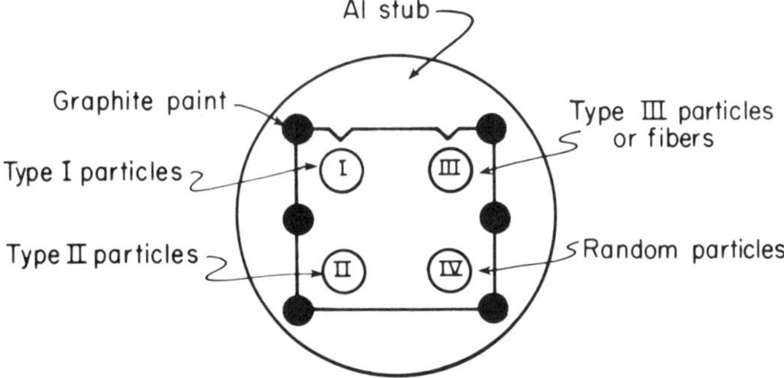

Figure 35 Location of particle types on SEM stub.

particles are randomly selected from pre-determined locations on the filter. The particles can be anchored by placing a small drop of methanol near each particle. As the methanol spreads, collodion from the coating travels with it to the particle and effectively holds the particles in place when the methanol evaporates. Following confirmation of the location of the particles on the stub by photomicrography, the stub is prepared for SEM/EDXRA study. Prior to EDXRA analysis the location of the particles is verified, a photograph taken and the particles labeled (Fig. 36). Photomicrographs of each particle are taken at the appropriate magnification which will permit observation of the surface characteristics.

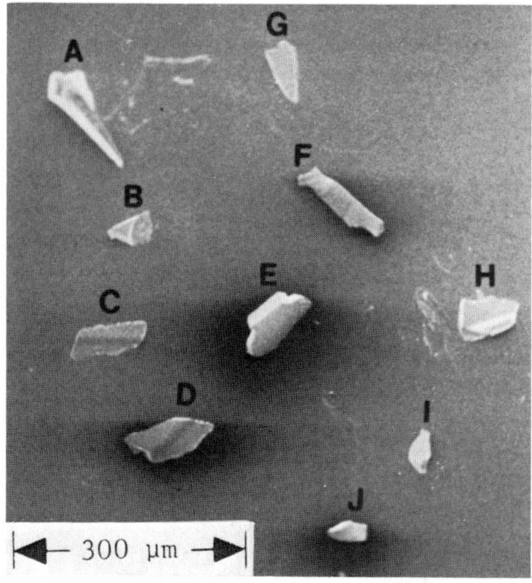

Figure 36 Labeling particles on SEM micrographs.

E. Preparation of Particles for Micro X-ray Powder Diffraction

Diffraction patterns can be obtained from either single crystals or a powder mixture. If x-ray diffraction data for a given compound have been determined and tabulated, then subsequent samples of that compound can be identified by comparison of the measured data with the tabulation. The ASTM data file lists powder diffraction data for over 20,000 compounds. Samples as small as 20 ng (6 particles for about 15 μm diameter) can be analyzed by x-ray powder diffraction. For samples containing fewer particles, diffraction patterns can be obtained only with prolonged exposure time. The diffraction lines on the x-ray film are measured and converted to the diffraction angles and d spacings using the Bragg equation:

$$n\lambda = 2d \sin \theta \tag{7}$$

where n = an integer, θ = wavelength of the x-rays, d = interplanar spacings, and λ = diffraction angle. The relative intensity of the diffraction lines is estimated, and the d spacings and their relative intensity pertaining to the unknown particles are then compared to those reported for substances suspected to be identical to the unknown sample. For utilization of the Bragg equation and the measurement of d spacings from diffraction lines, the reader is recommended to other texts [55,56].

F. Measurement of Refractive Index

The refractive index of any small particle may be determined microscopically by successively immersing the particle in liquids of known refractive indices until, in one such liquid, the particles become invisible. In this case, the refractive index of the invisible particle is identical to that of the liquid medium. In microscopical immersion methods, the liquid medium whose refractive index matches that of a given particle must be found empirically by trial and error. Since the procedure is described in detail elsewhere [10, 57,58], along with a method for recovering the particle, it will not be repeated here. However, two tests that expedite the matching process are by the central illumination method, commonly called the Becke test, and the oblique illumination method. Both procedures will identify whether the index of a given liquid medium is greater or less than that of a particle immersed therein. The procedure illustrated in Figure 37 can be used for determining refractive index.

G. Melting Point Determinations

Using a Mettler hot stage equipped with a hot stage controller permits, in addition to the determination of melting points, purity determinations, mixture analysis, composite diagram determination, polymorphism, and others. Using programmed heating rates, the phase changes preceding melting can be observed microscopically.

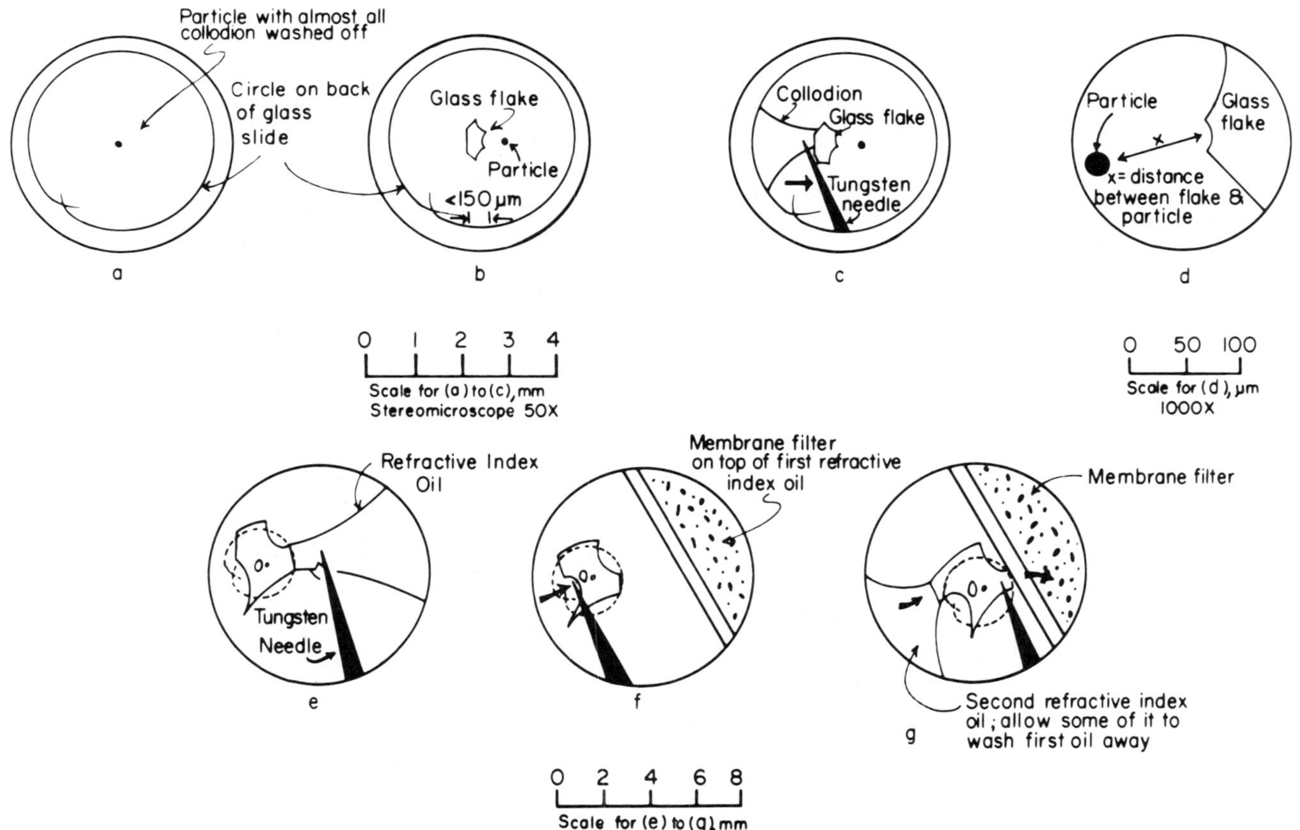

Figure 37 Mounting single particle for refractive index measurement. (From *Particle Atlas*, Vol. 1, p. 256.)

IX. PARTICLE IDENTIFICATION AND CHARACTERIZATION

A. Polarizing Microscopy

The physical and optical properties of particles are determined with a polarizing microscope. Such properties as shape, size, color, presence or absence of birefringence, and refractive index serve as identifying characteristics. A glossary of terms is necessary to describe the particles. For example, in describing the appearance, the particle can be a flake, which is a thin flattened particle, or a plate, which is also flattened but not as thin as a flake. When particles are thick and elongated, they are described as rods or small lumps. Chips are flat, smooth particles that are generally thinner and smaller than flakes or plates. The surface texture is important. The surface can be glassy, smooth, porous, or rough. The luster can be characteristic. A metallic luster is characteristic of metals in the compact state, adamantine is similar to that of diamond, vitreous resembles that of glass, resinous is similar to that of resins, greasy is seemingly unctuous, and silky resembles that of silk.

To describe and catalogue particles, a form similar to Table 7 should be used. The properties of two particle types are listed in the form. The use of such a form permits easy recording of data and serves to remind the analyst of all the observations that should be performed.

Table 7 Optical Properties Used to Classify Particle Types

Property	Type I[a]	Type II[b]
Estimated % by number	90	10
Shape and appearance	Polyhedral to subspherical grains	Irregular plates
Aggregation	None	None
Homogeneity	Homogeneous	Homogeneous
Surface texture	Smooth	Smooth
Transparency	Transparent	Opaque
Color-transmitted light	Colorless	Black
Color-reflected light	Colorless	White
Luster	Vitreous	Metallic
Brilliance	Glimmering	Dull
Pleochroism	None	None
Birefringence	Well-marked black crosses	None
Refractive index	1.5314	—
Solubility in 6 N HNO_3	Insoluble	Insoluble
Melting point	>300°C	>300°C

[a]Starch grains.
[b]Stainless steel.

To determine whether transparent particles are birefringent or isotropic, the particles are viewed between crossed polars. In this condition, isotropic substances become extinct; birefringent particles exhibit only four extinction positions, which are 90° apart. In other positions of the stage rotation, the birefringent particles remain with characteristic polarization colors.

Most of the identifying characteristics depend on the experience and ability of the microscopist for deciding on the exact nature of the particles being observed. Through experience with different types of particles, an increasing ability will develop in recognizing the identity of unknown particles. At least, a broad understanding of the morphological features of the unknown particles permits narrowing down the possible identity to a few substances.

In this recall of past experience, it is essential to have a collection of optical data of various substances, such as the *Particle Atlas*. The microscopist should attempt to solve the identification problem in terms of differentiating properties. For example, fragments of quartz and ground glass have the same appearance but different properties. Another example of similar morphology is that of corn starch and wheat starch. However, corn starch is polygonal, and between crossed polars, the crosses are perpendicular, but for wheat starch the grain is oval with the crosses shaped like two Ys joined in line at the tails.

B. SEM/EDXRA

The scanning electron microscope gives a topographical picture of small particles. Such information as particle size, shape, texture, and topography of the surface of the particulate sample can be obtained by this technique. In addition, agglomeration and purity can be detected directly, and the elemental composition can also be determined through the use of energy dispersive x-ray analysis (EDXRA).

Such features as conchoidal fracture, crystal habit, porosity, size, shape, and surface texture of the particle, which are observable in light microscopy, are also discernible through SEM. In addition, the microstructure of metals and the porosity of materials are more easily assessed by SEM. EDXRA involves the ionization of atoms in the particle by high-energy electrons and the resultant emission of characteristic x-rays from the elements present. The EDXRA directly measures the energy of the incident x-rays and presents the data as a spectrum of intensity versus energy. X-rays of all energies are detected simultaneously for elements of atomic number 12 or greater, so that a complete spectrum is obtained at once (Fig. 38). The EDXRA spectra for elements with atomic number less than 11 cannot be obtained because the energy of the x-rays is too low. Because of the depth of field and improved magnification and resolutions, micrographs of small particles obtained with the SEM provide greater morphological detail than the light microscope. In addition, the SEM equipped with an EDXRA attachment allows the semiquantitative determination of the elemental composition of even tiny particles. This elemental composition can differentiate the nature of two materials that possess the same morphological features, such as quartz and glass dust. However, the EDXRA spectrum of quartz contains only Si but that of ground glass usually contains Na, Al, Si, and Ca. Tables 8 and 9 list examples of particles identified by optical microscopy and SEM/EDXRA.

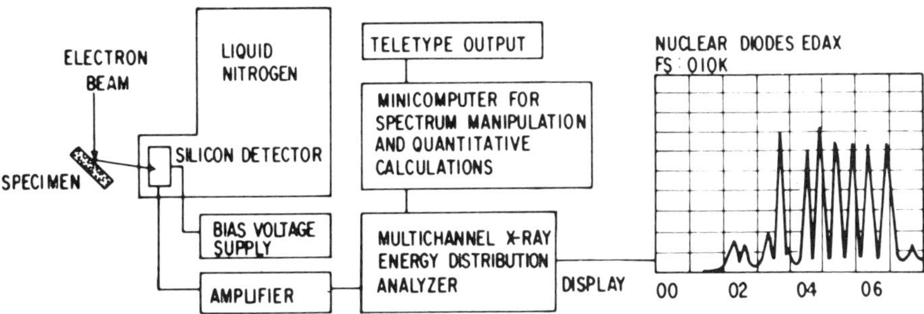

Figure 38 Diagram of energy dispersive x-ray analysis system.

C. Micro X-ray Powder Diffraction

Nearly every compound shows one or more metastable crystalline forms, each with distinctive properties. Diamond and graphite are identical chemically but easily differentiated by x-ray diffraction. Quartz and cristobalite are different forms of silica. Calcite and aragonite are both calcium carbonate. Using x-ray powder diffraction, the observed diffraction angles of a crystal can be converted to the values of interplanar spacings of the atoms in the crystal from the Bragg equation (7).

Through these procedures, crystalline materials can be identified. For example, crystals from a number of parenteral products were isolated and identified by optical microscopy, scanning electron microscopy, and energy dispersive x-ray analysis to be $BaSO_4$. X-ray powder diffraction conclusively confirmed the identification (see Table 10).

D. Other Microanalytical Methods

The transmission electron microscope (TEM) can be used to investigate particles when a greater depth of field and greater depth of focus are required. TEM makes use of electromagnetic waves of high-energy electrons [5]. The electrons of short wavelengths are diffracted through the particles and provide patterns similar to those obtained for x-ray diffraction. Microchemical tests under the light microscope can aid in the identification of small particles. Microchemical tests are best used to check specific entities, the preliminary identity of which has been arrived at by instrumental analytic methods. Additionally, confirmation requires the use of reference standards. The most generally useful microchemical tests are based on the morphology of precipitates formed by adding a reagent to an aqueous solution of the sample. In the sphere of inorganic qualitative analysis, the system developed by Chamot and Mason [59] is quite extensive.

In the realm of organic qualitative analysis, microchemical tests have been developed specifically for drug substances [60]. Another publication oriented toward organic compounds in general is the English translation of Behrens and Kley [61], which gives the conditions and results of organic reactions performed under the microscope.

Recently, a micro-Raman spectrometer (Microprobe MOLE, Instruments SA, Inc., Metuchin, NJ) became commercially available that can provide the composition of the particulate sample at the molecular scale. The sample

Table 8 Examples of Specific Identifying Characteristics

Substance	Identifying characteristics[a]
Glass	Glassy surface texture; equant shape, conchoidal fracture, transparent, sharp edges; refractive index ∿1.489 (Fig. 39a)
Corn starch grains	Polyhedral to subspherical grains, 8–15 μm in diameter; transparent, smooth surface texture; birefringent with characteristic black crosses between crossed polars; refractive index about 1.53 (Fig. 40a)
Stainless steel	Shape of thin flake; smooth surface texture; opaque under transmitted light and reflecting under incident light; metallic luster (Fig. 41a)
Rubber	Shape of irregular lumps; rough surface texture; opaque under transmitted light; resinous luster (Fig. 42a)
Coating of rubber closure	Irregular, translucent flakes; birefringent inclusions between crossed polars; different melting behavior of various portions of the particle mass (Fig. 43a)
Metallic mercury	Shape of liquid drops; when two or three particles are brought together with a sharp tungsten needle under a microscope, they readily mix with one another and form a single spherical particle; look opaque under transmitted light and black with a white spot in the center under incident vertical light (Fig. 44a)
Calcium sulfate dihydrate	Colorless, transparent, equant chips (Fig. 45a), exhibit birefringence under crossed polars; x-ray powder diffraction lines match those reported for calcium sulfate dihydrate crystals
Barium sulfate	Single or agglomerated well-formed, birefringent crystals of 8–30 μm in maximum linear dimension with symmetrical edges and smooth surfaces (Fig. 46a); x-ray powder diffraction lines match those reported for barium sulfate crystals

[a]For photomicrographs and descriptions of other particles, such as diatoms, pine pollen, cotton, Dacron (polyester), and asbestos fibers, the reader is referred to the *Particle Atlas*, Volume II.

Table 9 Examples of Particulate Samples That Can Be Identified by SEM/EDXRA Data

Substance	Identifying characteristics[a]
Glass	Glassy surface texture; equant shape, conchoidal fracture, sharp edges; EDXRA spectrum: Na, Al, *Si*, Cl, K, Ca, Ba (Fig. 39b and c)
Corn starch	Polyhedral to subspherical grains with smooth surface; EDXRA spectrum shows no major elements (Fig. 40b and c)
Stainless steel	Smooth surface texture; polished surface; platy shape; EDXRA spectrum: Cr, *Fe*, Ni (Fig. 41 b and c)
Rubber	Heterogeneous and rough texture; amorphous topography; EDXRA spectrum: Zn, *Al*, *Si*, S, Cl, K, Ba (Fig. 42b and c)
Coating of rubber closure	Rough surface texture, resinous luster; EDXRA spectrum shows a composition of Zn, Al, *Si*, S, Cl, K, Cu; the particles obtained by lightly scraping a rubber closure also have the same composition (Fig. 43b and c)
Metallic mercury	Spherical globules with smooth surface texture; EDXRA spectrum: characteristic peaks at 2.20, 9.99, and 11.82 keV (Fig. 44b and c)
Calcium sulfate dihydrate	Well-formed crystals with constant interfacial angles; EDXRA spectrum: a strong signal of *Ca* and *S* (Fig. 45b and c)
Barium sulfate	Well-formed crystals showing constant interfacial angles; smooth surface texture; EDXRA spectrum: a strong signal of *Ba* and *S* (Fig. 46b and c)

[a]For SEM micrographs and EDXRA spectra on asbestos fibers, the reader is referred to the *Particle Atlas*, Volume III.

to be analyzed is mounted on an ordinary microscope slide and illuminated by a laser beam. Molecular analysis of a specific particle within the sample area under microscopic examination can be determined by its Raman spectrum. This analytic methodology, which allows the qualitative localization of organic, inorganic, and biological samples at a microscopic scale, is based on an elastic scattering process by the molecules. Raman scattering requires a change in the molecular polarizability, and therefore molecules possessing a significant amount of symmetry will be Raman active.

By Raman spectroscopy, barium sulfate crystals have been characterized [8]. The spectra of $BaSO_4$ particles isolated from a parenteral product (Fig. 47a) and of known $BaSO_4$ crystals (Fig. 47b) exhibit characteristic peaks at 450 (455), 988, and 1135 cm^{-1}. The application of micro-Raman spectroscopy to the analysis of discrete fine particles (as small as 0.7 μm

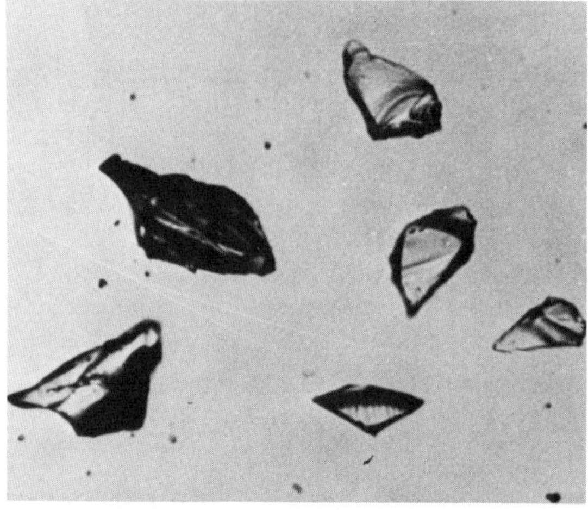

(a)

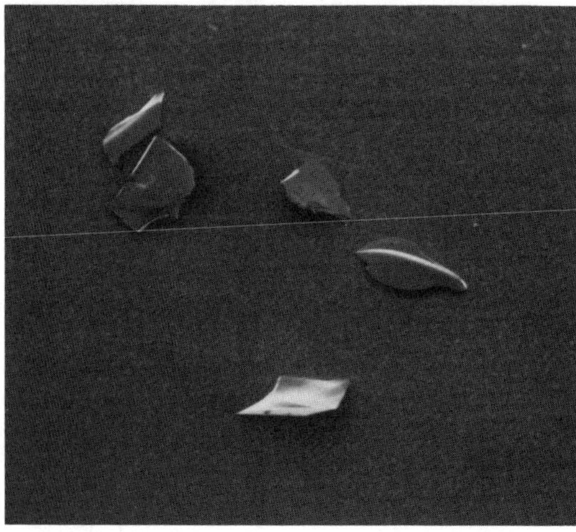

(b)

Figure 39 (a) Optical micrograph, (b) SEM micrograph, and (c) EDXRA spectrum of glass particles.

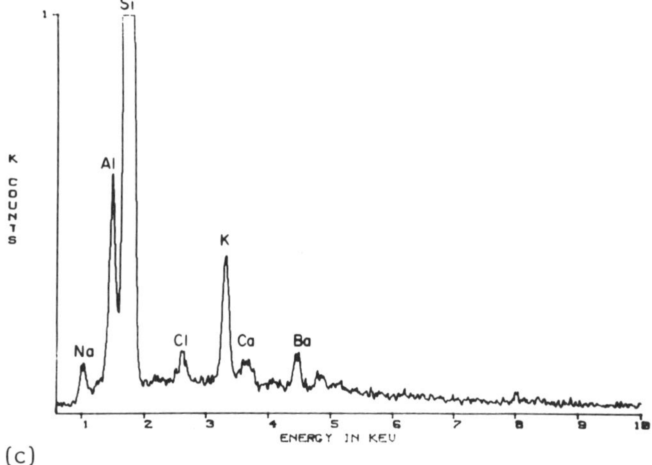

(c)

Figure 39 (continued)

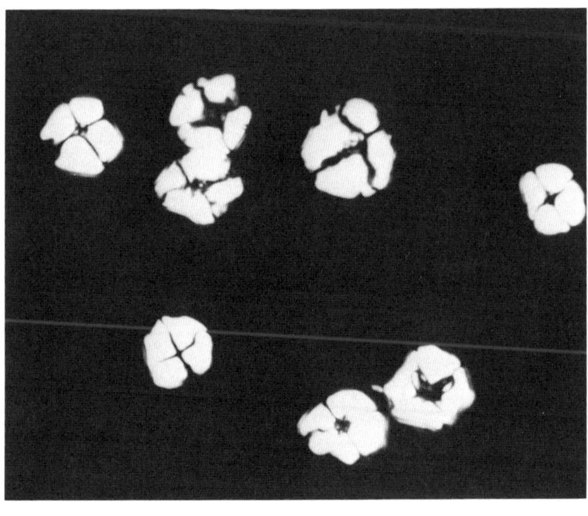

(a)

Figure 40 (a) Optical micrograph, (b) SEM micrograph, and (c) EDXRA spectrum of cornstarch.

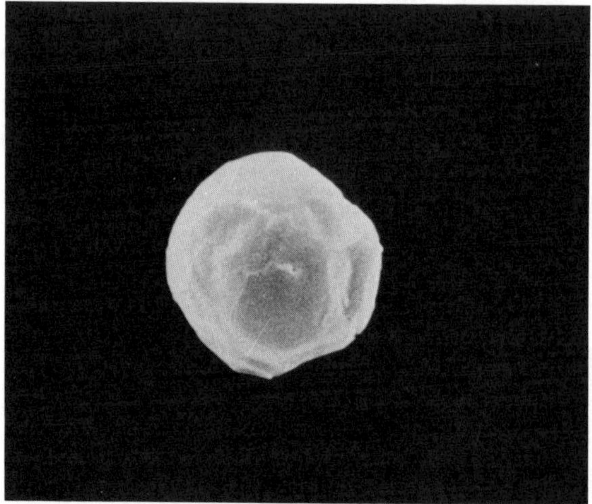

(b)

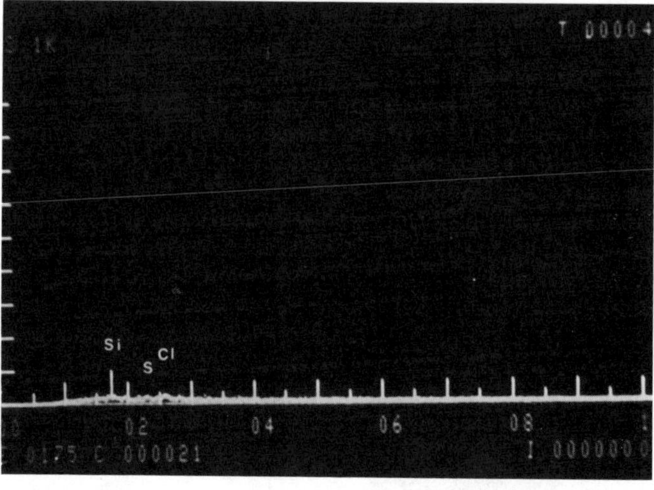

(c)

Figure 40 (continued)

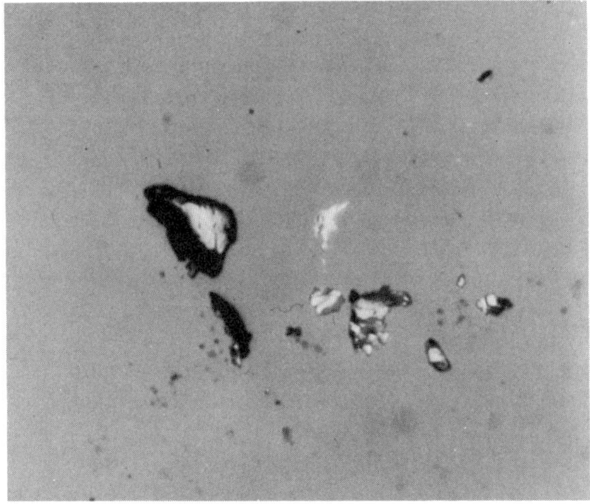

(a)

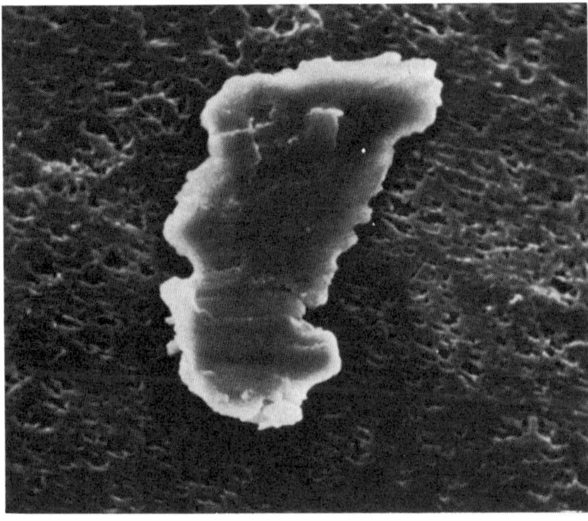

(b)

Figure 41 (a) Optical micrograph, (b) SEM micrograph, and (c) EDXRA spectrum of stainless steel.

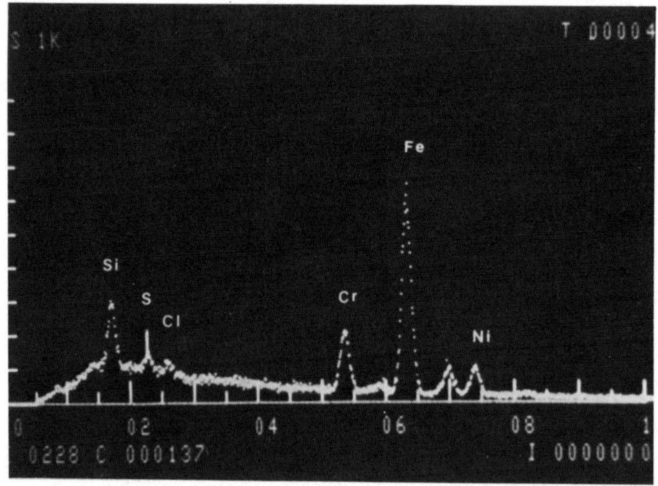

(c)

Figure 41 (continued)

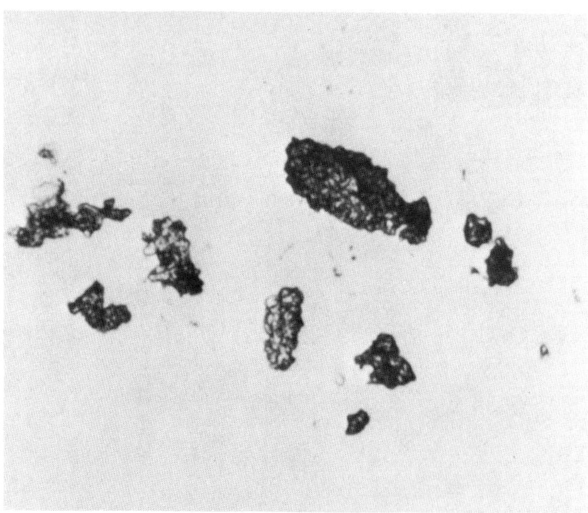

(a)

Figure 42 (a) Optical micrograph, (b) SEM micrograph, and (c) EDXRA spectrum of rubber.

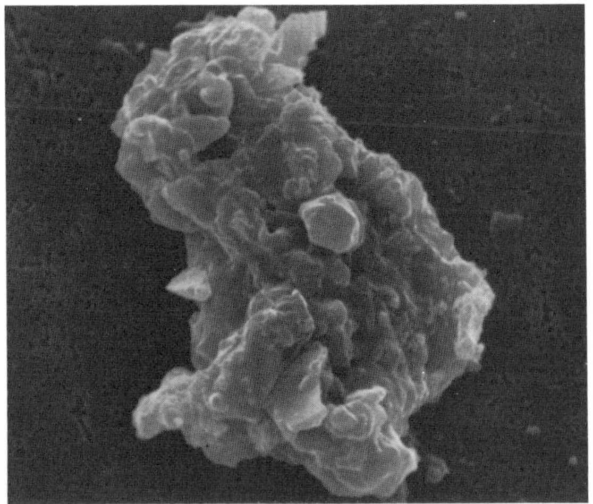

(b)

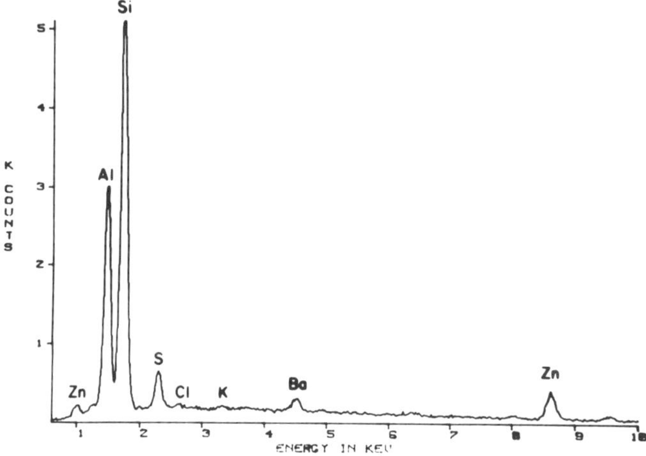

(c)

Figure 42 (continued)

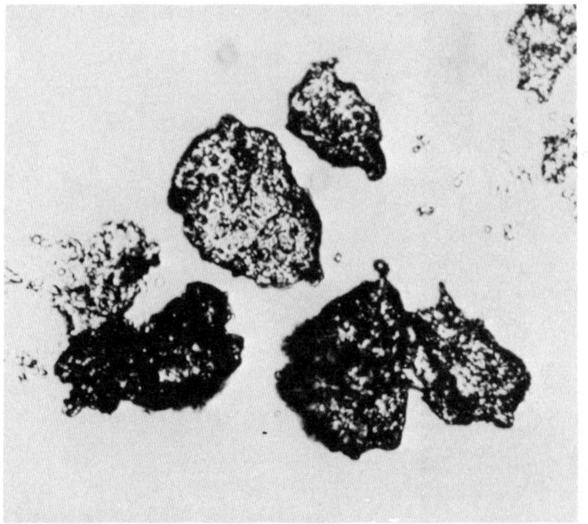

(a)

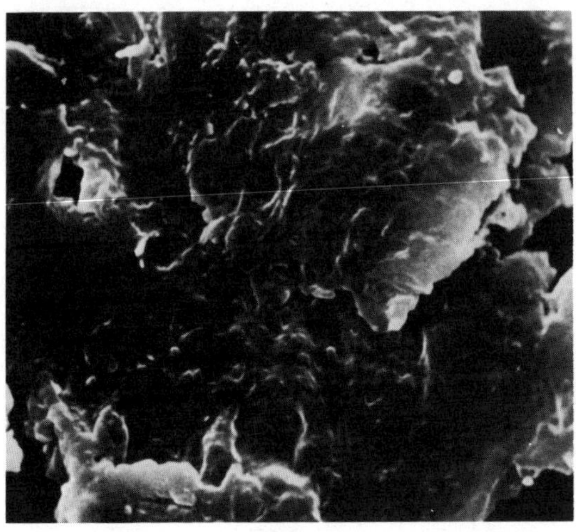

(b)

Figure 43 (a) Optical micrograph, (b) SEM micrograph, and (c) EDXRA spectrum of rubber closure coating.

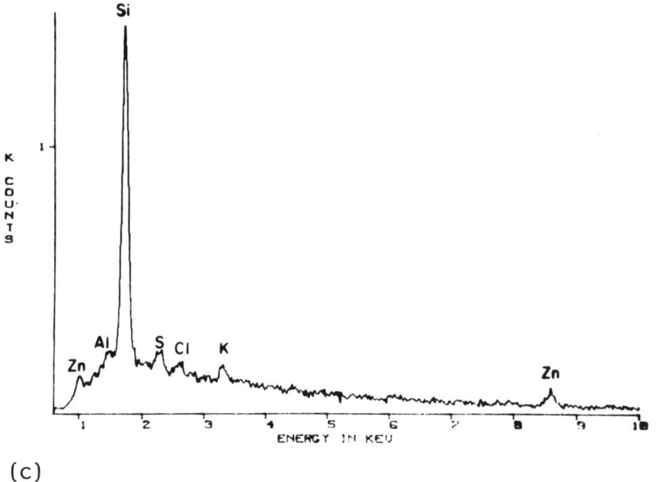

(c)

Figure 43 (continued)

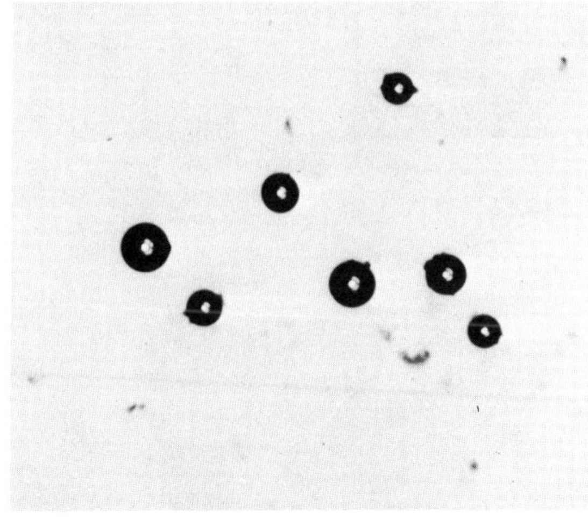

(a)

Figure 44 (a) Optical micrograph, (b) SEM micrograph, and (c) EDXRA spectrum of metallic mercury.

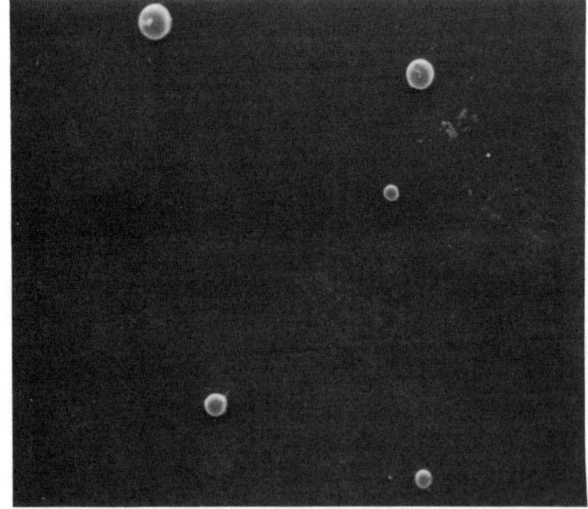

(b)

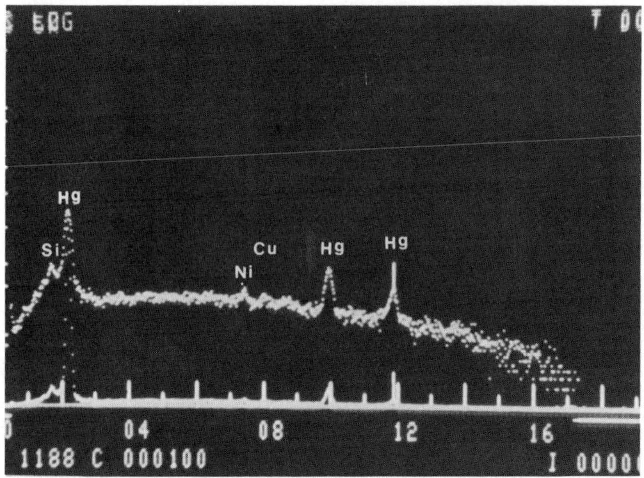

(c)

Figure 44 (continued)

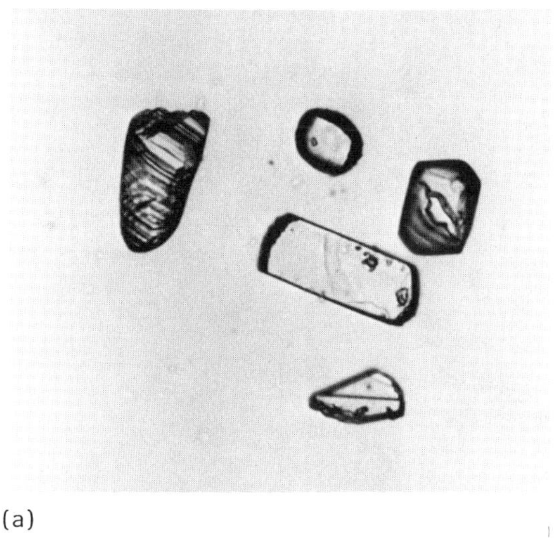

(a)

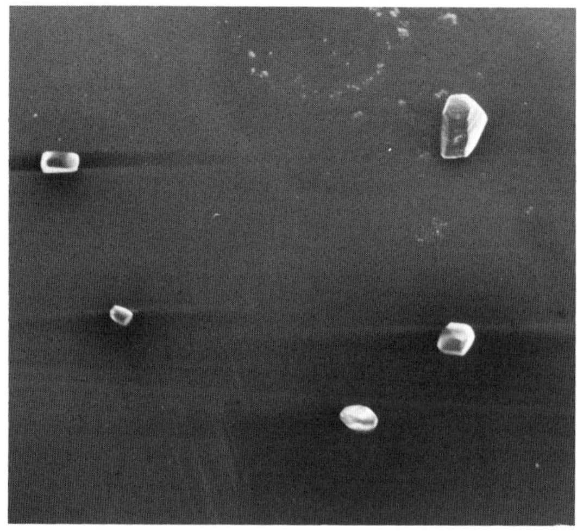

(b)

Figure 45 (a) Optical micrograph, (b) SEM micrograph, and (c) EDXRA spectrum of calcium sulfate.

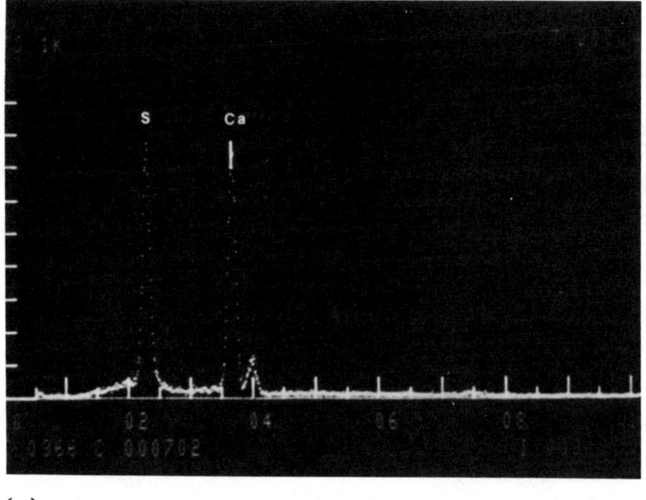

(c)

Figure 45 (continued)

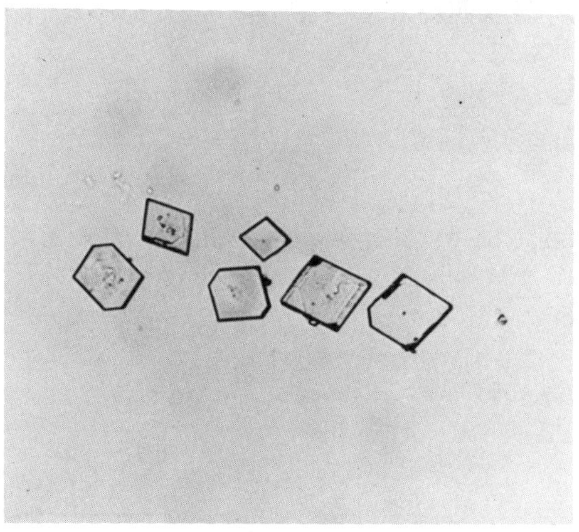

(a)

Figure 46 (a) Optical micrograph, (b) SEM micrograph, and (c) EDXRA spectrum of barium sulfate.

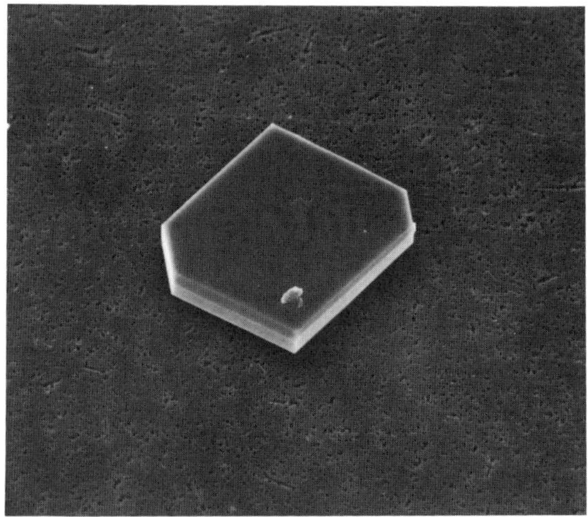

(b)

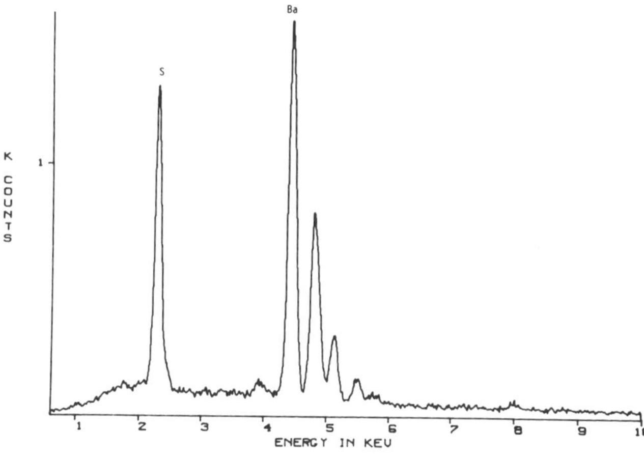

(c)

Figure 46 (continued)

Table 10 Comparison of d-Spacing Values of Particles from Atropine Sulfate Injection to a Reference and the Reported d-Spacing Values for $BaSO_4$[a]

d spacing for sample particles	d spacing for reference $BaSO_4$	Reported d spacing for $BaSO_4$
4.267 (25)	4.238 (25)	4.34 (36)
3.864 (50)	3.875 (50)	3.90 (57)
3.559 (10)	3.549 (10)	3.576 (31)
3.424 (100)	3.435 (100)	3.442 (100)
3.300 (50)	3.310 (50)	3.317 (67)
3.077 (100)	3.070 (100)	3.101 (97)
2.812 (50)	2.819 (50)	2.834 (50)
2.710 (50)	2.698 (50)	2.726 (47)
2.466 (10)	2.448 (10)	2.444 (2)
2.319 (10)	2.307 (10)	2.303 (6)
2.210 (10)	2.211 (25)	2.209 (27)
2.111 (100)	2.110 (100)	2.120 (80)
2.056 (10)	2.058 (25)	2.056 (23)
1.865 (10)	1.859 (10)	1.857 (16)
1.766 (10)	1.769 (10)	1.787 (3)
1.691 (10)	1.688 (10)	1.681 (7)
1.614 (10)	1.598 (10)	1.593 (8)
1.541 (10)	1.544 (10)	1.534 (18)

[a]The values in the parenthesis indicate the percentage relative intensity of diffraction lines corresponding to various d spacings.
Source: From X-ray powder data file 5-0488, ASTM Special Technical Publication 48-J, American Society for Testing Materials, Philadelphia, 1960, p. 622.

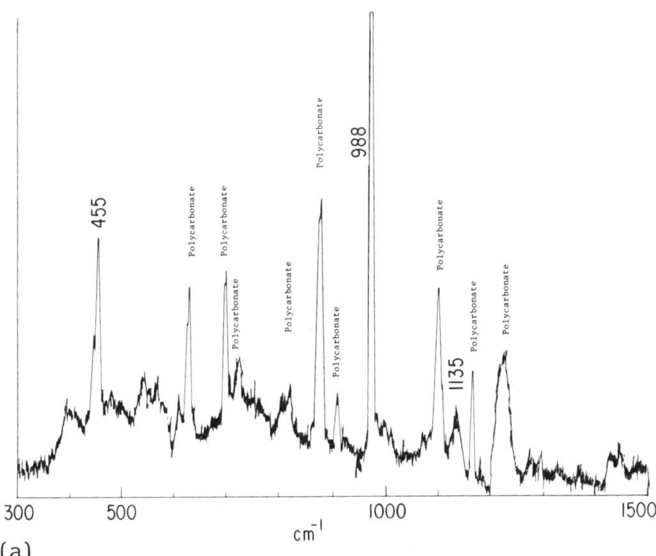

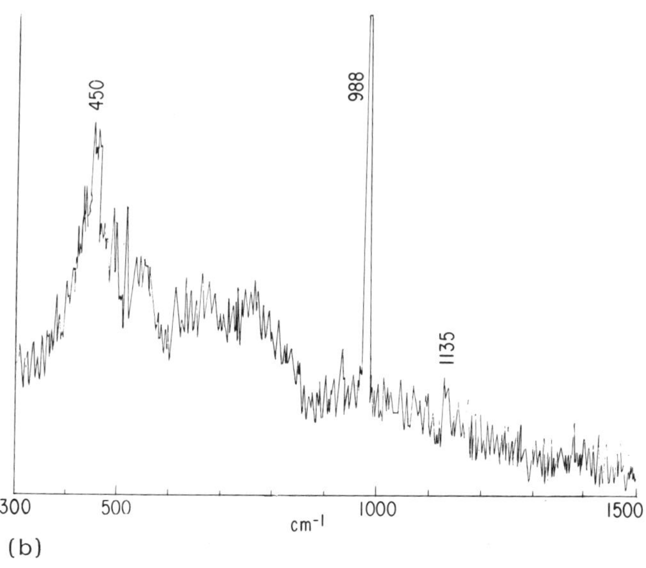

Figure 47 Raman spectra of (a) $BaSO_4$ crystal isolated from a parenteral product on a 0.45-μm polycarbonate filter. Peaks due to the crystal appear at 455, 988, and 1135 cm^{-1}. (b) Spectrum of reference $BaSO_4$ crystal on a glass slide showing peaks at 450, 988, and 1135 cm^{-1}.

in linear dimension) was reported by Rosasco et al. [62]. The single particles analyzed included thorium oxide (from 0.9 to about 40 μm), crystals of sodium nitrate, ammonium nitrate (0.7–20 μm), and polystyrene latex spheres (about 4 μm diameter).

X. ELIMINATION

Particulate contamination in parenteral medications can be minimized by exercising good manufacturing practices during manufacture and good hospital practices during administration. Control of particulates begins with the selection of the components, i.e., the container components and the ingredients, continues through the formulation phase and the establishment of standard procedures, and culminates in the various processing steps, i.e., cleaning components, compounding the solution, sterilization (filtration or terminal), and filling and stoppering. These procedures have been described in sufficient detail in other chapters comprising Volumes 1 and 2. However, filtration during filling into individual containers just prior to sealing is essential and has become standard practice in the industry. Although such filtration does not guarantee a particle-free solution at the time of administration to the patient, since other steps are required before complete closure of the container, it has proven to be successful in reducing the particulate burden and removing large particles.

Manufacturers of parenteral products have exercised strict procedures in preparing injectables with low particulate levels. The visible inspection of each container for particles ensures a high probability of elimination of product containing particles visible to the unaided eye. Nevertheless, the interactions that occur between solution and container components lead to the generation of particulates. More importantly, the administration of parenteral products in the clinical setting is vulnerable to contamination. Studies have shown in-use contamination rates between 4 and 15% [63–65]. To assure the delivery of a contaminant-free solution to the patient, whether such contamination is intrinsic or extrinsic, microbiological or particulate, good hospital practices must be exercised.

Comprehensive procedures have been recommended for compounding intravenous admixtures in hospitals [66,67] for the quality assurance in hospital-centralized intravenous admixture services [68]. Although such procedures are obligatory for the professional staff, they do not guarantee a contaminant-free product during administration. The only guarantee is to filter the solution as it enters the patient's circulation.

Several studies have demonstrated a significant reduction in the incidence of phlebitis in patients receiving filtered solutions [68–72], and the filtration of cardioplegic solutions in an isolated rat heart preparation prevented coronary vascular changes observed in unfiltered solutions [73]. Although particulate matter cannot be conclusively implicated as a cause of infusion phlebitis or coronary vascular changes, in-line filtration will protect the patient from the inadvertent administration of particulates, bacteria, and air. Figures 48 through 50 show the filtration of solutions in the hospital setting. Guidelines have been established recommending the use of a particulate retentive in-line filter for additives known to be typically heavily particulated, such as those requiring reconstitution, and whenever additives are introduced to an infusion solution [74].

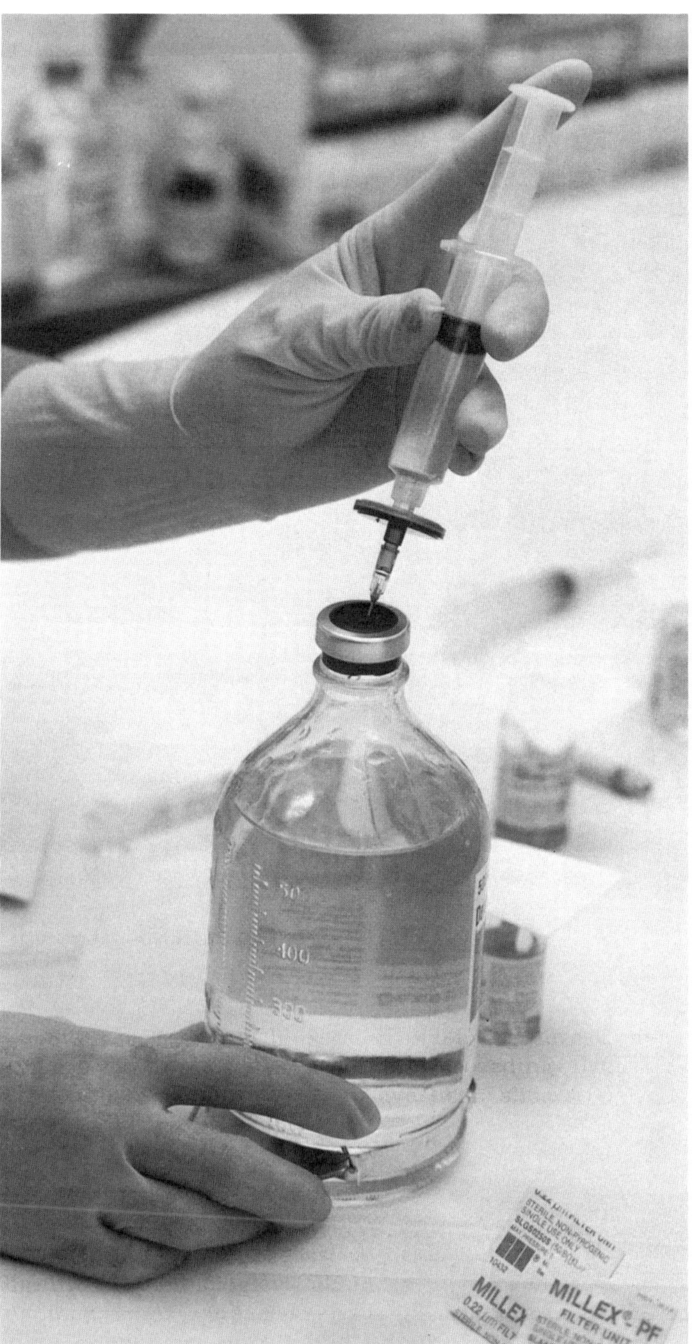

Figure 48 Transfer of an IV additive to an infusion solution using a 0.22-μm filter.

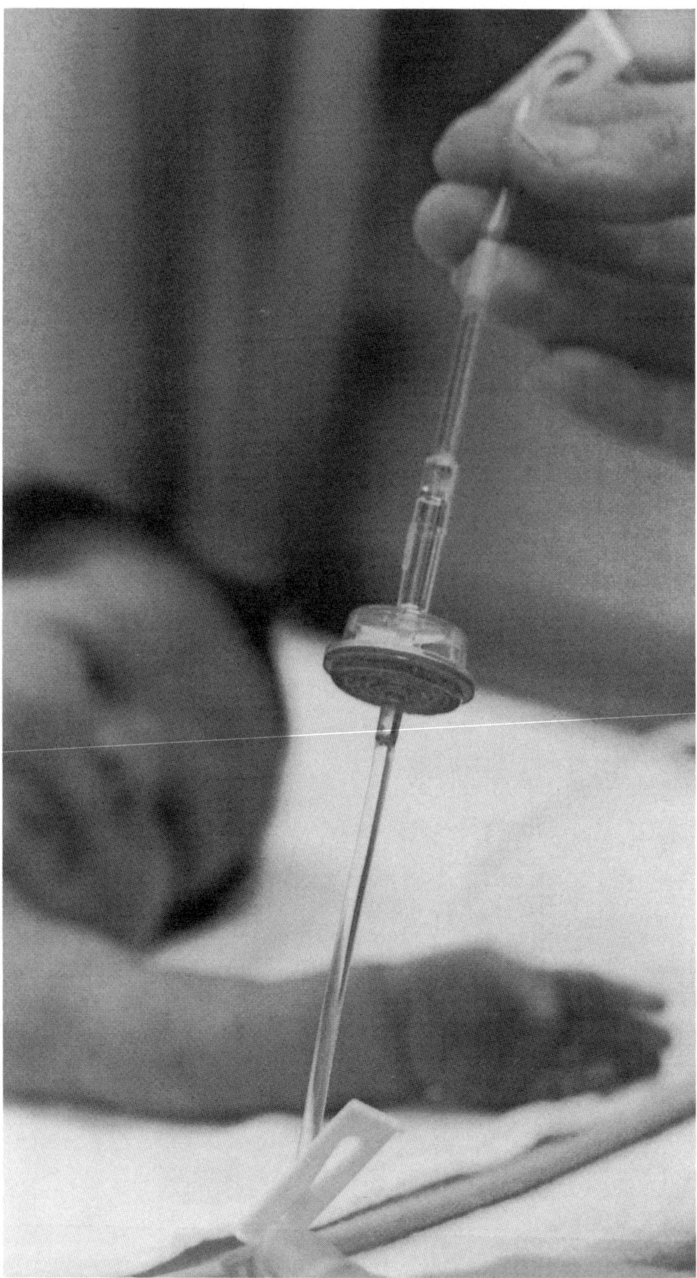

Figure 49 Administration of an IV solution to a patient using an in-line filter.

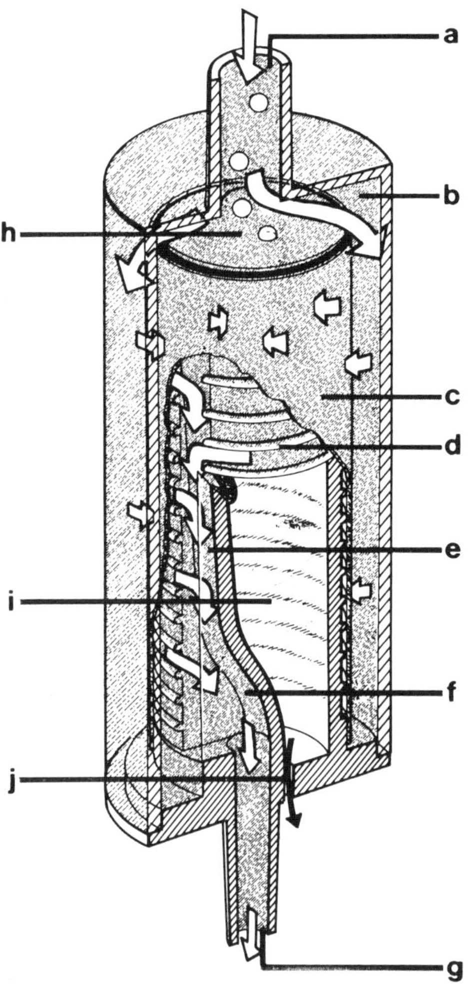

Figure 50 Diagram of the air-venting filter set. Fluid enters the inlet (a) of the upstream chamber (b) and is filtered through a hydrophilic membrane filter (c) that wraps around a center cylinder with circular ridge supports (d). The filtered fluid collects into a lengthwise grove (e) that leads to a passage inside the center cylinder (f) and exits by the outlet (g). Air in the administration system passes through the hydrophobic membrane filter (h) into an air compartment (i) inside the center cylinder and exits through an opening (j) to the atmosphere. (From the *American Journal of Hospital Pharmacy*, *36*:749–753, June 1979.)

XI. VISIBLE INSPECTION

The USP XXI revision extends the use of objective particulate standards to small volume parenteral solutions, but the zero defect standard for visible particulates remains the same for all parenterals: *every container whose contents show evidence of contamination with visible foreign material be rejected* [1]. Current GMP highlight the responsibility of each user to demonstrate and document the equivalence between a present process or device and a proposed successor. When an objective demonstration of equivalence to the human inspection for particulates in sealed sterile containers is attempted, some critical problems are encountered. Direct comparison of performance with calibrated standards is difficult, and calibrated particulate standards in sealed containers are still a future goal rather than a present reality. Utilization of destructive tests, i.e., membrane filtration and microscopic examination, add such a level of manipulative contamination as to make their use very difficult. The only available nondestructive visible particulate contamination inspection standard is the variable performance of the experienced parenteral product inspector. Recognizing the subjective nature of the visual inspection process, the Parenteral Drug Association published general guidelines for the visual inspection of parenteral products in final containers and in-line injection of container components [75].

Visible particulates are those that can be discerned with the unaided eye, although magnification can extend human visibility. A direct exploration of the visual threshold for the low-contrast particulates encountered in parenteral products was reported recently [76]. The findings (at 225 foot-candle illumination), summarized in Table 11, show that with unaided vision particles less than 50 μm are rarely seen, that 100 μm particles are detected 70% of the time and that particulates have to exceed 200 μm in diameter to be readily detected.

The reliability of visible inspection can be improved with a 3 diopter, 5 inch magnifying lens, which allows a 1.6 fold magnification. At a 225-foot candle (fc) illumination, the subvisible threshold can be reduced from

Table 11 Visibility of Low-Contrast Particulates Encountered in Parenteral Products[a]

	Diameter (μm)	
Visibility region	Unassisted vision	3-diopter lens
Subvisible	$50 \leqslant P$	$35 \leqslant P$
Proportionately visible	$50 < P < 200$	$35 < P < 130$
70% Manual rejection (reject zone boundary)	100	65
Visible	$P \geqslant 200$	$P \geqslant 130$

[a]Low-contrast spheroidal particulates with 225-fc illumination and white and black background.

50 to 35 μm. Similarly, the visible range is reduced from 50–200 μm to 35–130 μm. Table 11 shows that the 70% reject size is reduced to 65 μm and the secure rejection size is 130 μm for the magnified images.

An important assumption in the inspection for visual particulates is that the care exercised to achieve low visible particulate contamination will result in equally low contamination rates for subvisible particulates. This assumption does not of course embrace the problem of potential extractable and interaction products.

XII. MANUAL PARTICULATE INSPECTION

Manual particulate inspections are broadly separable into fully manual and semiautomated inspections. Of the procedures available, the fully manual inspection provides the best combination of security and discrimination.

Figure 51 shows a typical inspection booth used in manual inspections. A fundamental requirement in any visual particulate inspection is the illumination level utilized. This requirement has been extensively studied by the Illumination Engineering Society, and their recommendations are summarized in Table 12 [77]. A range of from 200 to 500 fc illumination is a prerequisite for particulate inspection. This can be achieved with a dual 20-W fluorescent fixture to provide open white enameled lighting. A selectable white-black background is used to optimize contrast, and the test containers are positioned approximately 8 in. below the center of the lamps in a region yielding an illumination of approximately 225 fc. A two-lamp ballast for the lighting fixture is required to reduce inspector fatigue. This results in a flicker rate of 240 per second; with a single lamp a flicker rate of 120 per second is visually perceptible.

Since the manual inspection procedure is affected by inspector fatigue, the lighting, booth and chair design, transport of incoming material and inspected material, container placement, and lens height adjustability must be carefully designed. Additionally, suitable rates must be achieved to make the process economically feasible. Pacers are therefore used to standardize the inspection time [78]. Inspection rates of 200 per hour for small blow-molded vials to 720 per hour for ampuls are achievable.

The inspection commences with container rotation to impart a swirling movement to the liquid contents. The swirling motion results in particulate movement, which the eye detects with better accuracy than it does stationary particles. The swirling motion required is brisk but below that at which cavitation (bubbling) results. The inspection commences coincidentally with the end of container swirling and starts from the container bottom where glass and other heavy fragments are to be found. The bottom first inspection is essential since the heavier fragments rub against the container inner surface and quickly become motionless. The inspection continues up through the body of the container and ends with a search of the meniscus for floating particles. The entire inspection sequence is performed with both white and black backgrounds, which are provided to assure adequate contrast for all particulates encountered.

A. Automatic Transport for Manual Inspection

The semiautomated inspection systems utilize machine transport and rotation of groups of containers into a lighted inspection zone usually provided with

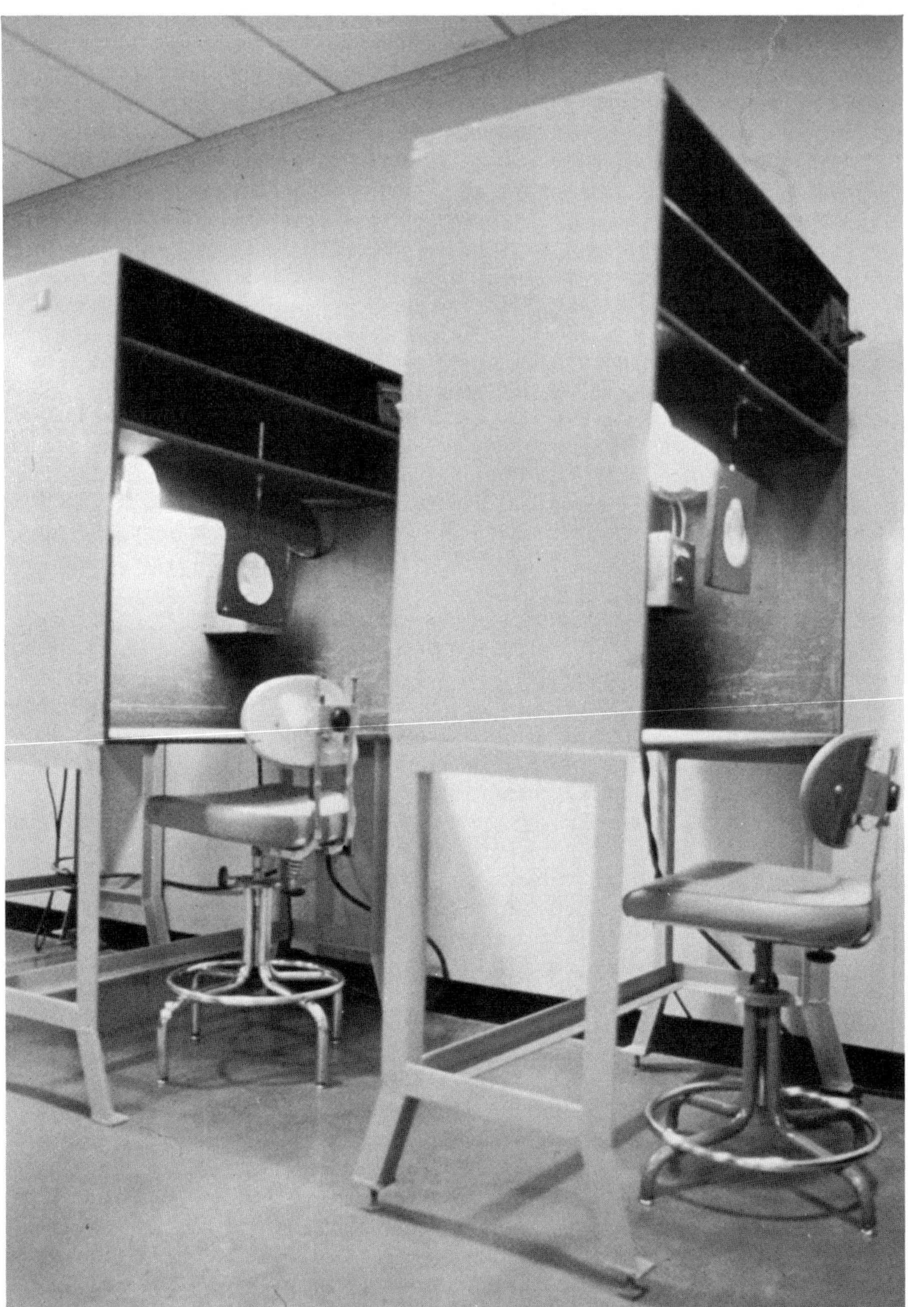

Figure 51 Standard visual inspection booth showing physical arrangements. (Courtesy Schering-Plough.)

Table 12 IES Lighting Recommendations for Visual Tasks of Varying Difficulty

Visual task	Recommended range of illuminance (fc)		
	Min.	Mid	High
High contrast or large size	20	30	50
Medium contrast or small size	50	75	100
Low contrast or very small size	100	150	200
Low contrast and very small size over prolonged period	200	300	500
Exacting task over very prolonged period	500	750	1000
Very special visual task of extremely low contrast and small size	1000	1500	2000

Source: From *IES Lighting Handbook*, 1981 reference volume, Section A-3, Table 1.

a 3-diopter magnifying lens. Reject sorting is effected by actuation of a pushbutton corresponding to the position of the container under inspection. Since there is no alternation of visual inspection background, as in the fully manual inspection, the lighting selection is a compromise between those used for low- and high-contrast particulates. Although the inspection transport system can index at a speed of 120 containers per minute, security equivalent to the fully manual inspection method is generally attained at inspection speeds approximately 40% higher than those of the manual method. Modern representatives of this type of inspection system are the Production Equipment, Inc., Model VIS, shown in Figure 52, and the Seidenader Equipment Co. Model V90, shown in Figure 53. Figure 54 shows a TV camera-assisted inspection system with a magnified vial image on the monitor screen. This system operates at a capacity of 1000 vials per hour.

Essential for the on-line inspection of a product is a rate that matches the production rate for the product. This requirement is often met by adding manual or semiautomated inspection stations on a conveyorized distribution and packout system. In some cases, on-line particulate inspections have been utilized in which container rotation or inversion to achieve particulate movement is not included. Since the human eye is more sensitive to particulate movement detection than to size detection quality of inspection can be compromised for speed.

B. Manual Inspection Training Programs

Training programs differ from company to company. However, the principal components of each are essentially the same. The initial phase of training consists of having individuals or small groups of "trainees" duplicate the inspection techniques, i.e., hand movements and mental concentration, of

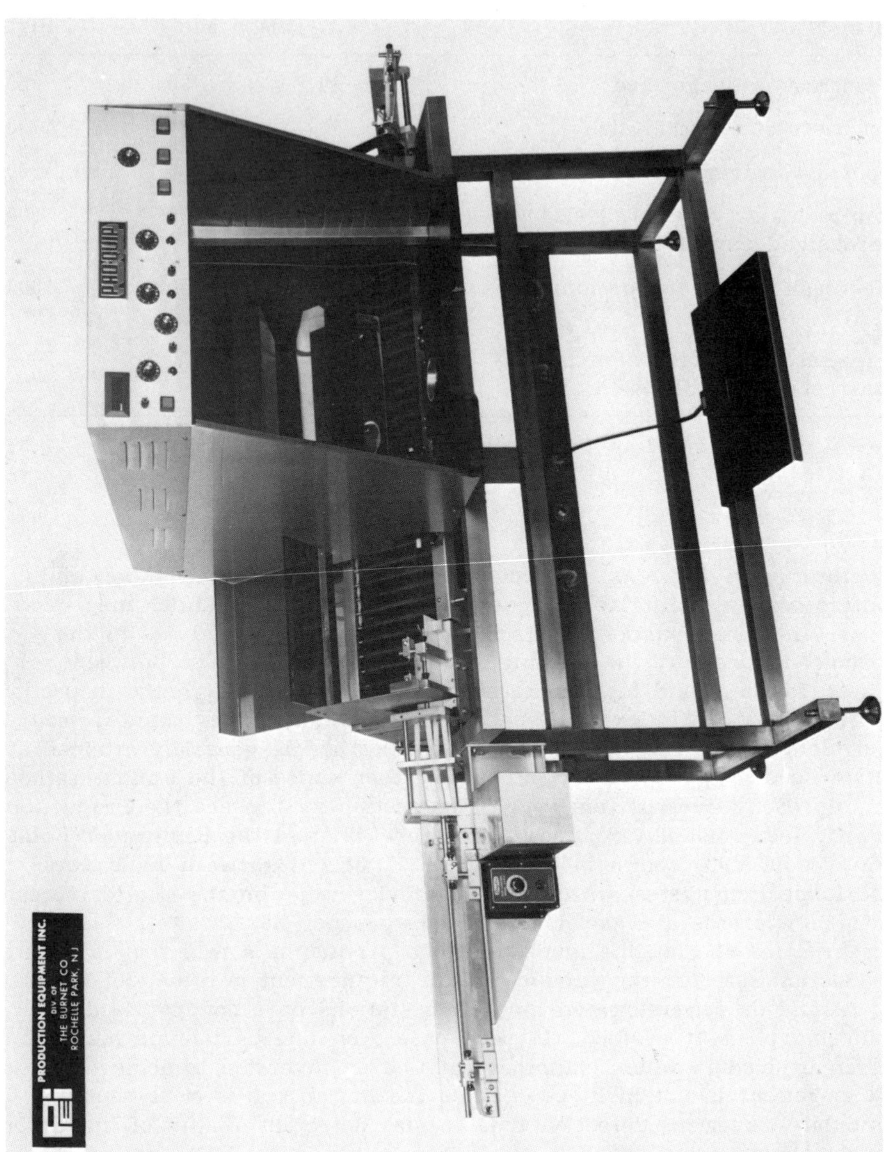

Figure 52 Production Equipment, Inc. Model VIS semiautomated inspection system.

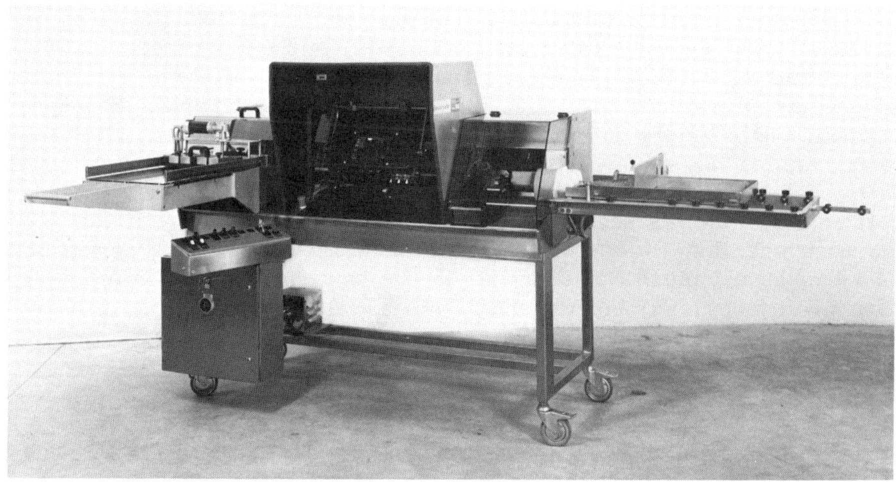

Figure 53 Seidenader Equipment, Inc. semiautomated inspection system.

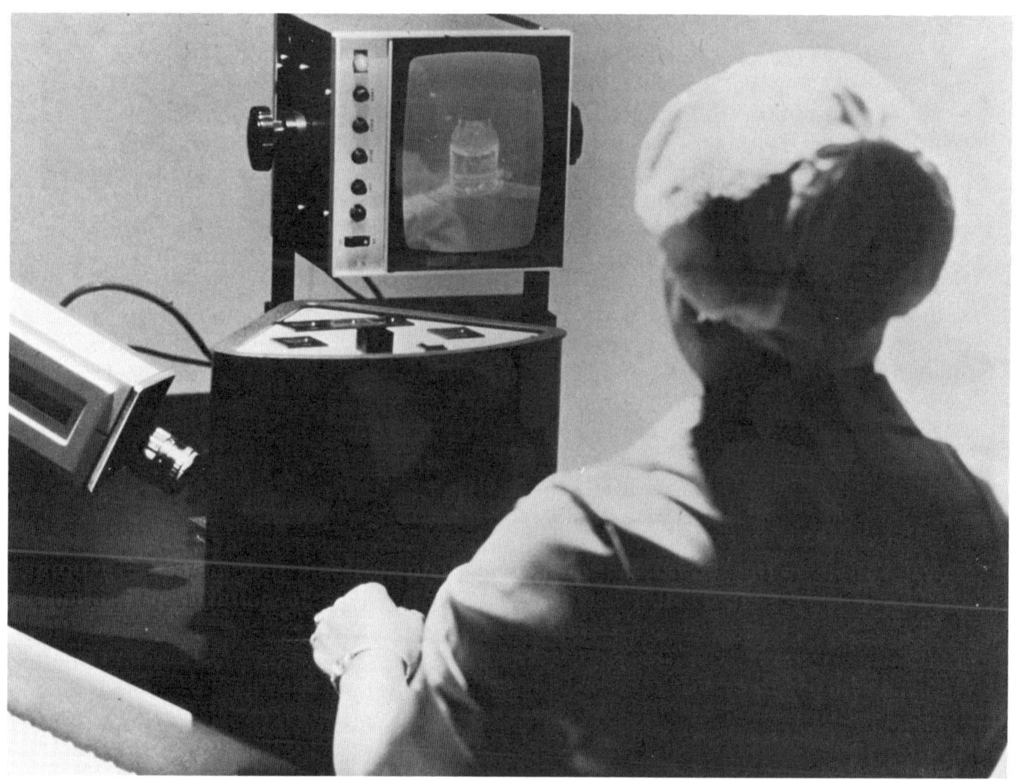

Figure 54 TV-assisted inspection system showing an enlarged view of a vial in test position. (Courtesy Schering-Plough.)

skilled inspectors using preselected reject samples. The test group of rejects is selected by the skilled inspection staff and categorized into "bad-bad" and "gray zone" rejects. The second phase of training utilizes actual production material with 100% reinspection by an experienced inspector. When a satisfactory level of proficiency has been achieved, the third phase of training commences. This third phase is actually a monitoring phase to assure adherence to the established quality levels over a period of 6–12 weeks. This is accomplished through a critical review of the quality assurance inspections of the trainees' work. A training period of 12–14 weeks is usually required to attain the essential attributes of inspection proficiency, manual dexterity, and social responsibility.

XIII. AUTOMATED INSPECTION SYSTEMS

Progress toward an automated inspection system was, until recently, hampered by the complexity and reliability of the available electronics. Another, even more significant factor was the lack of any effective inspection evaluation methodology. Several semiautomated transport devices equipped with lights and means to rotate the containers being inspected were marketed. These systems all used a human decision maker, and it was often questionable whether these devices improved the security and objectivity of the particulate inspection procedure.

In 1968, the Parenteral Drug Association, aware of the continuing need for an effective, cost-efficient particulate inspection system, commissioned the Emhart Corporation to develop a system based upon a TV camera and a memory that stored reduced screen images. An evaluation of one of the first machines [79] was based upon the use of three ampul groups standardized by manual inspection into three categories: good-good, gray zone, and bad-bad. Major difficulties were encountered with the magnetostrictive memory, and sufficient validation methodology was lacking.

A successor to the original Emhart design using more modern technology is currently manufactured by the Lakso Corporation. In 1978, Schipper and Gaines [80] published a comparison of performance between the improved Lakso inspection device and a group of eight manual inspectors. The investigators selected inspection replicability and reject rate as their evaluation criteria. The samples used in this evaluation were "good, "bad," and randomly selected from production material. Cohen's κ statistic was used to evaluate the consistency of the manual and machine inspections. This statistic corrects the raw scores for chance agreement. Cohen's Q test was used to investigate reject rate variations for bias.

The major advantages of automation of the particulate inspection procedure include elimination of both the laborious training requirement and human performance variability and an increased productivity resulting in improved cost effectiveness. Three automated particulate inspection systems are currently available. They are the Brevetti, Eisai, and Takeda machines. These high-speed systems (Figs. 55 through 57) make use of forward scattered light to improve small particulate detectability. However, the electronics of inspection systems produced by each system are unique. Eisai uses a combination of phototransistors and fiber optics and a second inspection station with frontal illumination to more securely detect opaque and black particulates. Brevetti uses a line array of photodetectors with the capability to accurately measure fill height in the container. Takeda masks

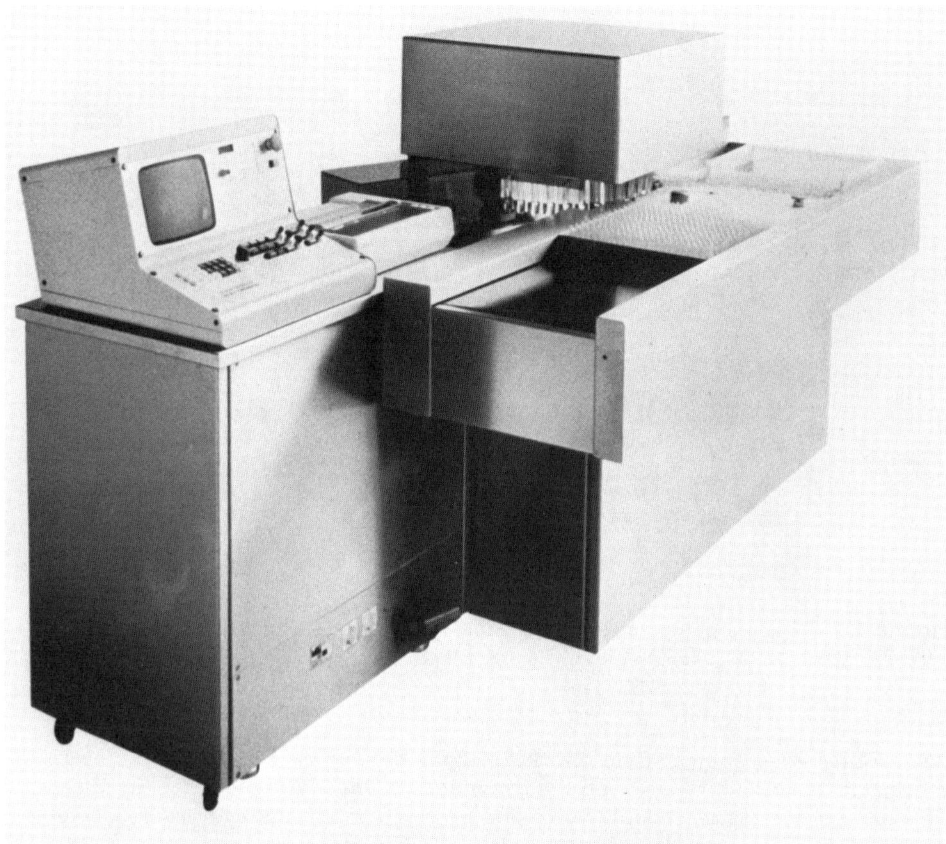

Figure 55 High-speed automated Brevetti particulate inspection system.

the container bottom and meniscus areas in an electronically segmented vidicon camera that processes multiple container images in parallel.

Knapp and Kushner have reported on the machine inspection developments beginning with semiautomated systems and progressing to fully automatic high-speed inspection systems [76,81–85]. In parallel with their device development, they approached particulate inspection of parenteral products as a scientific discipline whose fundamental problems were addressed in a well-established literature. Using two simple numerics to evaluate both human and machine inspection performance, these researchers quantified inspection security and discrimination in an accept/reject decision.

The methodology presented began with a review of the performance of the skilled manual inspector in determining the presence of production particulates in parenteral containers. When the results obtained by senior inspectors were examined, it was found that, although reject rates could be matched with high precision, the actual containers rejected differed markedly between inspectors and as widely for serial inspections by the same inspector, as shown in the Venn diagram of Figure 58. With this Venn diagram in view, it can be seen that any consistency test operating on the type of data shown could not yield meaningful results. The key to

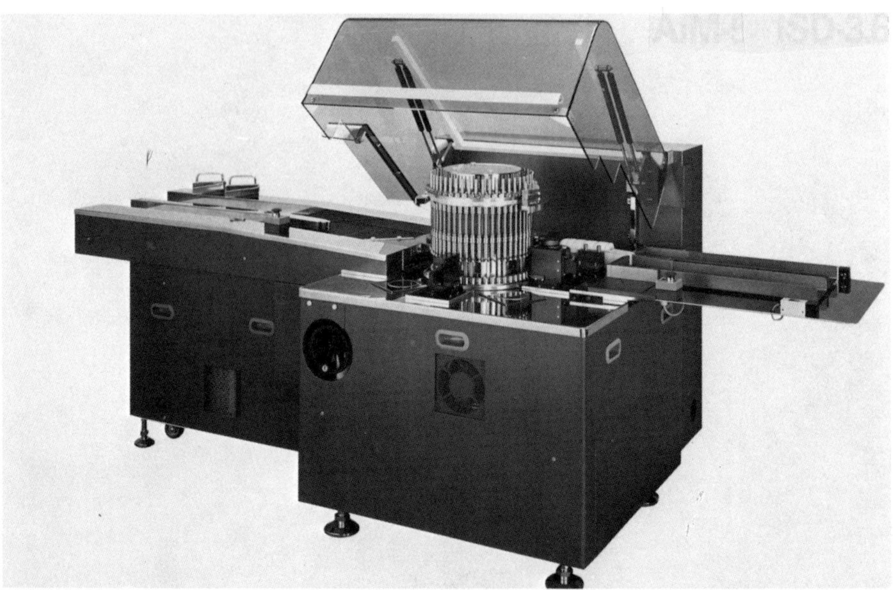

Figure 56 High-speed, automated Eisai particulate inspection system. AIM-277SD-6, AIM-578SD-4.5, AIM-581SD-3.6.

the problem was found when the individual behavior of each container in multiple inspections was carefully examined. The data recorded in this examination were the accept/reject history of each serially numbered container in each inspection. The number of rejections divided by the total number of inspections for each container was used as the experimentally determined container reject rate. The data are summarized into groups of equal rejection probability and graphically illustrated in Figure 59. This distribution establishes particulate inspection as a probabilistic rather than a deterministic process. It also indicates that visual quality judgment is a graded response rather than a yes/no characteristic as originally believed.

When senior inspectors with unlimited inspection time inspected containers in each group, a proportionality between particulate size and reject rate was established for particulates of equal contrast. Knowing the number of containers in each rejection probability group permits a simple computation of the average rejection contribution. This is simply the product of the rejection probability for the group multiplied by the number of containers in the group. The sum of the average rejection contributions from all probability groups determines the average quantity rejected and thus the reject rate.

Since visual quality judgments have a continuous graded characteristic, Knapp and Kushner proposed definitions for the categories good-good, gray zone, and bad-bad. These definitions and the operational relationships employed in validations are summarized in Table 13. The reject zone efficiency (RZE) is the average rejection probability for all containers manually defined to be in the "reject zone." Matching or exceeding this key parameter is the only requirement for validation of an automated inspection system. The discrimination parameter (RAG) is seen to be the undesired reject rate in the accept and gray zones.

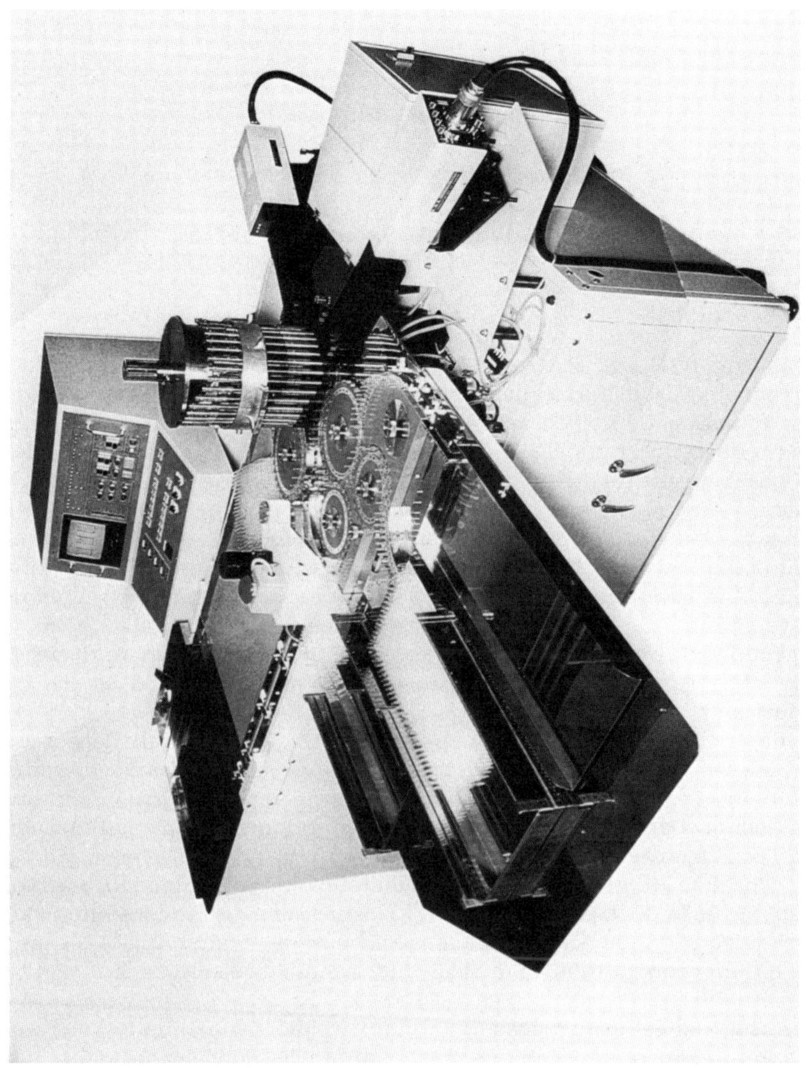

Figure 57 High-speed automated Takeda particulate inspection system.

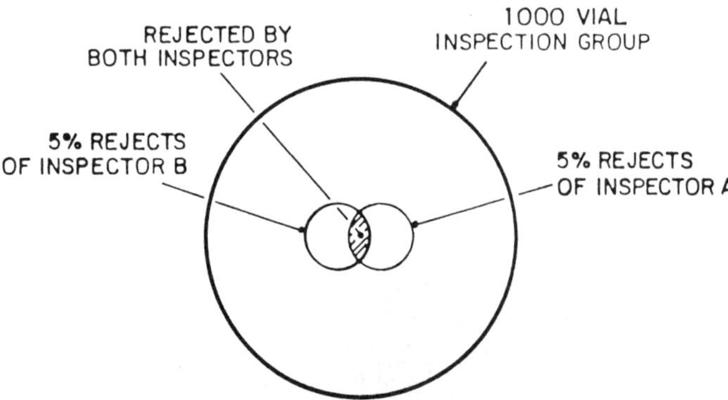

Figure 58 Venn diagram showing paradox resulting from the visual inspection for particulates.

Calculating RZE and RAG for each inspector and using these values as plotting coordinates has also been shown to be an effective method for the dynamic evaluation of inspector performance, as shown in Figure 60. The horizontal axis represents RZE, the inspection security parameter; the vertical axis represents RAG, the undesired reject rate in the accept and gray zones. The rectangles indicate the 95% confidence limits around each mean, shown as a dot. Inspector identity is coded numerically.

It can be seen that the 23 inspectors in Figure 60 are divided into three separable groupings: a low inspection security and low undesired reject rate group, a high security, high undesired reject rate group, and a mean group exhibiting the desired balance of security and undesired reject rate. The capability of this mean group was established as the inspection performance yardstick.

The determination of manual inspection performance equivalent security in a machine inspection is attained by first determining which containers are located in the reject zone by the standard manual method. The average rejection probability for this group of containers is calculated and compared to their average rejection probability in the alternative or automated system. The use of group averages facilitates use of standard statistics, which can be used to compute the 95% measurement confidence intervals usually required. This simple sequence of actions transformed the unrelated detection probabilities in human and machine rejections into a tractable problem.

Since the inspection process was shown to be probabilistic, the number of inspections required to achieve the desired 95% confidence limits was investigated. To avoid continued discussions with staff statisticians, a set of tables yielding the required number of trials was generated that satisfy both the null hypothesis and the alternate hypothesis. In general, the higher the RZE and the lower the number of sequential inspections employed, the lower the number of test group inspections were required to achieve the desired confidence limits. This relationship is shown in Table 14 for

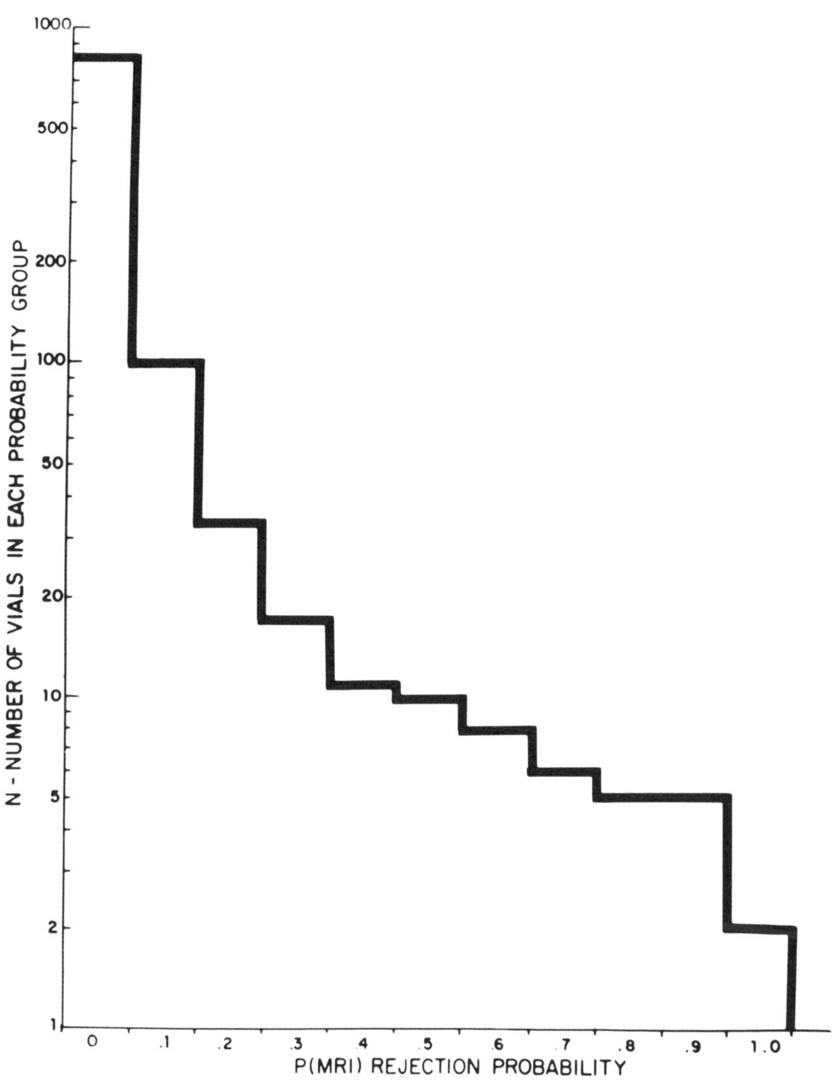

Figure 59 Histogram of container population distribution as a function of each container's rejection probability, 1000 vial randomly selected test group. Standard 17-sec paced manual inspection.

Table 13 Definitions and Operational Relationships Used to Achieve Efficient Comparisons and Validations of Particulate Inspection Systems and Techniques

	Zone		
	Accept	Gray	Reject
Single inspection rejection probability	0–0.3	0.3–0.7	0.7–1.0
Population	AZN AGN = (AZN + GZN)	GZN	RZN
Average quantity rejected	AGR = number of accept and gray zone containers rejected in a single inspection		RZR = number of reject zone containers rejected in a single inspection
Average rejection probability	$RAG = \frac{AGR}{AGN}$		$RZE = \frac{RZR}{RZN}$

joint manual and machine RZE of 0.80, 0.85, and 0.90. In Table 15, for an assumed RZE of 60, i.e., 60 containers in the manually defined reject zone, the number of test group inspections required have been calculated to show that the labor and time expenditure required for a secure validation using the methodology described is indeed modest. In 1983, an evaluation of a semiautomated inspection system utilizing the RZE or reject zone efficiency parameter for selected combinations of inspection speed and lighting revealed that a slower manual inspection rate was more secure and cost effective than the operating conditions selected for the semiautomated system [86].

Particulate contamination in parenteral products will continue to be of concern to regulatory agencies, the industry, and the medical profession. This chapter has addressed the important aspects of particulate matter, but to cover the subject thoroughly would require a textbook. Nevertheless, there remains an urgent need for research into the clinical significance and hazards, improved methods of monitoring and identification, and adherence to elimination procedures. Finally, although the industry has a serious obligation to provide particle-free products, hospitals must exercise good hospital practices in order to safeguard patients.

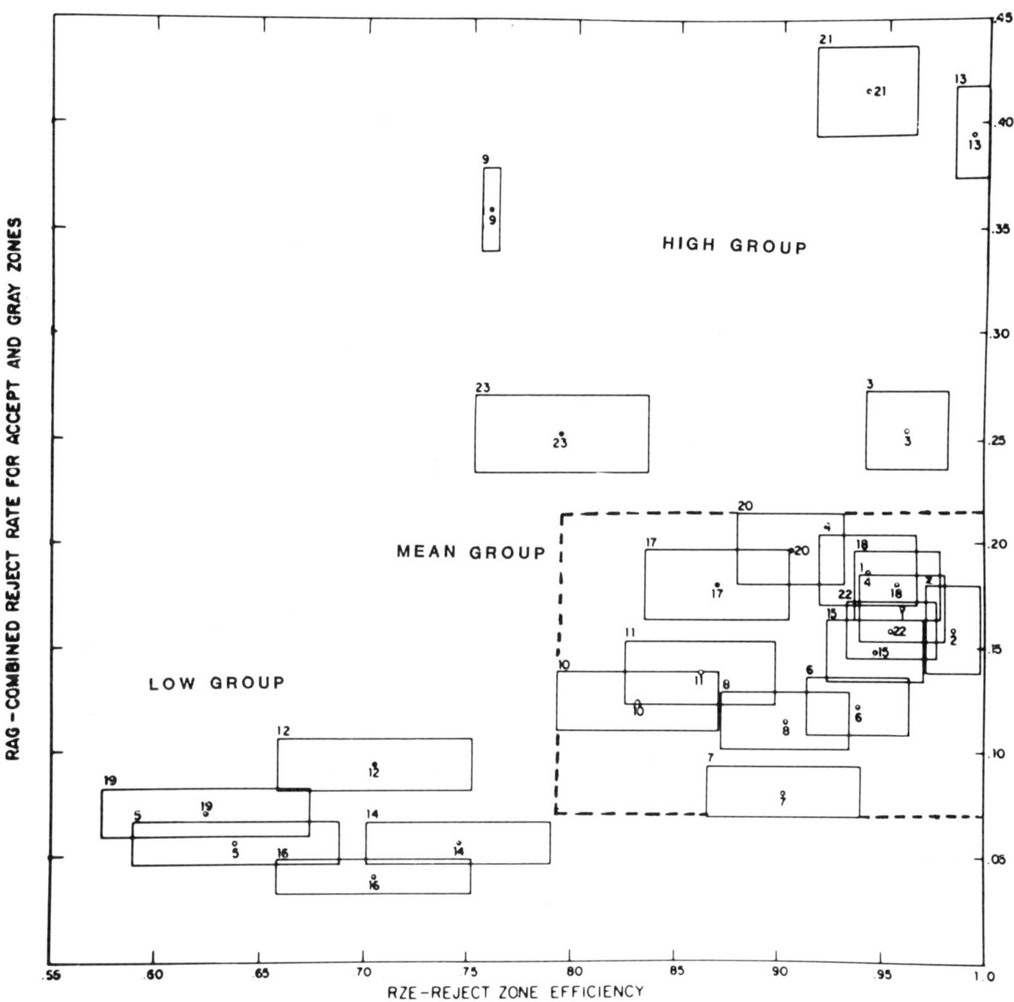

Figure 60 Dynamic selection of visual inspectors through a graph in which the joint security and discrimination achieved by each in particulate inspections is used as a selection criterion.

Table 14 Total Reject Zone Container Inspections Required for 95% Confidence Limit Validations[a]

Total reject zone container inspections, manual/alternate	$N = RZN \times 1$ (for 95% confidence limits)		
1/1	1385	1104	779
2/1	2618	2223	1754
2/2	3546	3190	2525
2/3	4327	4188	3563
RZE	0.80	0.85	0.90

[a]Case of equal manual and machine RZE of 0.80, 0.85, and 0.90.

Table 15 Number of Test Group Inspections Required for an Assumed Reject Zone Group of 60 Containers[a]

Test group inspections, manual/alternate	Number of inspections (for 95% confidence limits, RZN = 60)		
1/1	23	18	13
2/1	44	37	29
2/2	59	53	42
2/3	72	70	59
RZE	0.80	0.85	0.90

[a]To obtain the number of test group inspections required for 95% confidence limit validations from the data of Table 14, each entry is divided by the number of reject zone containers in the test group. Table 15 results when a 60-container reject zone population is assumed.

ACKNOWLEDGMENTS

The authors wish to acknowledge the generous contributions of information and valuable advice of Dr. Hans G. Schroeder, Brunswick Technetics, San Diego, California, and George Schwartzman, Sun City Center, Florida.

REFERENCES

1. Particulate matter. In *United States Pharmacopeia*/National Formulary, 21 ed., Mack Publishing Co., 1985.
2. W. B. Mead, Particles in intravenous fluids. *N. Engl. J. Med.*, 287:1152 (1972); *ibid.*, 292:1355 (1974).
3. T. C. Lyon, J. D. Beasley, and D. E. Cutright, Particulate contamination of dextran for intravenous use: An in vitro and in vivo study. *Milit. Med.*, 466–469, June (1974).
4. R. J. Sturgeon, N. K. Athanikar, H. A. Harbison, R. S. Henry, R. W. Jurgens, and A. D. Welco, Degradation of dextrose during heating under simulated sterilization. *J. Parent. Drug Assoc.*, 34: 175 (1980).
5. J. Y. Masuda and J. H. Beckerman, Particulate matter in commercial antibiotic injectable products. *Am. J. Hosp. Pharm.*, 30:72 (1973).
6. T. Rebagay, R. Rapp, B. Bivins, and P. P. DeLuca, Residues in antiobiotic preparations. I. Scanning electron microscopic studies of surface topography. *Am. J. Hosp. Pharm.*, 33:433 (1976).
7. T. Rebagay, H. G. Schroeder, and P. P. DeLuca, Residues in antibiotic preparations. II. Effect of pH on the nature and level of particulate matter in sodium cephalothin intravenous solution. *Am. J. Hosp. Pharm.*, 33:433–448, May (1976).
8. S. Boddapati, L. D. Butler, S. Im, and P. P. DeLuca, Identification of subvisible crystals of barium sulfate in parenteral solutions. *J. Pharm. Sci.*, 69:608 (1980).
9. L. Ernerot, I. Helstein, and E. Sandell, Some factors influencing the measured content of particulate matter in infusion fluids. *Acta Pharm. Suec.*, 1:501 (1970).
10. P. P. DeLuca, S. Boddapati, and S. Im, Guidelines for the identification of particles in parenterals. *FDA Bylines*, 10:111–165 (1980).
11. H. G. Schroeder, G. H. Simmons, and P. P. DeLuca, Distribution of subvisible microspheres after intravenous administration to dogs. *J. Pharm. Sci.*, 67:504 (1978).
12. M. Kanke, G. H. Simmons, B. A. Bivins, and P. P. DeLuca, Clearance of Ce-141 labeled microspheres from the blood and distribution in specific organs following intravenous and intraarterial administration in dogs. *J. Pharm. Sci.*, 69:755 July (1980).
13. L. V. Gardner and D. E. Cummings, The reaction of fine and medium sized quartz and aluminum oxide particles, silicotic cirrhosis of the liver. *Am. J. Pathol.*, 9:751 (1933).
14. E. J. King, H. Stantial, and M. Dolan, The biochemistry of silica acid. III. The excretion of silicic acid. *Biochem. J.*, 27:1007 (1933).
15. J. H. Brewer and J. H. Dunning, An in-vitro and in-vivo study of glass particles in ampuls. *J. Am. Pharm. Assoc.*, 36:287 (1947).
16. W. Von Glahn and J. W. Hall, The reaction produced in the pulmonary arteries by emboli of cotton fibers. *Am. J. Pathol.*, 25:575 (1949).

17. B. E. Konwaler, Pulmonary emboli of cotton fibers. *Am. J. Clin. Pathol.*, 20:385 (1950).
18. E. J. Bruning, Uber Entstehung und Bedeutung Interarterieller Fremdkorperembolien der Kindlichen Lunge. *Virchovs Arch.*, 327:460 (1955).
19. W. E. Stehbens and H. W. Florey, The behavior of intravenously injected particles observed in chambers in rabbits ears. *Q. J. Exp. Physiol.*, 45:252 (1960).
20. J. J. McNamara, M. D. Molot, and J. R. Stremple, Screen filtration pressure in combat casualties. *Am. Surg.*, 173:334 (1970).
21. S. Sarrut and C. Nezelof, Une complication de la therapeutique intraveineuse. *Presse Med.*, 68:375 (1960).
22. H. Cravioto, I. Feigen, and J. Silberman, Foreign body emboli following cerebral angiography. *Arch. Neurol.*, 3:711 (1960).
23. R. C. Drews, Use of Millipore filters in opthalmic surgery. *Am. J. Ophthal.*, 50:1 (1960).
24. N. S. Jaffe, Safeguards in cataract surgery. *South. Med. J.*, 61: 859–863 (1968).
25. J. M. Garvan and B. W. Gunner, Intravenous fluids: A solution containing such particles must not be used. *Med. J. Aust.*, 2:140 (1963).
26. J. M. Garvan and B. W. Gunner, The harmful effects of particles in intravenous solutions. *Med. J. Aust.*, 2:1–6 (1964).
27. J. M. Garvan and B. W. Gunner, Particulate contamination of intravenous fluids. *Br. J. Clin. Pract.*, 25:119–121 (1971).
28. A. M. Jonas, Potentially hazardous effects of introducing particulate matter into the vascular system of man and animals. Proceedings, FDA Symposium on Safety of Large Volume Parenteral Solutions, Washington, D.C., July 1966, pp. 23–27.
29. S. Turco and N. M. Davis, Clinical significance of particulate matter: A review of the literature. *Hosp. Pharm.*, 8:137 (1973).
30. W. H. Johnston and J. Waisman, Pulmonary cornstarch granulomas in drug user. *Arch. Pathol.*, 92:196 (1971).
31. W. E. Atlee, Talc and cornstarch emboli in eyes of drug abusers. *JAMA*, 219:49, January (1972).
32. S. Richman and R. D. Harris, Acute pulmonary edema associated with Librium abuse. *Radiology*, 103:57, April (1972).
33. A. E. Yeakel, Lethal air embolism from plastic bloodstorage containers. *JAMA*, 204:175, April (1968).
34. E. P. Holt, W. R. Webb, W. A. Cook, and M. O. Unal, Air embolism. *Ann. Thorac. Surg.*, 2:551 (1966).
35. T. F. Downham and D. P. Ramos, Non-allergic adverse reactions to aqueous procaine penicillin. *Mich. Med.*, 72:223 (1973).
36. R. C. Bell, Sudden death following injection of procaine penicillin. *Lancet*, 1:13 (1954).
37. J. E. Galpin, A. W. Chow, T. T. Yoshikawa, and L. B. Guze, Pseudoanaphylactin reactions from inadvertent infusion of procaine penicillin G. *Ann. Intern. Med.*, 81:358 (1974).
38. H. G. Schroeder, B. A. Bivins, G. P. Sherman, and P. P. DeLuca, Physiological effects of subvisible microspheres administered intravenously to beagle dogs. *J. Pharm. Sci.*, 67:508, April (1978).
39. J. D. Slack, M. Kanke, G. H. Simmons, and P. P. DeLuca, Acute hemodynamic effects and distribution kinetics of various sizes of microspheres. *J. Pharm. Sci.*, 70:660–664, June (1981).

40. M. Kanke, I. J. Sniecinski, and P. P. DeLuca, Interaction of microspheres with blood constituents. I. Uptake of polystyrene spheres by monocytes and granulocytes and effect on immune responsiveness of lymphocytes. *J. Parent. Sci. Technol.*, Nov./Dec. (1983).
41. J. Kreuter, U. Taeuber, and V. Illi, Distribution and elimination of poly(methyl-2-^{14}C methacrylate) nanoparticle radioactivity after injection in rats and mice. *J. Pharm. Sci.*, 68:1442 (1979).
42. D. Leu, B. Manthey, J. Kreuter, P. Speiser, and P. P. DeLuca, Distribution and elimination of coated poly(methyl-2-^{14}C-methacrylate) nanoparticles after IV injection in rats. *J. Pharm. Sci.*, 73:1433–1437 (1984).
43. G. Schwartzmann, Particulate matter as viewed by the FDA. *Bull. Parent. Drug Assoc.*, 31:161 (1977).
44. I. Vessey and C. E. Kendall, Determination of particulate matter in intravenous fluids. *Analyst*, 91:273–279 (1966).
45. Safety of Large Volume Parenteral Solutions, FDA/HEW, Washington, D.C., July 1966.
46. Y. S. Lim, S. Turco, and N. M. Davis, Particulate matter in small-volume parenterals as determined by two methods. *Am. J. Hosp. Pharm.*, 30:518–525 (1973).
47. G. H. Hopkins and R. W. Young, Correlation of microscopic with instrumental particle counts. *Bull. Parent. Drug Assoc.*, 28:15–25 (1974).
48. W. H. Thomas and Y. K. Lee, Particles in intravenous solutions. *Acta Pharm. Suec.*, 11:495–503 (1974).
49. G. F. Archambault and A. W. Dodds, Microscopical light-testing procedure for large volume parenterals. Proceedings, FDA Symposium on Safety of Large Volume Parent4ral Solutions, Washington, D.C., 1966, p. 15.
50. L. D. Carver, Light blockage by particles as a measurement tool. *Ann. N.Y. Acad. Sci.*, 158:710–721 (1969).
51. U.S. Pharmacopeia XIX, First Supplement, USP-NF 1975, p. 56.
52. Particulate matter in injections. In *United States Pharmacopeia/* National Formulary, 21 ed., 1985 Mack Publishing Co., p. 1257.
53. T. V. Rebagay, H. G. Schroeder, S. Im, and P. P. DeLuca, Particulate matter monitoring. I. Evaluation of some membrane filters for particulate matter monitoring. *Bull. Parent. Drug Assoc.*, 31:57–69 (1977).
54. H. G. Schroeder and P. P. DeLuca, Theoretical aspects of particulate matter monitoring by microscopic and instrumental methods. *J. Parent. Drug Assoc.*, 34:3, 183 (1980).
55. W. C. McCrone et al., *The Particle Atlas*, 2nd ed., Vols. I–IV (1973), Vols. V–VI (1978). Ann Arbor Science Publishers, Ann Arbor, Michigan.
56. L. V. Azaroff and M. J. Buerger, *The Powder Method in X-ray Crystallography*. McGraw-Hill, New York, 1958, pp. 56–78, 181–209.
57. N. H. Hartshorne and A. Stuart, *Practical Optical Crystallography*. American Elsevier, New York, 1964.
58. E. E. Wahlstrom, *Optical Crystallography*, 3rd ed. John Wiley & Sons, New York, 1966, pp. 66–70.
59. E. M. Chamot and C. W. Mason, *Handbook of Chemical Microscopy*, Vol. II. John Wiley & Sons, New York, 1940.

60. C. C. Fulton, *Modern Microchemical Tests for Drugs*. Wiley-Interscience, New York, 1969.
61. T. H. Behrens and P. Kley, *Organische Mikrochemische Analyse*. L. Voss, Leipzig. English Translation by R. Stevens. Microscope Publications, London, 1969.
62. G. J. Rosasco, E. J. Etz, and W. A. Cassatt, *Appl. Spectr.*, 29: 396 (1975).
63. D. G. Maki, R. L. Anderson, and J. A. Shylman, In-use contamination of intravenous infusion fluid. *Appl. Microbiol.*, 28:778–784 (1974).
64. S. Rusmin, P. P. DeLuca, R. P. Rapp, and B. Bivins, Microbial assessment of a clinical investigation on filtration and infusion phlebitis. *Bull. Parent. Drug Assoc.*, 31, February (1977).
65. R. Ravin, J. Bahr, F. Luscomb, et al., Program for bacterial surveillance of intravenous admixtures. *Am. J. Hosp. Pharm.*, 31: 340–347 (1974).
66. National Coordinating Committee on Large Volume Parenterals, Recommended methods for compounding intravenous admixtures in hospitals. *Am. J. Hosp. Pharm.*, 32:261 (1975).
67. K. Avis and M. Akers, Sterile Preparation for the Hospital Pharmacist. Ann Arbor Publishing, Ann Arbor, Michigan, 1981.
68. P. Ryan, R. P. Rapp, et al., In-line final filtration—a method of minimizing the risk of bacterial, fungal and particulate contamination of intravenous therapy. *Bull. Parent. Drug Assoc.*, 27:1 (1973).
69. P. P. DeLuca, R. P. Rapp, et al., Filtration and infusion phlebitis: A double-blind prospective clinical study. *Am. J. Hosp. Pharm.*, 32:1001–1007, October (1975).
70. R. R. Maddox, D. R. Rush, R. P. Rapp, et al., Double blind study to investigate methods to prevent cephalothin induced phlebitis. *Am. J. Hosp. Pharm.*, 34:29–34 (1977).
71. W. E. Evans, L. F. Barbor, and J. V. Simone, Double blind evaluation of 5-micron final filtration to reduce postinfusion phlebitis. *Am. J. Hosp. Pharm.*, 33:1160–1163 (1976).
72. W. J. Rusho and J. N. Baer, Effect of filtration on complication of post-operative intravenous therapy. *Am. J. Hosp. Pharm.*, 36: 1355–1356 (1979).
73. L. A. Robinson, M. V. Braimbridge, and D. J. Hearse, The potential hazard of particulate contamination of cardioplegic solutions. *J. Thorac. Cardiovasc. Surg.*, 87:48–58 (1984).
74. National Coordinating Committee on Large Volume Parenterals, Problems and benefits of in-line filtration. *Infusion*, 4:13–17 (1980).
75. W. E. Hamlin, General guidelines for the visual inspection of parenteral products in final containers and in-line inspection of container components. PDA Research Committee Task Group 3 report. *J. Parent. Drug Assoc.*, 32(2):63–66 (1978).
76. J. Z. Knapp, J. C. Zeiss, B. J. Thompson, J. S. Crane, and P. Dunn, Inventory and measurement of particulates in sealed sterile containers. *J. Parent. Sci. Technol.*, 37(5):170–179 (1983).
77. I.E.S. Lighting Handbook, Reference Volume, Section A-3, Table 1, 1981, I.E.S. of North America, New York.
78. M. Sokol and N. Kirsch, The pacing of mechanized pharmaceutical production operations. *Bull. Parent. Drug Assoc.*, 18:13–19 (1964).
79. P. R. Rosanen and R. C. Louer, Ampul inspection using Autoskan equipment. *Bull. Parent. Drug Assoc.*, 27:246 (1973).

80. D. Schipper and R. Gaines, Comparison of optical electronic inspection and manual inspection. *Bull. Parent. Drug Assoc.*, 32:119 (1978).
81. J. Z. Knapp, H. K. Kushner, and L. R. Abramson, Particulate inspection of parenteral products: An assessment. *J. Parent. Sci. Technol.*, 35(5):176–189 (1981).
82. J. Z. Knapp and H. K. Kushner, Generalized methodology for evaluation of parenteral inspection procedures. *J. Parent. Drug Assoc.*, 34(1):14–61 (1980).
83. J. Z. Knapp and H. K. Kushner, Implementation and automation of a particulate detection system for parenteral products. *J. Parent. Drug Assoc.*, 34(5):369–393 (1980).
84. J. Z. Knapp, H. K. Kushner, and L. R. Abramson, Automated particulate detection of ampuls using the probabilistic particulate detection model. *J. Parent. Sci. Technol.*, 35(1):21–35 (1981).
85. J. Z. Knapp and H. K. Kushner, Particulate inspection of parenteral products: From biophysics to automation. *J. Parent. Sci. Technol.*, 36(3):121–127 (1982).
86. C. H. Rothrock, R. Gaines, and T. Greer, Evaluating different inspection parameters. *J. Parent. Sci. Technol.*, 37(2):64–67 (1983).

7

Environmental Control in Parenteral Drug Manufacturing

Franco DeVecchi

Veco International, Inc., Farmington Hills, Michigan

I. INTRODUCTION

Environmental control is a major concern in parenteral drug manufacturing. There is substantial evidence establishing a direct relationship between the level of environmental control and the final quality of the product. Environmental factors must be considered in each of the following activities:

a. Facility design and construction
b. Equipment design and construction
c. Plant layout (flow of materials and personnel)

Each production phase has its specific environmental control requirements, and knowledge of the product, materials, and personnel flow is required for adequate design of each phase. A production facility is generally divided into the following areas corresponding to the different production phases:

Warehouse area for raw materials and finished product
Washing area for cleaning and preparation of product containers and accessories
Drug preparation area for the mixing, preparation, and filtration of active drug ingredients
Sterilization area
Product filling area
Final packaging area

There are existing guidelines that define environmental control requirements in some of the areas described above, for example, the "Proposed Good Manufacturing Practices for Large Volume Parenterals" published by the Food and Drug Administration in the Federal Register.[1] Other groups and associations, such as the Society of Clean Room Engineers of Switzerland,[2] the American Society for Testing and Materials[3] (Subcommittee VIII-D 22), the General Services Administration[4] (Federal Standard 209-B), and the American Association for Contamination Control,[5] have developed their own guidelines. However helpful these guidelines, none of them can be used as a standard industrywide, since environmental factors vary from process to process. It appears that there are no fixed parameters in terms of environmental factors that apply to the wide variety of processes and applications involved in parenteral drug manufacturing. Recent experience shows that the parameters defined by existing guidelines may not always provide an adequately controlled production environment.

To determine the adequacy of an environmental control system, there must be a performance evaluation. This evaluation depends on the point of view of those designing, building, and operating the system. Ideally, the requirements of each discipline should be satisfied, but economic factors typically have priority. A principle commonly applied in this case is that each discipline must allow some deviation from optimum to effect economic operation. In general terms, this can be applied if and when those aspects that are eliminated or restricted do not compromise the quality of the product being manufactured.

The environmental control system has two basic components, hardware and software. The hardware component of the system is defined as all the mechanical, electrical, and electronic systems and devices performing operations related to the environmental control system. The software component of the system is defined as the documents containing information on the operation, maintenance, control, and monitoring of the environmental control system. The correct combination of these two components is required for a system that is to provide continuous environmental quality within the pre-established ranges. The only way to properly design and construct a hardware-software system is to use the advice of those who have an intrinsic knowledge of the specific manufacturing process. Wherever possible, hardware should be used to reduce the dependency on software, since hardware performance has variables that are easy to monitor and control, whereas software has as many variables as the personnel who develop and apply it.

This chapter develops the idea that environmental control in a production facility should be centered on the control of cleanliness, which means control of airborne contamination, both viable (microorganisms) and nonviable. Cleanliness is not, of course, the only environmental factor to be controlled. Other factors, such as temperature, humidity, lighting, and special product and personnel requirements, should also be considered. As this chapter will point out, many of these factors are related in one way or another to contamination control.

II. TEMPERATURE AND HUMIDITY

Temperature control is required primarily to offer a comfortable working environment. Temperatures in the 68–74°F (19–23°C) range are considered acceptable. Lower temperatures are selected as a normal practice in manufacturing environments where special garments are used.

Heating, ventilation, and air conditioning (HVAC) systems are employed for temperature control within a manufacturing environment. Certain areas of the manufacturing process, like those where autoclaves and dry heat sterilization tunnels and ovens are located, provide higher heat loads to a system. Underestimation of these items can cause an improperly designed system that may not only cause discomfort for the working personnel but also result in higher contamination levels due to the increase in perspiration.

Humidity control, in most cases, is also a comfort requirement. However, the manufacturing process might also demand specific relative humidity levels. Relative humidity comfort levels are in the 45–55% range, whereas manufacturing process requirements can vary widely. Some products are manufactured in controlled environments with a relative humidity range of only 15–30%. This is the case with many freeze-dried materials.

Normal humidity levels can be easily achieved with air conditioning systems. Air dryers can be used to maintain lower than normal humidity levels. The majority of air dryers operate under the absorption principle and use a chemical compound for the assimilation of the water. These machines provide a continuous flow of dry air to the controlled environment by regenerating the desiccant in one part of the machine and dehumidifying the air in another. Comprehensive calculations are required to size these machines. All sources of water, such as personnel, materials, and air, must be considered. Controlled spaces requiring humidity control should be built with vapor-proof barrier materials to ensure the minimum of water migration.

III. CLEANLINESS

The parameters for cleanliness dictate the design of an environmental control system in a parenteral drug manufacturing facility. The system is primarily designed to prevent and control contamination from reaching the product at specific stages during the manufacturing process. Contamination can be defined as the presence of any undesirable element in a process or product. The relativity of this definition can be illustrated by the following example: cardboard is a material widely used for packaging pharmaceutical products. Nevertheless, cardboard can be considered a contaminant when present in washing, preparation, and filling areas.

Not only the nature but also the amount of the material can define its position as a contaminant. Certain quantities of particles of any nature can be accepted within a controlled environment if the quantities do not exceed designated amounts. For instance, in an aseptic filling operation, the quality of air is acceptable if and when the number of particles greater than or equal to 0.5-μm does not exceed 100 ft^{-3} of air. Thus, when defining contamination, it is important to indicate the type, nature, and limiting amount of each contaminant.

Knowledge of the sources of contamination is important. For critically controlled[6] environments, the sources of product contamination are

a. Personnel
b. Air
c. Equipment and materials used in manufacturing

A. Personnel as a Source of Contamination

Operating personnel are the number-one source of contaminants. A study presented at a NASA symposium[7] shows the typical particle count analysis in a clean room (Fig. 1). This demonstrates a relationship between the presence of personnel and the contamination level. Furthermore, Figure 1 shows that contamination emission levels can vary with the physical activity of personnel. The study reported that a group of surgeons under the auspices of NASA developed a full bacterial pattern of the human body and concluded that "bacterial contamination does not come from the skin itself, but comes from the sebaceous glands. Contamination on the hands and skin is mostly of the transient type and can only be eliminated for very short periods of time until the emissions of the glandular contamination reach them.

Clearly, it is very important to implement measures that will prevent or minimize contamination from personnel. These measures should include

a. Careful selection of operating personnel for critical areas
b. Comprehensive audiovisual training of personnel
c. Routine verification of manufacturing procedures
d. Periodic retesting and retraining of personnel
e. Constant supervision of personnel activity
f. Proper selection of clean room garments and proper gowning techniques

All the measures just mentioned are important, but one that has special relevance is the proper selection of clean room garments. The garments should actually filter out all contaminants carried or emitted by personnel that might be transferred to the product. At the same time, the fabric used should allow perspiration to evaporate. Garments made of continuous fibers or filaments (such as synthetic fibers) are recommended for use in clean rooms. Short fibers of animal or vegetable origin (such as wool or

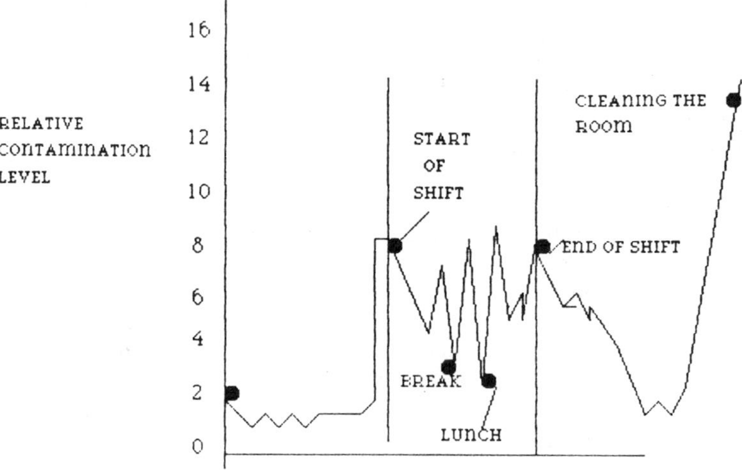

Figure 1 Relationship between personnel presence and contamination in a clean room.

cotton) can be too easily released and thus are a potential source of contamination. Mechanical and thermal resistance also should be considered in selecting the type of fabric to be used in the garments, since frequent washing and sterilization procedures will have a definite impact on the service life of any garment. The estimated life of a garment ranges from one-time usage (for disposables) to 6 months (for those made with a combination of natural and synthetic fibers).

Once the type of garment is selected, procedures should be established to ensure that the garment is affording the proper protection. The integrity of the garment should be checked prior to each use. Torn or stained garments should never be worn in critical operations. Maximum recycling periods should be determined for each garment, and a record should be kept to assure that the garment is disposed of at the end of its approved lifecycle.

Proper garment size is important to assure comfort and proper use of the garment during an operation. Incorrect size could leave body parts exposed to the critical environment and thus increase the risk of contamination. Washing and sterilization procedures should be carefully monitored, and materials should be tested for sterility according to a sampling plan; critical locations, such as the shoulders, axillae, and inner thigh, must be selected for sampling. If an outside cleaning and sterilization service or a uniform laundry service is used, a record and description of their washing, sterilization, control, and testing procedures should be required.

Disposable garments have been in use in recent years, and these should conform to the same type of requirements as reusable garments. Consideration of mechanical resistance is important, and technical specifications should assure that no fibers will be released.

B. Air as a Source of Contamination

The second largest source of contaminants is usually the air introduced into the controlled environment. Contaminants in the air can be divided into two main groups: those in solid phase and those in liquid phase.

In the solid phase, there are such contaminants as soils of all types, minerals, metals, vegetable fibers, synthetic materials, all the biological materials (for example, skin cells, hair, and bacteria), fumes from incomplete combustion, and vapors from oxidation of metals. Contaminants in the liquid phase can include sprays of all kinds, condensed vapors, and chemical vapors.

All these contaminants form part of a natural aerosol, or suspension of small particles. The natural aerosol has a concentration of suspended particles in the range of $10^2 - 10^7$ cm^{-3}. These particles are from different origins and can be classified as viable or nonviable. The ratio of viable to nonviable particles is not a constant. It depends on the type of environment being considered. Some authors have established ratios ranging from 1 viable per 500 particles to 1 viable per 20,000 particles.

Depending on the location where an air sample is taken, the concentration of viable particles, or microorganisms, varies. In populated areas, it could be 15,000 particles cm^{-3}. The microorganism concentration can increase or decrease depending on the type and number of industries located in a specific environment. Table 1 shows a typical microbiological pattern in an urban metropolis.

Table 1 Typical Microbiological Pattern in an Urban Metropolis

Concentration of microorganisms (m^{-3})	Location
4000–20,000	Typical apartment (interior)
3,250,000–8,000,000	Airport
9,000,000	Show room (trade show)
550,000,000	Telephone speaker

A great variety and quantity of microorganisms can sustain their growth in the air, and of course they are not all pathogenic. The ratio of pathogenic to nonpathogenic is related to the population concentration and to the level of sanitary conditions prevailing in the area.

It is also important to mention that the concentration of any type of particulate contamination can be affected by the climatic conditions. For example, a factor such as a dense layer of smog will alter the biological equilibrium, due to the decrease in ultraviolet radiations (which destroy microorganisms). Thus, the microorganism content of the airborne contamination increases.

Because of its importance in providing clean environments, the control of airborne contamination will be treated in detail in the remainder of this chapter.

C. Airborne Contamination Control

To prevent airborne contaminants from penetrating the clean or aseptic environment, all air supplied for that environment should be filtered. The level and type of filtration needed depend on the level of cleanliness required.

As a universal method for cleanliness classification, several industries have adopted a standard designated as Federal Standard 209-B, published by the United States General Services Administration. This standard classifies cleanliness according to the number of particles 0.5 μm or larger per cubic foot of air. (See Fig. 2.) This concentration is determined by sampling at a specific location and at a specific time.

The maximum number of particles (0.5 μm or larger) defines the class at which the specific environment is operating. The selected particle size and number of particles is arbitrary, and it was originally based on the ability of the particle counters[8] to measure accurately and constantly particles that are 0.5 μm or larger. These instruments are discussed further in a later section of this chapter.

New particle counting techniques currently available allow measurement and counting of smaller particles, and certain industries with a need of particle control in low ranges (around 0.1 μm), such as the microelectronics and semicondustor industries, have included in their definition of cleanliness new environmental classifications based on that level of particle size.

Until 1984, the classification started with "class 100," defining cleanliness only for those environments that had concentrations less than 100

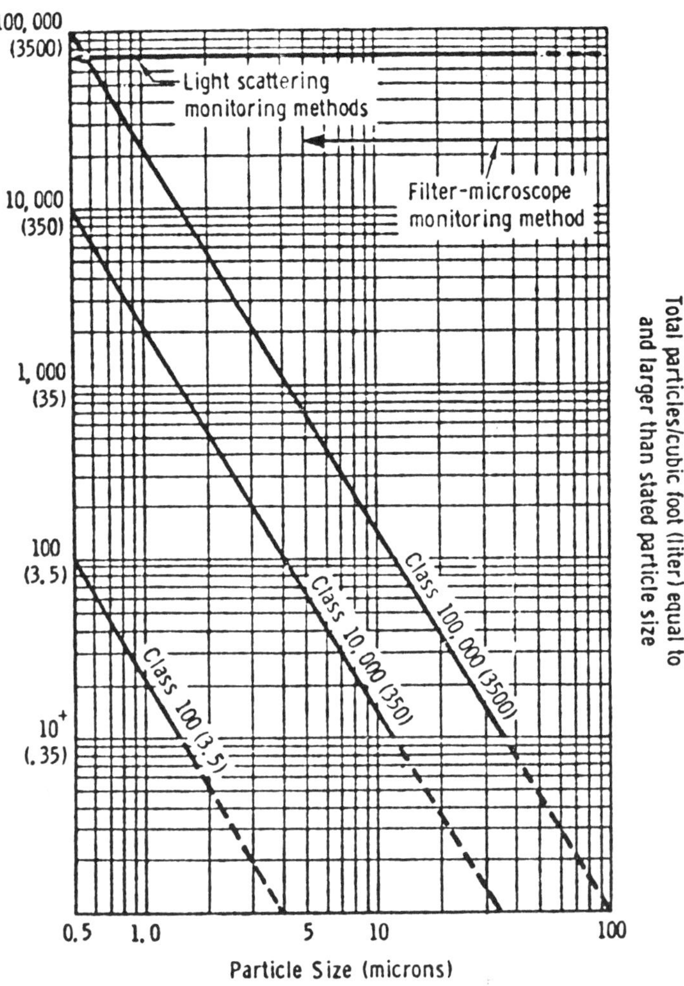

Figure 2 Particle size distribution curves.

particles (0.5 μm and larger) per cubic foot. Lower classifications were only used for internal purposes by those needing it for their manufacturing processes. New classifications are being proposed for a future revision of Federal Standard 209-B.

Nevertheless, such classifications as class 10 and class 1, if ever approved, will have very little or no impact on parenteral drug manufacturing operations. Critical operations, such as filling and compounding of sterile products, are currently successfully achieved under cleanliness conditions as defined by class 100. Numerous tests consisting of filling nutrient media under class 100 conditions and then incubating the media confirm that the cleanliness conditions offered at this level are sufficient to assure no viable contamination with the current manufacturing methods.

1. *Aerosol Behavior*

To control airborne contamination effectively, it is important to know the behavior of the particles traveling in the airstream. These particles are subject to various physical forces:

a. Gravitational forces: settling action forced by gravity
b. Electrostatic forces: particle attraction due to difference in electrical charge
c. Frictional forces: rubbing of particles against each other
d. Inertial forces: particle tendency to follow the airflow
e. Diffusion forces: particles in continuous and disorganized motion (Brownian motion)
f. Thermal forces: kinetic energy change forced by differences in temperature of the air masses

Each of these forces has a direct impact on the design and selection of systems for air contamination control. For example, since particles are attracted by gravitational forces with the attractive force proportional to the specific mass of the particle, the larger the particle, the faster it will settle, or be attracted toward the floor; this principle is applied in the design and use of large dust collectors. That diffusion forces have a greater impact on small than on large particles is a principle applied in the design and use of high-efficiency filters (to be discussed later). Table 2 compares the action of gravitational and diffusion forces and particles of various sizes.

The following results were obtained in a University of Minnesota study on typical particle size distribution in air:

> Particles of 0.5 micron and smaller represent only about 2% of the weight, but they account for about 59% of the number of particles floating in the air. Large particles, 10 microns and larger, are not frequently found in the environment or suspended in the air, due to their heavy weight and gravitational forces acting on them; they tend to settle down.[9]

2. *Air Filtration*

The main method of obtaining adequate clean air in today's production areas is air filtration. The existence of various types of air filters, each with different design, construction, and efficiency, poses a continuous

Table 2 Action of Gravitational and Diffusion Forces and Particles of Various Sizes

Diameter of particle (μm)	Settling speed (cm/sec)	Diffusion speed (cm/sec)
0.1	2.24×10^{-4}	1.68×10^{-3}
0.5	3.47×10^{-3}	5.92×10^{-4}
1	1.28×10^{-2}	4.02×10^{-4}
5	3.02×10^{-1}	1.74×10^{-4}
10	1.21	1.23×10^{-4}

Source: Smithsonian meterological tables, W. G. Frank.

problem in selecting adequate filtration stages to purify the air to evaluate its quality. An understanding of the characteristics of the filters will lead to adequate design of an air filtration system.

Filter Classification

Air filters retain particles by various collection methods. As already indicated, these methods take into consideration the various theories on particle and aerosol behavior. According to the type of collection method used, air filters can be classified as sieving or dynamic.

The sieving filter uses fibrous media with porosity smaller than the retained or stranded contaminants. This is considered the most elementary type of air filtration. This retentive action also occurs in all the filters operating under the dynamic principle. Because of the high operational cost and limited applicability of sieving filters, few filters use this collection method exclusively.

The filtration mechanism of a dynamic filter involves a combination of various effects.

Inertial impaction. When the air flows and encounters randomly oriented obstacles, particles traveling in the airstream must change direction if they are to follow the stream. Because of the inertial forces, this cannot happen quickly enough and the particle impacts a fiber. The effectiveness of the inertial impaction is increased by increasing the airstream's velocity and by decreasing the fiber's diameter. This effect is more evident on particles larger than 1 μm.

Direct impaction. Those particles of negligible mass are likely to be trapped not by inertial impaction but by the action of electrostatic forces or direct impact. The efficiency of this method varies inversely with the fiber's and particle's diameters. This effect is most operative on particles with diameters in the range of 0.5–1 μm.

Diffusion. Retention by diffusion takes place with very small particles in the range of 0.2–0.3 μm. The particles are captured by taking advantage of their disorganized motion (Brownian motion), and retention effectiveness is a function of Avogadro's number, the air velocity, and the particle's diameter. As the particles move in a disorganized fashion, they are trapped by the randomly oriented microfibers that constitute the filter.

Electrostatic. Particles can be retained by controlling the polarity of the filter medium, using the action of the electrostatic forces. These attractive forces vary inversely with the air velocity and the dimensions of the particle.

To select a filtration system using the appropriate collection methods, it is necessary to evaluate the level of airborne contamination surrounding the manufacturing facility, as this will have a direct effect on the particle burden to be controlled by the filtration system. It is also necessary to determine the operative characteristics of each filter.

Evaluation of Air Filter Systems

To select the proper filter system, the following operative characteristics of each filter must be evaluated:

a. Airflow resistance
b. Collection efficiency and rating method
c. Service life
d. Arrestance

Evaluating Airflow Resistance. The optimum filter should provide the highest efficiency with the lowest resistance to the airflow. This is a fundamental consideration in times when energy costs escalate so rapidly, since at a higher airflow resistance more power is required to move air through the filter and the system.

Airflow resistance is measured in inches of water column height by using a water manometer. The instrument has two ports: one is located upstream from the filter to be tested and the other, downstream. The reading will show the difference in static pressure from one side to the other, indicating the total resistance to the flow of air. This is also known as pressure drop. The pressure drop is proportional to the efficiency of the filter and to the airflow. The smaller the particle that is intended to be filtered out, the higher is the airflow resistance. The same occurs with the air volume: as the air volume increases for a given filter, the pressure loss increases. The airflow volume and filter efficiency together determine the resistance to the airflow. This is important for the selection of the blowers and air handling equipment, which are discussed later in the chapter.

Evaluating Filter Efficiency. Air filter efficiency is described by the percentage of particles that are retained by the filter; this is called the filter's collection efficiency. (For high-efficiency filters, the percentage of particles penetrating the filter is sometimes given; this percentage of penetration is 100% minus the collection efficiency.)

Different tests and methods for filter efficiency evaluation have been developed. No one test is applicable to all filters. It is important to know which filter is being used before selecting the method for evaluation, since methods of testing efficiency are directly related to the type of filtration mechanisms used. The methods can be divided into three basic groups, depending on the type of challenge presented to the filter.

Methods that use synthetic dust composed of precise mixtures of different types of particles of different sizes are known as granulometric methods. They are used for filters employing the sieving effect, with capability of retaining particles in the 15–20 μm range. These filters are used as a primary filtration stage in commercial and industrial heating, ventilation, and air conditioning. An example of this method is the AFI test.[10]

Methods that use atmospheric air without any artificial addition of dust, such as the ASHRAE 52–76 test,[11] which is a colorimetric test used to determine the efficiency of intermediate air filters with capability of retaining particles in the 2- to 3-μm range. These are the filters used as an intermediate filtration stage, typically as prefilters for high-efficiency filters.

Methods employing an aerosol with particles of uniform size and weight, such as the DOP[12] test, which uses a photometric detection device. This test is used for high-efficiency filters, which are capable of retaining particles in the submicrometer range (0.3 μm and larger). These filters are used as a final filtration stage in aseptically controlled environments.

Table 3 summarizes the three tests just mentioned.

Evaluating Service Life. The life of a filter is directly proportional to its capacity to retain contaminants. At the time a filter is selected, there is no way to forecast accurately how long it will be useful. Most filtration systems are set up in stages to extend the life of the higher efficiency filters. For example, environments with no stringent air quality requirements, such as offices and laboratories, commonly use a two-stage filtration system. This consists of one rough filter (metallic or similar) capable of retaining large particles 15 μm and larger (90% AFI efficiency) and a second filter capable of retaining particles 4 μm and larger (85–90% ASHRAE efficiency). Nonaseptic controlled environments typically have three stages: a primary filter (90% AFI), an intermediate filter (90–95% ASHRAE), and a final stage high-efficiency filter (95–99.97% DOP efficiency). Many times, these filtration systems are installed in one package at the air handling unit (see HVAC). Aseptic controlled environments usually have three stages consisting of rough (90% AFI), intermediate (90–95% ASHRAE), and final (99.97% DOP and up) filters discharging directly into the controlled environment.

Table 3 Filter Efficiency Evaluation Tests

Test	Challenge	Filter type	Filter material
AFI (granulometric)	Dust	Low efficiency	Natural fibers, metal, nonwoven fibers
ASHRAE 70-72 (colorimetric)	Atmospheric air	Medium efficiency	Fiberglass, synthetic fibers
DOP (photometric)	DOP aerosol	High efficiency	Microfiber glass

As a filter gets dirtier, the passage of the air becomes more difficult, so the pressure drop increases. The remaining service life of a filter is predicted by monitoring this pressure drop increase. Most filter manufacturers specify the differential pressure range indicative of the useful life of a filter.

With adequate prefiltration (ASHRAE 85–95%), the service life of final, or high-efficiency filters (99.97% DOP and up) can be extended to 3 years of continuous use. Filter service life will vary depending on the source of incoming air. The typical life expectancy for an intermediate bag filter with 100% new air in an urban metropolis is approximately 3 months. Primary filters are normally washable so they can be used indefinitely.

Evaluating Arrestance. Arrestance is defined as the capacity of the filter to retain dust. The filter design is the factor that determines the arrestance of the filter, and this generally is a function of the amount of filter medium used (in square feet or square meters) and the way the medium is pleated. The more medium a filter has, the higher its dust-loading capacity, or arrestance. The higher is the arrestance, the more dust the filter can retain before the pressure drop buildup is unacceptable. This means a longer service life for the filter. High arrestance is the typical design objective for intermediate bag filters and for accordion-pleated intermediate and final, or high-efficiency, filters.

In this discussion of air filter evaluation, three types of filters—primary, intermediate, and final, or high-efficiency—have been mentioned. Because of the importance of high-efficiency filters in environmental control in aseptic and controlled manufacturing rooms, this chapter will now describe such filters and their testing in some detail.

3. *High-Efficiency Particulate Air (HEPA) Filter*

The HEPA filter is a disposable, extended-media dry-type filter in a rigid frame. It has capabilities of retaining particles as small as 0.3 μm with a minimum efficiency of 99.97%. The HEPA filter, sometimes called the "absolute" filter, was developed by the U.S. Chemical Corps for the air masks used in chemical warfare. The filter medium consists of extremely fine (0.1 μm diameter) glass fibers. The medium's glass-fiber content is as high as 99%, leaving 1% for binders. Most of the microglass filter media on the market have fire-retardant and waterproof properties.

This superfine glass medium gives the HEPA filter distinctive filtration capabilities. It allows the retention of small particles due to the principle of Brownian diffusion. It also provides the interception by inertial effect of particles of intermediate size (impacted against the fiber by means of sudden changes of air directionality). Finally, it provides the sieving effect for large particles, the most elementary form of air filtration.

New generations of ultra-high-efficiency filters are now available with 99.99% retention of particles at the 0.1-μm level. The current designation of those filters is ultra penetration air filters (ULPA) and very efficient particle air filters (VEPA).

HEPA Filter Construction

To form a HEPA filter, the filter medium is pleated in an accordionlike fashion. Every pleat is spaced, by using a corrugated separator in most cases, and then bonded with an adhesive to a frame. The separator prevents the narrowing of the air passage due to the expansion or other movement of the filter medium. This allows the maximum airflow with a minimum of pressure. Thus, the basic components of a HEPA filter are

Frame
Filter medium
Separators
Adhesive
Gasket

Frame selection is based on filter application. Possible frame materials are particle board, plastic, or metal (galvanized or stainless steel or anodized aluminum). Particle board has been widely used by the industry with excellent results, although there is some concern about the possibility of particle release from this material. Generally, if the filter passes the DOP test and, once installed, provides class 100 air, it can be assumed that the filter will operate safely during the service life. Normally, only defective particle board frames represent a risk of contamination. Metallic frames, of course, are free from particle emissions. However, mechanical stresses will be induced into the metal frame by changes in temperature or by mechanical flexing, forcing the medium, the adhesives, and the rest of the components to react accordingly. Plastic frames have only recently been introduced. Some of the electrostatic properties of plastic materials need to be considered, due to the attraction, retention, and possible quick release of settled particles along the frame. Frame selection, in general, is based on chemical or fire resistance, since in normal operation any of the above-mentioned materials offers satisfactory results.

Most HEPA filter media in use today are manufactured with glass microfibers. Air velocities through the media are in the range of 5–12 ft/min. Media can be made to sustain temperatures from 4 to 250°C.

HEPA filter separators may be made of heavy kraft paper, aluminum alloy, plastic, glass, or asbestos. Because of their mechanical resistance, aluminum separators are preferred by the pharmaceutical industry. Also, aluminum separators show surface particle contamination more easily than do kraft paper separators. Recently, minipleat absolute filters and "separatorless" filters have been introduced. In these, the glass filter medium itself is used as a separator—either by having the glass medium molded (Flanders[13]), or by adding a glass paper ribbon (Astrocel II[14] or Vecopleat 90[15]). Other filters use a glass string (Filtra[16]). The elimination or reduction of the number of separators increases the amount of medium, thereby increasing the amount of airflow per square foot of filter. This reduces the amount of space required to process a given air volume.

The adhesives are used in the HEPA filter to bond the frame and the glass medium. The ideal adhesive is one that has a high-solid, low-solvent content. Any adhesive that has the potential of leaving solvent or air bubbles trapped could in time create a leakage problem not evident at the time of the factory testing. Rubber-based adhesives, in general, have a low content of solids (30% maximum). Before filter testing, it is necessary to verify if the adhesive has cured, meaning that the solvent has evaporated. Hot-melt adhesives represent one of the best alternatives for filters operating at temperatures below 150°F. Polyurethane foams also represent a good alternative, since their solid content is high. In a foam, cell control and the control of mechanical resistance are important. Some foams will dry with time, reducing their mechanical resistance and releasing particles due to impact and air erosion. Silicate adhesives, generally used in high-temperature filters, should be carefully selected to assure no particle-release action with time.

Most of the gaskets currently in use in the HEPA filter are made of close-cell neoprene foam. Alternate gasket materials, such as Teflon or molded urethanes, should assure resilience that is equivalent to or better than that of close-cell neoprene.

Testing of HEPA Filters

HEPA filter media are generally tested according to MLT-STD-L-51079B, Sec. 4.2.1.1.[17] The testing method uses a challenge of monodisperse aerosol of dioctylphthalate (DOP) of 0.3-μm diameter particles.[18] To assure the aerosol's particle size and concentration, special devices are used to generate the aerosol. Depending on the desired particle-size control, the aerosol can be generated either by hot or by cold methods. Depending on which generation method is used, the test is called the "hot DOP test" or the "cold DOP test."[19] The hot DOP test assesses the efficiency of the HEPA filter to retain particles of 0.3 μm, and the cold DOP test assesses the integrity of the filter.[20]

Efficiency Testing: The Hot DOP Test. HEPA filter efficiency testing is used mostly by manufacturers of the filter media and by manufacturers of the finished filter. Efficiency is tested by introducing thermally generated DOP aerosol into the medium or filter at the rated airflow (cubic feet per minute; liters per minute). An aerosol photometer then measures aerosol concentrations upstream and downstream to obtain the difference.

The photometer[21] principle of operation consists of a chamber containing a photocell and a light source (with the photocell shielded from the light source). Once the filtered aerosol is introduced into the chamber, usually at a rate of 1 ft^3/min, particles present in the aerosol refract the light and are detected by the photocell. The unit is calibrated to a voltage representing 100% concentration of the aerosol (80–120 μg/liter). The change in the electrical impulse (from the 100% concentration) is registered and the difference expresses the percentage of penetration. For example, a HEPA filter with a collection efficiency of 99.97% has a penetration of 100% − 99.97%, or 0.03%.

Since this test uses a thermally generated DOP aerosol as a challenge to the filter, it is customary to designate the test as a hot DOP test.

Integrity Testing: The Cold DOP Test. A similar test is used for verification of the filter integrity (leak testing or pinhole detection), but this test differs from the integrity test in the complexity of the aerosol generator and in the portability of the photometer employed. The aerosol in this case is air generated by mechanical means: pressurized air is pumped into a vessel containing room temperature DOP,[22] and the pressurized mixture is then released through a nozzle (Laskin nozzle) with a calibrated orifice. The concentration and particle size of the DOP aerosol will vary.[22] The content of 0.3-micron particles could range from 20% to 30%, and the rest of the particles could be larger or smaller. This type of test is used to assess not only the integrity of the filter medium but also the integrity of the filter seals and the adhesives used in framing the filter.

Cross-Contamination: Differential Pressure Control. Each manufacturing space should maintain its environmental integrity irrespective of the rest of the facility. Environmental pressurization with pressure control is a means used to prevent cross-contamination between environments. To pressurize an environment, outside air must be added to the environment in quantities sufficient to ensure an overflow to the adjacent environments. To achieve differential pressure control, predetermined air-flow patterns are established, creating a waterfall effect, with critical operations at the high-pressure level and less critical or noncritical operations at the low pressure level.

Differential pressures among various environments will be relative to the measured environments. (See Fig. 3.) If the source of outside air for various environments is a common one, the relative pressures will be maintained even if there are flow fluctuations from the source. If there are several independent sources of outside air, then differential pressures among the environments will vary as the inputs and outputs of the relative sources vary.

To maintain pressurization, all potential air leaks must be considered. Permanent openings, such as the ones needed for dry heat sterilizers or conveyors, should have a constant airflow from critically controlled environments. Recommended air velocities through openings range from 80 to 150 ft/min.

Opening doors alters the pressurization of a room. To minimize this effect, several concepts have been tried. (See Fig. 4.) Complex systems

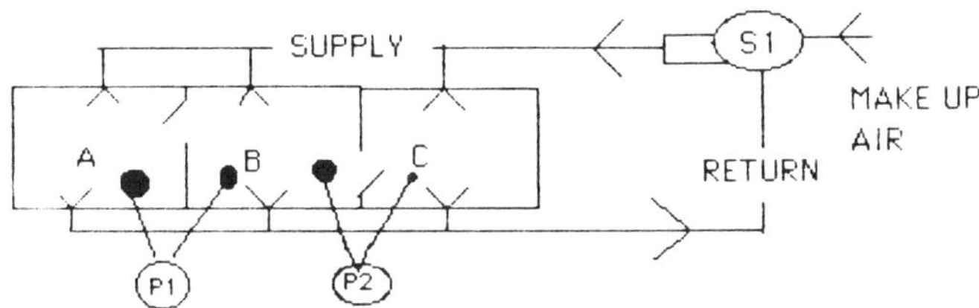

P1=PRESSURE ROOM A VS. ROOM B =DIFFERENTIAL PRESSURE
P2=PRESSURE ROOM B VS ROOM C= DIFFERENTIAL PRESSURE
ROOMS A,B,C HAVE A COMMON SUPPLY SOURCE S1
IF VOLUME IN SOURCE S1 CHANGES P1 AND P2 WILL NOT.

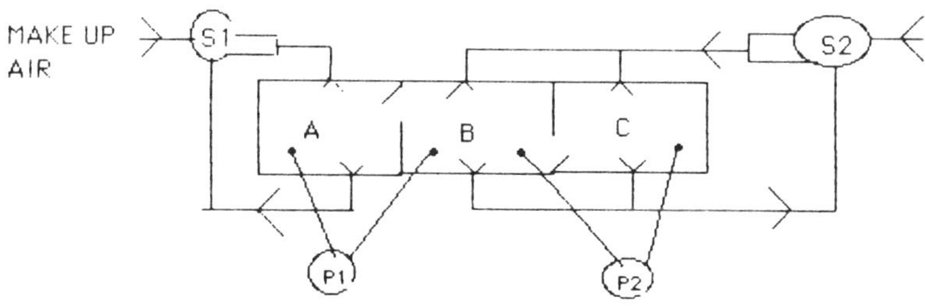

P1=PRESSURE ROOM A VS. B
P2=PRESSURE ROOM B VS C
ROOMS B AND C HAVE A COMMON SOURCE
ROOM A HAS AN INDEPENDENT SOURCE
P1 AND P2 VARY AS S2 AND S1 VARY

Figure 3 Differential pressures among various environments and sources.

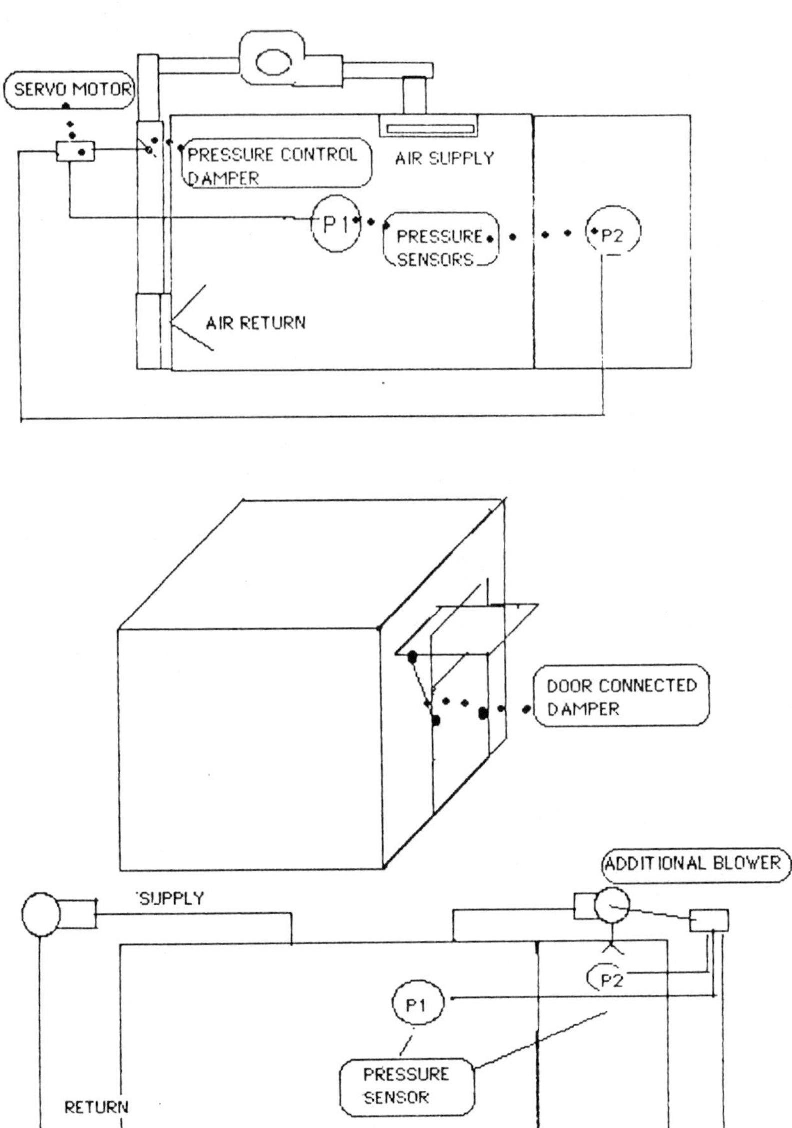

Figure 4 Room pressurization with doors opened.

supply additional air to the controlled environment when the door is opened. This involves a series of sensors that constantly monitor the pressure and activate the appropriate control devices. This method is accurate but expensive.

Other methods employ a damper mechanism consisting of bleeding ports in the structure that become deactivated when doors are opened. This method is acceptable but not very reliable due to the slow response of the damper mechanism. Still other methods involve the use of a permanent opening above or at the side of a door. This assures a constant flow of air, so when the door is opened, the flow is evenly distributed along the door and the opening. For such a method, balancing the air system is difficult. Once balance is achieved, it is a reliable method.

Most systems control pressure loss due to door openings by controlling the return air in every room. As a room's door is opened, air is allowed to flow through the door to the less pressurized environment, but at the same time the room's return dampers close until the appropriate pressure level is again reached. For this system, a complex network of sensing and monitoring devices is required.

For each method of controlling pressure loss, the system's response time is a determinant factor. In most cases, the opening of a door is limited to a very short time span, not giving the system enough time to respond. Adequate door-closing devices do more for pressurization control than does a complex control system. The methods of control just described become more critical at those facilities where the door opening time exceeds 30 sec.

Differential pressure ranges have been suggested by the Institute of Environmental Sciences and by the United States health authorities (FDA).[23] The former recommends 0.01 in. water gage and the latter recommends 0.05 in. water gage pressure differential from the critical to the less critical environment. Neither of these values is mandatory or recommended industry-wide. The only requirement is that the selected value be maintained continuously. If the selected value is too low, the stability of the system is seriously compromised.

E. Ventilation

Ventilation requirements for a controlled environment are determined by the number of people working in the environment, the number of air changes per hour required to achieve the desired level of cleanliness, the amount of air added for pressurization, and the nature of the manufacturing process. A minimum of 30–40 ft^3/min of fresh air per person is required for sustaining life. The volume requirements increase as other oxygen-consuming operations (such as those employing open flames) are conducted in the controlled environment. In those cases, a calculation must be made to determine the amount of oxygen used in any oxidation operation, and this amount must be added to the makeup of new air requirements.

One of the primary functions of the ventilation system is to provide enough capacity to ensure an adequate level of cleanliness. This capacity is commonly defined by the "number of air changes per hour" or by the "recirculation ratio" of the system. Every time the same volume of air is recirculated through a filter, the airborne particulate contamination level is proportionately decreased as a function of the efficiency of the filter.

Given enough time, if the air from an unoccupied enclosure is constantly recirculated through an air filter and if there are no sources of new contamination, then all contaminant particles are eventually eliminated. This is known as the dilution principle. An example can illustrate this.

> A room has an original particle count in the 0.3-μm level of 100,000. The recirculation ratio of the ventilation system is 100%, meaning the air is 100% recirculated through a HEPA filter. This HEPA filter has an efficiency of 99.97% on particles of 0.03-μm. After how many passages through the filter will the particles be eliminated?

In this example, it is assumed that there is no additional contribution of contaminants by the process. Therefore, it is a straightforward calculation.

The filter inefficiency level or penetration is 100% − 99.97%, or 0.03%. Then the first passage leaves 100,000 × 0.0003, or 30 particles, and the second passage leaves 30 × 0.0003, or 0.009 particles, which is virtually no particles in the room.

Nevertheless, calculating the required number of air changes per hour for a desired level of cleanliness is not simple, since there usually are factors constantly contributing new contaminants to a room. This must be taken into account in designing the ventilation system. To calculate the cleanliness level obtained by a ventilation system with a given recirculation ratio, the following formula may be used. The formula expresses the expected cleanliness level as a function of filter efficiency, recirculation ratio, total airflow, average room contamination, and both outside and inside air contamination:

$$C = \frac{S}{Q} + (1 - X)\ (1 - NP)\ (1 - NF)C_{oa}$$

where:

C = expected cleanliness level

S = contaminants generated in the room (of designated particle size)

X = recirculation ratio

Q = total airflow per hour (from ventialation system)

NP = prefiltered efficiency at a certain particle size (%)

NF = final filter efficiency at designated particle size (%)

C_{oa} = particle contamination from outside air (of designated size)

The following example can clarify the use of this formula.

> A room has an internal contamination level of 10 million 0.5-μm particles per cubic foot of air. The outside air contamination level at the same particle size is 4×10^7 ft^{-3} of air. The total airflow is 800 ft^3/min. The recirculation ratio is 90%. Prefilter efficiency for 0.5-μm particles and larger is 80%, and the final filter efficiency at the same level is 99.97%.

To calculate the expected cleanliness level, the following values can be substituted in the formula:

$S = 10,000,000$

$C_{oa} = 40,000,000$

$Q = 800 \times 60$

$NP = 0.80$

$NF = 0.9997$

$X = 0.9$

This equation is obtained:

$$C = 10,000,000/800 \times 60(\text{hr}) + (1 - 0.9)(1 - 0.80)(1 - 0.9997)(40,000,000)$$
$$= 448.3 \text{ particles} \quad (\text{of } 0.5\ \mu\text{m and larger}) \text{ per ft}^3 \text{ air}$$

If in the previous example the recirculation ratio had been only 60% but the rest of the conditions had been the same, the calculated C value would have been 1168.

In the original example, if the total airflow had been increased from 800 to 2000 ft^3/min, the resulting value of C would have been 323.3 particles.

These substitutions show the importance of establishing a system's correct total airflow and recirculation ratio. Increasing the recirculation ratio X speeds up cleanup more significantly than does increasing the total airflow Q.

It is important to realize that the expression "number of air changes per hour" (used earlier to describe ventilation capacity) does not mean replacement of a room's *entire* volume of air a certain number of times. If this (a full replacement of air) had been the case in the original example, the value of X (percentage of recirculated air, or recirculation ratio) would have been zero. Substituting this X value in the formula, we would have obtained the C value 2608. This value is noticeably greater than those obtained with 90 or 60% recirculation. The only way to achieve high environmental quality with a total air replacement, which is often the case when working with explosive mixtures, is by using serial filtration. In that case, the final efficiency of the filtration system is equivalent to the summation of the individual filter's efficiencies.

The amount of air ventilation required to achieve a desired cleanliness level in an environment is also influenced by any additional sources of clean air. For example, the use of laminar-flow devices (to be described later) introduces large volumes of recirculated clean air to the environment. This reduces the need for clean air from the ventilation system. In this case, the total airflow Q is the sum of the total airflow from ventilation air plus the air from the laminar-flow units. The X value, which is the recirculation ratio, typically exceeds 100% when laminar-flow units are used.

Another factor influencing the required amount of air ventilation is the presence of exhaust hoods used to remove toxic or dangerous gases. Where hoods are used, the ventilation system should provide enough air to replace the exhausted air. It is important to maintain a balanced air system.

F. Clean Rooms

Critical operations, meaning those where sterile products, containers, or closures are exposed to air, should be conducted in a strictly controlled environment. This type of environment is designated as a clean room, aseptic room, or sterile room. The last designation should be avoided due to the impossibility of creating a 100% viable-free environment.

A clean room is defined as a specially isolated environment strictly controlled with respect to airborne particles, temperature, humidity, air pressure, airflow, air motion, and lighting.

Isolation is one of the most important concepts. The ASHRAE *Guide and Data Book* (1971)[24] defines three isolation categories:

Direct isolation. Employed when the product is to be protected from contamination generated by an external source. In this case, the cleanliness level is dictated only by the product.

Reverse isolation. Employed when the product generates contamination, and the service equipment and personnel must be protected. In the case of working with biohazardous materials, special care has to be given to the exhausted air.

Mutual isolation. Employed when the product is to be protected, as in direct isolation, and when control is also required for the contamination generated by the product (as in the manufacture of some vaccines). Mutual isolation is also applicable when two products are to be protected from the contaminating effects of each other.

In general, parenteral drug manufacturing requirements usually fall into the first or the third category. The level of toxicity risk to the operator and to the outside environment determines the applicability of the third category.

Clean rooms can be classified by the type of air filtration used. A *conventional clean room* is an isolated environment in which air is supplied to the enclosure through terminal HEPA filter modules that are located in the ceiling or walls and cover at least 30% or the cross-sectional area. In this circumstance, air delivered to the room is of a turbulent nature.

A *laminar-flow room* is one in which a HEPA-filtered air mass moves in parallel flow lines with uniform velocity and minimum eddies. In a laminar-flow system, the air is introduced evenly from HEPA filter panels covering one entire surface of the room (ceiling or walls) and returned into the opposite surface of the room. The air velocity across the room is held in the range of 60–150 ft/min. Because the system utilizes a uniform air mass at low velocity, the air acts almost as a noncompressible fluid, so it is aerodynamic and unidirectional. Its motion is in a stratified pattern, thus creating a turbulence-free environment and providing good contamination control.[25]

A laminar-flow room is classified according to the direction of its airflow: it is called a vertical-flow, or downflow, room when the airstream is perpendicular to the floor, and a horizontal-flow, or cross-flow, room when the air travels parallel to the floor. (See Fig. 5.)

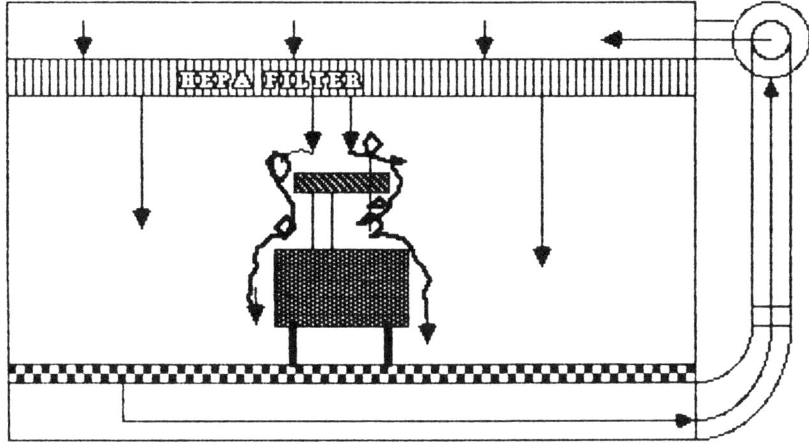

Figure 5 Vertical laminar-flow clean room.

A vertical-flow room offers a continuous clean air shower. Contamination generated in the area will be swept down and exhausted through a perforated floor. This type of room will not allow any cross-contamination from one side of the room to the other in any direction.

In a horizontal-flow room, contamination generated at the filter face will be exhausted across the room at the opposite wall. (See Fig. 6.) This room offers continuous particle removal across the entire room. This type of room will not allow cross-contamination of operations taking place perpendicular to the airflow, but in operations taking place parallel to the airflow, downstream contamination can occur, which is one of the limitations on the use of this type of room.

A clean room can also consist of a conventional clean room together with laminar-flow workbenches or modules. In this system, HEPA filters installed at the ceiling of the room filter air for pressurization, heating, cooling, and ventilation. A relatively small portion of the ceiling is covered with these filters; therefore the air is introduced in a turbulent manner. To

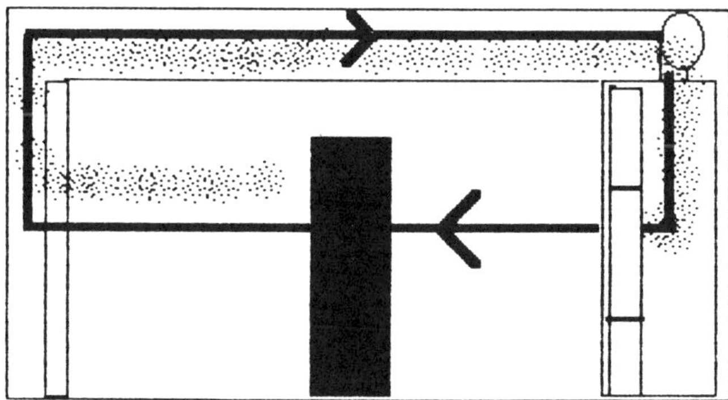

Figure 6 Horizontal laminar flow.

provide the degree of cleanliness required for any aseptic filling operation, laminar-flow work stations, to be described in the next section, are placed directly above or in front of this critical part of the process.

1. *Laminar-Flow Work Stations*

The concept of contamination control by laminar flow can be applicable to independent work stations as well as to entire rooms. Laminar-flow work stations are used to provide class 100 conditions at those locations where critical operations are performed.

A work station can be designed to operate in a vertical or horizontal modality. (See Fig. 7.) Selection of airflow direction is, in general, based on the following considerations.

a. As a general rule, to prevent turbulence, if most of the operational movements in the controlled environment are vertical, the selected system should blow air horizontally. If most of the operational movements are horizontal, the selected flow should be vertical.
b. The rule just stated is acceptable when there is only one type of motion taking place, or when all operations are executed at the same level or plane. In the case of the parenteral drug industry, this rule is difficult to apply, since most of the filling machines used in critical areas

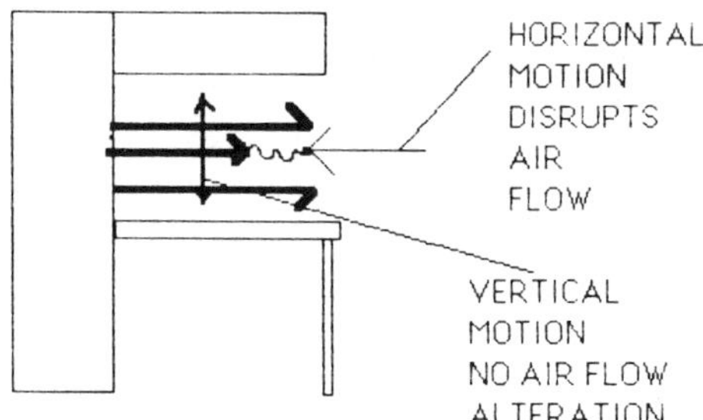

EFFECT OF MOTION ON A HORIZONTAL LAMINAR FLOW HOOD.

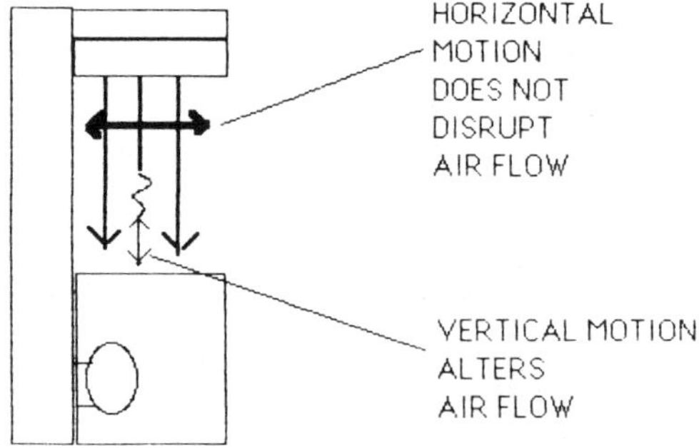

EFFECT OF MOTION INSIDE A VERTICAL LAMINAR HOOD

Figure 7 Motion inside laminar-flow hood.

have displacements in the three planes. To make an adequate selection of airflow direction, careful consideration should be given to the machine profile so the selected airflow pattern encounters a minimum of obstructions prior to coming in contact with the critical areas.

A laminar-flow system for a work station consists of a main frame that holds a HEPA filter, a plenum, and a blower capable of maintaining a cross-face velocity of 100 ft/min (±20%). In a vertical-flow station, the air is confined by permanent partitions, by vinyl curtains, or by the most recent and innovative device, the Kleen-Edge,[26] which contains the air by using a clean-air curtain. (See Fig. 8.)

2. Particle Disposition in Laminar-Flow Conditions

An understanding of the particle deposition concept in laminar-flow conditions is important for the proper design of laminar-flow rooms and clean workbenches. There are two possible conditions for particle deposition (see Fig. 9):

When an obstruction breaks the airstream, the shape of the obstructing object and the airflow direction generate turbulence. (Because of this, careful consideration should be given to the laminar airflow direction

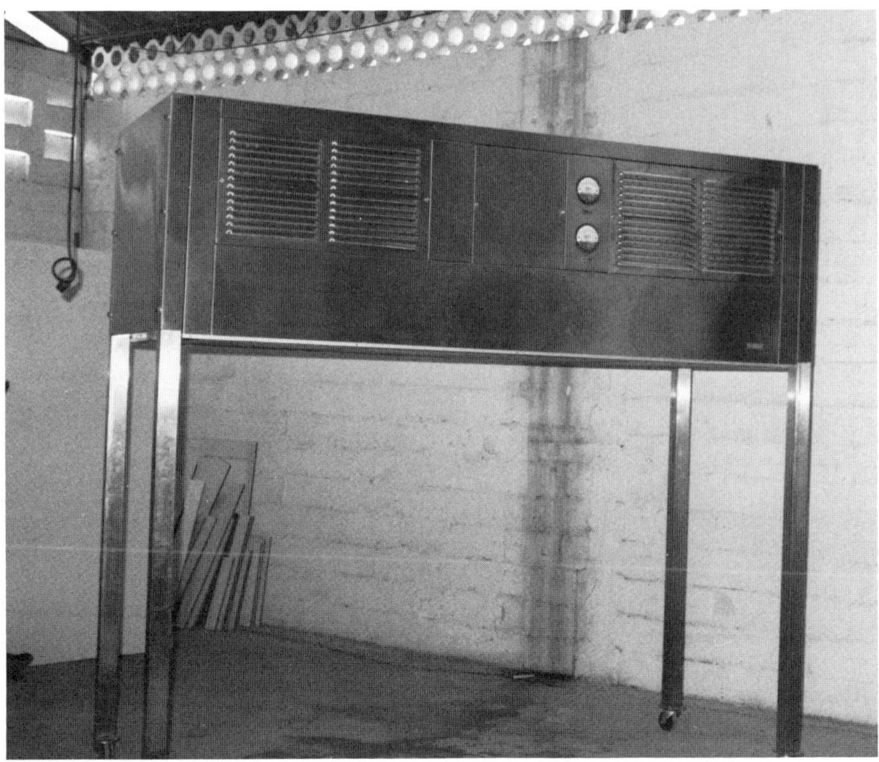

Figure 8 Vertical flow system with air curtains (Kleen-edge). (Courtesy of Veco International, Inc.)

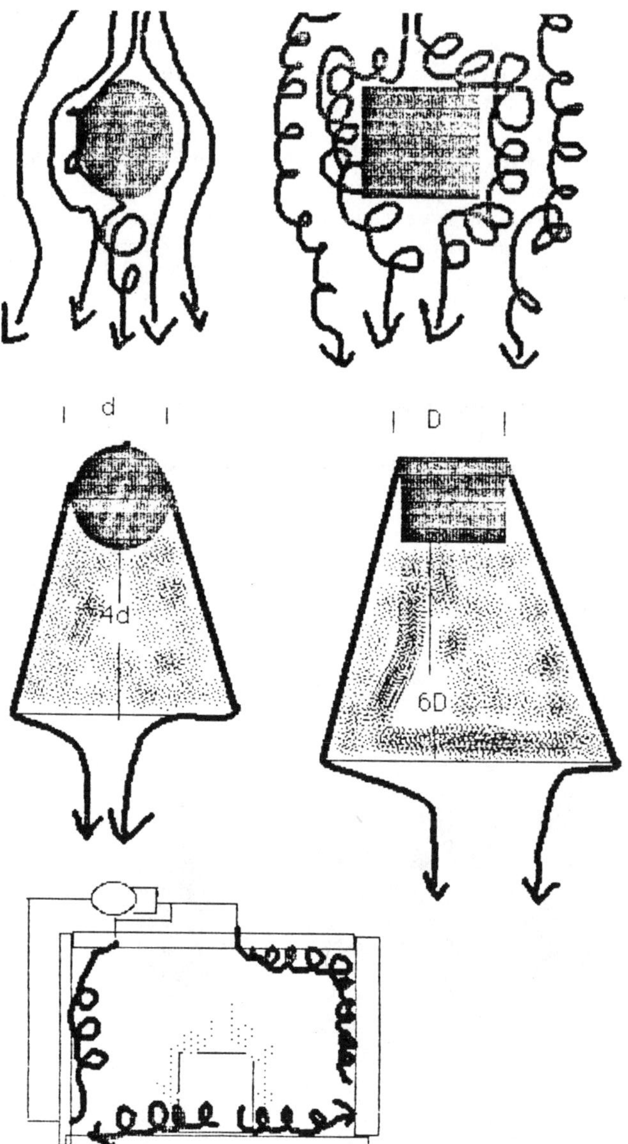

Figure 9 Particle deposition in laminar flow.

and to the aerodynamics of the objects that interfere with the airflow before it reaches critical areas.) Also, whenever there is a void, there is always a zero-velocity area, creating eddy currents that mean turbulence and cross-contamination problems. Generally, the turbulent zone will prevail for a distance equivalent to four to six times the diameter or length of the void, or zero-velocity area. After that distance, the flow will recover. Particles trapped in the eddy current are not eliminated and can re-enter the critical areas, increasing the cross-contamination risk. This process is called re-entrainment.

Due to frictional drag and viscosity, particles can drop on surfaces parallel to the airstream, which are areas of virtually zero velocity. These particles can later be re-entrained. In the case of a class 100 room, this disposition of particles occurs particularly along the walls or, in the case of vertical-flow laminar work stations, along the sides of the vinyl curtains or directive panels.

3. *Advantages of Laminar-Flow Systems*

Some of the characteristics that make laminar flow the best selection in contamination control systems are the following.

a. Laminar flow has the characteristic of transporting particles less than or equal to 15 μm at the same speed as the air, thereby helping to remove those particles that constitute the largest group of airborne contaminants.
b. Laminar-flow devices use HEPA filters that provide the lowest contamination level possible at present.
c. HEPA filter efficiency is 99.97% for particles 0.3 μm and larger. Most bacterial forms have dimensions above 0.5 μm. As explained before, HEPA filters operate under the diffusion principle, and as stated, the diffusion forces have a greater effect on submicrometer-range particles. If the dimensions of some of the viruses are considered, it is likely that they will be trapped by the action of this force.
d. Even if laminarity is altered by obstacles breaking the stream lines, it recovers some distance behind the object.
e. Laminar-flow systems, due to their high recirculation ratio, provide the best cleaning and recovering capabilities of any air filtration system available.
f. Laminar-flow systems produce a uniform air distribution, facilitating control over turbulence.
g. Laminar-flow systems are the only ones that consistently provide class 100 or better cleanliness levels.

4. *Heating, Ventilation, and Air Conditioning Systems*

Heating, ventilation, and air conditioning systems are an integral part of clean room design. The primary purpose of an HVAC system is to provide a specific set of environmental conditions required for the manufacturing process. The established requirements can be met by several combinations of equipment and systems. An important point during the design stages is to match the equipment and system claims with the actual performance desired for that combination.

There are several components in an HVAC system. In general, they can be grouped as follows:

Air moving equipment (blowers, fans, and so on)
Air cooling and heating systems
Air distribution network
Air filtration equipment
Control systems (temperature, humidity, pressure, and air volume)
Monitoring and alarm devices

Air Handling Unit

An air handling unit can be described as the core of the heating, ventilation, and air conditioning central system. This piece of hardware houses the supply and return fans, the heating and cooling coils, the humidifiers, and some stages of air filtration, as well as a series of control devices that regulate the performance of every one of the components within the unit.

Central systems used for controlled areas normally employ air-to-air or air-to-water cooling systems. Design generalizations are difficult because of the many types of systems and facilities existing. As a rule, most of the critical environments have a dedicated air handling system (including all the components required for humidity, temperature, cleanliness, and pressurization control). This is not to say that the heating and cooling media cannot be centrally generated. One of the reasons for the use of dedicated systems is that critical areas are generally in isolated spaces within a larger building in which requirements for cleanliness and other environmental control parameters have been established. Therefore, heating and cooling requirements within the controlled environment are not affected in a serious manner by conditions outside the building, allowing a better, more precise, and economical environmental control.

Heating and cooling requirements are calculated based on the proposed use of the controlled environment. These parameters determine the size, type, and nature of the hardware to be used in the air handling unit. Oversize or undersize could result in inadequate performance of the system.

Compared with air handling units used in commercial systems, the units designed to service a clean environment must meet some additional requirements. Their control systems governing the airflow, temperature, and humidity usually are designed within closer tolerances. Also, any insulation materials must be carefully selected and installed to prevent cross-contamination or medium migration, and fresh air filtration devices must be selected and installed to provide a low particle burden to the system, regardless of the type of final filtration used.

Air Distribution Network

"An air distribution network is a structural assembly whose primary function is to convey air between specific points." This is the definition used by the Sheet Metal and Air Conditioning Contractors, National Association (SMACNA).[27] Design of an air distribution network is determined by the air volumes and total pressures handled by it.

In terms of operational pressure and velocity, air ducts are classified as follows:

High pressure: 3 in. water gage and up
Low pressure: 0–2 in. water gage

The operational pressure is determined by the frictional drag losses caused by the air in motion as well as by the losses caused by obstacles to the free path, such as grilles, air filters, and coils. Design of seals and reinforcements and selection of sheet metal thickness should be based on the desired operational pressure of the system. Systems can have a combination of high- and low-pressure components and, therefore, various construction methods throughout, depending on the points of delivery along the system.

Adequate design for an air distribution network must consider the following factors:

a. Dimensional stability
b. Integrity at specified air volumes and pressures
c. Vibration
d. Noise (transmission and generation)
e. Exposure to damage
f. Support

If all these factors are not considered, it could create problems regarding the adequacy and integrity of the controlled environment. Therefore, qualification specifications should be verified during construction.

Insulation. Particle-releasing materials are not allowable in the air path. Insulation and acoustical liners should only be applied to the exterior of the duct work. If inner liners are used, as is the case in some air handling units, they should be totally sealed, and the nature and qualifications of the procedure should be documented. No asbestos-containing material should be permitted as an insulating, sealing, or adhesive agent.

Flexible Ducts. Certain applications require the advantage and versatility of flexible ducts. Integrity of the air distribution network is a major concern in the selection of adequate material. Factory-fabricated flexible ducts for air conditioning applications are of the following types:

a. Spiral wire-reinforced fabric duct
b. Spiral band-reinforced fabric duct
c. Flexible metal duct
d. Factory insulated and acoustical duct

The preferred type for controlled environment applications is the flexible metal duct with an insulated jacket and a vapor barrier. Fabric ducts are not an adequate choice due to their damage risk and potential particle-releasing action.

Flexible duct is usually limited to short distances to minimize problems involving air tightness and continuity of the vapor barrier. This type of duct should be consistent with the overall design of the duct work. Generally speaking, flexible materials are suitable only for low-pressure systems.

Air Diffusers. The air can be delivered to the controlled environment from the air distribution network by a diffuser. The function of this device is to distribute the air throughout the room. Air delivery can be at low or high velocities and with or without a final filtration. Low-velocity diffusers are used for those environments in which turbulence is considered a potential threat to the environment. Generally, those are rooms with contamination levels less than or equal to 10,000 particles of 0.5 μm or larger per cubic foot of air. These environments typically utilize low-velocity

HEPA air filters, which are terminal filter units. These units have no control over the direction of the air.

High-velocity diffusers are used mostly for comfort to create a turbulent environment to assure proper temperature control. Turbulence is generated by delivering the air at high speeds in a directional fashion, creating eddy currents along the directed air path. This type of diffuser is usually avoided in controlled spaces because turbulence represents a potential for cross-contamination. Also, the construction of this type of diffuser does not facilitate adequate cleaning and sanitizing.

Return Louvers and Grilles. Louvers and grilles return the air to the air distribution network. Adequate louver or grille selection for specific locations depends on various factors:

a. Interaction with architectural components
b. Interaction with machinery and equipment
c. Volume of air to be removed
d. Ideal airflow patterns
c. Nature and type of sanitizing procedures

An air return has a limited influence on airflow direction. Air velocities drop off dramatically at a short distance from the exhaust grille. (See Fig. 10.) At a distance equivalent to the diameter of the opening of the return air grille, the velocity of the air is only 10% of its velocity in the return air duct. Low and uniformly distributed openings along the base of the controlled environment are preferred. This minimizes the effects of turbulence created by frictional drag losses created by the air contact at floor level. Return grilles sometimes house prefilters designed to prevent contaminants from entering the duct work and to control the undesired effects of backflow, which is potentially present in some installations when the systems are not fully operational. (If no booster exhaust is used, the airborne contaminant can re-enter the clean space as a result of changes in system pressure.)

Obstructions to air returns caused by equipment or personnel could alter the airflow patterns. Thus, layouts used during the design and qualification stages must be maintained. This is particularly important in those installations equipped with partial or total laminar-flow equipment, to assure proper usage of the laminar-flow properties.

Construction of louvers, grilles, and diffusers should facilitate adequate cleaning and sanitation procedures. The installation should guarantee the integrity and continuity of the air distribution network as well as of the controlled environments. Leaks in joints at the connecting points of diffusers and of return grilles jeopardize the adequacy of the operation.

Control

The combination of equipment designed to provide the necessary balance of environmental conditions must include a control system. A control system provides feedback consisting of a continuous analysis of the conditions prevailing in the controlled environment. It continuously compares resultant conditions with the expected, pre-established conditions and triggers adjustments necessary for adequate balance.

The degree and complexity of the control system is based on the type of process, the size of the facility, the type of systems used for energy

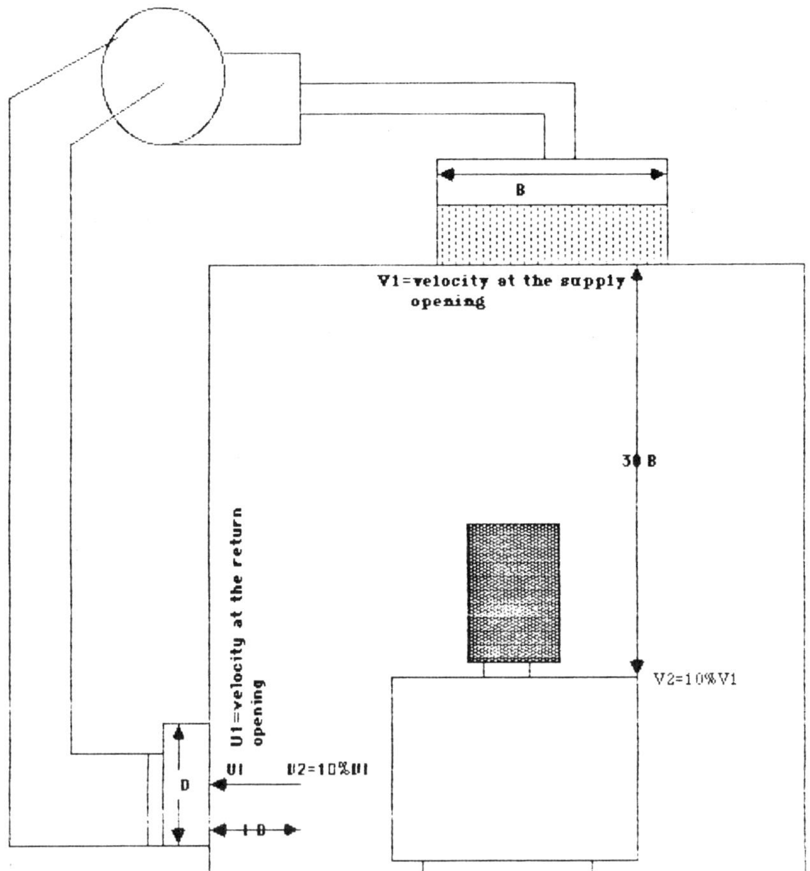

Figure 10 Effect of distance and velocity in an air return. Velocities are expressed as percentage of opening velocity.

conservation, the safety devices required for the process, and regulations of local or federal authorities.

Control devices can be activated and control reactions transmitted by pneumatic or electrical energy. Selection of control devices is based on such factors as cost, reactive speed, availability, accuracy, service precision, and performance.

The most common control devices used in a clean room are thermostats and humidistats. Thermostats control all the heating and cooling devices, and humidistats control humidification and dehumidification, as required. These temperature and humidity controls employ such devices as thermocouples, mercury-operated devices, hot-wired thermosensors, and gold-plated mirrors.

Devices used for controlling pressure and air volume work closely with the other equipment used for environmental control, such as duct work, dampers, and air handling devices. Depending on the type of system, several sensing stations are located within the room and up- and downstream of the air distribution network, to assure the proper pressure differentials among the various rooms. The required reaction time of these controls should be determined by the allowable recovery time of a critical enclosure. That is, if a pressurization control takes too long to react after a depressurization action, such as the opening of a door, the integrity of the enclosure could be in jeopardy. Control system complexity and the cost of the pressurization and volume control devices vary with such things as the air volumes handled and the desired control accuracies and reactive speeds. The control devices can be electromechanical, electropneumatic, or electronic (transducers).

Sequencing and calibration of controls are customary procedures in any new installation. Accurate verification of these procedures, of equipment, and of recording methods is an integral part of maintaining the environment.

Monitoring and Alarm Devices

Monitoring devices provide continuous information with respect to a specific environmental condition. Unlike the control devices, these do not operate or adjust any other devices. Monitoring devices can be permanently installed to service the clean room or controlled environment, or they can be brought into it as required. For convenience and a more effective operation, a continuous monitoring system should either be installed at the controlled environment or placed in an adjacent, easy-to-access location.

Alarm devices are used to alert the users of the system to deviation from the standard operational parameters. Two levels of alarms are typically established for the critically controlled environments in a parenteral drug manufacturing operation. The first is designated as alert level. This indicates that the system is approaching unsatisfactory conditions. For example, if the temperature level is set at 70°F and the specified range is ±3°F, an alert level can be set at 72°F. At this point, those responsible for the system should investigate why the system is behaving as it is and determine if a corrective procedure is required. When the facility is operating at alert levels, manufacturing operations can continue. The second level of alarm is designated as action level. At this point, the system is completely out of range; manufacturing operations must be stopped, and corrective action must be taken.

IV. SYSTEM QUALIFICATION AND VALIDATION

Verification of the operational characteristics prior to commissioning an environmental control system is defined as qualification of the system. The series of testing and verification procedures used to provide assurances of the system's proper and continuous operation is defined as validation. Environmental performance tests are required for both the qualification and validation procedures.

Environmental system validation consists of challenging the system as a whole and comparing the results with the expected operational parameters. If the results of three consecutive tests are within the specified range, the system can be considered valid. Once all systems are validated, the facility can be certified.

A. Environmental Performance Testing

To verify that all the components of an environmental control system function properly, a sequence of performance tests should be conducted:

a. Airflow and uniformity test
b. Temperature control test
c. Humidity control test
d. Pressurization control test
e. HEPA filter leak test
f. Airborne particle count test
g. Enclosure induction leak test
h. Airflow patterns test
i. Particle dispersion test
j. Recovery test
k. Airborne microbial sampling on critically controlled environments
l. Surface sampling[28]

Detailed information on these tests is given in the appendix. Most of them are performance tests required for the validation of the environment. The test sequencing indicated is the one typically used. These tests should be executed in "at-rest" and "operational" conditions, and some of the tests[29] should be repeated at least three times in operational conditions to verify the ability of the system(s) to perform continuously within the specified parameters. An at-rest facility is a facility that is complete, has all equipment installed but not operating, and is without personnel. An operational facility is a facility in normal operation with all services functional, with equipment operating, and with personnel present.

Performance tests executed in at-rest conditions serve as baseline information. After the tests are repeated in operational conditions, the baseline information helps to determine the degree to which the environment is affected by the manufacturing process. It is after this analysis that certain procedures, equipment, and methods may be changed.

B. Stress Testing

Testing should also be done under stress conditions representing possible but unlikely situations. This determines the ability of the environmental control system to remain stable. Stress conditions are predetermined by the particular system's design. For example, in a clean or aseptic environment composed of several rooms with doors to a common access corridor and gowning area, a stress condition might be when all doors are opened at the same time and left open until the pressure differentials among critical and noncritical environments go outside the pre-established safe range. Testing to determine the span of time between the doors' opening and the pressure differentials going out of specification determines the boundaries within which the system can operate safely. This result can be used to determine action levels in case of the actual occurrence of such a condition. Other stress testing, such as operating with the doors open in a clean room while the room's particle count is being taken, can be used to determine the potential effect of door openings for various lengths of time during operation. Stress testing is also used to determine the ability to recover the prespecified conditions after such an occurrence as power failure. Stress testing is also an effective means for validating and qualifying the environmental control system.

Reporting Form Sample:

DATE:________________ STANDARD OPERATING PROCEDURE No.__________

LOCATION____

PERSON PERFORMING THE TEST____

STARTING TIME_____________ FINISHING TIME_____________

EQUIPMENT, SERIAL NUMBER, AND CALIBRATION DATE:

____

____

____

____

TEMPERATURE IN THE ROOM_________ °F HUMIDITY__________%

DESIGN CONDITIONS TO BE TESTED FOR:

____

____

____

TESTING LOCATIONS:________________ATTACHED DRAWING No.__________

ACTUAL CONDITIONS:

____

____

____

ACCEPTANCE OR REJECTION STATEMENT:

____

____

____

SIGNATURES:

PERSON CONDUCTING THE TEST:_________________________ DATE:_______

SUPERVISOR____ DATE:_______

REVIEWED BY____ DATE:_______

Figure 11 Reporting form sample.

C. Measuring Instruments

Measuring instruments are integral parts of environmental performance evaluation. A description of some of these instruments is given in some of the sections of this chapter as well as in the appendix.

Every measuring device involves a comparison against a reference standard. This process is known as calibration. Compliance with calibration requirements should be verified before starting any testing procedure. On many occasions, testing services are contracted with outside vendors. In those cases, careful consideration must be given to the equipment that will be used. Equipment used by certification companies is subjected to continuous handling, which could alter adjustments and cause divergent results from the standardization. Therefore, it is recommended that those instruments required for performance testing be owned or at least operated by the parenteral drug manufacturer.

D. Reporting Forms

Reporting forms for validation purposes should provide a complete record of each test. (See Fig. 11.) The following information is usually contained in a reporting form:

Date when the test was conducted
Start and Finish time
Location of the test
List of testing equipment, serial numbers, and last calibration date
List of the design conditions to be tested for
At least two signatures of those involved in the test and of those responsible for the testing procedure
Diagrams showing the testing locations

This list can be made as comprehensive as the user requires.

V. APPENDIX[30]

A. Air Flow and Uniformity Test

1. *Purpose*

a. Demonstrate that the air system is balanced and capable of delivering sufficient air volumes to maintain a minimum cross-sectional velocity under the HEPA terminal filter modules of at least 90 ft/min measured 6 in. downstream of the filters.
b. Verify air velocities before the air encounters an obstruction.
c. Verify horizontal and vertical air velocity components at the point the clean air reaches an obstacle or a surface 40 in. above the floor, whichever occurs first.

2. *Equipment*

Use a hot-wire anemometer and stand and a Pitot tube.[31]

3. Method

a. These tests are to be executed by approved personnel in every room where a HEPA terminal filter module is installed.
b. Draw a grid on the floor as indicated by the room's diagram.
c. Measure and record the velocity at the center of each grid at the specified heights (Fig. 12).
d. Allow no objects within 10 ft of the anemometer, except for built-in equipment. Minimize the number of people present during the at-rest testing.
e. Measurements should be taken for a minimum of 15 sec.
f. Record the pressure readings (in inches) from the manometer connected to the module's plenum.

4. Acceptance

Measured clean air velocity shall be higher than 90 ft/min and not exceeding 150 ft/min at 6 in. downstream from filter face. Velocity differences within the same plenum should not vary more than 25%. These are suggested, not mandatory, values.

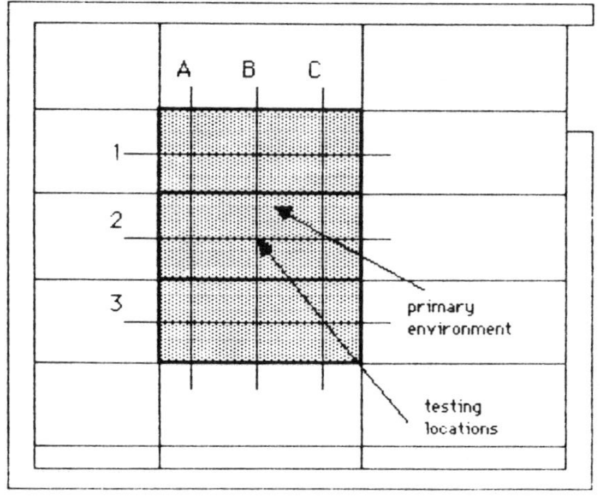

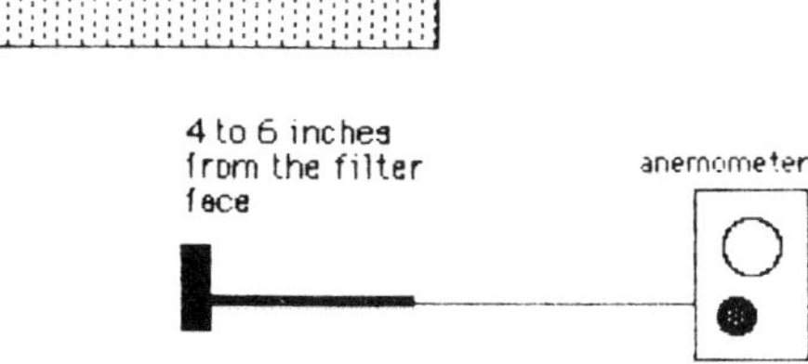

Figure 12 Airflow uniformity test in a primary environment.

B. Temperature Control Test

1. Purpose

Demonstrate the ability of the air handling system to control temperature at 75°F (±10%) all year round.

2. Equipment

Use a calibrated dry bulb thermometer,[32] thermoanemometer,[33] or thermocouples and recorder.

3. Method

a. Air conditioning systems are to be in continuous operation for at least 24 hr prior to performing these tests. All lights in the sterile core are to be on during the testing as well as during the 24-hr preconditioning period.
b. Measure and record temperatures at 15-min intervals for a period of 2 hr at each of the indicated locations for each room.
c. The test should be repeated for at-rest and operational conditions.

4. Acceptance

The system shall be capable of maintaining a dry bulb temperature of 72°F (±10%) all year, with the specified occupancy and heat generation design levels.

C. Humidity Control Test

1. Purpose

Demonstrate the capability of the air handling system to control humidity at the specified level for each room.

2. Equipment

Use dry bulb and wet bulb thermometers, and an automatic humidity recorder.

3. Method

a. Execute this test after all the balancing procedures have been concluded.
b. Measure and record humidities for the conditions and locations specified for every room under at-rest and operational conditions.
c. Operate the system for at least 6 hr prior to the start of the test.
d. Record water temperatures at the beginning and end of the test, if possible.

4. Acceptance

The relative humidity at each grid point shall be equal to the specified levels and tolerance limits indicated on each recording form. Typical accepted values are 50 ± 10%. If these levels are attained, the system is acceptable.

D. Pressurization Control Test

1. *Purpose*

Demonstrate the capability of the system to control pressure levels within the specified limits.

2. *Equipment*

Use an air pressure gage[34] with resolution of 0.01 in. of water.

3. *Method*

a. All HVAC and laminar-flow systems are to be in continuous operation when performing these tests.
b. To avoid unexpected changes in pressure and to establish a baseline, all doors in the sterile facility must be closed and no traffic is to be allowed through the facility during this test.
c. Pressure readings are taken with the high- and low-pressure tubing at the following locations (refer to each room's diagram).
d. The following stress conditions as indicated in the matrix in Figure 13 should be simulated while monitoring pressures at the locations delineated in step c.

4. *Acceptance*

a. Pressure differentials should be as indicated in the design conditions at all times under at-rest conditions.
b. Pressure differentials should be maintained as indicated in design conditions under standard simulated operating conditions.
c. Pressure differentials should be above 0.02 in. of water at the primary environments when stress conditions occur.
d. The system will not be acceptable if, at any time during normal operational, at-rest, or stress conditions, the pressure in the primary environments becomes less than zero, or negative.

Note: The final balancing report will become part of the validation documentation.

	Test 1	Test 2	Test 3	Test 4
Gowning	Closed	Open	Closed	Closed
Ancillary	Closed	Closed	Open	Closed
Primary (room)	Closed	Open	Open	Open
Corridor	Closed	Closed	Open	Closed

Figure 13

E. HEPA Filter Leak Test

1. *Purpose*

Ensure against HEPA filter failure due to damage during installation or operation.

2. *Equipment*

DOP polydisperse aerosol is generated by blowing air through liquid dioctylphthalate (DOP) at room temperature. The approximate light scattering mean-droplet-size distribution of the aerosol is as follows:

99% + smaller than 3.0 μm
95% + smaller than 1.5 μm
92% + smaller than 1.0 μm
50% + smaller than 0.72 μm
25% + smaller than 0.45 μm
11% + smaller than 0.35 μm

The DOP aerosol generator is compressed air operated, equipped with Laskin-type nozzles as described in USA Standard N-5.11. The aerosol photometer is a light-scattering type with a threshold sensitivity of at least 10^{-3} μg/liter. Capable of measuring concentrations in the range of 80–120 μg/liter and having air sampling flow rate of 1 ft^3 (±10%) per minute. This instrument is to be calibrated by the manufacturer after every 100 hr of use.

3. *Method*

a. This test is performed only by certified personnel, who introduce DOP aerosol upstream of the filter through a test port and search for leaks downstream with an aerosol photometer.
b. Filter testing is to be performed after operational air velocities have been verified and adjusted where necessary.
c. Align the aerosol photometer.
d. Position the aerosol generator such that DOP aerosol will be introduced into the airstream upstream of the HEPA filters.
e. Open the appropriate number of nozzles until a DOP challenge concentration of 100 μg/liter of air is reached. This challenge concentration is measured upstream of the HEPA filter and is evidenced by a reading between 4 and 5 on the logarithmic scale of the aerosol photometer.
f. Scan each filter by holding the photometer probe approximately 1 in. from the filter face and passing the probe in slightly overlapping strokes, at a traverse rate of not more than 10 ft/min, so that the entire face is sampled.
g. Make separate passes with the photometer probe around the entire periphery of the filter, along the bond between the filter medium and the frame, and along all other joints in the installation through which leakage might bypass the filter medium.

4. *Acceptance*

a. An unacceptable leak is defined as 0.01% of the reference calibration curve.

b. Leaks are sealed using silicone sealant (DOP or 3M weatherstrip adhesive) by caulking a 1–2 in. area around the leak parallel to the medium and between the separators. The sealant is forced over the filter medium between the separators and smoothed flush with the separators. The filter is then rechecked for leaks as specified above.

c. The extent of filter face obscured at any one point by patching materials is limited to 5% of the filter area, so that the resulting void in the airstream will be filled in before reaching the work area. If more is sealed, the filter must be rejected and a new one installed.

F. Airborne Particle Count Test

1. *Purpose*

Establish that, at critical work locations within clean rooms, a count of less than 100 particles (0.5 μm and larger) per cubic foot of air is maintained.

2. *Equipment*

Use a light-scattering particle counter, as described in the American Society for Testing Materials Standard F50-69.

3. *Method*

a. These tests are performed by authorized personnel after the HEPA filter leak tests and air velocity tests are completed.

b. To first obtain baseline data with the room in static conditions, perform the following tests with operational personnel absent and the equipment at rest.
Using the particle counter, count particles of 0.5 μm and larger at heights of 40 in. in the center of each grid shown on the test report (Fig. 14).
If the particle count is less than 50 ft^{-3} of air, four additional counts at this location are taken to place these particle counts within a 50% confidence interval.

c. After completion of these tests, if the HEPA air filtration modules are operating within accepted limits, repeat step b with operational personnel present and the fill equipment running. If at any time there is a deviation from accepted parameters, the various components of the systems in operation are reviewed, repaired, or adjusted until the desired conditions are achieved.

4. *Acceptance*

a. The air systems can be considered validated when the results of three consecutive sets of tests are within accepted operational parameters.

b. At any of the designated critical locations (a critical location is where any sterilized product or material is exposed to the working environment), the particle count shall not exceed 100 particles of 0.5 μm and larger per cubic foot of air.

5. *Ancillary Environment Acceptance Level*

The same test should be repeated at ancillary environments. Ancillary environment shall not exceed a particle count of 100,000 particles of 0.5 μm

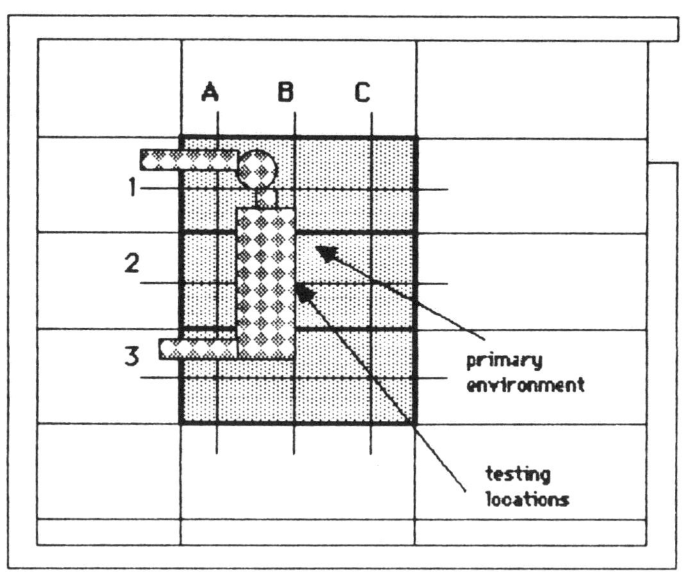

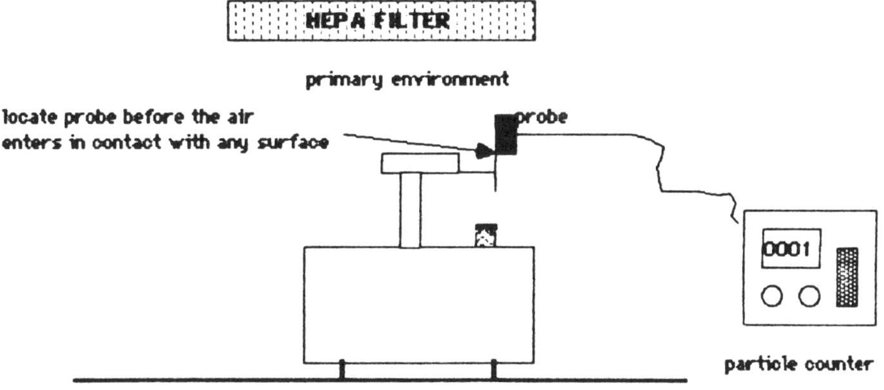

Figure 14 Particle count test.

and larger per cubic foot of air in order to be considered acceptable by current regulations. It is common practice to design and operate ancillary environments at levels not exceeding 10,000 particles of 0.5 μm and larger per cubic foot of air. This is to provide additional protection to the final product while it is processed at the critical area.

Table 4 summarizes the contamination sources and the suggested control methods. A review of these prior to executing the above procedures is recommended.

Table 5 provides the cleanliness class definition as established in Federal Standard 209-B.

Table 6 provides a guideline of cleanliness levels required for a typical manufacturing operation.

Note: Particle counters measure and count particles 0.1 μm and larger. There is a relationship between the particle size and the sample flow: the smaller the particle intended to be measured, the lower the flow.

Typical particle counters for clean room testing (Royco, Climet, Met-one, and Kratel) measure and count particles down to 0.3 μm with flow rates from 0.1 ft^3/min to 1 ft^3/min. The high sampling flow rate of 1 ft^3/min makes it possible to scan HEPA filter installations. These instruments use regular white light as a source inside the sensing chamber, limiting their use to measuring only particles 0.3 μm and larger.

Lasers and modern electronics have made it possible to measure and count particles down to 0.1 μm, but at a very low sampling flow rate of 0.01 ft^3/min. These instruments are used to classify ultraclean rooms (class 10).

Another instrument currently in use is the condensation nucleus counter (CNC). This instrument can count particles independent of the size. Particles are measured by condensing alcohol in them to make them grow, making it impossible for the photometer to then count the particles. Particle size evaluation is typically made by another instrument, such as a dynamic particle size analyzer. Due to the complexity of these instruments, their use has been limited to research installations and a few very specialized clean rooms.

Clean rooms used in parenteral drug manufacturing can be classified accurately with the white light particle counters, with a particle count range of 0.5 μm and larger and a sampling flow rate of 0.1–1 ft^3/min. The rest of the instruments described above are used for classifying class 10 and class 1 rooms and for other unique applications.

E. Enclosure Induction Leak Test

1. *Purpose*

This test is performed to determine if there is intrusion of unfiltered air into the clean work areas from outside the clean room enclosure through joints and cracks in the walls or ceiling, for example (other than from the pressurized air supply system), and to determine unfiltered air intrusion into the clean room through open doorways.

2. *Equipment*

Use the optical particle counter.

Table 4 Contamination Sources and Control

Source	Control
People	Total body covering in critical areas and partial covering in noncritical areas.
	Adequate personnel flow and restricted access to aseptic and critical environments
	Adequate equipment location to avoid excess handling of materials and provide minimum movement of personnel
	Limits on numbers of personnel in critical environments
	Adequate operating procedures for personnel
Process	Adequate cleaning and sterilization procedures and equipment
	Barriers and separation between high-risk and low-risk operations
	Protective laminar-flow equipment
	Adequate process equipment designed for operation in critical areas; proper covers and barriers to contain contamination from moving parts
	Adequate operating procedures to assure proper handling, cleaning, and sterilization of machinery and equipment
	Adequate standards for equipment and construction material selection
	Adequate selection of manufacturing environments
	Adequate vacuum cleaning devices for powder or contaminant generation operations
Materials	Adequate material control and selection
	Adequate sterilization and filtration procedures
	Adequate handling of material procedures and equipment
	Adequate control and testing methods to assure cleanliness levels and sterility
Air	Adequate air filtration systems
	Adequate monitoring of air cleanliness levels
	Adequate air system validation procedures
	Adequate maintenance procedures

Table 5 Air Cleanliness Classes

	Maximum number of particles			
	0.5 μm		5 μm	
Class	ft^{-3}	$liter^{-1}$	ft^{-3}	$liter^{-1}$
100	100	3.5	—	—
10,000	10,000	350	65	2.3
100,000	100,000	3,500	700	25

Source: From Federal Standard 209B, GSA.

3. *Method*

a. Measure the concentration outside the clean room enclosure immediately adjacent to the surface of doorway to be evaluated. This concentration should be at least 100,000 particles of 0.5 μm or larger per cubic foot. If the concentration is less, generate an aerosol to increase the concentration.
b. To check for construction joint leakage, scan all joint areas at a distance of 6 in. away at a speed of approximately 10 in./min.
c. To check for intrusion of open doorways, measure the concentration inside the enclosure at 10 in. from the open door.
d. Repeat the same test in front of any openings, such as pass-throughs or electrical outlets, and in front of any opening connecting with the outside.
e. Repeat this test while opening and closing clean room entrance doors.

4. *Acceptance*

No construction joint leaks or intrusion through open doors should exceed 0.1% of the measured external concentration.

Table 6 Guideline of Cleanliness Levels Required During Manufacturing of a Parenteral Drug

Operation	Class	Cleanliness level (particles 0.5 μm/ft^3 and larger)
Warehousing	—	—
Preparation	100,000	No more than 100,000
Filtration	100,000	No more than 100,000
Filling area	100,000 or better	No more than 100,000
Filling line (point of use)	100	No more than 100

Note: Figure 15 shows a particle counter like the one used for this and other cleanliness assessment procedures.

H. Airflow Patterns Test

1. *Purpose*

Determine airflow interaction with machinery and equipment in a critical area protected with a laminar-flow clean air system. Determine the airflow patterns during fill line operation. Select and improve the flow pattern that generates the minimum turbulence and best washing capabilities.

2. *Equipment*

Use a white visible or yellow smoke generator,[35] anemometer, and 35 mm camera, or videotape machines.

3. *Procedure*

a. Verify that the laminar-flow devices in the sterile core are operational.
b. Check air velocities at 6 in. from the filter face to ensure that the device is operating within the specified laminar flow velocity (90 ft/min or above).
c. Verify that the ventilation and air conditioning systems are operating and balanced.
d. If the system operates according to the specified operating parameters, begin to generate white visible smoke at the critical locations. (A critical location is defined as any area where sterilized product or material is exposed to the working environment.)

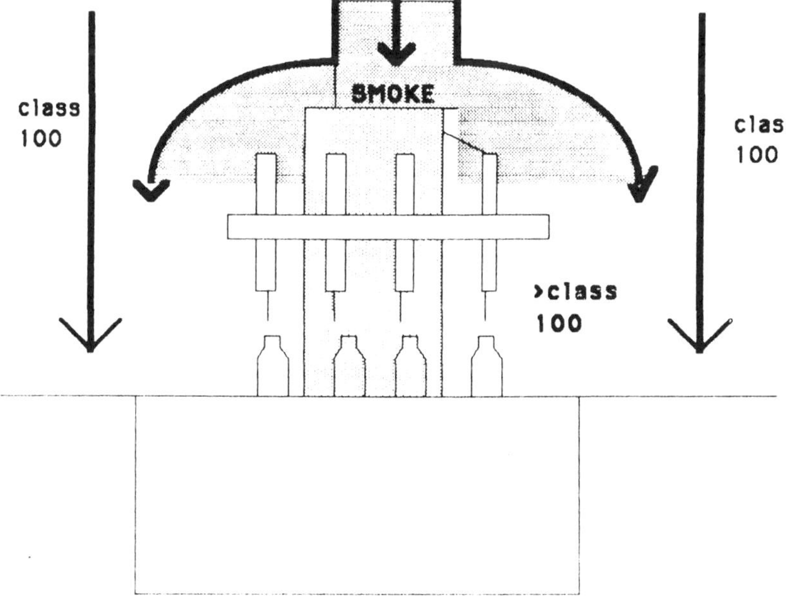

Figure 15 Particle dispersion and recovery test.

e. Generate white smoke inside and over each component that forms part of the line (to avoid damage to the materials or equipment, ocver them tightly with plastic). Film the smoke as it travels through each critical area of the machine.
f. Smoke should flow through these critical areas. If the air does return (backflows) because of turbulence, the system cannot be accepted and must be rebalanced or adjusted. Slight turbulence, due to equipment configuration, is not significant as long as the air does not return to the critical areas.
g. If the system passes the test in step f, continue to film while the smoke is generated and an operator enters the protected area. If the smoke backflows to the critical working area at any point during this operation, procedures must be established to prevent cross-contamination and re-entry into these areas. If the unit passes, proceed to step h.
h. Determine if the generated turbulence can carry contaminants from other areas to critical points of the line. If so, adjust the airflow to ensure a minimum of turbulence and rapid cleaning. If the turbulence cannot be stopped, a different aerodynamic pattern must be found. (Covers and diffusers can be used over the filling equipment.) If turbulence carries contaminants from any area to the critical areas, the system should be re-evaluated and analyzed in terms of the filling, capping, and laminar-flow equipment.

4. *Acceptance*

If the results of steps f, g, and h are unsatisfactory, the laminar-flow system cannot be validated, and the rest of the validation tests should not be carried out until a satisfactory operation has been reached. Otherwise, the system is valid and can be certified. Should corrective changes be necessary, the changes are made, recorded, and the validation process repeated.

I. Particle Dispersion Test

1. *Purpose*

The purpose of these tests is to verify the parallelism of airflow throughout the work zone and the capability of the clean room to limit the dispersion (Fig. 15).

These tests may be applied at the discretion of the buyer when deemed necessary.

2. *Equipment*

Use a visual smoke generator, particle counter, and hot-wire anemometer.

3. *Method*

a. Perform this test after completion of the air velocity uniformity tests.
b. Divide the work zone into 2 × 2 ft grids of equal area.
c. Set up smoke generator, with outlet tube pointing in the direction of airflow and located at the center of a grid area at the work zone entrance plane.
d. If smoke is introduced with air pressure, adjust it to provide a smoke outlet velocity equal to the room air velocity at that point.

e. Operate particle counter with the sample tube at normal work level and at a point remote from the smoke source. Verify that the counter indicates particle concentrations less than 100 particles of 0.5 μm or larger per cubic foot.
f. Move the sample tube in toward the smoke source from all directions at this level to the point where particle counts show a sudden and rapid rise to high levels (10^6 ft^{-3}). This defines the envelope of dispersion away from the smoke source and demonstrates the airflow parallelism control of the room.
g. Repeat for all grid areas. Prepare a diagram showing grid areas and corresponding dispersion envelopes.

4. Acceptance

The degree to which dispersion away from the smoke source is confined and the regularity of the pattern (indication of directional drift in one direction) is a matter of the configuration of the line. It is recommended that dispersion should not extend beyond 2 ft radially from the point of smoke source: i.e., at 2 ft away from generation point, particle count should be less than 100 particles of 0.5 μm and larger per cubic foot.

Note: Figure 16 shows the airflow patterns on a table while under a Kleen-edge laminar airflow module.

J. Recovery Test

1. Purpose

Determine the capabilities of the system to recover from internally generated contamination.

2. Equipment

Use a visual smoke generator, particle counter, and hot-wire anemometer.

3. Method

a. With smoke generation output tube located at a predesignated location, generate smoke for 1–2 min and shut off.
b. Wait 2 min, and then advance the sample tube of the particle counter to a point directly under the smoke source and at the level of the work zone. Record the count of particles 0.5 μm or larger. If the count is not 100 particles or less ft^{-3}, repeat test with wait interval increased in steps of $\frac{1}{2}$ min until counts are less than 100 ft^{-3}.
c. Repeat for all grid areas, recording recovery time for each grid area.

4. Acceptance

The recovery time should not be more than 2 min.

K. Airborne Microbial Sampling on Critically Controlled Environments

1. Purpose

To determine the airborne microbial contamination level.

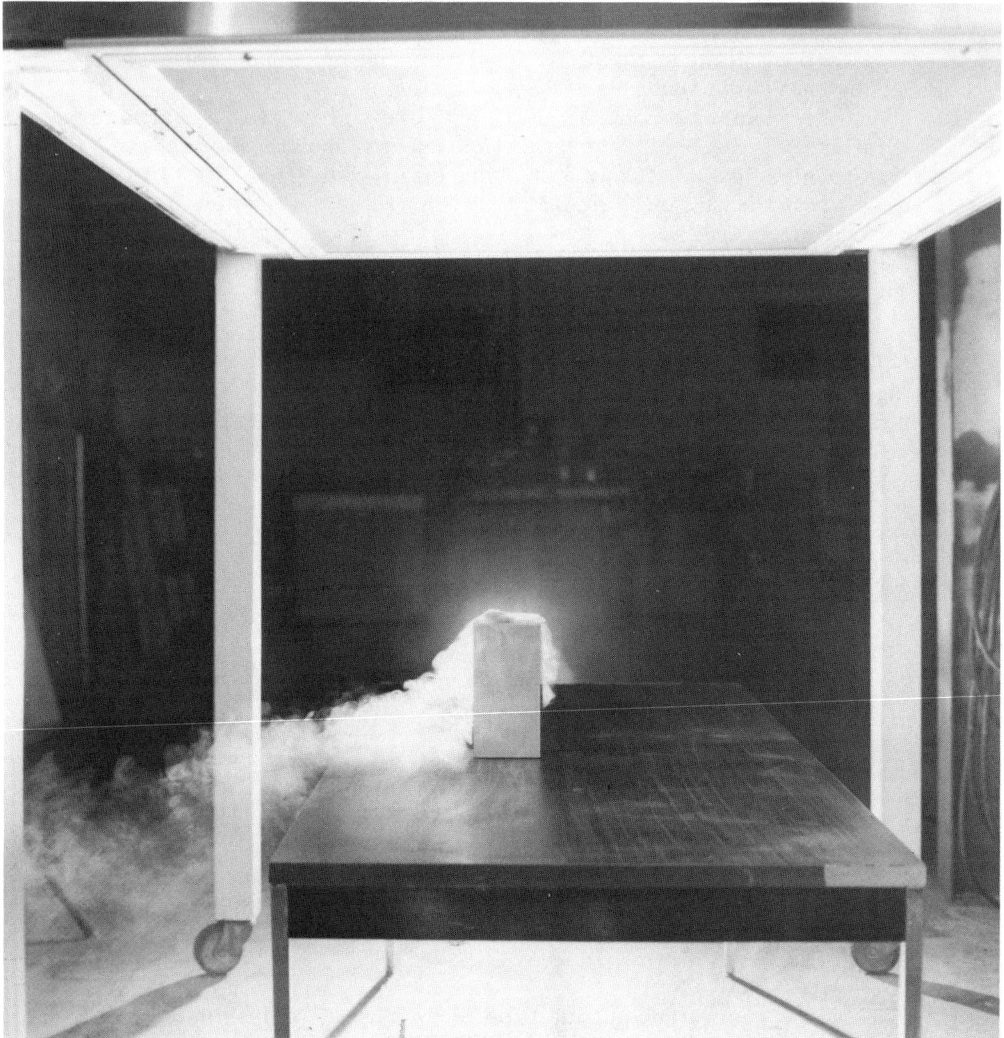

Figure 16

2. Equipment

Use a solid surface impactor with a rotating collection surface and/or staged plates (Anderson-Slit).

3. Method

a. After proceeding with calibration and indications given in the operating manual, follow steps b through f.
b. Aseptically prepared collection plates are placed in the sampling apparatus. Petri dishes used must be sterilized prior to filling. Verify the adequacy of petri dish dimensions so the operational characteristics are maintained according to the manufacturer's specifications. (Plastic petri dishes are not recommended, because static charges are likely to be present in plastic and to reduce the collection efficiency.)

c. Any general-purpose, solid bacteriological medium, such as trypticase-soy agar or blood agar, can be used. Selective media are not recommended, since they inhibit the repair and growth of injured or stressed cells.
d. Verify the air sampling rate, time, and location of the plate before starting the sampling. Sampling time should be 20 min at every location. After the sampling is completed, remove the collection plate(s), cover, and identify them. Identification should include date, sampling instrument number, location, and plate number.
e. Plates then are taken to an incubator and maintained inverted, to prevent condensation drop, for a period of 18–24 hr at 35°C.
f. After incubation, the number of colonies on each plate is counted, using a standard bacterial counter.

4. *Acceptance*

The total number of colonies from sample plates in the same location divided by the time in minutes (assuming a sample of a cubic foot per minute) will give the number of viable particles per cubic foot of air sampled. This number should not exceed 0.1, assuming the accepted microbiological theory that each colony represents a single particle, and the correlation to the class 100 laminar-flow conditions in a controlled environment. This criterion has also been established by relating the number of colonies per liter of air, limiting that amount to 0.0035 colonies in a class 100 environment.

Note: Fallout sampling is not an acceptable method to determine the microbial environmental quality of laminar-flow devices. Due to the airflow patterns over petri dishes, a minimal percentage of air comes in contact with the culture media, rendering the test invalid. The only way to assure adequate contact is by drawing the air by mechanical force over the media.

Filtration devices that employ membrane filters are also used with some drawbacks; after filtration, the filter must be agitated to remove all particles, and this could result in damage to the cells, causing loss of some organisms. Blending the membrane with liquid medium is a better technique for a more representative analysis.

Table 7 provides the NASA (National Aeronautics and Space Administration) proposed limit of microorganisms in accordance with cleanliness level classification.

Table 7 Number of Live Organisms as Proposed by NASA STD NH135430 and MSFC-STD-246

	Live organisms	
Class	ft^{-3}	$liter^{-1}$
100	0.1	0.0035
10,000	0.5	0.0176
100,000	2.5	0.0884

Source: From NASA *Handbook for Biological Engineers*, Washington, D.C., Technical Information Services.

L. Surface Sampling

1. *Purpose*

Determine the microbial contamination level on surfaces.

2. *Equipment*

Use a rodac plate (nutrient agar culture medium).

3. *Method*

a. Press the rodac plate directly against the surface to be sampled. Incubate until colonies are developed. Use this technique for flat and smooth surfaces, such as tables, floor, and walls.
b. This technique is to be used after decontamination procedures. Agar media left on surfaces could present a problem. Therefore, decontamination procedures should immediately follow sampling.
c. Identify every plate, indicating the exact location where the sample was taken. Room landmarks should be noted for present and future referencing.

4. *Acceptance*

Maximum number of colonies per square foot should not exceed 100. This is an arbitrary number set by NASA.

BIBLIOGRAPHY

Agnew, B., *Laminar Flow-Clean Room Handbook*. Los Angeles, Agnew-Higgins, 1965.

American Conference of Governmental Industrial Hygienist, *Industrial Ventilation*. Ann Arbor, Michigan, Edwards Brothers, 1980.

ASHRAE, *Guide and Data Book*. New York, American Society of Heating, Refrigerating, and Air Conditioning Engineers, 1971.

Department of Defense, *Military Specification Filter, Particulate High-Efficiency, Fire Resistance*. MIL-F-51068C, June 8, 1970.

DeVecchi, F., *Training Personnel to Work in Sterile Environments*. Los Angeles, Pharmaceutical Technology, 1978.

DeVecchi, F., *Clean Room Analysis*. Pharm Tech Conference Proceedings, 1981.

DeVecchi, F., *Air Systems Validation*. Center for Professional Advancement, Course Notes, 1982.

Dimmick, R. L., and Wolochow, H., *Problems of Measuring Numbers of Microbes in Occupied Spaces*. Institute of Environmental Sciences, 1981 proceedings.

Federal Standard 209-B, *Clean Room and Work-Station Requirements*. Washington, D.C., GSA, 1966.

Food and Drug Administration, *Current Good Manufacturing Practice in Manufacture, Processing, Packing or Holding*. Federal Register, Feb. 13, 1976.

Fuscaldo, A., Erlick, B. J., and Hindman, *Laboratory Safety*. New York, Academic Press, 1980.

McCrone, W., Draftz, R., and Delly, J. G., *The Particle Analyst*. Ann Arbor, Michigan, Ann Arbor Science Publishers, 1968.

NASA, *Symposium on Clean Room Technology in Surgery Suites.* St. Louis, Midwest Research Institute, 1971.

NASA, *Handbook for Biological Engineers.* Washington, D.C., Technical Information Services.

U.S. Air Force, *Technical Order 00-25-203: Standard and Guidelines for Design and Operation of Clean Rooms and Clean Work Stations.* Washington, D.C., Technical Information Services, 1963.

NOTES

1. Food and Drug Administration, Federal Register. Friday, February 13, 1976.
2. Society of Clean Room Engineers of Switzerland, P.O. Box 239, CH. 8032, Zurich, Switzerland.
3. American Society for Testing and Materials, 1916 Race St., Philadelphia, PA 19103.
4. General Services Administration, Specifications Activity, Printed Materials Supply Division, Building 197, Naval Weapons Plant, Washington, D.C. 20407.
5. Formerly the American Association for Contamination Control. Refer to Institute of Environmental Sciences, 940 East Northwest Highway, Mount Prospect, IL 60056.
6. A "controlled" environment has moderate contamination control requirements. This means the level of airborne contaminants is specifically defined by size, range, nature, or concentration, but there is no need for strict control over contaminants generated by personnel, materials, equipment, and so on. Comfort conditions are provided for operations personnel. A "critically controlled" environment has strict contamination control requirements in which not only air supply but also materials, equipment, and personnel are regulated to control airborne contamination within a defined cleanliness level. A critically controlled room is called a "clean room."
7. NASA (National Aeronautics and Space Administration) Symposium on Clean Room Technology in Surgery Suites. Paper by John A. Ulrich P.S., May 21, 1971. NASA contract NASW-1936, reprint MRI-1064.
8. A particle counter is a light-scattering instrument with display or recording means to count and size discrete particles in air, as defined by the American Society for Testing Materials, Standard F50-68. Instruments of this type have a sampling flow rate of at least 0.1 (and preferably 1.0) ft^3/min and a size discrimination capability for particles greater than or equal to 0.5 μm and less than or equal to 5.0 μm.
9. Fundamentals of Aerosol Science and Engineering for Contamination Control in Clean Rooms course. Benjamin H. Liv, University of Minnesota, Mechanical Engineering Department.
10. AFI: American Filter Institute.
11. ASHRAE: The American Society of Heating, Refrigerating, and Air Conditioning Engineers, Inc., 345 East 47 St., New York, NY 10017. Standard 52-76 provides means of comparing performance characteristics of one air-cleaning device with another. This standard does not provide any means to determine the cleanliness level expected for those environments served by the cleaning device.

12. DOP stands for diocytlphthalate. The DOP test is used to determine the integrity of high-efficiency air filters. The test procedures are defined by the Institute of Environmental Sciences *Recommended Practices for HEPA Filters*, No. IES-RP-CC-001-83-T. The test uses a heterogeneous dioctylphthalate aerosol having the following approximate light-scattering mean-droplet size: 99%, less than 3.0 μm; 50%, less than 0.7 μm; and 10%, less than 0.4 μm. The aerosol is generated by a mechanical aerosol generator.
13. Flanders Corporation, P.O. Box 1708, Washington, NC 27889.
14. Astrocel: registered trademark of American Air Filter Corporation, P.O. Box 35530, Louisville, KY 40232.
15. Vecopleat: registered trademark of VECO International, Inc., 24079 Research Drive, Farmington Hills, MI 48024.
16. Filtra Corporation, 104 Wagaraw Rd., Hawthorne, NJ 07506.
17. MLT-STD-L-51079B Sec. 4.2.1.1, *HEPA Filter Testing*. National Standards Association, 5161 River Road, Bethesda, MD 20816.
18. U.S. Army Edgewood Arsenal Document No. 136-175A; Instructions Manual for Installation, Operation, and Maintenance of Penetrometer Filter Testing DOP, Q107.
19. Recommended Practices for HEPA Filters, IES-RP-CC-001-83-T Section 9.3. Institute of Environmental Sciences, 940 East Northwest Highway, Mount Prospect, IL 60056.
20. A new test method has recently been introduced for the evaluation of ultra-high-efficiency filters (ULPA and VEPA) by using a condensation nucleus counter (CNE). The method is designated as ASTMF-91-70. The ULPA Filter has a minimum efficiency of 99.9995% on particles of 0.12 μm. The VEPA Air Filter has a minimum efficiency of 99.999% on particles of 0.3 μm.
21. A photometer is a light-scattering mass concentration indicator. Instruments of this type, with a threshold sensitivity of at least 10^{-3} mg/liter for 0.3-μm diameter DOP particles and capability of measuring concentrations over a range 105 times the threshold sensitivity, are suitable for scan testing. A linear readout photometer has a linear reading scale graduated from 0 to 100 with a range switch to vary the full scale response in multiples of 10, through at least four decades of response. The instrument should be capable of indicating 0.001% of a concentration that registers 100% on the highest range. A logarithmic readout photometer has a logarithmic response scale graduated from 0 to 5, covering the full range of instrument sensitivity without range switches. For this type of photometer, "one scale division" means the first intermediate scale division following the zero mark.
22. See note 12.
23. Institute of Environmental Sciences. Recommended practices for clean room design CRP-12. FDA proposed good manufacturing practices. Federal Register 2, 13, 1976.
24. ASHRAE. *Guide and Data Book*. New York, American Society of Heating, Refrigerating, and Air Conditioning Engineers, 1971.
25. The laminar air flow technology was developed in 1965 by Sandia Laboratories, Albuquerque, New Mexico, under a grant by the U.S. Atomic Energy Commission. As the requirements for miniaturization increased in the electronic field, the requirements for cleaner environ-

ments also increased. Laminar flow air technology has been in use in the pharmaceutical industry since the middle 1960s.

26. Kleen-Edge: registered trademark of VECO International, Inc., 24079 Research Drive, Farmington Hills, MI 48024.
27. SMACNA: Sheet Metal and Air Conditioning Contractors National Association, Inc., 8224 Old Courthouse Road, Tysons Corner, Vienna, VA 22180.
28. Tests 11 and 12 should be executed after tests 1–10 are satisfactory.
29. Tests 1–4, 6, and 11.
30. Adapted from the *Manual of Recommended Practices* (1984), Institute of Environmental Sciences, Mount Prospect, IL.
31. A Pitot tube is a device for measuring total velocity and static pressures of flowing fluid streams.
32. A dry/wet bulb thermometer is an instrument used to measure moisture in the air so the accurate dew point can be found.
33. A thermoanemometer (or hot-wire anemometer) is an instrument for measuring air velocities based on the convection cooling effect of airflow on a heated wire. Instruments of this type specifically designed for low air speeds ranging from about 25 to 300 ft/min are suitable for velocity measurements.
34. An air pressure gauge is an inclined manometer or magnehelic gauge capable of measuring 0.01–2.0 in. water gauge static pressure.
35. A smoke generator is a ventilation smoke tube pencil for generating visible smoke for air tracer studies.

8
Quality Assurance

Samir A. Hanna

Bristol-Myers Company, Syracuse, New York

I. INTRODUCTION

Quality assurance has as its objective the measurement of product attributes in order to assure that the product being manufactured conforms to its specifications. To assure production of the product with desired attributes requires testing during manufacture. The ultimate responsibility for the quality of a product rests with manufacturing personnel. However, the total control of quality requires an organized effort of the entire company to assure that every component and every step of the parenteral manufacturing process be regarded as critical and be performed according to the specified requirements that assure that the required quality is in the finished product.

The principles of quality assurance in manufacturing parenterals are basically the same as for the manufacture of any pharmaceutical. The quality of parenteral products is the sum of all factors that contribute directly or indirectly to the manufacture of products that are of acceptable quality, safety, and therapeutic effectiveness. These include product research and development, purchasing of materials, manufacturing, testing, inspection, labeling, release, storage, and distribution. End-product testing alone, although an important function to assess the acceptability of the finished product, will not ensure product quality.

II. QUALITY ASSURANCE SYSTEM

The ultimate objective of a quality assurance system is to establish confidence that the manufactured product has the desired high quality. Although manufacturing has prime responsibility for quality results, quality assurance must establish control points to monitor the quality of the parenteral product during processing as well as after completion. These control

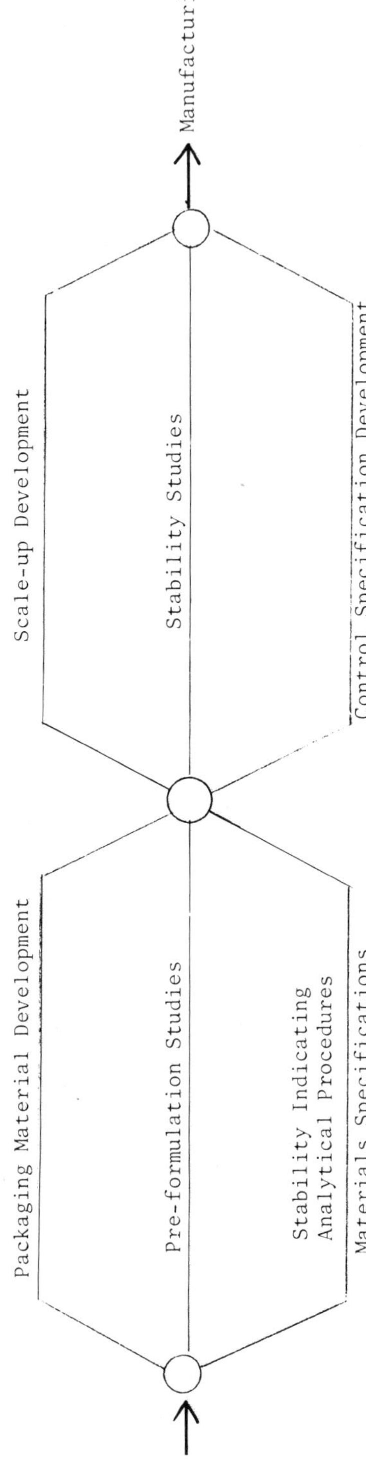

Figure 1 Quality assurance system for pharmaceutical research and development of parenteral products.

points include facilities for warehousing, manufacturing, filling, packaging, and storage; material control; manufacturing control of equipment, process steps, environmental and other auxiliary services as water, air, steam, inert gases, and vacuum; packaging and labeling control; finished product control; and marketed product monitoring.

A flowchart for a quality assurance system is diagrammed in Figures 1 and 2 for parenteral products in development and in manufacturing stages, respectively. These systems can vary in details from company to company and will depend on the nature and size of the manufacturing facility and on the types of parenteral dosage forms produced.

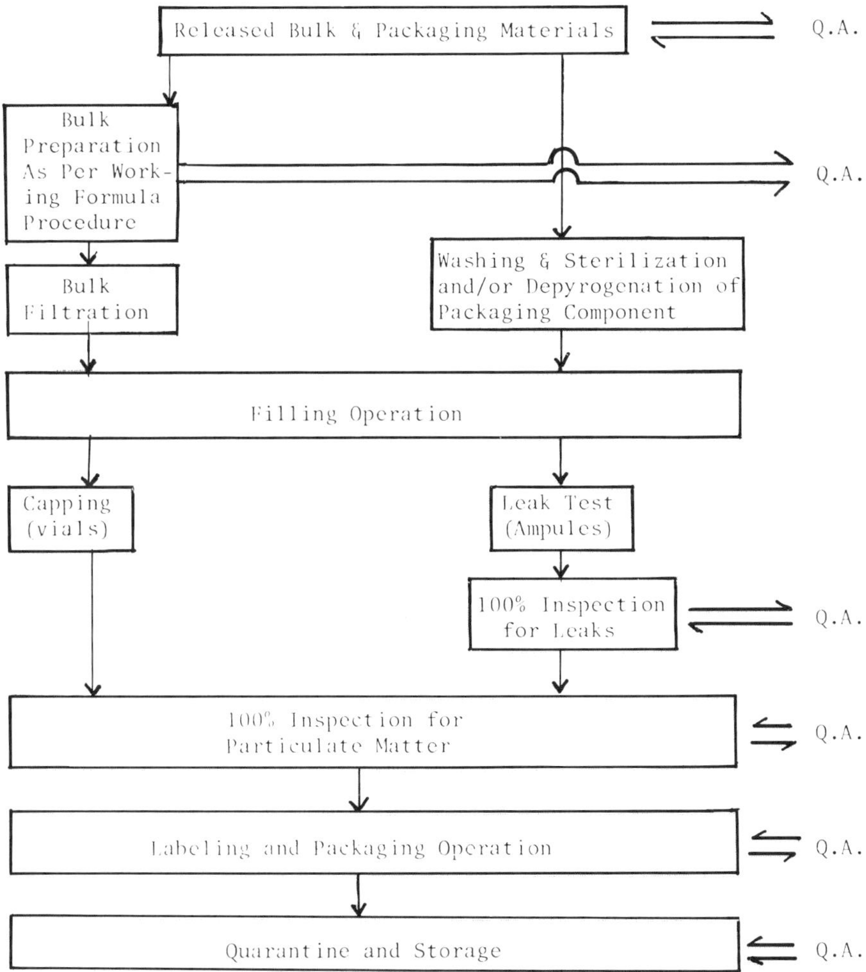

Figure 2 Quality assurance system for manufacturing of parenteral products.

III. RAW MATERIAL CONTROL

The storage conditions of raw materials for parenteral manufacturing, particularly hygroscopic substances, are important. Because of the great number of potential sources of contamination, strict sanitation of plant warehouse is an absolute necessity. Quality assurance should make periodic sanitation inspections and follow-up to assure that deficiencies are corrected.

An extensive and varied microbial flora is usually associated with raw materials from natural sources, for example, heparin and vegetable oils. Synthetic raw materials, on the other hand, are normally free or low in microbial contamination. Raw materials with abnormally high microbial contamination may have to be subjected to a sterilization procedure that may include heat treatment, radiation, or recrystallization from a bactericidal solvent, such as alcohol.

A. Sampling of Raw Materials

Samples of raw materials are to be collected in sterile containers using a disinfected or sterilized sampling "thief" or scoop, observing aseptic technique for microbiological analysis or clean container and clean technique for analytic laboratory. The number of containers to sample in a given lot can be determined by using MIL-STD-105D as shown in Table 1.

Samples are to be labeled as to lot number, receiving number, supplier, container size and type, name of raw material, and date of receipt. Samples are then submitted to quality assurance analytic and microbiological laboratories.

B. Chemical and Microbiological Attributes

In the development of raw material specifications, the analytic research and development chemist should strive for the following:

Ascertain which chemical, physical, and biological characteristics are critical for assuring reproducibility from lot to lot of raw materials to be used for evaluating each lot of raw material produced or purchased.

Establish the test methods and acceptable tolerance for the attributes to be evaluated.

Establish the supplier's ability to supply raw materials of consistent quality.

Good raw material specifications must be written in precise terminology, be complete, and provide details of test methods, type of test instruments to use, manner of sampling, and proper identification. Figure 3 lists general tests, limits, and other physical or chemical data for raw materials related to identity, purity, strength, and manner of quality assurance. Figure 4 provides a quality assurance monograph for ascorbic acid, USP, as an example of a specific raw material.

The current FDA Good Manufacturing Practices (GMP) covering raw material handling procedures are found in the Code of Federal Regulations, Title 21, Section 211.42. It simply states that "components" be received, sampled, tested, and stored in a reasonable way, that rejected material be disposed of, that samples of tested components be retained, and that

Table 1 Number of Containers of Raw Materials to Be Sampled per Lot

Inactive raw materials	
Containers	No. samples
1	All
2–8	2
9–15	3
16–90	5
91–150	8
151–280	13
281–500	20
501–1200	32
1201–3200	50

Active raw materials	
Containers	No. samples
1–5	All
6–10	6
11–18	7
19–28	8
29–100	9
>101	10

Empty vials, cartridge components, or stoppers		
Cases, rolls, or boxes (no. per lot)	Cases, rolls, or boxes (no. of samples)[a]	Units sample number
1–8	2	↓
9–15	3	↓
16–90	5	↓
91–150	8	↓
151–280	13	↓
281–500	20	↓
501–1200	32	↓
1201–3200	50	↓
3201–10,000	80	↓
10,001–35,000	125	315
35,001–150,000	200	500
150,001–500,000	315	1250
>500,001	500	1250

[a]Across pallet.

I. Raw material name
   A. Structural formula, molecular weight
   B. Chemical names
   C. Item number
   D. Date of issue
   E. Date of superseded monograph, if any, or new
   F. Signature of writer
   G. Signature of approval

II. Samples
   A. Safety requirement
   B. Sample plan and procedure
   C. Sample size and sample container to be used
   D. Reserve sample required

III. Retest program
   A. Retesting schedule
   B. Reanalysis to be performed to assure identity, strength, quality, and purity

IV. Specifications (wherever applicable)
   A. Description
   B. Solubility
   C. Identity
      1. Specific chemical tests: related alkaloids; organic nitrogenous bases; acid moiety or inorganic salt tests for sulfate, chloride, phosphate, sodium, and potassium; spot organic and inorganic chemical tests
      2. Infrared absorption
      3. Ultraviolet absorption
      4. Melting range
      5. Congealing point
      6. Boiling point or range
      7. Thin-layer, paper, liquid, or gas chromatography
   D. Color: either by direct measurement of color using Klett colorimeter or equivalent or by color comparison to a standard color material
   E. Powder fineness or density: a quick qualitative measurement of particle size of a bulk material
   F. Solvent: to ensure that the bulk material manufacturing process is under sufficient control to produce material essentially free of solvent residues
   G. Microbial count: a total microbial count of 100—1000 microorganisms per gram or milliliter is usually specified
   H. Sterility: some bulks must be sterile before processing, as in the case of parenteral antibiotic
   I. Pyrogen: all bulk materials to be used for parenteral manufacturing must be pyrogen free
   J. Safety test: to ensure that no change in manufacturing has occurred that would produce a product of significantly higher toxic properties than the reference material

Figure 3 Raw material quality assurance specification.

K. Purity and quality
   1. General: completeness of solution, pH, specific rotation, nonvolatile residue, ash, acid-insoluble ash, residue on ignition, loss on drying, water content, heavy metals, arsenic, lead, mercury, selenium, sulfate, chloride, carbonates, acid value, iodine value, saponification value
   2. Special quality tests: particle size, crystallinity characteristics, and polymorphic forms
   3. Special purity tests: for example, ferric in ferrous salts, peroxides and aldehydes in ether and related degradation products

L. Assay: calculated either on anhydrous or hydrous basis (μg/mg or in units)

V. Test procedures
   A. Compendial, USP or NF references
   B. Noncompendial, detailed analytic procedure; weights, dilutions, extractions, normality, reagents, instrumentation used; calculations

VI. Approved suppliers: list of prime suppliers and other approved alternative suppliers, if any

Figure 3 (continued)

appropriate records of these steps be maintained. In practice, the manufacturer will physically inspect and assign lot numbers for all raw materials received and will quarantine them until they are approved for use. Each raw material is sampled according to standard sampling procedures and is sent to the quality control laboratory for testing according to the written procedures (Fig. 4). If acceptable, it is moved to the release storage area and properly labeled to indicate the item number, name of material, lot number, date of release, reassay date, and signature of a quality assurance inspector. It is retested as necessary according to an established schedule to assure that it still conforms to specifications at time of use. Quality assurance should reserve samples from active and inactive raw materials that consist of at least twice the quantity necessary to perform all tests required to determine whether the material meets the established specification. These reserve samples should be retained for at least 5 years. Approved components shall be rotated in such a manner that the oldest stock is used first. Any raw material not meeting specifications must be isolated from the acceptable materials, labeled as rejected, and returned to the supplier or disposed of promptly. To verify the supplier's conformance to specifications, further supporting assurance by means of on-site periodic inspections is pertinent to the total quality of raw materials. This will assure that cross-contamination does not take place due to improperly cleaned equipment or poor housekeeping practices since contaminants may go undetected because specifications generally are not designed to control the presence of unrelated materials. In general, raw materials may be classified into two basic groups: those that are active or therapeutic ingredients, and those that are inactive, inert materials.

Item number	Date of issue	Superseded	Written by	Approved by

Sampling plan:
See Table 1

Preservation sample
4 oz

Retest program

Schedule	Tests
1 year	Identity specific-rotation Assay

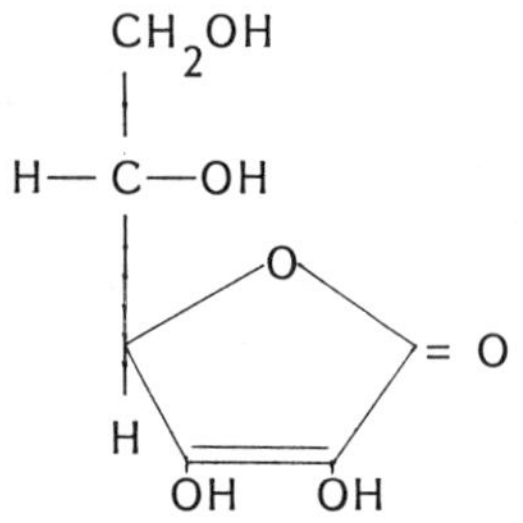

$C_6H_8O_6$ Mol. wt. 176.13 L-Ascorbic Acid

Specifications

Description	White or slightly yellow crystals or powder; on exposure to light gradually darkens; in the dry state, it is reasonably stable in air, but in solution rapidly oxidizes; melts at about 190°C
Solubility	Freely soluble in water; sparingly soluble in alcohol, insoluble in chloroform, ether, and benzene
Identification	
Infrared	The infrared absorption spectrum of a potassium bromide dispersion of it exhibits maxima only at the same wavelengths as that of a similar preparation of USP Ascorbic Acid RS.
Alkaline cupric tartrate	Color reduces slowly at room temperature but more readily upon heating
Specific-rotation	Between +20.5° and +21.5
Residue on ignition	NMT 0.1%
Heavy metals	NMT 0.002%
Assay	99.0—100.5% on anhydrous basis
Completeness of solution	10 g per 20 ml of water for injection is not less clear than an equal volume of water for injection examined similarly

Test Procedures: for all tests, see USP

Approved suppliers
1. Roche Laboratories, Division of Hoffman-LaRoche, Inc., Nutley, NJ
2. Pfizer, Inc., New York, NY

Figure 4 Ascorbic acid, USP.

1. Antibiotics

Antibiotics are one of the few drugs for which the official analytic method appears in the Code of Federal Regulations. The USP XXI and NF XVI refer to the Code of Federal Regulations for specifications and analytic methods given in the individual monographs for each antibiotic. The Code of Federal Regulations, Title 21, Chapter 1, Parts 436 to 436.517 and Parts 442 and 455, contains the analytic method specifications for all antibiotics approved for human use in the United States. The number of tests required varies from one antibiotic to another. The data in Table 2 provide the tests required by the Code of Federal Regulations for some antibiotics and antibiotics prepared as injections. Testing of antibiotics is generally performed by chemical, microbiological, or biological methods, or by all three methods. Caution must be exercised during antibiotic raw material sampling for testing to assure that it is not altered during the sampling procedure. The sample must be taken in a relatively dry atmosphere, relatively free from dust, and free from both chemical and microbial airborne contamination, and exposure must be reduced to a minimum during sampling. Special attention should be given to the assay for potency of antibiotic raw materials. Since the potency value in terms of micrograms per milligram obtained for this material is used in calculating the number of grams or kilograms required for the working formula procedures, it is recommended that at least two separate weighings of such antibiotic raw material powder be assayed on each of three different days (six different assays using six different weighings). If all the individual results are not within the normal distribution of the group or show too much variance, additional assays should be done until a mean potency is obtained with confidence limits of ±2.5% (or better) at $P = 0.05$.

2. Actives Other than Antibiotics

The current editions of the USP XXI and NF XVI contain monographs on most therapeutically active materials used in parenteral manufacturing. Since there is such a wide variance in the nature of the active ingredients used in parenteral manufacturing, it is impossible to summarize briefly the testing of those raw materials. One of the most important decisions to be made in raw material control is the degree of purity that will be maintained for each material. It is not uncommon to find an appreciable variation in the degree of purity between samples of the same raw material purchased from different commercial sources. The selection then must be one that results in the highest purity practical for each raw material, consistent with safety and efficacy of the final injectable dosage form. A typical raw material currently existing in a compendium has a purity requirement of generally not less than 97%. Its specification normally consists of its description, solubility, identification, melting range, loss on drying, residue on ignition, special heavy metal testing, specific impurities that are pertinent to the method of synthesis of each individual raw material, and assay. The methods of assay are usually chemical in nature. However, it should be indicated that the compendial testing of raw materials is intended to be the minimum testing required from the legal point of view. For certain injectable products, it may be necessary to obtain an active ingredient with a special specification far tighter than that of the comparable compendial standard. Raw materials cannot be adequately evaluated and controlled without special instrumental testing, such as spectrophotometry; infrared

Table 2 Tests for Some Parenteral Antibiotics

Antibiotic[a]	% Loss on drying	Moisture	pH	Crystal-linity	Iodo-metric assay	Hydroxyl-amine col. assay	Residue on ignition
Sterile ampicillin sodium and injection		(NMT) Not more than 2	8.0–10.0	X	X	X	
Sterile hetacillin potassium and injection		NMT 1	7.0–9.0	X			
Sterile dicloxacillin sodium monohydrate and injection		3.0–5.0 NMT 5	4.5–75	X	X	X	
Sterile tetracycline hydrochloride and injection	NMT 2		1.8–2.8	X			
Sterile cefotoxin sodium and injection		NMT 2	4.2–7.0	X		X	
Sterile cephalothin sodium and injection	NMT 1.5		4.5–7.0 6.0–8.5	X	X	X	
Sterile cephapirin sodium and injection		NMT 2		X	X	X	
Amikacin sulfate and injection		NMT 8.5	9.5–11.5 3.5–5.5				NMT 1

[a]Antibiotic raw materials used for injectable dosage forms manufacturing must conform to the standards listed in the CFR for each specific antibiotic.

[b]Potency is determined microbiologically using the diffusion plate assay and/or the turbidimetric assay.

[c]Iodometric and hydroxylamine colorimetric for most penicillins and cephalosporins as an alternative assay procedure. Column chromatography for tetracycline hydrochloride impurities. Ultraviolet spectrophotometry for tetracycline hydrochloride. Colorimetric for sterile hetacillin potassium. Nonaqueous titration for cephapirin.

Potency (%)	Sterility	Pyro-genicity	Safety	Special test	Micro-biological	Ident-ification	Specific rotation
90–115	X	X	X		Potency[b,c]	X	
90–120 as ampicillin	X	X	X		Potency[b,c]	X	
90–115	X	X	X	Organic chlorine and free chlorine content	Potency[b,c]	X	
90–115	X	X	X	Histamine or hista-minelike substances	Potency[b,c]	X	
90–120	X	X	X		Potency[b,c]	X	
90–115	X	X	X		Potency[b,c]	X	+129° ±5°
90–115	X	X	X		Potency[b,c]	X	
90–120	X	X	X		Potency[b]	X	(NLT) Not less than +97° and NMT +105°

spectrophotometry; potentiometric titrimetry; column, gas, paper, thin-layer, and high-pressure liquid chromatography; polarography; x-ray diffraction; x-ray fluorescence; spectrophotofluorometry; calorimetry; and radioactive tracer techniques. No less demanding are the tests required for microbiological assay, pharmacological assay, and safety testing. For certain parenteral products, even when highly purified and well-characterized raw materials are involved, specifications should include additional critical features, such as particle size, crystal shape, and the form, such as crystalline or amorphous. Any of these characteristics could have an effect on the safety or effectiveness of the final oral dosage form. It is a GMP requirement that all raw materials, active or inactive, be assigned a reassay date. Meaningful or indicative tests that would assure purity and potency are performed at reassay times to confirm continued suitability of each raw material.

IV. COMPONENT CONTROL

The microbial flora of parenteral packaging components is affected by its composition, transportation exposure, and storage conditions. Packaging components and closure systems used for parenteral filling have to be sterile and pyrogen free.

Glass containers and rubber stoppers, particularly those transported in cardboard boxes, often contain mold spores of *Penicillium* sp. and *Aspergillus* sp., and bacteria, such as *Bacillus* sp. and *Micrococcus* sp. Other packaging and closure system components, like aluminum, Teflon, metal foils, and other polymeric materials, all of which usually have a smooth impervious surface free from crevices or interstices, are usually free from microbial contamination.

Parenteral products are packaged and sealed in a variety of containers with different closure systems that comprise a wide range of chemical compounds. These include glass, various polymeric materials, and assorted elastomeric closures.

Most parenteral products today are in a liquid form, although a number of parenteral products must be packaged as powders until administered, at which time they are reconstituted into the proper liquid form. Commercially available packaging designs for parenteral products are glass single-dose ampuls sealed by fusion, glass single- or multiple-dose vials with elastomeric closure and aluminum overseal; glass or polymeric bottles of more than 50 ml for large volume intravenous administration, and cartridges of various designs and components that involve one or more of the above materials, plus the attached needle.

Parenteral containers intended to provide protection from light must meet the requirements for the USP light transmission test (Table 3). The light-resistant amber color of parenteral containers results from an interaction between iron and sulfur for greenish amber or iron and titanium for brownish amber.

A. Glass Containers

Glass is still the container of choice for small volume parenterals because of its chemical resistivity. Glass, particularly types I, II, and III suggested by the USP for parenteral use, resist the corroding action of water,

Table 3 Glass and Plastic Light Transmission Limits for Parenteral Containers

	Max. % light transmission at any wavelength between 290 and 450 nm (USP)	
Size	Flame sealed	Closure sealed
1	50	25
2	45	20
5	40	15
10	35	13
20	30	12
50 and more	15	10

acids, bases, and salts to varying degrees. Dry materials do not react chemically with glass. However, glass can be chemically active under certain conditions, for example, the formation of flakes in neutral saline solutions.

Table 4 lists the three glass types defined by the USP for use in parenteral products.

Parenteral containers made from glass tubing or molded glass are available. The molded glass, with its heavier wall weight, provides more protection against mechanical breakage.

Parenteral containers made of glass may be treated in order to reduce alkalinity or improve the inner surface. This is usually accomplished by sulfur dioxide hot gas treatment, glass annealing at higher temperature, or hydrofluoric acid washing.

Commercially available ampuls usually feature a scored or colored break design at the constriction of the neck that makes opening of the ampul easy. This easy-break feature will make the ampuls more vulnerable to breakage during manufacturing and transportation. A minimum and maximum break force range should be specified for each size of ampul. If a color identification band is used, then description and physical measurement specification and comparison to standard color band should be incorporated in the tests.

Incoming shipments of parenteral glass containers should be checked by the quality assurance department to assure that it meets the appropriate pre-established tests, as shown in Figures 5 and 6.

B. Polymeric Containers

During the past decade, more and more polymeric parenteral containers have been used, particularly for large volume intravenous fluid administration. Advantages claimed for the use of parenteral polymeric containers include reduction of particulate material, elimination or reduction of the possibility of airborne contamination or air embolism during administration,

Table 4 Identification of Glass Types Used in Parenterals

Type	Description	Major chemical composition		USP test	Limit size (ml)	0.02 N acid (ml)
		Component	% Avg.			
I	Borosilicate glass, highly resistant	SiO_2	80	Powdered glass	All	1.0
		Al_2O_3	5			
		Na_2O	7			
		K_2O	0.5			
		B_2O_3	12			
		CaO	1			
II	Sulfur dioxide-treated soda-lime glass, dealkanized inner surface	SiO_2	75	Water attack	100 or less	0.7
		Al_2O_3	2			
		Na_2O	10			
		K_2O	0.5			
		B_2O_3	3		Over 100	0.2
		CaO	10			
III	Soda-lime glass, somewhat average chemical resistance	SiO_2	75	Powdered glass	All	8.5
		Al_2O_3	2			
		Na_2O	15			
		K_2O	0.5			
		B_2O_3	3			
		CaO	12			

Item number	Date of issue	Superseded	Written by	Approved by

Sampling plan	Preservation sample	Retest program
See Table 1	None	2 years

Description 1-ml flint clear glass ampul, blue color break, and white identification band

Physical measurements	
Height	66.5—67.5 mm
Width, outer diameter	10.40—10.70 mm
Bulb, outer diameter	7.0—9.0 mm
Neck, outer diameter	5.7—6.9 mm
Body, height	21.0—22.0 mm
Color identification	White band, 0.5—1.5 mm wide at maximum bulk diameter
Color band	Blue band, 0.5—1.5 mm wide at approximately center of constriction

Visual properties
- Spikes or "bird-swings" (deformed melted glass rodlike shape extends between inner walls)
- Leaners out of plumb
- Missing identification band
- Color breaks positioned improperly
- Height inconsistency
- Free of blemishes or scratches

Chemical resistance	USP powdered glass test

Figure 5 Glass ampul, 1 ml.

reduction in breakage, economy in space during transportation and storage, simplified disposal, and a reduction in weight and noise that simplifies handling. However, polymeric parenteral containers are not necessarily totally inert and can present a number of problems to the development pharmacist. Problems that have occurred or may occur include permeation, leaching, sorption, chemical reaction, and instability of polymeric material used. Loss of drug potency and antimicrobial activity due to sorption has been reported. Cosolvent systems used to solubilize poorly soluble drugs can serve as extractants of polymer additives. Polymeric materials generally used in parenteral manufacturing are chemically related to polyolefin, vinyl resins, or polystyrene. Table 5 lists some of the characteristics of these plastics. Regardless of end use or fabrication method of the polymer, additives must be compounded or dry blended into the base resin. These additives can be classified as stabilizers, plasticizers, lubricants, colorants, fillers, impact modifiers, and processing aids. Not all polymer contain all these types of additives. Polyvinyl chlorides, polypropylenes, and polyethylenes possess good thermal stability and other desirable processing and packaging properties that make them the most commonly used polymers for parenteral products.

Item number	Date of issue	Superseded	Written by	Approved by

Sampling plan	Preservation sample	Retest program
See Table 1	None	2 years

Description	10-ml flint clear glass vial
Physical measurements	
Height	60—62 mm
Width, outer diameter	21.0—23.0 mm
Lip, height	4—5 mm
Neck, inside diameter	10.5—11.5 mm
Neck, outer diameter	15—16 mm
Seal test	
Visual properties	
Spikes or "bird-swings"	
Leaners out of plumb	
Height inconsistency	
Free of blemishes or scratches	
Chemical resistance	USP glass powder test

Figure 6 Glass vial, 10 ml.

Containers composed of plastic and intended for packaging products prepared for parenteral use must meet the USP requirements of biological and physiochemical tests for plastic containers. Without specifying the type of polymer, the USP divided plastic containers for parenteral use into six classes and three extraction temperatures, 50, 70, and 121°C. With the exception of the implantation test, the procedures are based on the use of extracts. It is required that the extraction conditions should not in any instance cause physical changes, such as fusion or melting of the plastic. Therefore, the class designation of a plastic must be accompanied by an

Table 5 Characteristics of Some Polymers Used in Parenteral Containers[a]

Polymer	Clarity	Permeability				Effect of laboratory reagents			
		O_2	N_2	CO_2	H_2O	W acid	S acid	W alkali	S alkali
Polyethylene	O	H	L	H	L	R	OAA	R	R
Polypropylene	T	H	L	H	L	R	OAA	—	R
Polyvinyl chloride	C	H	—	H	H	—	—	—	—
Polystyrene	C	H	L	H	H	—	OAA	—	—

[a]W = weak, S = strong; O = opaque, T = translucent, C = clear; L = low, H = high; R = resistant; OAA = oxidizing acids attack.

indication of the temperature of extraction, for example, class I-50 will represent a class I plastic extracted at 50°C. The systemic test by intravenous or intraperitoneal injection and the intracutaneous test of the USP biological test are designed to determine the biological response of animals—mice and rabbits—to plastics by the single-dose injection of specific extracts prepared from the sample. The implantation test is designed to evaluate the reaction of living tissue to the plastic by implantation of the sample itself into animal tissue. In the extraction tests it is important to use the specified weight and surface area for extraction at the stated temperature. In the implantation test the proper preparation and placement of samples under aseptic conditions are important. If a plastic is to be exposed to a cleansing or sterilization technique prior to its end use, then the tests are to be conducted on a sample prepared after being preconditioned by the same treatment.

The physicochemical tests are designed to measure some of the physical and chemical properties of plastic containers using an extract in water for injection. The tests include determination of nonvolatile residue, residue on ignition, heavy metals, and buffering capacity. Other physical and chemical test techniques utilized to identify and characterize polymers include infrared by attenuated total reflectance, ultraviolet spectrophotometry, nuclear magnetic resonance, differential scanning calorimetry, and thermogravimetric methods. For molecular weight or molecular weight distribution melt viscosity, gel permeation or exclusion chromatography is recommended. Table 6 lists the classification of plastics for biological tests as shown in USP.

Table 6 Classification of Plastics

Class						Test			
I	II	III	IV	V	VI	Sample	Animal	Dose	Procedure[a]
X	X	X	X	X	X	Sodium chloride	Mouse	50 ml/kg	SI, IV
X	X	X	X	X	X		Rabbit	0.2 ml/animal at each of 10 sites	IC
	X	X	X	X	X	1:20 Solution of alcohol in sodium chloride injection extract	Mouse	50 ml/kg	SI, IV
	X	X	X	X	X		Rabbit	0.2 ml/animal at each of 10 sites	IC
		X		X	X	Polyethylene glycol 400 extract	Mouse	10 g/kg	SI, IP
				X	X		Rabbit	0.2 ml/animal at each of 10 sites	IC
		X	X	X	X	Vegetable oil extract	Mouse	50 ml/kg	SI, IP
			X	X	X		Rabbit	0.2 ml/animal at each of 10 sites	IC
			X		X	Implant strip	Rabbit	Four strips per animal	IMP

[a]SI = systemic injection; IV = intravenous; IC = intracutaneous; IP = intraperitoneal; IMP = intramuscular implantation.

C. Elastomeric Closures

Elastomeric closure physical properties, flexibility, resilience, and elasticity give it the ability to adapt itself to depressions and crevices and to conform to contours by pushing tightly against the opposing sealing surface, preventing parenteral fluid flow through the interface or out the open end of a container. It does not merely serve as a closure but must also permit removal of the product when needed, by single or multiple penetration with a needle. This unique combination of properties permits elastomeric closures to be used for vials, large volume parenteral bottles, and different types of cartridges in a variety of shapes, thicknesses, sizes, and chemical compositions.

Considerable progress has been made in the past 25 years in elastomeric chemistry, and the development pharmacist can choose from a wide range of natural and synthetic elastomers with properties that vary in terms of moisture and gas permeation, oil and heat resistance, chemical resistance, coring, fragmentation, and acceptability for autoclaving.

Commercially available elastomeric closures can be divided chemically into saturated and unsaturated elastomers. Unsaturated elastomers are polyisoprene (natural and synthetic), polybutadiene, styrene and nitrile butadiene, and polychloroprene. Saturated elastomers include butyl, ethylene propylene and diene, and silicone. The perfect elastomeric closure has not yet been developed, but depending on the procedure used almost all elastomers contain polymer reinforcing agents or fillers, activators, and accelerators for curing, besides small quantities of antioxidants, waxes, plasticizers, pigments, and lubricants. The properties of the elastomeric closure depend not only upon these ingredients, but also on the processing procedure, cleansing procedures, contacting media, and conditions of storage. For such reasons, evaluation of the suitability of an elastomeric closure for a specific use should incorporate investigation of extractables using placebos and other suitable aqueous and organic solvents. Table 7 lists general characteristics of some elastomeric closures, and a suggested quality assurance specification is given in Figure 7.

Table 7 Characteristics of Some Elastomers Used for Parenteral Closures

Elastomer type	Physical properties	Age/heat resistance	Moisture transmission, vapor/gas	Oil resistance	
				Mineral	Vegetable
Polyisoprene	Very good	Poor	Poor	Poor	Poor
Polybutadiene	Very good	Poor	Poor	Poor	Good
Butyl	Fair	Good	Very good	Good	Good
Silicone	Fair	Very good	Poor	Poor	Poor
Nitrile butadiene	Good	Fair	Good	Very good	Good

Item number	Date of issue	Superseded	Written by	Approved by

Sampling plan	Preservation sample	Retest program	
See Table 1	None	Schedule	Tests
		I year	UV IR % ash extractable

Description	Gray elastomeric closure, dimensions in millimeters
Specific gravity (using analytic balance with side arm adapter)	1.15—1.25
Percentage ash	31—35
Ultraviolet absorption (methanolic extract)	Scan conforms to that of a reference standard
Infrared absorption	Scan conforms to that of a reference standard
Extractables by water for injection	Water extract is used for the determination of, reducing agents using 0.01 N iodine, heavy metals using colorimetric or atomic absorption, pH change potentiometrically, and total extractables by weight
Organic solvent, e.g., chloroform	Organic solvents extract is used for total extractable, UV, IR, and TLC screening
Safety test (if necessary)	USP XXI, p. 1198, biological test

Figure 7 Butyl elastomeric closure.

V. WATER CONTROL

A. Water System

Water is an ingredient in the vast majority of parenteral products. Water is used for washing, rinsing, and as a vehicle and is employed at some point in some sterilization processes. An adequate supply of water must be assured that will meet all criteria of quality for different needs in parenteral production from the feed water to the final step. A good water system design must consider equipment suitability, material selection, operational controls, component compatibility, construction practices, cleaning procedures, sanitary methods, sampling procedures, preventive maintenance, sterilization techniques, and compliance with control specifications. The quality aspects of a water system are affected by the quality of the raw or potable water, any processing it receives, and the distribution system. That microorganisms can exist in water means that the production of sterile water poses special problems of preparation, storage, and distribution.

The microbial and chemical quality of water is of great importance in parenteral products. Most raw or potable water used in pharmaceutical processes contains a wide variety of contaminating electrolytes, organic substances, gross particulate matter, dissolved gases, such as carbon dioxide, and microorganisms. Bacteria indigenous to fresh raw water include *Pseudomonas* sp., *Alcaligenes* sp., *Flavobacter* sp., *Chromobacter* sp., and *Serratia* sp. Bacteria that are introduced by soil erosion, rain, and decaying plant matter include *Bacillus subtilis*, *B. megaterium*, *Klebsiella aerogenes*, and *Enterobacter cloacae*. Bacteria that are introduced by sewage contamination include *Proteus* sp., *Escherichia coli* and other Enterobacteria, *Streptococcus faecalis*, and *Clostridium* sp. Stored water bacteria contamination include mainly gram-negative bacteria and other microorganisms, such as *Micrococcus* sp., *Cytophaga* sp., yeast, fungi, and *Actinomycetes*. The reliance on a sampling program as a means of monitoring the quality of the water is only practical if the sample is truly representative of the water quality. Sampling points, frequency of sampling, and type of testing should be considered from the standpoint of the water system size, capacity of equipment, type of equipment, and distribution system. Type and size of water treatment and pretreatment equipment and its operational characteristics have a direct effect on the chemical and microbial quality of water. Bacteria may gain access to a water distribution system at any outlet, such as a tap or sampling point, especially those fitted with a hose, if they are not regularly disconnected and disinfected. Microbial infection and chemical contamination may build up in any unused sections of pipeline "dead legs," booster pumps, and water meters. A standard water-sampling procedure for total microbial count is shown in Figure 8. Similar procedures without strict microbiological cleanliness are followed for water chemical testing. A suggested water-sampling program is shown in Table 8.

B. Drinking Water

The quality of water from the main supply varies with the source, the type of treatment it is subjected to, and the local authority. Essentially, it should be free from known pathogens and from fecal contamination, such as *E. coli*, but it may contain other microorganisms and meet certain chemical purity specification. When the supply is derived from surface waters, microorganisms are usually greater in number and faster growing than that of supplies from deep water sources, such as a well or spring. Due to the variabilities of source, temperature, season, organic level, and complexity of distribution systems, the bactericidal effect of the initial chlorine addition can be decreased and, if used, lead to less chemical contamination. Drinking water frequently contains significant levels of microorganisms and a variety of chemical impurities. Chemical and microbiological testing of drinking water usually includes pH, free chlorine, chloride, sulfate, ammonia, calcium and magnesium, carbon dioxide, heavy metals, oxidizable substances, total solids, and bacteriological purity for total microbial count and *E. coli*. United States Public Health Services regulations describe the testing procedures and limits for each locality.

1. Prepare sufficient number of 120-ml Pyrex sample containers according to the sampling program, and cap loosely.
2. For sample containers to be used for drinking water samples, add 0.1 ml of a 10% sodium thiosulfate solution to deactivate any residual chlorine.
3. Autoclave all sample containers at 121°C for 15 min.
4. Open sampling points like tap fixtures and allow water to run for not less than 500—1000 ml.
5. Hold the sample container by the base, and remove the screw cap, taking precautions not to touch the lip edge of the sample container.
6. Collect not less than 100 ml of the water sample, and immediately secure the cap to the sample container.
7. Label the sample container, source of water, sample point location, and number, type of water, and time and date sampled.
8. Transfer the sample within 1 hr of sampling to the microbiology laboratory.
9. Refrigerate the sample in the microbiology lab until testing within 24 hr of sampling.
10. Follow USP total aerobic microbial count test.

Figure 8 Water-sampling procedure.

C. Purified Water

Purified water is usually produced by passing the water through anion and cation exchange resin beds or reverse osmosis. It should be prepared from drinking water complying with the limits and requirements of the U.S. Public Health Services.

Ion-exchange treatment will remove dissolved ionic impurities. Deionization does nothing to improve the microbiological quality of the water. Ion-exchange beds that are not frequently regenerated with strong acid and alkali will contribute significantly to bacteriological contamination, leading often to pyrogenic problems. Ion-exchange equipment should be sized to ensure frequent regeneration independent of the chemical quality regeneration requirements, which usually take longer, thus encouraging the growth of bacteria and possible pyrogenic problems. Intermittent and low-flow conditions can be minimized by installing a recirculation cycle on the ion-exchange system. The flow rate of this system should approach the rated service flow of the ion-exchange system.

Reverse osmosis treatment will remove a large portion of the dissolved minerals, particulates, bacteria, viruses, and pyrogens. However, procedures must be carefully written to ensure that the reverse osmosis system is properly monitored, maintained, and sanitized on a regular basis as it has been shown that bacterial contamination can occur.

Table 8 Water Sampling Program

Location sample point	Test	Frequency
Raw water (potable water)	Microbial	Daily
	Chlorine residual	Daily
	Condictivity	Continuous
	Chemical, USP	Weekly
	pH	Daily
Carbon filter	Microbial	Daily
	Chlorine residual	Weekly
DI equipment	Conductivity	Continuous
	Total solids, USP	Daily
	pH	Daily
	Microbial	Daily
	Pyrogen	Weekly
	Chemical, USP	Weekly
	Resin analysis	6 Months
Reverse osmosis equipment	Microbial	Daily
	pH	Continuous
	Chlorine residual	Continuous
	Pyrogen	Daily
	Conductivity	Continuous
	Chemical, USP	Daily
	Feedwater hardness	Daily
Distillation equipment	Microbial	Daily
	pH	Daily
	Pyrogen	Daily
	Conductivity	Continuous inlet and outlet
	Chemical, USP	Daily
	Particulates	Weekly
Storage	Microbial	Daily
	pH	Daily
	Pyrogen	Daily
	Chemical, USP	Daily
Distribution use points	Microbial	Weekly
	Pyrogen	Weekly
	Conductivity	Weekly
	Chemical, USP	Weekly
	Particulates	Monthly
	pH	Weekly
Clean steam generator	Chemical, USP	Weekly

Chemical and microbiological testing of purified water includes determination of pH, chloride, sulfate, ammonia, calcium, carbon dioxide gas, heavy metals, oxidizable substances, total solids, and bacteriological purity for total microbial count and *E. coli*. Testing procedures and limits are shown in the USP.

D. Water for Injection

Water for injection is intended not only to conform to a high degree of chemical purity but also to be free from pyrogenic substances. Water for injection is prepared by distillation or reverse osmosis. Distillation is the most widely used and accepted method of producing sterile pyrogen-free water. As the water leaves the still, it is free of microorganisms, but contamination may occur as a result of a fault in the cooling system, heat exchanger design, vent filter installation, storage vessel, or the distribution system. The bacterial contaminants of distilled water are usually gram-negative bacteria. The heating and storing of water for injection at 80°C will prevent bacterial growth and the production of pyrogenic substances that accompany such growth. Certain drug components cannot be formulated at this temperature, and water has to be cooled before use, which may lead to microbial growth. In these cases, it is better to plan the production schedule so that storage for more than a few hours at room temperature is avoided, especially if the products cannot be terminally sterilized. Chemical and microbiological testing of water for injection include pH, chloride, sulfates, ammonia, calcium, carbon dioxide, heavy metals, oxidizable substances, total solids, and pyrogen. Testing procedures and limits are shown in the USP.

VI. MANUFACTURING CONTROL

The preparation of parenteral products cannot be isolated from the premises and conditions under which it is manufactured. To assure that parenteral products meet high standards of quality and purity, an effective system for maintaining the facilities where such products are manufactured is required. A successful sanitation program must be enforced within and outside areas leading to the parenteral manufacturing facilities. Floors, walls, and ceilings should be resistant to external forces, capable of being easily cleaned, and in good repair. An adequate air ventilation system, water system, proper temperature, and proper humidity are important factors.

The microbiological and chemical quality of parenteral products are influenced by the environment in which they are manufactured and by the materials used in their formulation. Unless terminally sterilized, the microflora of a finished parenteral product may represent the contaminants from the raw materials, equipment with which it was made, atmosphere, manufacturing personnel, or the final container or closure system into which it was packed.

A. Personnel

People are the mainstay of any plant housekeeping and sanitation program. The best design, the best layout, and the best materials are useless if the people who are involved in the parenteral manufacturing process are not trained in the function, operation, and control of parenteral production. An effective training program for parenteral production personnel should cover the responsibilities of their positions, gowning techniques, disinfection and cleaning procedures for their bodies, equipment, and clean rooms; disposal procedures; the working of the environment control system; the operation of the laminar-flow system; the procedure to follow in case of power failure and other emergencies; the operation of sterilization equipment; and airborne particle counting and microbial monitoring procedures. No personnel should be admitted into parenteral production areas when they are physically ill, especially when they are suffering from respiratory or gastrointestinal disorders. A personal biological control pattern for personnel working in the parenteral production area, especially filling rooms, that involves making fingerprints on culture plates and media filling of product units could be used to assess the effectiveness of a training program. All personnel involved in parenteral production should undergo periodic medical examinations and the medical findings compared with those recorded at previous examinations.

B. Facilities

Designing facilities for parenteral products is a complex undertaking demanding the coordinating efforts of diverse specialists from engineering, research, production, and quality assurance departments. Surfaces of walls, floors, and ceilings should be smooth and nonporous. Joints should be sealed by suitable caulking material. Heli-arc welding or another suitable procedure should be used to seal ultra-high-efficiency filter frames to duct work. Outlets and other penetrations should be internally sealed from the external environment by silicone rubber sealant. Epoxy coatings or cladding with laminated plastic is acceptable for most surface finishing to provide smooth, impervious, and washable walls, floors, and ceilings. Electrical cables and ducting for other services, like pipes, should be installed in deep cavity walls where they are accessible for maintenance, but where they do not collect dust or microorganisms. Molds are the most common microbial flora on walls, ceilings, and floors, and the species usually found are *Cladosporium* sp., *Aspergillus* sp., *Penicillium* sp., and *Auriobasidiomycetes* sp. Continuous airflow from high-pressure spaces to low-pressure areas with corresponding pressure drop distribution should be maintained and monitored between the filling and manufacturing areas. Manometers measuring air velocity and pressure drops across filters must be periodically checked. Temperature and humidity control, fan efficiency, condition of the air, and illumination levels should be monitored to assure compliance to specifications. The most common materials used for pipelines are stainless steel, glass, and plastic. Stainless steel is recommended for water systems. Pipes must be welded to form a continuous length and smooth internal surface to eliminate any pits or crevices at points of potential microbial growth. They must be sloped from the source to assure a continuous flow of water.

Filters should be examined for dirt buildup by monitoring for pressure drop periodically. A DOP (dioctylphthalate) aerosol test should be performed every 6 months to ensure that the final HEPA filters are properly sealed and free of leaks. Figures 9 through 13 show protocols for quality assurance testing for air velocity measurement, HEPA filter leak testing, temperature

Written by Approved by Superseded Date of issue

Procedure

1. Adjust fans, dampers, registers, and any other control devices to deliver the air quantities specified for each and every component of the air system.
2. Using a calibrated anemometer, measure the feet per minute (fpm) velocity during the steady portion of the cycle for:

   Supply air in cfm (fpm × area square ft)
   Static pressure
   Fresh air cfm
   Return velocity
   Discharge air at every supply outlet
3. A limit of ±10% of specification is usually accepted.

Figure 9 Air velocity measurement.

and humidity control tests, pressure differential measurement, and particle count tests, respectively.

Particle counts are needed to verify air cleanliness, and probes should be temporarily or permanently located at the critical working levels, like filling needles, and readings should be taken during normal working activity. Normal accepted maximum levels are 100 and 100,000 particles of 0.5 μm or larger per cubic foot of air for filling and all other parenteral manufacturing areas, respectively. Common methods for checking the microbial quality of the environment include the exposure of nutrient agar medium for a given period of time or drawing a measured quantity of air into a sampler with a vacuum pump and impinging it upon a nutrient agar medium. Samples should be taken as close to the working area as possible. The spore-forming bacteria *Bacillus* sp. and *Clostridium* sp., the nonsporing bacteria *Staphylococcus* sp. and *Streptococcus* sp., the molds *Aspergillus* sp. and *Mucor* sp., and the yeast *Rhodotorula* sp. are commonly found in untreated air environments. A microbial air count of less than 1 microorganisms per 1000 ft^3 of air should be maintained at the parenteral production filling areas.

C. Equipment

Prior to the start of any parenteral production step, the quality assurance personnel should ascertain that the proper equipment and tooling for each manufacturing stage are being used. Equipment must be identified by labels bearing name, dosage form, item number, and lot number. Weighing and measuring equipment used in production and quality assurance, such as balances and thermometers, should be calibrated and checked at suitable intervals by appropriate methods, and records of such tests should be maintained by quality assurance. An example of such a calibration method is given in Figure 14.

To reduce the risk of microbial contamination due to equipment mishandling, the following good manufacturing practices should be followed:

Written by | Approved by | Superseded | Date of issue

Reference: Photometer Scanning Method, Section 7, AACC STD

Procedure

1. Use polydisperse DOP aerosol generated by blowing air through liquid dioctylphthalate at room temperature into the airstream ahead of the HEPA filter to produce a uniform concentration.
2. Measure the upstream concentration immediately upstream of the HEPA filter.
3. Scan the filter by holding the light-scattering photometer probe not more than 1 in. from the filter face and passing the probe in slightly overlapping strokes across the filter face so that the entire face of the filter is sampled. Then, make separate passes around the entire periphery of the filter and along the band between filter media and frame and other joints in the installation.
4. Using a light-scattering photometer with a threshold sensitivity of not less than 10^{-3} micrograms per liter for 0.3 μm diameter DOP particles and capable of measuring concentrations in the range of 80–120 μg/liter, and an air ample flow rate of 1 ft^3 ± 10% per minute, the approximate light scattering mean droplet size distribution of the aerosol is

   99% smaller than 3 μm
   95% smaller than 1.5 μm
   92% smaller than 1 μm
   50% smaller than 0.72 μm
   25% smaller than 0.45 μm
   11% smaller than 0.36 μm
5. A linear readout light-scattering photometer reading more than 0.01% is considered unacceptable.
6. A HEPA filter should have an efficiency of 99.97% to particles 0.3 μm and larger. Most of the known viable contaminants will be above those limits.

Figure 10 HEPA filter leak test.

all equipment should be dismantled and cleaned after each lot; coupling nuts on pipework and valves should be taken apart and the parts cleaned after each lot; the product should be protected from any lubricant used on moving parts; agitator blades, preferably of one piece with the shaft, should be cleaned after each lot; a separate sampling outlet should be installed on the bulk tank beside the runoff value to avoid the risk of microbial growth; a new set of filters must be used for each lot; and all surfaces in direct contact with the product should be smooth, continuous, and free from pits with all junctions rounded or coved and the welds polished with no dead ends.

Written by	Approved by	Superseded	Date of issue

Procedure

1. The air conditioning system shall be in continuous operation for a period of at least 24 hr.
2. During the test, all the lights and equipment in the test area should be turned on and operational personnel should be present.
3. Read simultaneously the temperature and humidity every 15 min for a period of 2 hr using dry and wet bulb thermometers and sling psychrometer.
4. Take different readings at different locations in the area, especially the air inlet and outlets next to each module.
5. Set thermostats and humidistats to the upper limit (75°F and 55–60% RH), the lower limit (65°F and 40–50% RH), and the operational temperatures (68°F and 50% RH). Initial temperatures and humidities and the time required for the area to reach the control level at the various locations in the area are recorded.
6. The upper and lower levels achieved at every testing location will give the operational performance data of the air system. If the deviation from the control points exceeds the tolerances for the system, proper corrective action should be taken. The out-of-tolerance variances could be indicative of inadequate air distribution or improper airflow pressure differentials.

Figure 11 Temperature and humidity measurement.

Written by	Approved by	Superseded	Date of issue

Procedure

1. Verify the airflow pattern using a visible smoke generator.
2. Measure the differential pressure among the various areas in parenteral manufacturing with the use of a calibrated manometer.
3. First obtain base data for each area with minimum activity, then normal data with normal activity, including number of people, equipment in operation, and so on.
4. Take readings from various points at the openings of each area.
5. A positive pressure differential should always be kept between clean and nonclean areas, especially those that are adjacent to and connected by wall openings for conveyors.

Figure 12 Pressure differential measurement.

Written by	Approved by	Superseded	Date of issue

Procedure

1. Calibrate the light-scattering particle counter and its recorder every 6 months.
2. Measure particle counts at various points in the parenteral production area as close as possible to the filling area.
3. Take the particle count without operational personnel first to obtain a threshold level, then a second reading with personnel and other equipment in operation to obtain the operational level.
4. Collect not less than 1 cfm air volume at each sampling location.
5. At any location, if the particle count is 10 particles of 0.5 μm or larger per cubic foot of air, then repeat the readings at least five times and record the average.
6. Record the particle count data at the hour of readings, day, location sampled, and average number of readings used at each point.
7. Maximum of 100 or 100,000 particles of 0.5 μm diameter and larger per cubic foot of air at filling points and all other parenteral manufacturing areas, respectively, are acceptable.

Figure 13 Particle count measurement.

Written by	Superseded	Date of issue	Approved by

Procedure

1. Employ suitable USP melting point standards for the range of the thermometer to be tested.
2. Use USP method class I to determine the actual melting range of the standards.
3. Tag the thermometer with date calibrated, next calibration, temperature correction, and signature of the person conducting the calibration test.
4. Check the thermometer every 3 months.

Figure 14 Thermometer calibration procedure.

D. Compounding

A working formula card and procedure should be prepared for each batch size of injectable produced. To attempt expansion or reduction of a batch size of a parenteral product by manual calculations at the time of production cannot be considered good practice. Quality assurance must review and check the working formula card and procedures for each production batch before, during, and after production operation for

Signature and dating when issued by a responsible production person
Proper identification by name and dosage form, item number, lot number, effective date of document, and reference to a superseded version (if any), amount, lot, code number, and release date of each of raw material utilized
Initialing each step by two of the operators involved
Calculations of both active and inactive materials, especially if there were any corrections for 100% potencies for actives used
Reassay dates of components used
Starting and finishing times of each operation
Equipment to be used, record of its cleanliness, and specifications of its setup
Proper labeling of release components and equipment indicating product name, strength, size, lot number, and item number

Only released, properly labeled raw materials are allowed in the manufacturing area. Quality assurance should check and verify that the temperature, humidity, microbial monitoring, airborne particulates, and pressure differential in the manufacturing area are within the specified limits. Quality assurance should verify and document the use of proper equipment, the proper addition of ingredients, proper mixing time, proper drying time, and proper filter type and size. At certain points, samples are to be taken for the analytic and microbiological laboratories for potency assay and any other testing necessary to ensure batch uniformity. In-process released bulk materials waiting for filling should be labeled with product name, item number, lot number, size, strength, gross, and tare and net weight or volume of contents.

VII. FILLING AND SEALING CONTROL

Good manufacturing practices require that in-process quality assurance testing be adequately planned throughout all stages of manufacturing. The number of samples taken for testing and the type of testing are obviously dependent upon the size of the batch and the type of parenteral product. If deviation from specified limits occurs, the necessary corrective action is taken and recorded and a resample is taken and tested to determine whether the quality attribute of the parenteral product is now within limits. In some instances, as in the case of volume checking, if the deviation is excessive all injectables produced prior to the corrective action must be isolated, accounted for, and rejected.

A variable group of tests, including checking for volume for solutions and weight variation for powders, are widely used for in-process parenteral production control. The USP recommends certain excess volumes that are sufficient to permit withdrawal and administration of the labeled volumes of liquids (Table 9).

A. Control Charts

The use of control charts is increasingly becoming an essential part of any quality assurance operation. Figure 15 represents a graphic control chart of the data presented in Table 10. Control charts may be classified as portraying attributes or variables. Variable charts are based on the normal distribution; attribute charts are based on binomial distribution. Variable charts are applied when actual numerical measurements of quality attributes are available; attribute charts refer to some other attributes of quality that are present or absent in which each sample inspected is tested to determine whether it conforms to the requirements. Variable charts, or the $\overline{X}$,R (mean and range) charts are undoubtedly the most generally used charts in the quality assurance of parenterals. The most common and usual application of variable charts in parenteral manufacture is in particulate matter and volume control. Routinely, in-process results are plotted on a control chart so that a complete picture of any possible fluctuation during the entire filling operation can be readily detected. The control limits or process capability can be determined by sampling, measuring, and recording results in subgroups that cover the filling operation. The range within each subgroup, that is, the absolute number difference between the lowest and highest individual injectable reading and the average range, is calculated for the total number of groups. The average injectable reading plots can detect movements toward limits that will allow making necessary corrections before limit values are exceeded. Although the subgroup's sample range plots will allow the monitoring of the sample range trend, an increase in sample range values or general high variability indicates possible control problems. In

Table 9 Volume in Container[a]

	Recommended excess volume	
Labeled size	Mobile vehicle	Viscous vehicle
0.5 ml	0.10 ml	0.12 ml
1.0 ml	0.10 ml	0.15 ml
2.0 ml	0.15 ml	0.25 ml
5.0 ml	0.30 ml	0.50 ml
10.0 ml	0.50 ml	0.70 ml
20.0 ml	0.60 ml	0.90 ml
30.0 ml	0.80 ml	1.20 ml
50.0 ml or more	2%	3%

[a]For test procedure, see USP.

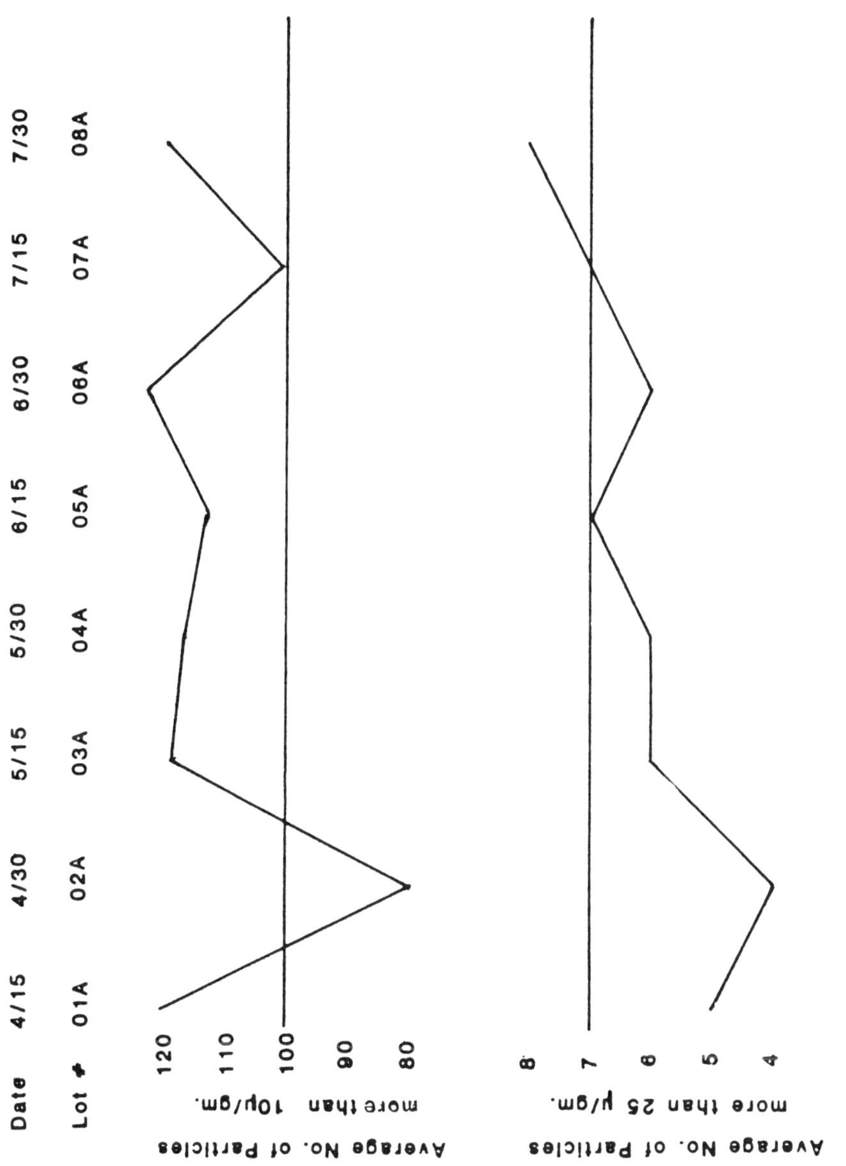

Figure 15 Sterile sodium ampicillin injection, particulate matter.

Table 10 Sterile Sodium Ampicillin Injection Particulate Matter Monitoring[a]

Lot	01A	02A	03A	04A	05A	06A	07A	08A
Date	4/15	4/30	5/15	5/30	6/15	6/30	7/15	7/30
No. particles >10 μm/g	80	90	115	105	205	80	65	55
	100	140	110	120	95	205	45	155
	200	115	85	210	135	55	45	105
	140	210	80	75	50	115	230	90
	90	75	210	80	85	165	120	200
Avg/g	122	80	120	118	114	124	101	121
No. particles >25 μm/g	5	8	4	3	7	2	4	7
	4	2	9	5	8	2	9	1
	7	3	2	8	2	7	10	12
	4	4	6	6	11	7	4	11
	5	3	10	9	2	12	8	9
Avg/g	5	4	6	6	7	6	7	8

[a]Limits: NMT 125 average particles per gram of >10 μm and NMT 10 average particles per gram of >25 μm.

the above-mentioned example, all average numbers of particles per gram are within the established limits and no corrective action is required.

B. Particulate Matter

Parenteral products possess special quality requirements in addition to those of any other pharmaceutical product. Parenteral products must be sterile, pyrogen free, and free of visible particulate matter. The USP requires that care should be exercised in the preparation of all products intended for injection, to prevent contamination within microorganisms and foreign material. Good manufacturing practice requires that each final container of injection be subjected individually to a physical inspection, whenever the nature of the container permits. Particulate matter in parenteral products, especially when its route of administration is intravenous, has been shown to be injurious to humans. Test procedures and standards for the limits of particulate matter in large and small volume parenteral products have been established by the USP. Each particulate matter laboratory should validate its facilities, personnel, equipment, reagents, and techniques before accepting any results by running reference standards and spiked samples with known different concentrations of particulate matters. There has been no successful solution to the problem of particulate matter. Apparently, this is due to a number of factors, including the complex nature of drugs (active and inactive), variety of component materials used to package parenteral products, different manufacturing equipment, level of environmental controls, and human activity. Additionally, there is as yet no ideal method for analysis and identification of particulate matter.

Particulate matter encompasses many different materials: cotton, glass, rubber and its constituents, plastic, tissues, insect fragments, undissolved drugs, bacterial contamination, lint, hair, paint, plant fragments, metals, dust, paper fragments, wax or oil droplets, and other unidentified materials.

Detection and measurement for particulate matter are either nondestructive or destructive. Particles of about 50 μm and larger can be detected by visual examination against a black and white background with a light providing an intensity of illumination between 100 and 350 footcandles (fc). The visual examination technique is qualitative and leads to considerable subjective variation and operator fatigue. For the latter reason, the inspectors should not be allowed to inspect for more than 3 hr consecutively without a break. Depending on the operating costs, the manual handling of injectables for 100% visual inspection can be mechanized to save much expensive labor time. One inspector's output using the automated machine, for example, may be 2800–4200 h^{-1}, depending on the container size and product type, compared with a manual output of 750–900 h^{-1}.

Destructive particulate matter measurement includes Coulter counter, Royco liquid counter, HIAC particle counter, and filtration followed by microscopic examination. The Coulter counter instrument operates on the basis of electrical resistance, so the solution being tested must be an electrolyte. The instrument is capable of detecting particles from 1 μm. The liquid Royco/HIAC particulate counter counts and sizes particles based on the light blockage principle and is capable of detecting particles from 0.5 to 9000 μm. This instrument needs periodic calibration. The filtration and microscopic examination technique consists of filtering the solution through a membrane filter; then the particles are detected, identified, sized, and counted on the membrane. This is a very tedious method and requires much skill by the microscopist.

The process of identifying particulate matter in parenteral products, although complex, is an important step in assuring a quality product. By identifying particulate matter, quality assurance may be able to trace it back to its source, and necessary corrective action or improvement can be taken.

The process of identification of particulate matter in parenteral products by microscopy includes

- Visual inspection
- Filtration and isolation of particles
- Microscopic examination
- Separation and isolation of sufficient number of each particulate type
- Examination of the physical and optical properties by polarized light microscope; if such properties can identify the particles, then specific analytic testing can be used to confirm the identification
- Scanning electron microscopy and/or energy dispersive x-ray analysis to obtain elemental composition of particles
- Micro x-ray powder diffraction for crystallinity identification
- Micro chemical tests to confirm or determine functional groups
- Mass spectroscopy to elucidate structure formula and/or molecular weight

C. Filtration

The next step in parenteral manufacturing after compounding and before filling is usually filtration, which can be for clarification or sterilization. Whether or not the parenteral product is to be autoclaved in its final containers, it is preferable, whenever possible, to filter the solution to remove any particulate matter prior to filling. Several filter media can be used for clarification and sterilization, including cellulose esters, synthetic polymers, microfilaments, polycarbonates, silver, unglazed porcelain, fritted glass, diatomaceous earth, and stainless steel. They are commercially available as disk or cartridge filters. Examples of quality assurance specifications for disk and cartridge filters are shown in Figures 16 and 17.

A typical filter consists of a meshwork of millions of microcapillary pores of uniform size ranging from 8 to 0.22 μm, the latter considered capable of removing microorganisms. A bacterial challenge test is usually carried by the filter manufacturer to ascertain the bacterial retention of the filter. Usually such bacterial challenge test is performed using *Pseudomonas diminuta* (ATCC 19146) at concentrations of 10^6–10^7 organisms cm^{-3} at 40 psi. Prefilters of 5 μm and larger pores should be used for highly particulate-contaminated solutions before sterile filtration.

The integrity and proper placement of a filter in a holder can be checked by nondestructive tests used to predict the functional performance of the filter, such as the bubble point test, diffusion test, and forward flow test. Depending on the filter porosity, each size, disk or cartridge, has a characteristic bubble point that should be supplied by the filter manufacturer's protocol. The bubble point test is the differential gas pressure at which a fluid is displaced form the pores of a wetted filter under specified test conditions. The bubble point test is used as an in-process quality assurance

Written by	Approved by	Superseded	Date of issue

Description	White color free of any visual defects, 293 ± 1 mm in diameter, 59 ± 1 mm center hole and 150 ± 2 nm thickness.
Identity	Moisten a small disk of filter paper with a drop of freshly prepared 1:1 mixture or 20% v/v aqueous morpholine solution and 5% w/v aqueous sodium nitroferricyanide solution. Place a portion of the disk filter under test in a micro test tube, and cover the mouth of the test tube with the treated filter paper. Carefully heat the test tube over a small flame. A blue stain on the reagent-treated filter paper will indicate the presence of cellulose.
Extractables	NMT 0.5% by weight using methanol.
Biological safety	Meets USP biological safety test for plastics, class II −50°C (see Table 6).
Flow characteristics	NLT 15 ml min^{-1} cm^{-2} at vacuum of 27.5 in. of mercury using water.
Integrity	≤0.5 ml min^{-1}/0.5 ft^{-2} at 40 psig ≥50 psig bubble point using water.

Figure 16 Cellulose ester disk filter specifications.

Written by	Approved by	Superseded	Date of issue
Description	Tan pleated cartridge, 10 ± 0.1 in. length, 3.0 ± 0.03 in. in diameter		
Identity IR	Conform to reference standard scan.		
Extractables	NMT 0.5% by weight using ethanol.		
Biological safety	Meets USP biological safety test for plastics, class VI--121°C (see Table 6).		
Flow characteristics	4.7 psi pressure drop at 25°C at 10 liters/min using water.		
Integrity test	≤8 ml min^{-1}/10 $in.^{-1}$ water-wetted cartridge at 40 psig.		

Figure 17 Nylon 66 cartridge filter specifications.

Written by	Approved by	Superseded	Date of issue

Procedure

1. Aseptically assemble the filter per the production working instruction.
2. If test is being performed prior to sterile filtration, stop, and wait until the filter is cool.
3. Connect filter inlet to wetting fluid, and place the hose into a sidearm flask inclined at about 45°.
4. Open inlet hose gradually to wetting fluid.
5. Wet filter thoroughly by opening the vent to allow fluid to flow for 5—10 min. For aqueous solutions with hydrophobic filters, use the recommended supplier organic solvent followed by water.
6. Close inlet valve. Apply about one-third the recommended bubble point pressure.
7. Continue pressure until flow is reduced to a steady dropwise rate coming from the sidearm flask. Adjust the pressure to 80% of the recommended bubble point pressure.
8. Increase the pressure gradually until flow increases to more than 10 times the original flow. Record pressure versus volume. The bubble point is the pressure at which the volume or the flow increased dramatically.
9. The filter must have a bubble point greater than that specified by the supplier to pass the test.

Figure 18 Bubble point integrity test.

procedure and should be performed before and after sterile filtration to assure the integrity of the filter. A suggested bubble point test procedure is shown in Figure 18.

D. Integrity of Seal

Hermetically sealed ampuls for a single-dose parenteral product are routinely tested for proper sealing through the leaker test. The leaker test is intended to detect an incomplete seal, capillary pores, or tiny cracks in ampuls so that they may be discarded.

Leaker tests are performed by producing either a negative or a positive pressure with an incompletely sealed ampul. In the first test, the ampuls are entirely immersed in a dye solution, usually 1% aqueous methylene blue solution, in a vacuum chamber. A vacuum of not less than 27 in. of mercury is then sharply released after 10 min, and this procedure is repeated three times. This treatment will cause the dye to penetrate any small opening in ampuls and color the contents; these can then be easily identified and removed by visual inspection. In the second test, the ampuls are immersed in a dye bath, usually 1% aqueous FD&C red no. 1 solution, and subjected to a short autoclave cycle followed by visual inspection to remove any colored ampuls. A modification of this test is performed by immersing the ampuls immediately after sterilization, and while still hot, into a dye bath; then the colored ampuls are removed by visual inspection. Methylene blue dye should be replaced with another suitable dye when performing the leaker test for strong reducing agent drugs like ascorbic acid injections. These methods do not lend themselves to rubber-stoppered containers, where reliance is placed upon the elasticity of the rubber fitting snugly against the side of the opening of the container, eliminating the need for a leaker test.

VIII. PACKAGING CONTROL

A. Compendial Requirements

The USP includes certain requirements for the packaging and labeling of parenteral products, as follows.

a. The volume of injection in single-dose containers is defined as that specified for parenteral administration at one time and is limited to a volume of 1 liter.
b. Parenterals intended for intraspinal, intracisternal, or peridural administration are packaged only in single-dose containers.
c. No multiple-dose container shall contain a volume of injection more than sufficient to permit the withdrawal and administration of 30 ml, unless an individual monograph specifies otherwise.
d. Containers for injections packaged for use as irrigation solutions may be designed to empty rapidly, may contain a volume in excess of 1 liter, and are exempt from the foregoing requirements relating to packaging.
e. Injections intended for veterinary use are so labeled and are exempt from the packaging requirements concerning the limitation to single-dose containers and to volume of multiple-dose containers.
f. The label states the name of the preparation, the percentage content of drug of a liquid preparation, the amount of active ingredient of a dry

preparation, the volume of liquid to be added to prepare an injection or suspension from a dry preparation, the route of administration, storage conditions, lot number, expiration date, and name of manufacturer or distributor.

g. The container label is so arranged that a sufficient area of the container remains uncovered for its full length or circumference to permit inspection of the contents.
h. The label must state the name of the vehicle and the concentration of each constituent, if it is a mixture, and the names and preparations of all substances added to increase the stability or usefulness.
i. Preparations labeled for use as irrigating solutions must bear on the label statements that they are not intended for intravenous injection.

B. Quality Assurance During Packaging Operation

If the quality control laboratory analysis confirms that the product has complied with specifications and that quality assurance audit of manufacturing operations was satisfactory, the bulk parenteral product is released to the packaging department and production control is notified. Production control issues a packaging form that carries the name of the injectable product, item number, lot number, number of labels, inserts, packaging materials to be used, operations to be performed, and the quantity to be packaged. A copy of this form is sent to the supervisor of label control, which in turn will count out the required number of labels and inserts. Since labels and inserts may be spoiled during the packaging operation, a definite number in excess of that actually required is usually issued. However, all labels and inserts must be accounted for at the end of the operation, and unused labels and inserts must be accounted for before their destruction. If the lot number and expiration date of the parenteral product are not going to be printed directly on the line, the labels are run through a printing machine that imprints the lot number and expiration date. The labels are recounted and placed in a separate container with proper identification for future transfer to the packaging department. Packaging department then requests, according to the packaging form, the product to be packaged and all packaging components, such as labels, inserts, bottles, caps, seals, cartons, and shipping cases. Quality assurance inspects and verifies all packaging components and equipment to be used for packaging operation to ensure that it has the proper identification, that the line has been thoroughly cleaned, and that all materials from the previous packaging operation have been completely removed. Packaging operations should be performed with adequate physical segregation from product to product. Injectables of similar size should not be scheduled on the neighboring packaging lines at the same time. Quality assurance should periodically inspect the packaging line and check filled and labeled containers for compliance with written specification, e.g., absence of foreign drugs and labels, adequacy of the containers and closure system, and accuracy of labeling. Some packaging operations, especially those using high-speed equipment, are fitted with automated testing equipment to check each container for fill and label placement. Alternatively, an operator may visually inspect all packages fed into the final cartons. Proper reconciliation and disposition of the unused and wasted labels should occur at the end of the packaging operation.

Quality assurance should examine specific sample numbers per specific time from each phase of packing and labeling operation for the following defects.

Label: incorrect identification band, incorrect or missing code bars; incorrect color; whether it is loose or torn, soiled or defaced; and registration
Printing: lot number/expiration date, whether it is wrong or missing, illegible or mislocated; lot number on shipper missing; printing missing or skips; incorrect shipping label; and smeared printing
Insert: whether it is missing, incorrect, torn, dirty, or poorly folded
Intermediate shipper: labeling requirements and physical appearance requirements
Outer shipper: whether it is soiled internally or externally; incorrect top; and incorrect count

A proper action level and acceptable quality level (AQL) categories should be assigned to each defect according to its effect on the quality of the parenteral product, ranging from fatal, critical, major to minor defects.

Quality assurance should select finished preservation samples at random from each lot. The preservation samples should consist of at least twice the quantity necessary to perform all tests required to determine whether the product meets its established specification. These preservation samples should be retained for at least 2 years after the expiration date and stored in their original package under conditions consistent with product labeling.

Quality assurance should also select a finished sample and send it to the analytical control laboratory for final testing, which is usually an identification test.

IX. FINISHED PRODUCT CONTROL

A. Sampling Procedure

Sampling procedures of finished parenteral products can be based either on attribute inspection that grades the product as defective or nondefective or inspection by variables for percentage defective. The focal point of any sampling plan is the acceptable quality level. The second important step is to decide on the inspection level of the sampling plan, which will determine the relationship between the lot size and the sample size (N/n). The principal purpose of the sampling plan is to assure that parenterals produced are of quality at least as good as the designated AQL. This means that as long as the parenterals fraction defective (r) is less than the AQL designated for a specific production procedure, then a large percentage of the lots of parenterals produced will be accepted. Sampling procedures for inspection by variables for percentage defective may be used if a quality characteristic can be continuously measured and is known to be normally distributed, such as mean of the sample or the mean and standard deviation of the sample. The assumption of a specific distributional form is a special feature of variable sampling. A separate plan must be employed for each quality characteristic that is being inspected or a common sampling plan is used, but the allowable number of defects varies for each quality characteristic; that is, no critical defects are allowed (c), but some minor defects are allowed. Also, the fraction defective yielded by a given process mean and standard deviation should be calculated to assure a normal distribution of sample statistics.

For practical purposes, MIL-STD-414 for inspection by variables for percentage defective and MIL-STD-105D for inspection by attributes for defective or nondefective products are often used to design a sample plan.

In parenteral manufacturing, sampling procedures for inspection by attributes are generally used, for the following reasons.

Variables sampling, as compared with attributes sampling, requires more mathematical understanding and clerical calculation.
Switching procedures from different inspection levels in variables sampling are more cumbersome.
For large lot sizes, which is the case in parenteral manufacturing, producer's risk is larger in variables sampling than in attributes sampling plan.
The smaller sample size required by variables sampling sometimes costs more, depending on the type of quantitative test performed, than a large sample size required by a comparable attributes plan because of the precise measurements required by the variable plan.
Variables data can be converted to attributes data, but the reverse is not possible.

There are three types of attributes sampling plans: single sampling, double sampling, and multiple sampling.

1. Single-Sampling Plan

A single-sampling plan specifies the sample size that should be taken from each lot of injectables and the number of defective units that cannot be exceeded in this sample. For example, a sample of 100 (n) is taken from a lot; if 2 (c) or fewer defective units are found, the lot is accepted. The discriminatory power of a sampling plan is explained by its operating characteristic (OC) curve. This curve serves to show how the probability of accepting a lot will vary with the quality of the sample of injectable inspected. The operating characteristic curves for a single sampling plan that gives the probability of accepting a lot from a randomly operating process turning out products of average quality at various defective levels for samples of different sizes and different acceptance numbers are given in Figure 19.

From this figure, the OC curve of the above-mentioned example of single-sampling plan, n = 100 and c = 2, shows that if the injectable quality (percentage defective) is 5, the probability of lot acceptance is 12; if it is 1, the probability of acceptance is 92. Again, Figure 19 shows that OC curves vary with the number of n as c in this example is kept proportional to n. This example shows that the precision of a sampling plan increased with the size of a sample (n). The three OC curves for sampling plan n = 100, c = 2; n = 100, c = 1; and n = 100, c = 0 illustrate that a plan varies with the acceptance number alone (c). The smaller the c, the tighter is the plan; as c is increased, the plan becomes more lax and the OC curve is raised. The schematic instructions for a single-sampling plan are shown in Figure 20.

2. Double-Sampling Plan

The first sample is smaller than a comparable single-sample plan. The second sample size is generally twice the size of the first. Consequently, if the lot is accepted or rejected on the first sample, there may be a considerable savings in total inspection cost. If the results of the first sample fall within the acceptance and rejection values, a second sample is taken. The results of the two samples are combined and compared with the final

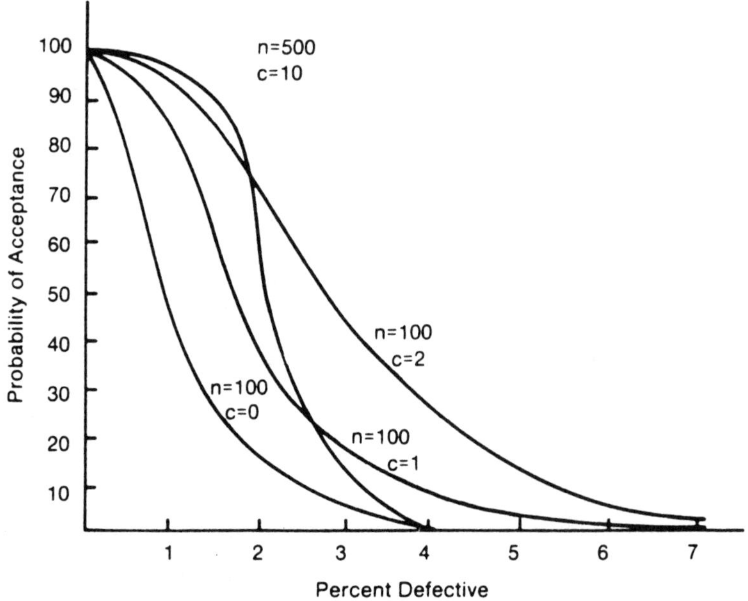

Figure 19 Operating characteristics curves for sampling plan for samples of different sizes and different acceptance numbers.

acceptance or rejection values. For example, a first sample of 50 ($n_1 = 50$) is taken from a lot, if 2 ($c_1 = 2$) or fewer defective units are found, the lot is accepted; if 7 or more defective units are found, the lot is rejected. If the number of defective units is 3 but not more than 6 ($c_2 = 6$), a second sample of 100 ($n_2 = 100$) is taken; if in the combined sample ($n_1 + n_2 = 150$) the number of defective units is 6 or less, the lot is accepted; if 7 or more defective units are found, the lot is rejected. Operating characteristic curves of double-sampling plans showing the probability of acceptance

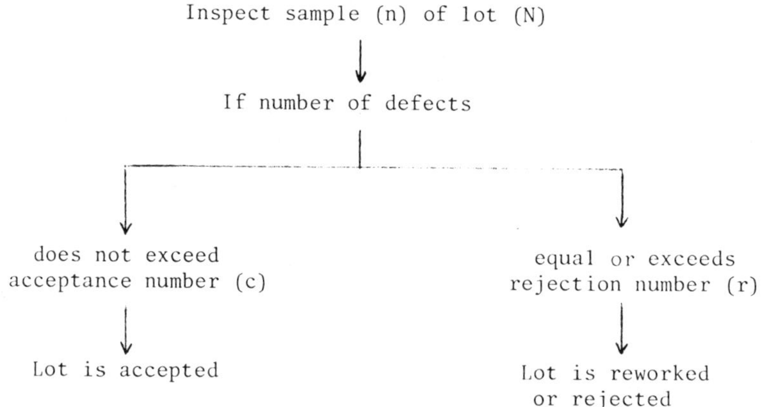

Figure 20 Schematic instructions for MIL-STD-105D single-sample plan.

or rejection on the first sample and combined first and second samples for the above-mentioned example are shown in Figure 21. Curve II in this figure gives the principal operating characteristic curve for the plan, since it gives the probability of final acceptance. The difference between curve II and curve I gives the probability of acceptance on the second sample; the difference between curve II and curve III gives the probability of rejection on the second sample. To illustrate, for the previously mentioned example, for a lot of injectables with a fraction defective of 5, the probability of acceptance on the second sample is 59 and the probability of final acceptance is 63.5. The schematic instructions for double-sampling plan are shown in Figure 22.

3. *Multiple-Sampling Plans*

This plan allows for more than two samples when necessary for a final decision. For standardized sampling, the plan is tied to a maximum of seven equal samples. For nonstandardized sampling, the sample size may vary between inspection checks depending on the proximity of the sample results to the acceptance or rejection values. For example, in a multiple standardized sampling plan, if from a given lot the cumulative sample sizes, acceptances, and rejection numbers of 20, 40, 60, 80, 100, 120, and 140; 0, 1, 3, 5, 8, 9, and 10; 4, 5, 6, 8, 10, 11, and 12 are assigned, respectively, the lot is rejected if the number of defective units at any sampling stage equals or exceeds the rejection number. If not, the multiple

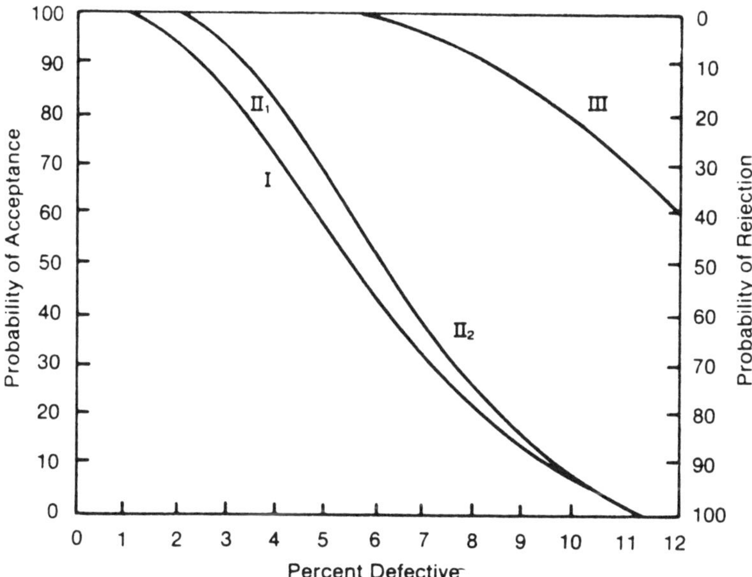

Figure 21 Operating characteristic curves of double-sampling plan: (I) probability of acceptance on first sample (left scale); (II) probability of acceptance on combined samples (left scale); (II_2) probability of rejection on combined samples (right scale); (III) probability of rejection on first sample (right scale).

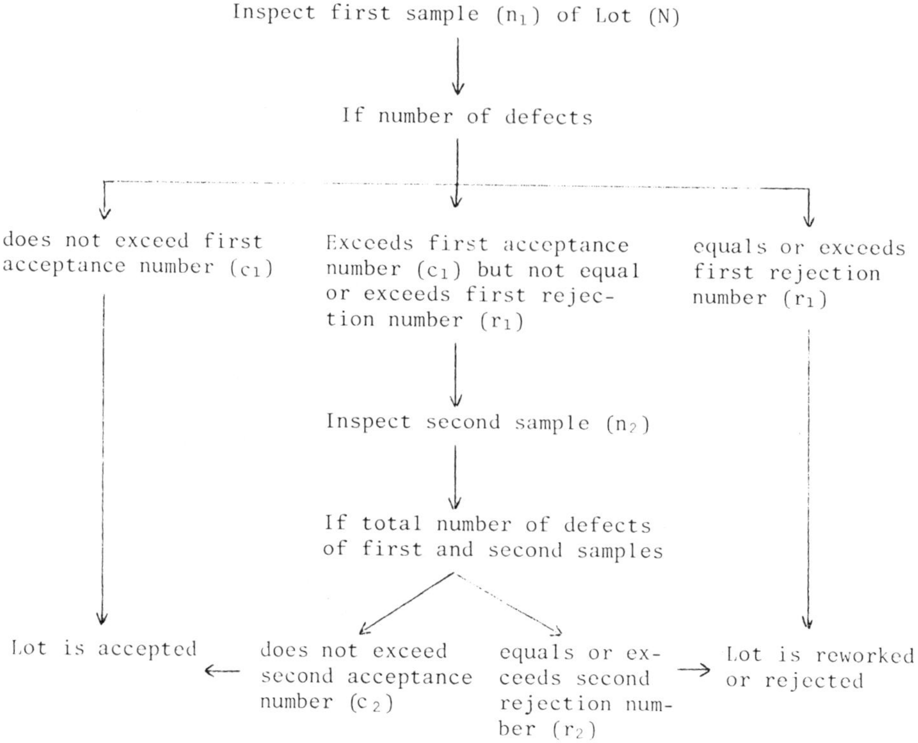

Figure 22 Schematic instructions for MIL-STD-105D double-sampling plan.

sampling procedure continues until at least the seventh sample is taken when a decision to accept or reject the lot is to be make. The schematic instructions for multiple sampling plan are shown in Figure 23.

Military standard sampling procedures for inspection by attributes (MIL-STD-105D) was issued by the U.S. Government in 1963. The focal point of MIL-STD-105D is the acceptable quality level. In applying MIL-STD-105D it is necessary also to decide on the inspection level. This determines the relationship between the lot size and the sample size. For a specified AQL and inspection level and a given lot size, MIL-STD-105D gives a reduced, a normal, or a tightened sampling plan. The switch from the normal plan to the tightened plan is made if two of five consecutive lots have been rejected on original inspection. Switching back from tightened to normal plans is made if five consecutive lots have been accepted on original inspection. Switching from normal to reduced sampling plan is made if ten consecutive lots have been accepted on original normal inspection and the total number of defectives is less than a value set forth in a special table. Figure 24 shows the operation characteristic curves for both normal and tightened plans for a single sampling plan with an AQL of 1% and sampling size of 50 (n = 50). If the lot has a fraction defective of 1, the probability of acceptance on the normal inspection is 92.5; if the tightened inspection is used, this probability will decrease to 82.

The construction of a sampling plan normally requires four quality standards be specified: acceptable quality level, unacceptable quality level

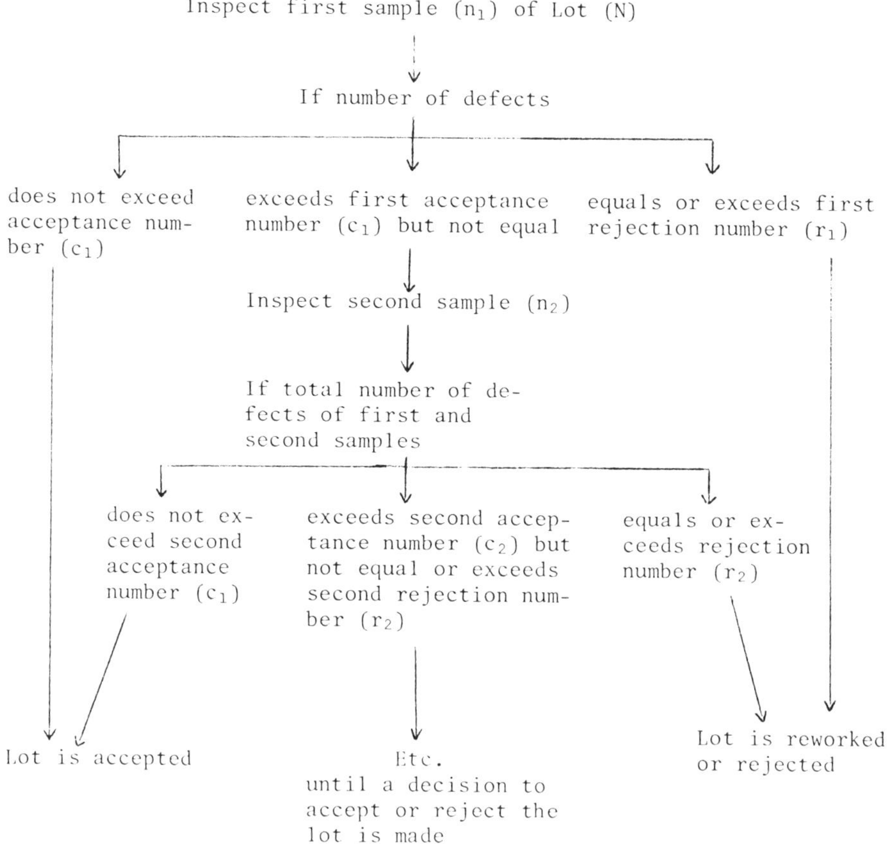

Figure 23 Schematic instructions for MIL-STD-105D multiple sampling plan.

(UQL), producer's risk (α), which is the probability of rejecting good quality, and consumer's risk (β), which is the probability of accepting poor quality. Figure 25 defines these parameters for projections for a sampling plan. The usual approach is the determination of desirable AQL, UAL, α, and β subsequent computation of sample size and acceptable values by applying the tables of MIL-STD-105D. For low-dosage or highly toxic parenterals, as in the case of digoxin or warfarin sodium injections, it is desirable that the AQL and UAL be kept close together and α and β be very small; consequently, a large sample will be required for a suitable sampling plan. Conversely, the plan will call for very few samples if the AQL and UQL are quite far apart and α and β are large, as in the case of sterile water for injection. For example, a lot of 50,000 ampuls is required to contain no more than 1% defective ampuls and the single normal inspection level of MIL-STD-105D is used. Entering Table I of MIL-STD-105D (Table 11), find letter N under column II for the general inspection levels for lot size of 35,000–150,000. Entering Table II-A (Table 12), find the sample size of 500 and at an AQL 1, 10 for acceptance and 11 for rejection.

In practice, this means that a 500-ampul sample is taken from the lot at random and tested; the lot is accepted if 10 or fewer are defective and

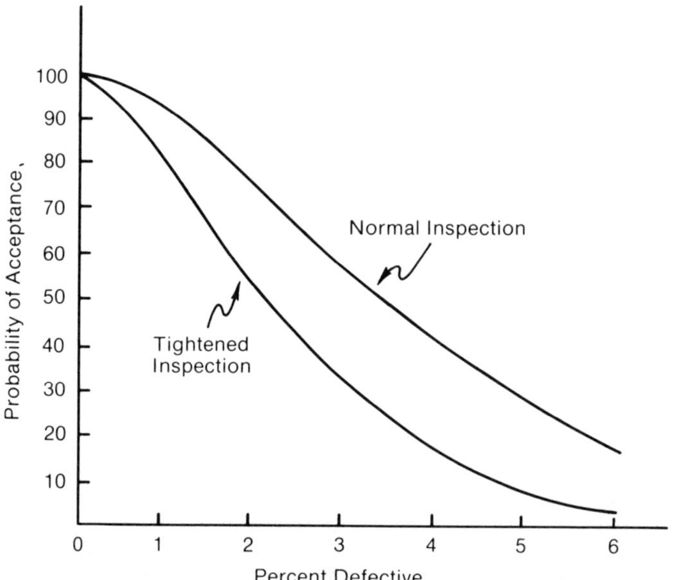

Figure 24 Operating characteristic curves for a MIL-STD-105D single-sampling plan.

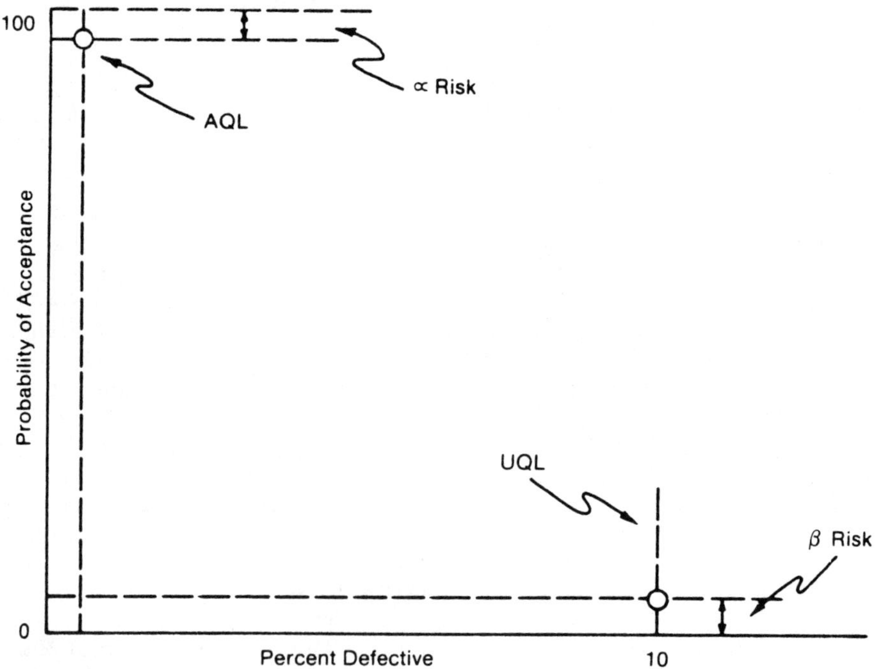

Figure 25 Parameters defining projection for a sampling plan.

Table 11 Sample Size Code Letters

Lot or batch size	Special inspection levels				General inspection levels		
	S-1	S-2	S-3	S-4	I	II	III
2–8	A	A	A	A	A	A	B
9–15	A	A	A	A	A	B	C
16–25	A	A	B	B	B	C	D
26–50	A	B	B	C	C	D	E
51–90	B	B	C	C	C	E	F
91–150	B	B	C	D	D	F	G
151–280	B	C	D	E	E	G	H
281–500	B	C	D	E	F	H	J
501–1200	C	C	E	F	G	J	K
1201–3200	C	D	E	G	H	K	L
3201–10,000	C	D	F	G	J	L	M
10,001–35,000	C	D	F	H	K	M	N
35,001–150,000	D	E	G	J	L	N	P
150,001–500,000	D	E	G	J	M	P	Q
500,001 and over	D	E	H	K	N	Q	R

Source: From Military Standard, Sampling Procedures and Tables for Inspection by Attributes, U.S. Dept. of Defense, MIL-STD-105D, 1963.

rejected if 11 or more are defective. If tightened inspection is used for the sample example, it would call for a sample size code of P for the general inspection level III. From Table II-B (Table 13), a sample size of 800 would now have to be used, instead of 500, and at an AQL 1, 12 for acceptance and 13 for rejection. On the other hand, if reduced inspection is to be used for the same example, it would call for a sample size code of L for the general inspection level I. From Table II-C (Table 14), a sample size of only 80 will be required and at an AQL 1, 2 for acceptance and 5 for rejection.

To examine the kind of sampling job one accomplishes with these three sampling plans, one has to examine the OC curves for code letters N, P, and L at an AQL level of 1.0% defective in the same MIL-STD-105D. These curves indicate that, at sampling size code letter N, one would accept lots containing 3.0% defectives 12% of the time. At a sample size code letter P, however, one would accept lots with 3% defectives only 2% of the time. In reduced inspection, with a sample size code letter L, one would accept lots with 3% defectives 46% of the time.

MIL-STD-105D gives four additional special inspection levels—S-1, S-2, S-3, and S-4—which may be used when relatively small sample sizes are necessary, such as might be the case with costly destructive testing.

Table 12 Master Table for Normal Inspection

Sample size code letter	Sample size	Acceptable quality levels (normal inspection, single sampling)																									
		0.010	0.015	0.025	0.040	0.065	0.10	0.15	0.25	0.40	0.65	1.0	1.5	2.5	4.0	6.5	10	15	25	40	65	100	150	250	400	650	1000
		A R	A R	A R	A R	A R	A R	A R	A R	A R	A R	A R	A R	A R	A R	A R	A R	A R	A R	A R	A R	A R	A R	A R	A R	A R	A R
A	2	↓	↓	↓	↓	↓	↓	↓	↓	↓	↓	↓	↓	↓	↓	0 1	↓	↓	1 2	2 3	3 4	5 6	7 8	10 11	14 15	21 22	30 31
B	3	↓	↓	↓	↓	↓	↓	↓	↓	↓	↓	↓	↓	↓	0 1	↑	↓	1 2	2 3	3 4	5 6	7 8	10 11	14 15	21 22	30 31	44 45
C	5	↓	↓	↓	↓	↓	↓	↓	↓	↓	↓	↓	↓	0 1	↑	↓	1 2	3 3	3 4	5 6	7 8	10 11	13 15	21 22	30 31	44 45	↑
D	8	↓	↓	↓	↓	↓	↓	↓	↓	↓	↓	↓	0 1	↑	↓	1 2	2 3	3 4	5 6	7 8	10 11	↑	↑	↑	↑	↑	↑
E	13	↓	↓	↓	↓	↓	↓	↓	↓	↓	↓	0 1	↑	↓	1 2	2 3	3 4	5 6	7 8	10 11	14 15	↑	↑	↑	↑	↑	↑
F	20	↓	↓	↓	↓	↓	↓	↓	↓	↓	0 1	↑	↓	1 2	2 3	3 4	5 6	7 8	10 11	14 15	21 22	↑	↑	↑	↑	↑	↑
G	32	↓	↓	↓	↓	↓	↓	↓	↓	0 1	↑	↓	1 2	2 3	3 4	5 6	7 8	10 11	14 15	21 22	↑	↑	↑	↑	↑	↑	↑
H	50	↓	↓	↓	↓	↓	↓	↓	0 1	↑	↓	1 2	2 3	3 4	5 6	7 8	10 11	14 15	21 22	↑	↑	↑	↑	↑	↑	↑	↑
J	80	↓	↓	↓	↓	↓	↓	0 1	↑	↓	1 2	2 3	3 4	5 6	7 8	10 11	14 15	21 22	↑	↑	↑	↑	↑	↑	↑	↑	↑
K	125	↓	↓	↓	↓	↓	0 1	↑	↓	1 2	2 3	3 4	5 6	7 8	10 11	14 15	21 22	↑	↑	↑	↑	↑	↑	↑	↑	↑	↑
L	200	↓	↓	↓	↓	0 1	↑	↓	1 2	2 3	3 4	5 6	7 8	10 11	14 15	21 22	↑	↑	↑	↑	↑	↑	↑	↑	↑	↑	↑
M	315	↓	↓	↓	0 1	↑	↓	1 2	2 3	3 4	5 6	7 8	10 11	14 15	21 22	↑	↑	↑	↑	↑	↑	↑	↑	↑	↑	↑	↑
N	500	↓	↓	0 1	↑	↓	1 2	2 3	3 4	5 6	7 8	10 11	14 15	21 22	↑	↑	↑	↑	↑	↑	↑	↑	↑	↑	↑	↑	↑
P	800	↓	0 1	↑	↓	1 2	2 3	3 4	5 6	7 8	10 11	14 15	21 22	↑	↑	↑	↑	↑	↑	↑	↑	↑	↑	↑	↑	↑	↑
Q	1250	0 1	↑	↓	1 2	2 3	3 4	5 6	7 8	10 11	14 15	21 22	↑	↑	↑	↑	↑	↑	↑	↑	↑	↑	↑	↑	↑	↑	↑
R	2000	↑	↑	1 2	2 3	3 4	5 6	7 8	10 11	14 15	21 22	↑	↑	↑	↑	↑	↑	↑	↑	↑	↑	↑	↑	↑	↑	↑	↑

A = Acceptance number.
R = Rejection number.
↓ = Use first sampling plan below arrow. If sample size equals or exceeds lot or batch size, do 100% inspection.
↑ = Use first sampling plan above arrow.
Source: Mil. Std. 105D.

Table 13 Master Table for Tightened Inspection

Sample size code letter	Sample size	Acceptable quality levels (tightened inspection, single sampling)																									
		0.010	0.015	0.025	0.040	0.065	0.10	0.15	0.25	0.40	0.65	1.0	1.5	2.5	4.0	6.5	10	15	25	40	65	100	150	250	400	650	1000
		A R	A R	A R	A R	A R	A R	A R	A R	A R	A R	A R	A R	A R	A R	A R	A R	A R	A R	A R	A R	A R	A R	A R	A R	A R	A R
A	2	↓	↓	↓	↓	↓	↓	↓	↓	↓	↓	↓	↓	↓	↓	↓	↓	↓	↓	1 2	2 3	3 4	5 6	8 9	12 13	18 19	27 28
B	3	↓	↓	↓	↓	↓	↓	↓	↓	↓	↓	↓	↓	↓	↓	0 1	↓	↓	1 2	2 3	3 4	5 6	8 9	12 13	18 19	27 28	41 42
C	5	↓	↓	↓	↓	↓	↓	↓	↓	↓	↓	↓	↓	↓	0 1	↓	↓	1 2	2 3	3 4	5 6	8 9	12 13	18 19	27 28	41 42	↑
D	8	↓	↓	↓	↓	↓	↓	↓	↓	↓	↓	↓	↓	0 1	↓	↓	1 2	2 3	3 4	5 6	8 9	12 13	18 19	27 28	41 42	↑	↑
E	13	↓	↓	↓	↓	↓	↓	↓	↓	↓	↓	↓	0 1	↓	↓	1 2	2 3	3 4	5 6	8 9	12 13	18 19	27 28	41 42	↑	↑	↑
F	20	↓	↓	↓	↓	↓	↓	↓	↓	↓	↓	0 1	↓	↓	1 2	2 3	3 4	5 6	8 9	12 13	18 19		↑	↑	↑	↑	↑
G	32	↓	↓	↓	↓	↓	↓	↓	↓	↓	0 1	↓	↓	1 2	2 3	3 4	5 6	8 9	12 13	18 19	↑	↑	↑	↑	↑	↑	↑
H	50	↓	↓	↓	↓	↓	↓	↓	↓	0 1	↓	↓	1 2	2 3	3 4	5 6	8 9	12 13	18 19	↑	↑	↑	↑	↑	↑	↑	↑
J	80	↓	↓	↓	↓	↓	↓	↓	0 1	↓	↓	1 2	2 3	3 4	5 6	8 9	12 13	18 19	↑	↑	↑	↑	↑	↑	↑	↑	↑
K	125	↓	↓	↓	↓	↓	↓	0 1	↓	↓	1 2	2 3	3 4	5 6	8 9	12 13	18 19	↑	↑	↑	↑	↑	↑	↑	↑	↑	↑
L	200	↓	↓	↓	↓	↓	0 1	↓	↓	1 2	2 3	3 4	5 6	8 9	12 13	18 19	↑	↑	↑	↑	↑	↑	↑	↑	↑	↑	↑
M	315	↓	↓	↓	↓	0 1	↓	↓	1 2	2 3	3 4	5 6	8 9	12 13	18 19	↑	↑	↑	↑	↑	↑	↑	↑	↑	↑	↑	↑
N	500	↓	↓	↓	0 1	↓	↓	1 2	2 3	3 4	5 6	8 9	12 13	18 19	↑	↑	↑	↑	↑	↑	↑	↑	↑	↑	↑	↑	↑
P	800	↓	↓	0 1	↓	↓	1 2	2 3	3 4	5 6	8 9	12 13	18 19	↑	↑	↑	↑	↑	↑	↑	↑	↑	↑	↑	↑	↑	↑
Q	1250	↓	0 1	↓	↓	1 2	3 3	3 4	5 6	8 9	12 13	18 19	↑	↑	↑	↑	↑	↑	↑	↑	↑	↑	↑	↑	↑	↑	↑
R	2000	0 1	↑	↓	1 2	2 3	3 4	5 6	8 9	12 13	18 19	↑	↑	↑	↑	↑	↑	↑	↑	↑	↑	↑	↑	↑	↑	↑	↑
S	3150		↑	1 2								↑	↑	↑	↑	↑	↑	↑	↑	↑	↑	↑	↑	↑	↑	↑	↑

A = Acceptance number.
R = Rejection number.
↓ = Use first sampling plan below arrow. If sample size equals or exceeds lot or batch size, do 100% inspection.
↑ = Use first sampling plan above arrow.
Source: Mil. Std. 105D.

Table 14 Master Table for Reduced Inspection

Sample size code letter	Sample size	Acceptable quality levels (reduced inspection,* single sampling)																									
		0.010	0.015	0.025	0.040	0.065	0.10	0.15	0.25	0.40	0.65	1.0	1.5	2.5	4.0	6.5	10	15	25	40	65	100	150	250	400	650	1000
		A R	A R	A R	A R	A R	A R	A R	A R	A R	A R	A R	A R	A R	A R	A R	A R	A R	A R	A R	A R	A R	A R	A R	A R	A R	A R
A	2	↓	↓	↓	↓	↓	↓	↓	↓	↓	↓	↓	↓	↓	↓	0 1	↓	↓	1 2	2 3	3 4	5 6	7 8	10 11	14 15	21 22	30 31
B	2	↓	↓	↓	↓	↓	↓	↓	↓	↓	↓	↓	↓	↓	0 1	↑	↓	0 2	1 3	2 4	3 5	5 6	7 8	10 11	14 15	21 22	30 31
C	2	↓	↓	↓	↓	↓	↓	↓	↓	↓	↓	↓	↓	0 1	↑	↓	0 2	1 3	1 4	2 5	3 6	5 8	7 10	10 13	14 17	21 24	↑
D	3	↓	↓	↓	↓	↓	↓	↓	↓	↓	↓	↓	0 1	↑	↓	0 2	1 3	1 4	2 5	3 6	5 8	7 10	10 13	14 17	21 24	↑	↑
E	5	↓	↓	↓	↓	↓	↓	↓	↓	↓	↓	0 1	↑	↓	0 2	1 3	1 4	2 5	3 6	5 8	7 10	10 13	14 17	21 24	↑	↑	↑
F	8	↓	↓	↓	↓	↓	↓	↓	↓	↓	0 1	↑	↓	0 2	1 3	1 4	2 5	3 6	5 8	7 10	10 13	↑	↑	↑	↑	↑	↑
G	13	↓	↓	↓	↓	↓	↓	↓	↓	0 1	↑	↓	0 2	1 3	1 4	2 5	3 6	5 8	7 10	10 13	↑	↑	↑	↑	↑	↑	↑
H	20	↓	↓	↓	↓	↓	↓	↓	0 1	↑	↓	0 2	1 3	1 4	2 5	3 6	5 8	7 10	10 13	↑	↑	↑	↑	↑	↑	↑	↑
J	32	↓	↓	↓	↓	↓	↓	0 1	↑	↓	0 2	1 3	1 4	2 5	3 6	5 8	7 10	10 13	↑	↑	↑	↑	↑	↑	↑	↑	↑
K	50	↓	↓	↓	↓	↓	0 1	↑	↓	0 2	1 3	1 4	2 5	3 6	5 8	7 10	10 13	↑	↑	↑	↑	↑	↑	↑	↑	↑	↑
L	80	↓	↓	↓	↓	0 1	↑	↓	0 2	1 3	1 4	2 5	3 6	5 8	7 10	10 13	↑	↑	↑	↑	↑	↑	↑	↑	↑	↑	↑
M	125	↓	↓	↓	0 1	↑	↓	0 2	1 3	1 4	2 5	3 6	5 8	7 10	10 13	↑	↑	↑	↑	↑	↑	↑	↑	↑	↑	↑	↑
N	200	↓	↓	0 1	↑	↓	0 2	1 3	1 4	2 5	3 6	5 8	7 10	10 13	↑	↑	↑	↑	↑	↑	↑	↑	↑	↑	↑	↑	↑
P	315	↓	0 1	↑	↓	0 2	1 3	1 4	2 5	3 6	5 8	7 10	10 13	↑	↑	↑	↑	↑	↑	↑	↑	↑	↑	↑	↑	↑	↑
Q	500	0 1	↑	↓	0 2	1 3	1 4	2 5	3 6	5 8	7 10	10 13	↑	↑	↑	↑	↑	↑	↑	↑	↑	↑	↑	↑	↑	↑	↑
R	800	↑	↑	0.2	1.3	1 4	2 5	3 6	5 8	7 10	10 13	↑	↑	↑	↑	↑	↑	↑	↑	↑	↑	↑	↑	↑	↑	↑	↑

*If the acceptance number has been exceeded, but the rejection number has not been reached, accept the lot, but reinstate normal inspection.
A = Acceptance number.
R = Rejection number.
↓ = Use first sampling plan below arrow.
↑ = Use first sampling plan above arrow.

In summary, the steps necessary for the use of MIL-STD-105D are as follows.

Choose the AQL.
Choose the inspection level.
Determine lot size.
Find sample size code letter from the table.
Choose the type of sample plan, and find its table.
Use the tightened or reduced inspection table for the same type of plan whenever it is required.

A continuous sampling plan with in-process testing clearly can yield more valuable information on the homogenity of the production procedure to increase the opportunity to detect and correct any production difficulties. Such testing is facilitated by the fact that the entire lot is accessible and the sample may be obtained entirely at random. Actually, the same procedures described before for sampling plans may be applied to continuous sampling as well.

B. Specification

Final testing of parenteral products is made in the analytical and microbiological quality control laboratories. These tests are designed to determine compliance with specifications. Thus, the testing of the finished product for compliance with a predetermined standard prior to release of the parenteral products and subsequent distribution is a critical factor in quality assurance. The purpose of establishing these specifications and standards is to assure that each injection contains the amount of drug claimed on the label, that all the drug in each injection is available for complete absorption, that the drug is stable in the formulation in its specific final container for its expected shelf life, and that the injections themselves contain no toxic foreign substances. Normally, the design of test parameters, procedures, and specifications is done during product development. It is a good manufacturing practice to base such parameters on experience developed during processing of several pilot and production batches. Furthermore, the results of these studies should be subjected to statistical analysis in order to appraise correctly the precision and accuracy of each procedure for each characteristic. In the long run, with additional production experience, it is possible that specification be modified for perfection and upgrading of product specification. The various disciplines of quality control testing of injectables can be clearly understood from the quality control attributes outlined in Figure 26.

C. Reconciliation

When the parenteral manufacturing process has been completed, the theoretical yields to be expected from the formulation at different stages of manufacture and the accountability calculations are checked for comparison with the practical and permissible yield limits. Such information is recorded on appropriate forms, as shown in Figure 27, and any discrepancy must be reconciled if beyond process allowable variation.

Finished product name, strength, and size

Description

Identification

Volume check

pH

Particulate matter
- HIAC
- Halsey

Turbidity

Color

Moisture

Weight variation for sterile solids

Content uniformity for sterile solids

Sterility

Pyrogenicity

Safety

Additives, if any

Trace penicillin test, if needed

Degradation products and/or impurities

Assay

Figure 26 Parenteral finished product quality assurance specification.

D. Auditing

Good manufacturing practices require that the manufacturing process be adequately documented throughout all stages of the operation. The history of each batch, from the starting materials, equipment used, and personnel involved in production and control until packaging is completed, should be recorded. Reserve samples are to be stored for at least 2 years beyond the labeled expiration date of each product. The areas of record keeping are

Individual components, raw materials, and packaging
Master formula card
Batch production
Container and labeling
Packaging and labeling operation
Laboratory control testing, in-process and finished
Proper signing and dating by at least two individuals independently for each operation in the proper spaces
Reconciliation of materials supplied with amount of injectables produced, taking into account allowable loss limits

Product name Strength Size Lot # Code #

I. Container accountability
   A. Containers issued to parenteral production
   B. Finished containers filled
   C. Excess containers returned to warehouse
   D. Samples
      1. Quality assurance
      2. Preservation
      3. Stability
   E. Rejects
   F. Containers accountability = B + C + D + E = X; deviation = $[(A - X)/A] \times 100 = \pm \%$.

II. Bulk accountability
   A. Weight or volume of bulk prepared
   B. Filled quantity = units sealed × average fill
   C. Samples
      1. Quality assurance
      2. Machine setup
      3. Other
   D. Bulk accountability = B + C = X; deviation = $[(A - X)/A] \times 100 = \pm \%$.

Prepared by Date
Checked by Date
Quality assurance Date

Figure 27 Parenteral product accountability.

Before quality assurance releases the product for distribution, it should evaluate the complete batch records of all in-process tests and controls and all tests of the final product to determine whether they conform to specifications.

A summary example of a quality assurance audit of a parenteral product to assure correct in-process operations is as follows.

a. Approval of bulk parenteral for filling: lot number strength, size, signatures, working formula card and procedure, filtration record, sterilization record, and corrections
b. Approval of filled product for packaging: lot number, strength, size, signature, working formula card and procedure, biological control report, environmental control report, filtration record, sterilization record, labeling, packaging forms, volume check, and visual inspection
c. Approval of finished product in stock: lot number, strength, size, signatures, working formula card and procedure, analytic and microbiological results, biological control report, environmental control report, filtration and sterilization record, packaging and labeling inspection, reconciliation record, line clearance, and release for stock

E. Complaints

Good manufacturing practice regulations stipulate that quality assurance must record in a special file any complaints regarding the quality of a drug, including any change in its physical characteristics. Quality assurance must investigate thoroughly each complaint and route specimens, or in some instances preservation and/or stability samples, to respective laboratories for appropriate testing. Appropriate measurement should be taken, recorded, and filed with the original complaint. Reports of injuries or adverse reactions resulting from the use of a drug should be forwarded to the appropriate authorities. All complaint records should be retained for at least 2 years after distribution of the drug has been completed, or 1 year after the product's expiration date, whichever is shorter.

BIBLIOGRAPHY

Black, S. S., *Disinfection, Sterilization and Preservation*. Lea & Febiger, Philadelphia, 2nd Ed., 1977.

Feigenbaum, A. V., *Total Quality Control*. McGraw-Hill, New York, 1961.

Graves, M. J., *Parenteral Products*. William Heinemann Medical Books, London, 1973.

Griffin, R. C., and Sacharon, S., *Drug and Cosmetic Packaging*. Noyes Data Corp., Park Ridge, New Jersey, 1975.

Hoover, J. E., *Dispensing of Medication*. Mack Publishing Co., Easton, Pennsylvania, 8th Ed., 1976.

Peldzar, Jr., M. J., Reid, R. D., and Chan, E. C. S., *Microbiology*. McGraw-Hill, New York, 1977.

Turco, S., and King, R. E., *Sterile Dosage Forms*. Lea & Febiger, Philadelphia, 2nd Ed., 1979.

The United States Pharmacopeia/National Formulary, 21st Ed./16th Ed., Mack Publishing Co., 1985.

9

Federal Regulation of Parenterals

Jonas L. Bassen*

Consultant
Bowie, Maryland

Bernard T. Loftus†

Consultant
Fairfax, Virginia

I. INTRODUCTION

This chapter presents an overview of the federal regulation of drugs, with particular emphasis on parenteral drug products and their regulation. The text explains the regulatory process in some detail.

The basic federal statute (there are others) governing the regulation of drug products is the Federal Food, Drug, and Cosmetic Act of 1938 (the Act). The congress entitled the legislation, "An act to prohibit the movement in interstate commerce of adulterated and misbranded food, drugs, devices, and cosmetics, and for other purposes." The courts in the ensuing years have further developed that congressional intent, and they have discussed some of the other purposes. The Supreme Court has said[1] that the Act as a whole was designed primarily to protect consumers from dangerous products. Its purpose was to safeguard the consumer by applying the Act to articles from the moment of their introduction into interstate commerce all the way to the moment of their delivery to the ultimate consumer. This interpretation of the Act's intent necessarily includes, in the health team, to carry out the purposes of the Act, not only the enforcement people employed by the U.S. Food and Drug Administration (FDA), the agency that administers the Act, but also the entire team of health professionals who are involved with drug products. The latter includes scientists who do the research and development to create a drug product, the clinical investigators who test the developing product in small patient populations, and the physicians, nurses, pharmacists, and technicians who play

**Former affiliation*: Director, Division of Industry Liaison, Bureau of Drugs, U.S. Food and Drug Administration, Washington, D.C. (Retired)
†*Former affiliation:* Director, Division of Drug Manufacturing, Bureau of Drugs, U.S. Food and Drug Administration, Washington, D.C. (Retired)

important and respective roles in the chain of events in which a drug product ultimately finds its way to the actual patient.

In another case,[2] the Supreme Court said that the purposes of the Act touch phases of the lives and health of people, which, in the circumstances of modern industrialism, are largely beyond self-protection.

With respect to parenteral drug products, much has been learned since 1970. This knowledge is reflected in great improvements in the processing of the products as well as in their handling all the way to the patient's bedside. It is also reflected in the more vigorous regulatory activities of the FDA in the area of parenteral drugs.

II. HISTORY OF FEDERAL DRUG REGULATION

A. Parenterals in the Food and Drugs Act of 1906

The National Food and Drugs Act of 1906 included within the meaning of the term "drug" any substance or mixture of substances intended to be used for the cure, mitigation, or prevention of disease of humans or other animals. More particularly, it included all medicines and preparations recognized in the United States Pharmacopeia or National Formulary for internal or external use, and it deemed a drug to be adulterated if it were sold under or by a name recognized in the Pharmacopeia or National Formulary that differed from the standard of strength, quality, or purity determined by the tests laid down by either of these two official compendia. Thus began a long and still continuing regulatory partnership between the private standard-setting organizations and the agency that ultimately became the Food and Drug Administration. The ninth revision of the *U.S. Pharmacopeia*, published in 1916, contained the first standards for sterile preparations. These included sterilized distilled water and two parenteral sterile solutions: solution of hypophysis (solution of the pituitary body), and physiological solution of sodium chloride. USP IX also introduced a chapter on sterilization, to encourage the production of preparations that would be free of microorganisms.

It was some time after the publication of USP IX before parenteral drugs came into routine medical use. This was because of the prevalence of pyrogenic reactions to the sterile solutions prepared in hospitals. Early investigations by Siebert and Fantus on pyrogens encouraged Baxter and others to explore commercial production of intravenous solutions in about 1930. Sterile, pyrogen-free, vacuum-packed glass containers of several basic intravenous solutions were soon introduced. Pyrogenicity problems continued, however, largely associated with the reuse of administration equipment in hospitals. After World War II, when commercial disposable administration sets were introduced, pyrogenic reactions in hospitals decreased dramatically.

The increased use of parenteral medications was reflected in the inclusion of 26 monographs in NF VI, which became effective in 1936. NF VI general chapter on ampuls reflected an expansion from two pages in NF V to more than nine pages in NF VI. The NF VI also introduced a definition and standard for clarity of ampuls.

The inadequacies of the 1906 Act in controlling the safety and quality of drugs, particularly the absence of any premarket clinical or toxicological testing requirements, were poignantly demonstrated by a major tragedy, the "elixir of sulfanilamide" disaster. This tragic event resulted in over 100 deaths. In its rush to place an oral sulfanilamide preparation on the market (there were injectable forms), a company had included diethylene glycol, a deadly poison, in its formulation as a solvent. The elixir was not tested for toxicity before it was released to the market. This episode happened at a time when Congress was deliberating on new food, drug, and cosmetic legislation. It hastened the passage of the Federal Food, Drug, and Cosmetic Act on June 25, 1938, and the repeal of the 1906 Act.

B. Role of the Compendia Under the 1938 Act

Most of the drug provisions of the 1938 Act were new and without precedent, but one important feature that was carried over was the recognition of the USP and NF as official compendia. The status of compendial tests and monographs was strengthened, and they served as the basis for enforcement of the strength, quality, and purity of official drugs. In 1944, a section of the Department of Labor-Federal Security Appropriation Act made it possible for the FDA to cooperate with associations and scientific societies in the revision of the *U.S. Pharmacopeia* in the development of methods of analysis and mechanical and physical tests necessary to carry out the work of the FDA[3]. Actually, such cooperation took place only on an informal basis, and it was not until 1977 that the FDA established a formal liaison unit with budgeted funds to work on revisions of the USP.

C. Major Features of the Basic Statute, 1938 Act as Enacted

1. *Definitions*

The second chapter of the act defines certain terms used repeatedly in this text. The definitions are quoted directly from the Act.

> Drug
>
> Section 201(g)(1):
>
> The term "drug" means (A) articles recognized in the official United States Pharmacopeia, official Homeopathic Pharmacopeia of the United States, or official National Formulary, or any supplement to any of them; and (B) articles intended for use in the diagnosis, cure, mitigation, treatment, or prevention of disease in man or other animals; and (C) articles (other than food) intended to affect the structure of any function of the body of man or other animals; and (D) articles intended for use as a component of any articles specified in clause (A), (B), or (C); but does not include devices or their components, parts, or accessories.
>
> Label
>
> Section 201(k):
>
> The term "label" means a display of written, printed, or graphic matter upon the immediate container of any article; and a requirement made by or under authority of this Act that any word,

statement, or other information appear on the label shall not be considered to be complied with unless such word, statement, or other information also appears on the outside container or wrapper, if any there be, of the retail package of such article, or is easily legible through the outside container or wrapper.

Labeling

Section 201(m):

The term "labeling" means all labels and other written, printed, or graphic matter (1) upon any article or any of its containers or wrappers, or (2) accompanying such article.

New Drug

Section 201(p):

The term "new drug" means—(1) Any drug (except a new animal drug or an animal feed bearing or containing a new animal drug) the composition of which is such that such drug is not generally recognized, among experts qualified by scientific training and experience to evaluate the safety and effectiveness of drugs, as safe and effective for use under the conditions prescribed, recommended, or suggested in the labeling thereof, except that such a drug not so recognized shall not be deemed to be a "new drug" if at any time prior to the enactment of this Act it was subject to the Food and Drugs Act of June 30, 1906, as amended, and if at such time its labeling contained the same representations concerning the conditions of its use; or (2) Any drug (except a new animal drug or an animal feed bearing or containing a new animal drug) the composition of which is such that such drug, as a result of investigations to determine its safety and effectiveness for use under such conditions, has become so recognized, but which has not, otherwise than in such investigations, been used to a material extent or for a material time under such conditions.

2. *Prohibited Acts and Penalties*

Since the Act's authority rests on the commerce clause of the U.S. Constitution, its prohibitions are contingent on the offending article's having been somehow associated with interstate commerce. Thus (with a few exceptions), the article must have been introduced into or delivered for introduction into interstate commerce. Or, an article that was legal when it entered interstate commerce might become illegal afterward. In the food area, the 1950 Oleomargarine Amendment to the Act declared that adulterated or misbranded oleomargarine in public eating places constituted a burden on interstate commerce and gave the FDA the authority to act against such illegal margarine whether or not it entered interstate commerce. The 1976 Devices Amendment, in a bolder vein, provided that in any action to enforce the requirements of the Act with respect to a device, the connection with interstate commerce required for jurisdiction would be presumed to exist. For pharmaceuticals, including parenteral drug products, as of this writing, the FDA must still prove interstate commerce before it may act in the courts.

The Act prohibits the introduction or the delivery for introduction into interstate commerce of adulterated or misbranded drugs and new drugs in violation of the requirements of the new drugs section. It prohibits the adulteration or misbranding of a drug in interstate commerce, and the alteration, mutilation, destruction, obliteration, or removal of the whole or any part of the labeling of, or the doing of any other act with respect to a drug if such act is done while the drug is held for sale after shipment in interstate commerce and results in the drug being adulterated or misbranded. The courts have interpreted these prohibitions very broadly so that, in effect, if an ingredient of a drug product has some interstate commerce ramification the drug product itself is considered to be in interstate commerce. Further, if someone does any act with respect to a drug before it reaches the ultimate consumer that causes it to be adulterated or misbranded, e.g., if a pharmacist dispenses a prescription drug without the authority of a licensed practitioner, the FDA has jurisdiction over that act.

The Act even prohibits the receipt in interstate commerce of a drug that is adulterated or misbranded, but it protects a dealer who has received a valid guaranty from a vendor. The giving of a false guaranty is prohibited. The law also protects a dealer who received an adulterated or misbranded drug in good faith.

Refusal to permit inspection is prohibited, as is failure of a manufacturer to register with the FDA or failure to list products with the FDA. The revealing of any method or process that, as a trade secret, is entitled to protection is prohibited if such information was obtained under the various authorities of the Act.

It is prohibited to use in any labeling or advertising any representation or suggestion that the drug product has been approved under the new drug section of the Act, and no reference to FDA inspections is permitted in labeling, advertising, or other sales-promotion material. Prescription drug manufacturers are prohibited from failing to furnish licensed practitioners who submit written requests copies of all printed matter included in any package in which that drug is distributed, or copies of such other printed matter as is approved by the FDA.

The 1906 Food and Drugs Act made it compulsory for the agency (then the Bureau of Chemistry of the U.S. Department of Agriculture) to refer to the appropriate U.S. Attorney for criminal prosecution all violations of that Act after giving the party involved an opportunity to be heard. There were no exceptions. If it appeared that any provisions of that Act had been violated by that party, the U.S. Attorney was obliged to cause appropriate proceedings to be commenced and prosecuted in the proper courts of the United States, without delay, for the enforcement of the penalties provided by the Act. Although this "no exceptions" congressional mandate to prosecute was by no means enforced to the letter, it did flood the courts with minor litigation. The 1938 Act gave the FDA more discretion. It contained a proviso that the FDA did not have to prosecute "minor" violations (a term the Act did not define) whenever it believed that the public interest would be adequately served by a suitable written notice or warning. There have always been officials in the agency who believe in rigid, go to court every time, law enforcement; and there have always been other officials who prefer, when it is possible and in the public interest to do so, to use the threat of the sanctions of the Act, rather than the actual sanctions themselves, as wedges to persuade the industry to correct problems. There are persuasive arguments for both schools of thought. In practice, the FDA uses its best judgment, which is obviously influenced by which of the two schools of thought is in the ascendancy in the agency at the time. Very few violations are criminally prosecuted.

Most criminal violations of the Act are misdemeanors and as such cannot be punished by more than a year in jail; they also carry maximum penalties of $1000. But, longer jail sentences and larger fines can be awarded if the case involves more than one count. If the violation is committed with the intent to defraud or mislead, it is a felony punishable by a maximum of 3 years in prison or a fine of not more than $10,000, or both, for each count. The Act provides the same felony penalties in the situation where a person has been convicted of an earlier violation of its requirements. So for practical purposes, even though it is a legal misdemeanor, conviction in a criminal case is a serious matter because upon the second conviction the person involved becomes a felon. Convicted felons lose some of their legal rights, including the right to vote. They can be proceeded against by their professional associations or the State Boards that license them and may be expelled from their associations, or they may lose the license to practice their professions.

The Act provides for seizure of adulterated or misbranded drugs and of drugs that are in violation of the requirements of the new drug section. Seizures have diminished in number in recent years because of the success of the FDA recall program. But, there will always be a need for the FDA to act to remove violative drug products from the market when the private firms or persons responsible for those products are unwilling or unable to do it.

The Act conveys broad seizure powers exercised through the U.S. District Courts. There are no legal limits to the numbers of seizures that can be made of adulterated drugs and violative new drugs. Generally, if the FDA is alleging a product is misbranded, there can be no more than one case under litigation unless the FDA has been successful in a previous proceeding involving the same alleged misbranding. Even in misbranding cases in which there has been no previous adjudication, multiple seizures can be made if there is a finding that there is probable cause to believe from facts found, without hearing, that the misbranded article is dangerous to health or that its labeling is fraudulent, or would be in a material respect misleading, leading to the injury or damage of the purchaser or consumer.

In seizure actions, as in all court actions initiated by the FDA, action is taken in the name of the United States. The government is asking the court to seize and condemn the goods. Since the parties involved are the United States and the seized goods, and the goods cannot act for themselves, the owner or the owner's agent may appear and file a claim of owner and an answer to the charges. On demand of either party, any issue of fact must be tried by jury. The Act provides for some consolidations of cases if seizures have taken place in different court jurisdictions. The claimant is entitled to samples of the seized goods and a copy of the analysis on which the government based its case. If, upon trial, the claimant prevails, the seized goods are released. If the government prevails, the goods are condemned. They may be ordered destroyed, or the court can release them to the claimant under bond to be brought into compliance under FDA supervision. Condemned new drugs must be destroyed. If the seized goods had been imported and the adulteration or misbranding did not occur after importation, they can be exported under certain rigid conditions.

The 1938 Act also included provisions for injunction proceedings giving the U.S. District Courts the authority to restrain most of the violations prescribed by the Act. The FDA has used the injunction provisions of the Act with great effect in situations in which serious danger to health or fraudulent situation had to be stopped immediately. The tremendous advantage of injunctions in regulatory problems involving adulterated drug products, particularly so when injectable drug products are involved and there is a sterility problem or a pyrogen problem, is that the FDA has the opportunity to request the court to order the manufacturing plant involved to close down temporarily until its processes are corrected to the point where the plant can produce sterile and nonpyrogenic drug products. Sometimes (not always), U.S. District Courts will order recalls of adulterated or misbranded drug products. In this way, massive amounts of violative products can be purged quickly from the market. The Act itself does not provide for recalls. The authority cited by the FDA in requesting the courts to order recall is the broad discretionary power of the court itself. Some federal judges do not believe they have such authority and will not order recalls.

3. *Adulteration Provisions*

The legal concept "adulterated" is approached two ways in the Act: from the evidence of laboratory examination of drug products, and from evidence of objectionable conditions observed during manufacturing or holding of the product.

A drug product is deemed adulterated if it is filthy, putrid, or decomposed, in whole or in part; if its strength differs from or its purity or quality falls below what it is supposed to be; or if some other substance has been mixed or packed with it, or substituted wholly for it, in such a way as to reduce its quality or strength. These are all adulterations in the dictionary sense; they are proved by the evidence obtained from the laboratory examination of samples. For example, filth, such as fly parts, has been found in vials of injectible drug products. For another example, laboratory examinations sometimes establish that the amount of an active ingredient present in a vial or ampul is less than the amount declared on the label and less than the lower limit permitted for that ingredient in its specifications. Such laboratory results indicate that there may have been a formulation problem or possibly a stability problem, but they do not prove either. However, they do prove adulteration.

The Act deems a drug product adulterated if its name is recognized in an "official compendium" (*U.S. Pharmacopeia*, National Formulary, or Homeopathic Pharmacopeia of the United States), and its strength differs from, or its quality or purity falls below the standards set forth in that compendium. Again, the proof of adulteration is obtained from the examination of samples. A manufacturer of an injectable drug product is not required by the Act to use the tests or methods of assay exactly as they are set forth in the *U.S. Pharmacopeia* (for example). Indeed, the manufacturer does not have to use them at all, but may use any methods if it can be proved that their results are equal to or better than the compendial tests and methods; but the products released to the market must pass those compendial tests and assays if they are sampled and tested by the FDA. If not, they are deemed adulterated.

The Act regards drugs as adulterated if they are produced under objectionable conditions, which cannot always, if at all, be demonstrated by laboratory examinations of samples of finished products. If, for example, an injectable drug product has been prepared, packed, or held under insanitary conditions whereby it may have been contaminated with filth or whereby it may have been rendered injurious to health, it is adulterated as a matter of law. The FDA laboratory may examine 100 samples and not find evidences of the rodent or insect filth that the investigator observed, or may not find any evidence whatsoever of the rodenticide that was being carelessly used. The proof in such cases is the inspectional evidence of the actual objectionable manufacturing or storage situation. In the same vein, the Act says a drug is deemed adulterated if the methods used in, or the facilities or controls used for, its manufacture, processing, packing, or holding do not conform to or are not operated or administered in conformity with current good manufacturing practice to assure that the drug meets the requirements of the Act as to safety and has the identity and strength and meets the quality and purity characteristics that it purports or is represented to possess. This is the so-called good manufacturing practice (GMP) provision of the Act. Again, the proof in such a case is the inspectional evidence. More often than not in such situations, the FDA will not collect samples at all (although they have the option to do so), and if they do collect samples they usually hold them as exhibits without laboratory examination. Under the GMP section, current manufacturing practice and good manufacturing practice are inseparable. What is current is not necessarily good. The law always requires what is both good and current, but not necessarily "best." This is important to consider in the parenterals industry because technology develops so swiftly that firms are constantly acquiring better equipment, but not necessarily concomitantly improving their processes. The FDA is the arbiter of what is or is not acceptable GMP, subject to review by the courts. Every parenteral drug manufacturer must produce products in conformity with the requirements of FDA current good manufacturing practice regulations for drug products.

One cannot sample and examine parenteral drug products for sterility on the same statistical bases on which one examines most other dosage forms. Sterility must be proved by validation and control of the manufacturing process. In recent years, the FDA has initiated numerous court actions in which the agency charged that parenteral drugs were adulterated within the meaning of the GMP adulteration section of the Act because there was a lack of assurance that the drugs were sterile or that they were nonpyrogenic.

4. *Misbranded Drugs*

The Act contains two broad labeling requirements, together with a number of more specific requirements. Failure to comply with any of them would result in a drug's being misbranded. The broad requirements are that a drug's labeling may not be false or misleading in any particular and that a drug's labeling must bear adequate directions for use and adequate warnings against unsafe use. Prescription drug labels (and this includes all parenteral drugs except insulin, which is legally an over-the-counter drug) must bear the legend: "Caution: Federal law prohibits dispensing without a prescription."

Other specific labeling requirements mandate that official drugs must be packaged and labeled as prescribed in the official compendia, and that when a product bears the name of an official drug, but differs from one or more of the compendia's requirements, its label must reveal wherein it differs from the official standard. Also, drugs subject to deterioration must bear special precautionary labeling.

5. *New Drugs*

This section of the statute prohibited the introduction into interstate commerce of any new drug unless an application filed in accordance with the regulations was effective. A new drug application (NDA) under the basic Act automatically became effective on the day 60 after filing, unless prior to that date the FDA found the drug to be unsafe and notified the applicant in writing to this effect. If the FDA determined that a new drug was unsafe, it had the burden to sustain its decision and the applicant could appeal the denial to a U.S. District Court. The new drug section directed the FDA to promulgate regulations exempting from its requirements investigational drugs shipped to experts qualified by education and training to investigate the safety of drugs. The early investigational new drug regulations simply required a label on the investigational drug: "Caution: New drug limited by federal law to investigational use," plus some simple record keeping and a statement that the investigator had the facilities to conduct the investigation and would make the records of the investigation available for inspection by an FDA employee. Sponsors were not required to notify the FDA that investigational drugs were being tested on humans.

D. Amendments to the Basic Statute

The insulin amendment, which was passed by Congress in December 1941, required certification by the FDA of all batches of the injectable, insulin, before marketing. Speedy passage of this amendment, in a record time of 3 days, was due to the fact that the insulin patents would expire by year end. Insulin had been regulated under a licensing system conducted by the University of Toronto. The University had a batch-testing system in effect for many years. Upon expiration of the patents any manufacturer, however ill equipped, could have manufactured insulin, unless appropriate authority was given to the FDA to control its potency and purity.

1. *Antibiotic Certification*

The tremendous demand during and immediately after World War II for penicillin and other antibiotics produced by novel production processes, with frequent sterility failures, required government control to assure their safety and potency. Although these were new drugs and could have been controlled under the new drug section of the Act, it was generally accepted that stricter controls were needed. Congress passed an amendment in 1945 placing drugs containing penicillin (and later added streptomycin, chlortetracycline, chloramphenicol, and bacitracin) as antibiotics requiring batch certification for sterility, purity, and potency. Fees were to be charged the manufacturers and others for the certification service. The statute directed the FDA to promulgate regulations governing fees, methods of assay, standards of identity, strength, quality and purity, and other particulars sufficient to set up the certification service. Applicants for certification of new antibiotics were required to submit data showing safety and effectiveness, and all applicants were required to have adequate manufacturing and other controls. Antibiotics were the first new drugs to require proof of efficacy as well as safety. Recognition of the inextricable relationship between safety and efficacy foreshadowed the requirement of proof of efficacy in the Drug Amendments of 1962.

2. *Durham-Humphrey Amendment*

This 1951 amendment defined three categories of prescription drugs and distinguished them from over the counter (OTC) drugs. It provided pharmacists with specific guidance on dispensing prescription drugs. Labels of prescription drugs were required to bear the statement, "Caution: Federal law prohibits dispensing without prescription." Failure of the label to bear this statement caused a drug to be misbranded. Drugs requiring a prescription were those intended for use by humans that were

Habit-forming and are specifically named in the statute[4]

Not safe for self-medication because of their toxicity or other potential harmful effect, or the method of use, or the collateral measures necessary for their use are only safe under the supervision of a practitioner licensed by law to administer such drugs

"New drugs" limited to prescription use under a new drug application (NDA)

3. *Drug Amendments of 1962*

Legislation to amend the drug provisions of the Act was pending in Congress when a major therapeutic disaster, the thalidomide tragedy in 1961, finally speeded passage of these sweeping amendments. A key concept of these amendments was that the FDA should have the authority to prevent the marketing of unsafe and ineffective drugs, rather than having to wait until defective drugs were shipped in interstate commerce before legal action could be taken to remove them from the market. The extensive changes in the drug provisions may be summarized as follows.

Proof of effectiveness as well as safety was now required before "new drugs" could be marketed. Adequate and well-controlled investigations conducted by experts qualified to evaluate the effectiveness of the drug under the conditions of use prescribed, recommended, or suggested in the labeling or proposed labeling were the only types of evidence to be used in approval of new drugs.

A retroactive requirement was added for proof of effectiveness for all new drugs deemed approved only for safety between 1938 and 1962. Manufacturers were given 2 years to submit proof of effectiveness before such drugs could be ordered off the market. Evaluation of proof of effectiveness for uses claimed in the labeling proved to be a gargantuan project beyond the resources of the FDA. Thus the FDA contracted with the National Academy of Sciences and the National Research Council (NAS/NRC) in 1966 to review the efficacy of over 4000 "deemed approved" new drugs for efficacy of label claims. This drug efficacy study and its implementation, which became known as drug efficacy study implementation (DESI) has probably had a greater impact on the marketing of drugs, including parenteral dosage forms, than any other type of regulatory action ever undertaken by the FDA.

New drug review was changed so that it became an approval, a positive action by the FDA. The FDA now had 180 days (or additional time as agreed between the sponsor and the FDA) for initial consideration of the application. A hearing procedure was provided in case the FDA would indicate the drug was not approvable or did not act within 180 days.

Requirements on investigational drugs were strengthened. The FDA was given specific authority to issue regulations requiring submission of reports of preclinical tests, including animal tests, adequate to justify proposed clinical testing.

Reports were required by the manufacturer on experience with new drugs and antibiotics already on the market, as was prompt reporting to the FDA when the manufacturer learned of anything that affected safety and efficacy.

Previously approved NDAs would be withdrawn on the basis of new evidence that manufacturing controls were inadequate or the NDA holder failed to maintain required records or submit required reports of experiences with the drug.

A requirement was added that all drug firms must operate under current good manufacturing practice and failure to do so would render the drugs manufactured therein adulterated.

Inspection authority over those establishments manufacturing, repacking, or holding prescription drugs was strengthened by requiring FDA access to all records, files, processes, or facilities that have a bearing in determining whether there may be a violation with respect to such drugs.

For the first time, registration was required of all domestic drug-manufacturing establishments as well as inspection at least once every 2 years.

Batch certification of all human antibiotics was provided for.

Labeling requirements were changed so that, in the case of prescription drugs, the quantity of all active ingredients must appear, both on the label and in the labeling. This had been a requirement for parenteral drugs prior to 1962. The FDA was given authority to standardize drug names.

Prescription drug advertising was required to show the established name, the quantitative formula to the same extent as required on the label, and a true and nonmisleading brief summary of adverse effects, contraindications, efficacy, and other information for the guidance of physicians.

E. Regulations and the Rule-Making Process

To simplify an explanation of this process, it may be viewed as consisting of three parts: first, the statutory authority; second, the promulgation of regulations; and third, administrative review.

1. *Statutory Authority*

To implement the provisions of the Federal Food, Drug and Cosmetic Act, Congress delegated to the FDA through the Secretary of Health, Education and Welfare broad authority to promulgate regulations for the efficient enforcement of the Act under Section 701(a). The exceptions to this authority are those provisions of the Act that are cited in Section 701(e). These include several drug provisions relating to certain types of adulteration and misbranding. Regulations issued under Section 701(e) require an opportunity for a public hearing under formal rule-making procedures, referred to as an evidentiary public hearing. Regulations promulgated under Section 701(a) on the contrary are subject only to notice and comment or informal rule making under the provisions of the Administrative Procedures Act.[5]

Some sections of the Act mandate regulations to be promulgated to implement a statutory provision. For example, under Section 502 relating to misbranding of drugs, a drug in package form is deemed misbranded unless its label contains, among other requirements, an accurate statement of the quantity of contents in terms of weight, measure, or numerical count. Realizing that there may be some variations that are reasonable, the statute contains a proviso that the Secretary shall prescribe regulations setting forth such exceptions. Thus, a regulation was promulgated wherein the declaration of net contents in the case of large volume parenterals may be embossed on the glass container instead of on the label.[6]

Some provisions not only mandate regulations but indicate their scope. For example, certification of antibiotic regulations specifies that they shall prescribe standards of identity and of strength, quality, and purity, methods of assay, and so on, but also say that the tests to be required should be those that can provide accurate results in the shortest period of time.

A number of provisions contain no statutory guidance on the issuance of regulations. The FDA must then determine whether the issuance of regulations is necessary for the efficient enforcement of the Act. Guidance may come from the legislative history on that particular section as disclosed in the debate and conference report on the legislation. For example, in considering quality manufacturing controls during the debates on the legislation that resulted in the passage of the Drug Amendments of 1962, there was a consensus that regulations defining minimum standards were essential. There was a difference of opinion whether the regulations should be promulgated under existing Section 701(a) or 701(e). The preamble to the 1978 revision of the drug current good manufacturing practice (CGMP) regulations discusses this and concludes that it was the intent of Congress to issue such regulations under Section 701(a).[7] These regulations implement Section 501(a)(2)(B), which defines a drug as adulterated unless it is manufactured, packed, or held under current good manufacturing practice. Since these general regulations must reflect "current" good manufacturing practice, they must be updated to keep pace with advances in pharmaceutical manufacturing. Issuance of additional CGMP regulations for specific classes of drugs, such as large volume parenterals and compressed medical gases, are considered by the FDA on the basis of the need for efficient enforcement. Guidelines, rather than regulations, may be adequate in some cases. When there is no statutory authority in the Act, as in the case of recall of drugs, the FDA can only issue guidelines.

2. *Promulgation of Regulations*

FDA authority to promulgate CGMP regulations is based on various provisions of the Act as noted earlier. However, the procedures the FDA must follow in rule making have been shaped by two laws, the Federal Register Act of 1935 and the Administrative Procedure Act of 1946. Congress passed the Federal Register Act to simplify the problem of keeping the public informed of the large number of regulations issued by Federal agencies during the "New Deal" era of the 1930s. The *Federal Register* was designated as the official publication for all regulations.[8] Publication of a regulation in the *Federal Register* fulfills only part of the requirements. The final regulations are then codified by part and section under Title 21 of the Code of Federal Regulations (CFR). These volumes are revised annually as of April to incorporate regulations published in the *Federal Register* during the preceding 12 months.[9] The Administrative Procedures Act (APA) added several legal requirements to the rule-making process. It introduced as a general requirement the element of public participation into rule making. With certain exceptions, all rules must first be published as proposals in the *Federal Register*, and at least 30 days must be allowed for public comment before a rule can become final. This "notice and comment" type of rule making is referred to as informal rule making, in contrast to formal rule making requiring evidentiary public hearings.

The FDA has implemented the APA with administrative practices and procedures regulations consolidated under Parts 10 through 20 of Chapter 1 of 21 CFR. To encourage public participation in its rule making and other administrative proceedings, the FDA has explained when and how interested parties may petition the Commissioner to issue, amend, or revoke a regulation or order. Prescribed formats are established. The one most frequently used is aptly titled "Citizen Petition." Specialized formats for petitions requesting an administrative reconsideration of action or administrative stay of action are described in Part 10. This is particularly helpful to health professionals who are knowledgeable in the technical aspects of some regulations but not in the procedural aspects.

FDA administrative practices and procedures regulations describe informal rule making it follows under its authority to promulgate regulations under Section 701(a) for efficient enforcement of the Act. Although the rule permits any interested party to propose a regulation, most regulations are proposed by the Commissioner. A notice of proposed rule making is published in the *Federal Register* using a format prescribed by an executive order designed to improve the quality of federal regulations. The format requires, among other items, a summary of the substance of the document in the first paragraph in easily understandable terms; relevant dates, e.g., closing date for comments; name, address, and phone number of the FDA contact; supplementary information in the form of a preamble summarizing the proposals and the facts and policy underlying it; the statutory authority; the exact terms of the regulation itself; and whether an environmental impact statement is needed and an identifying docket number. Comments are to be submitted to the FDA hearing clerk in a standard format, usually within 60 days of publication of the proposal.

Final regulations are promulgated based on a review of all comments, although the commissioner may decide to issue a new proposal. The basis for the final regulation must be solely on the administrative record. Publication in the *Federal Register* must be in a prescribed format, similar to that for the proposal. However, the supplementary information in the preamble will contain a summary of each type of comment submitted on the proposal with the commissioner's conclusions. The exposition of the commissioner's rationale for accepting or rejecting a comment is most enlightening to those who must comply with a regulation as to FDA interpretation of specific points. After publication of the final regulation, interested parties may petition for administrative review of part or the entire rule.

3. *Substantive or Interpretive*

There has been controversy over the legal status of regulations promulgated under Section 701(a). In the proposed CGMP regulations, Section 210 states that the regulations are in fact substantive, so that failure to comply with any section of the CGMP shall render a drug to be adulterated under Section 501(a)(2)(B) of the Act, and thus regulatory action could be taken against the drug and person(s) responsible for the adulteration.[10] The commissioner, in the preamble to the final regulations, cited a number of recent court decisions upholding his view that the CGMP are substantive, binding regulations. The commissioner invited a challenge through judicial review to those holding other views. If the regulations are determined to be only interpretive, then in any court case, the FDA would have to establish that its regulations are in accord with current good manufacturing practice.

4. *Guidelines*

The rule-making provisions of the Administrative Procedure Act exempt interpretive rules and statements of policy from the notice and comment requirements to implement a statutory requirement of a law. The former, referred to by the FDA as guidelines, may be published in the *Federal Register* without notice and comment, or only a notice of the availability may be published. In case of guidelines of major significance, the FDA has chosen to publish them as proposals with opportunity for comment. Thus, the FDA proposed comprehensive guidelines on the recall of drugs and other regulated products in 1976 and subsequently published a final regulation under Sections 7.1 through 7.59, in the FR of June 16, 1978. The preamble contains an extensive review of the voluntary nature of the regulation after considering the lack of clear statutory authority to enforce recalls. When guidelines are not published in the *Federal Register*, the *Federal Register* will carry a notice of their availability. The FDA Dockets Management Branch has established a file of all guidelines that are not published in the *Federal Register*. The 21 CFR 10.90(b)(1) contains a comprehensive exposition on guidelines. A portion defining guidelines follows:

> Guidelines establish principles or practices of general applicability and do not include decisions or advice on particular situations. Guidelines relate to performance characteristics, preclinical and clinical test procedures, manufacturing practices, product standards, scientific protocols, compliance criteria, ingredient specifications, labeling, or other technical or policy criteria. Guidelines state procedures or standards of general applicability that are not legal requirements but are acceptable to FDA for a subject matter which falls within the laws administered by the Commissioner.

In view of the broad definition of guidelines, the FDA has considerable latitude in deciding whether to issue a guideline or a regulation under 701(a) in a given situation to carry out its obligation for efficient enforcement of the Act.

5. *Other Acts and/or Executive Orders Affecting Regulations*

Rule making by all federal agencies has been affected by a requirement of the National Environmental Policy Act (NEPA) that an environmental impact statement shall be prepared and filed for every major agency action that might affect the quality of the human environment. The FDA has issued implementing regulations as to the format and other aspects of environmental impact statements under the Act.[11] An environmental impact analysis is required to explain why no environmental impact statement is required for specific regulations on NDA or other submissions.

The FDA "Good laboratory practice for non clinical laboratory studies" regulations[12] have had an impact on regulations of other agencies, such as the Environmental Protection Agency (EPA), which also requires filing of nonclinical laboratory studies under its regulation of pesticides. In March 1978, the FDA and the EPA entered into a formal agreement whereby the FDA would perform laboratory inspections for the EPA and both the FDA and the EPA would share information on inspectional findings and compliance activities on nonclinical laboratory studies.

6. *Economic Impact*

Improving Government Regulations

Several recent presidential orders in both the Carter and Reagan administrations[13] have attempted to improve federal regulations and to limit unnecessary regulation so that they do not impose burdens on the economy, on individuals, and on state and local governments. Agencies are required to prepare regulatory analyses for significant regulations that include a determination of the economic impact as defined by certain criteria. Agencies are also required to publish semiannually in the *Federal Register* an agenda of significant regulations under development or review. These agenda are helpful to industry in their planning.

7. *Administrative Review*

Some sections of the Act provide for administrative review. However, the FDA in its administrative practices and procedures regulations provides for administrative review of all regulations. The FDA introduced some new mechanisms for administrative review, such as a "Public hearing before a public board of inquiry," somewhat like a science court of appeals; and a "Public hearing before a public advisory committee," in addition to the traditional "Formal evidentiary public hearing." The objective of these procedures is to provide varied means to parties objecting to FDA decisions to exhaust administrative remedies before seeking judicial review.

A recent regulation involving parenteral drugs, which resulted in a request for administrative review, is summarized below. This was a request for an administrative stay of part of a final regulation on "Large volume parenteral drugs in plastic containers, compatibility studies," published in the *Federal Register* of December 5, 1978. The original proposal was published in the *Federal Register* of November 7, 1974. The preamble cited the public health need for determining whether there was a hazard from the leaching of components in plastic containers into drugs commonly added to large volume parenterals (LVP) by requiring compatibility studies on 36 commonly used additive drugs. Since all large volume parenterals in plastic containers were new drugs and required new drug approval, the FDA cited a provision of the new drug section of the Act as a basis for the new regulation. The proposal would have required that all holders of NDAs for LVPs in plastic conduct compatibility studies for the 36 additives and submit status reports at specified intervals after the study protocols were approved by the FDA. Additionally, the proposal would have required that labeling of all LVPs in plastic bear the prominently placed warning, namely,

> Additive may be incompatible. Those additives known to be incompatible should not be used. Consult with pharmacist, if available. If in the informed judgment of the physician, it is deemed advisable to introduce additives to this solution, use aseptic technique. Thorough and careful mixing of any additive is mandatory. Do not store solutions containing additives.

The FDA published a final rule in the *Federal Register* of December 15, 1978, 4 years after publication of the proposed regulation. Five comments were received on the proposal. The preamble in the final rule summarized these comments and the commissioner's conclusions. Minor changes were made in the wording and timing of status reports, as well as allowing NDA holders to phrase the warning statement as long as it conveyed the message. However, the final rule added two new requirements, namely, that after February 13, 1979, all new drug applications for a large volume parenteral drug in a plastic immediate container must contain results of compatibility studies, and that holders of new drug applications for large volume parenterals in plastic may put new labeling into use without advance approval of the FDA [310.509(g) and (h)]. Holders of previously approved NDAs would be allowed to continue marketing while compatibility studies were being conducted up to a period of 2 years. Five petitions were filed for an administrative stay of action under 21 CFR 10.35, pointing out that there had been no opportunity to comment on the new provisions and that these new provisions were patently unfair to those filing new drug applications as against holders of existing new drug applications. Additionally, since the new requirements were not part of the administrative record, there had been no opportunity to comment before the new requirements were finalized. On March 13, 1979, the commissioner published an order in the *Federal Register* staying the two sections. He has not reproposed them.

III. MAJOR REGULATIONS AFFECTING PARENTERALS

The FDA rule-making process distinguishes among several types of regulations: procedural, technical, mandated by statute, and guidelines. Many affect parenteral drugs. However, those discussed in detail herein are characterized by having a special type of regulatory control. Three major regulations with different types of regulatory controls are new drugs with premarket clearance requirements; antibiotic and insulin certification combining premarket clearance and batch certification; and current good manufacturing practice with inspection-compliance controls. These major regulations and their controls are not static. The FDA responds to new situations by revising these regulations, usually belatedly, and also by changing its enforcement approach. Thus in 1982 (FR 9/7/82, p. 39155), the FDA amended the antibiotic and new animal drug regulations to exempt all classes of antibiotic drugs from batch certification requirements.[14]

A. New Drug Regulations

The new drug section of the Act, Section 505, prohibits the introduction into interstate commerce of any new drug unless an application pursuant to these regulations has been approved by the FDA as demonstrating the safety and efficacy of the drug for the claims and conditions in its labeling. This is not an application in the ordinary sense, since NDAs usually comprise many volumes of data, including, by reference, data acquired during the investigational drug phase under an exemption for investigational use.

1. *Investigational Drugs*

Since a new drug may require extensive preclinical and/or clinical investigation by qualified investigators in the United States and foreign countries, the Act provided for promulgating regulations exempting new drugs shipped in interstate commerce for investigational use from the prohibition under the new drug regulations. Prior to beginning testing in human subjects, the sponsor of a new drug must file a Form 1571, notice of claimed investigational exemption (IND), with the FDA. The sponsor must wait 30 days after FDA receipt of the application before proceeding with clinical testing. The FDA must notify the sponsor if it questions the advisability of initiating clinical tests, according to the plans and protocols in the FD-1571. The FD-1571 is a most comprehensive listing of information on all aspects of the investigational use of the drug, beginning with its chemistry, manufacture, and identity and purity; animal studies with a statement that such studies have been conducted in conformity with FDA good laboratory practice (GLP) nonclinical laboratory studies regulations; training and experience of investigators and individuals who will monitor the clinical studies; and the plans and protocols for various phases of clinical studies beginning with clinical pharmacology to establish efficacy. Additionally, the sponsor must file an FD-1752 attesting to the investigators' qualifications and details on the conduct of the experimental project and the requirement to report significant adverse findings to the FDA. A statement, FD-1753, must be signed by the investigator(s) signifying they understand their obligations under the regulations.

Before a new drug sponsor undertakes the very extensive clinical studies to establish safety and efficacy, there is a need for some understanding between the FDA and the sponsor as to the type of protocols that will satisfy the "substantial evidence" requirement for well-controlled studies. Although the general principles of clinical testing will be applicable to most therapeutic classes of drugs, many classes will require special consideration in the design of clinical trials. To assist sponsors as well as its own evaluators, the FDA started the publication in 1977 of a series of clinical guidelines for different classes of drugs.[15] In preparing these guidelines, the FDA was assisted by the experts on its various advisory committees, as well as by industry pharmacologists. Small volume parenterals represent dosage forms included in many different drug classes, and clinical trials would be conducted on the basis of the guideline for the particular therapeutic class. There are no clinical guidelines for large volume parenterals per se. Clinical guidelines provide sponsors with the FDA opinion as to an acceptable experimental design, but following a guideline will not guarantee acceptance of the study.

The FDA has developed a plan for initiating end-of-phase II conferences between sponsors and the reviewing division in the Center for Drugs and Biologics, particularly for those new molecular entities that in its judgment represent a likely important therapeutic gain, as well as other types of drugs, based on its classification of drugs for review purposes. This was designed to speed approval of such therapeutic drugs. Phase II clinical investigation is intended to include early controlled clinical trials designed to demonstrate effectiveness and relative safety.[16]

2. *New Drug Application and Approval*

Sponsors of new drugs must submit a new drug application on Form 356-H-May 1985 for an original application or an abbreviated application (ANDA) or supplements to approved NDAs and ANDAs. For original applications, particularly for new chemical entities, the submission must include the information outlined in Form 356-H. This outline includes a large number of elements, the major ones being: (a) the chemistry of the drug and relationship to other chemistry or pharmacologically related drugs; (b) reference to any IND applications or any master file whose contents are incorporated in the application; (c) preclinical studies, if required; (d) clinical studies, including summary of the literature; (e) evaluation of safety and effectiveness; (f) copies of labels and all labeling; (g) composition of the drug; (h) description of the methods used in and the facilities and controls used for manufacturing; and (i) samples of the drug.

In practice, some of the elements listed in the FD-356H may be modified or waived, depending upon the classification of the drug, but all new drugs must be shown to be safe and effective.

3. *Postapproval Obligations*

Once an NDA is approved, the NDA holder must maintain certain records and make reports to the FDA of a number of conditions that come to a firm's attention that would raise questions as to the drug's safety and efficacy. These reports are to enable the FDA to determine if there are grounds for the withdrawal of the NDA, and the failure to make such reports is in itself grounds for withdrawal. The NDA holder must report promptly any mix-up in the drug or its labeling, any information concerning any change or deterioration of the drug, or any failure of distributed batches to meet the NDA specifications.

Whenever the holder of the NDA receives any information concerning toxicity, unexpected side effects, or failure to exhibit expected action, a report must be furnished the FDA within 15 working days. Periodic summaries of clinical experiences reported to the firm, as well as reports in the medical literature, are required to be reported on special reporting forms.

Another important condition is the prompt submission of all promotional advertising.

4. *NDA Supplements*

Supplements to NDAs are required for a variety of significant manufacturing changes, and approval of these changes must be obtained before they can be implemented. In some cases such changes are instigated by the FDA itself, as was the case in the large volume parenteral industry during the early 1970s when basic changes in manufacturing procedures were required.

Other changes requiring approval of a supplemental NDA are changes in labeling and in any mailing or promotional pieces following the initial promotion.

5. *Abbreviated New Drug Applications*

The ANDA procedure was instituted by the FDA in 1970 to permit the submission of an abbreviated new drug application (ANDA) for marketed drugs that were identical and related to pre-1962 drugs that had been deemed approved for safety and were reviewed under the drug efficacy study implementation (DESI) program and judged effective. ANDAs were designed to implement the DESI program and the requirements for approval of each reviewed drug were published in the Federal Register.

In 1981 the FDA announced its acceptance of ANDAs or paper NDAs for some post-1962 NDA'd drugs based upon literature references to well-controlled clinical studies, thus exempting such ANDAs from further clinical testing. With the passage of the Drug Price Competition and Patent Restoration Act of 1984 the ANDA process received statutory status, albeit with many complex provisions. Because of the complexity of the new regulations the Center for Drugs and Biologics has prepared guidance documents to assist ANDA sponsors. ANDAs require use of the new revised FD-356-H as with NDAs. However, there are parts of the contents listed on the back of the form which may be omitted. And in the case of parenterals bioavailability studies may be omitted.

B. Batch Certification

Batch certification represents the tightest type of regulation. Until the recent amendment of the antibiotic regulations, all antibiotic manufacturers were required to submit representative samples from each batch for certification by assays performed by FDA laboratories. The high level of compliance with antibiotic standards convinced the FDA that batch certification was no longer required to ensure the safety and efficacy of antibiotic drugs. The final regulation does contain a provision that batch certification may be reinstituted if the commissioner finds evidence that such controls are necessary in specific instances to ensure the safety and eficacy of that antibiotic drug(s).

Insulin products were the first drugs requiring batch certification following the passage of the 1938 Act. The concept of batch certification was adopted from the licensing system and batch testing by the University of Toronto, the holder of the insulin patents. The circumstances surrounding the passage of the amendment to the Act were detailed earlier in this chapter. Currently many novel forms of insulin are being developed, and this may be one reason for the continuation of batch certification.

C. Current Good Manufacturing Practice

The concept that the control of the quality of a drug can only be achieved through the application of adequate controls in the development and production stages by technically trained personnel was recognized by both the drug industry and the FDA before 1962. There was ample evidence to show that in such vital characteristics as sterility of parenteral solutions the chances of passing defective lots based upon relatively small sample sizes were too high. And the patient, usually in a debilitated condition, should not be exposed to such a risk. Congress, in passing the 1962 Amendments, adopted this concept by the simple expedient of adding another characteristic to the definition of adulteration under the Act, Section 501. Henceforth a drug shall be deemed to be adulterated

> . . . if it is a drug and the methods used in, or the facilities or controls used for its manufacture, processing or holding do not conform to or are not operated or administered in conformity with current good manufacturing practice to assure that such drug meets the requirements of this Act as to safety and has the identity and strength, and meets the quality and purity characteristics which it purports to possess.

To implement this requirement, the FDA was to issue regulations defining, for the first time, "current good manufacturing practice." The FDA issued the first CGMP regulations on June 20, 1963. One of the problems facing those drafting these regulations was how to determine what good practices were "current." An account of the circumstances surrounding their issuance[18] shows that, prior to publication for comment of the proposal in the *Federal Register* (FR), there was some consultation with industry scientists to assure that the practices proposed were indeed both good and current. This same account reviews a decade of FDA-industry experience with revisions of these general or umbrella CGMP regulations. The latest revisions of the CGMP regulations for human and veterinary drugs were published in the FR of September 29, 1978, and became effective on March 28, 1979. Because these regulations provide legal standards for controlling the quality of drugs, they should be of interest to all health professionals. They can also provide an insight into standard operating procedures that may serve those who are called upon to set up a quality control program on the handling and administration of parenterals in health care facilities. Unlike other regulations, regulatory controls are based primarily on inspections of establishments manufacturing, processing, packing, or holding human and veterinary drugs. To appreciate the scope of these regulations, it is desirable to consider

Provisions of the CGMP in terms of quality control concepts and their contribution to assurance of quality
Why revisions are necessary
Why specialized CGMPs have been proposed for LVPs and some provisions in the proposal
Comparisons of the general CGMPs with the LVPs proposals and the need for CGMPs for small volume parenterals

1. Provisions of the CGMP Regulations

Subpart A: General Provisions, Including Scope and Definitions

1. Traceability of a product is the basis for the definition of "lot number, control number or batch number," namely, "any distinctive combination of letters, numbers or symbols—from which the complete history of the manufacture, processing, packing, holding, and distributing of a batch or lot of drug product or other material can be determined."

2. "Acceptance criteria" should have an associated sampling plan as a basis for making a decision to accept or reject a lot or batch, according to product specifications.

3. Validation, a key word and concept in the evaluation of CGMP compliance, is unfortunately not defined in this or other subparts of the regulation. The word *validation* appears in five sections of the CGMP but in only one, 211.165(e) on validation of test methods, is there reference as to how such validation shall be accomplished. However, the FDA has attempted to explain its concept of validation in other documents. In March 1984 and again in September 1985, the FDA issued a draft for comment on its "Guideline on general principles of process validation." In all of these drafts, the FDA offered the following as one definition of process validation:

> Process validation is a documented program which provides a high degree of assurance that a specific process will consistently produce a product meeting its pre-determined specifications and quality attributes.

Although these draft documents [see later text for further discussion] apply to all drugs and devices, emphasis is given to validation of sterilization processes. Since parenterals are subjected to sterilization, the FDA compliance programs on large and small volume parenterals, as well as the proposed LVP regulations, have offered guidance as to what the agency considers adequate validation for these drug products.

Subpart B: Organization and Personnel

1. Responsibilities and authority of a quality control unit are to be spelled out in writing.

2. Personnel qualification for assigned functions and training in CGMP shall be conducted on a continuing basis.

3. Only authorized personnel shall enter those areas of the buildings and facilities designated as limited-access areas.

4. Consultants advising on CGMP shall be qualified, and records shall be maintained on their employment and qualifications.

Subpart C: Buildings and Facilities

1. Buildings—their size, construction, and operational areas—are to be designed so that they are suited to the types of products produced or held therein to prevent contamination or mix-ups.

2. Special operations require more detailed criteria as to the adequacy of the building and facilities. Thus, the requirements for aseptic processing must include

> Floors, walls, and ceilings of smooth, hard surfaces that are easily cleanable;
> Temperature and humidity controls;
> An air supply filtered through high-efficiency particulate filters under positive pressure, regardless of whether the flow is laminar or non-laminar;
> A system of monitoring environmental conditions;
> A system for cleaning and disinfecting the room and equipment to produce aseptic conditions.

3. Equipment for adequate* control over air pressure, microorganisms, dust, humidity, and temperature shall be provided when appropriate* for the manufacture, processing, packing, or holding of a drug product.

4. Sanitation shall be assured by requiring written procedures for cleaning and assigning responsibility of seeing that they are followed. Rodenticides, insecticides, or fumigating agents shall not be used unless registered and used in accordance with the Federal Insecticide, Fungicide and Rodenticide Act (FIFRA). Sanitation procedures shall apply to work performed by contractors.

Subpart D: Equipment

1. Adequacy of equipment design, size, and location should be validated.

2. Equipment cleaning and maintenance record keeping is essential.

Subpart E: Control of Components and Drug Product Containers and Closures

1. Take appropriate measures to establish suitable specifications, and assure conformance with the "specs" by proper records.

2. Retest components, drug product containers, and closures as necessary due to conditions or passage of time that might adversely affect them.

3. Assure that drug product containers and closures are not reactive, additive, or absorptive, so as to alter the strength, quality, or purity of the drug beyond the applicable specifications.

4. Enforce standards and specifications to ensure that such hazards as pyrogens are eliminated from containers and closures for parenterals.

Subpart F: Production and Process Controls

1. Provide written procedures and deviation control with approval by the quality control unit.

2. Validate process by process capability studies.

3. Control against microbiological contamination, including validation of the sterilization process.

4. Reprocessing must be based on procedures that will ensure that reprocessed batches will conform with *all* established standards, specifications, and product characteristics.

Subpart G: Packaging and Labeling Control

1. Provide written procedures and documentation to assure that every stage from the design, receipt, identification, storage, and handling of labeling and packaging and their application to the drug product is adequately controlled.

2. All prescription drug products and most OTC drug products shall have expiration dates on their labeling based on adequate stability studies. However, the commissioner proposed in a separate *Federal Register* document

---

*Such words as *adequate* and *appropriate* are used frequently in this and other sections of the CGMP. This puts the burden on the manufacturer of showing through data and performance records that the selections are "adequate" and "appropriate." Such flexibility is viewed by industry as a desirable attribute in the CGMP.

published at the same time as the CGMP final rule that certain OTC drug products be exempted from expiration dates. These included those OTC drug products used without dosage limitation, such as rubbing alcohol, provided that it could be shown that they are stable for at least 3 years. Drug products to be reconstituted at time of dispensing shall bear expiration information for both the reconstituted and unreconstituted products.

Subpart H: Holding and Distribution

1. There shall be written procedures to describe the warehousing. Where necessary to protect product, there shall be appropriate environmental controls.
2. There shall be written distribution procedures so that any recalls, if required, can be handled expeditiously.

Subpart I: Laboratory Controls

1. Any specifications, standards, sampling plans, test procedures, or other laboratory controls, such as stability testing, are to be approved by the quality control unit.
2. The laboratory controls required are specified.
3. Testing and release procedures are specified for the usual drug products and exceptions in the case of short-lived radiopharmaceutical parenterals where batches may be released prior to completion of sterility and/or pyrogen testing. Appropriate laboratory testing is provided for, as necessary, of each batch of drug product required to be free of objectionable microorganisms.
4. A written stability program based on studies conducted in the same container-closure system in which it will be marketed is required.
5. Products purporting to be sterile and/or pyrogen-free must be batch tested prior to release.
6. Reserve samples are required with specific retention times. However, large volume parenterals are exempted from the reserve sample requirement for sterility and pyrogen testing.

Subpart J: Records and Reports

1. Documentation through written procedures and records is now required for practically all operations. The items to be reported in a laboratory assay report are spelled out for the first time in the CGMP.
2. Complaints must be documented, and procedures must be followed in the investigation of complaints by quality control.

D. Proposed CGMP Regulations for Large Volume Parenterals

The preamble to the proposal to issue CGMP regulations for LVPs, published in the *Federal Register* of June 21, 1976, contains a lengthy explanation of why specific CGMPs are necessary for this class of drugs. The reasons given may be summarized as follows.

a. The critical risks to patients from an LVP product that is nonsterile, pyrogenic, or otherwise defective.
b. Failure of the LVP industry, comprising fewer than six companies, to meet what FDA considered good manufacturing practice, based on investigations following a massive recall in 1971 of one manufacturer's

products and a GMP survey in 1973 of all manufacturers. This survey adopted entirely new criteria for air quality, water quality, sterilization, and process controls, criteria of which the industry had previously not been made aware. Based on these new criteria, the FDA found all the manufacturers deficient. These deficiencies and the criteria were discussed with all LVP firms in individual conferences even though this was an industrywide problem. By requiring the firms to meet the new criteria, involving large and extensive improvements in plant and procedures, the FDA claimed it quickly raised all LVP suppliers to the level of current good manufacturing practice.

c. The FDA pointed out that imposing process standards for sterilization of LVPs had precedents in the precise standards for certain biologicals and for low-acid foods in hermetically sealed containers.
d. The proposed regulations supplement the general drug CGMPs, but where it is impossible to comply with the applicable section in both regulations, the specific LVP section supersedes the general one.

1. Key Points in Proposed LVP-CGMPs and Comments

A number of terms and conditions relating to LVPs are defined for the first time. The following examples are quoted from the proposal.

> Large volume parenteral means a terminally sterilized aqueous drug product packaged in a single dose container with a capacity of 100 milliliters or more and intended to be administered and used in man. It includes intravenous infusions, irrigating solutions, peritoneal dialysates, and blood collecting units with anticoagulant. The term, large volume parenteral, does not include any biological drug product subject to section 351 of the Public Health Service Act.
>
> Controlled environment area means any area in which the manufacture, processing, packing or holding of a large volume parenteral drug product occurs and in which environmental factors such as humidity, temperature, particulate and microbial quality of air must be controlled to assure that the drug product has the purity characteristics that it purports or is represented to possess.

Such areas include the weighing, mixing, or filling of LVPs, transfer area, and areas in which gowning occurs. The sections dealing with these areas are very specific as to their environmental requirements. For example, proposed §212.221 states

> Air in controlled environment areas shall have:
> (a) a per cubic foot particle count of not more than 100,000 in a size range of 0.5 microns and larger when measured by automatic counters or 700 particles in a size range of 5.0 microns or larger when measured by a manual microscopic method;
> (b) a temperature of 72°F ±5 or 22°C ±3;
> (c) a maximum relative humidity of 50% and a minimum of 30%;
> (d) a positive pressure differential of at least 0.05 inch of water with all doors closed in relation to a less clean adjacent area;
> (e) at least 20 air changes per hour

Under Definitions, §212.3, the term F_0 is defined as "the equivalent amount of time, in minutes at 121°C or 250°F, which has been delivered to a product by the sterilization process."

Subpart M is a separate part devoted to sterilization requirements. It states the minimal processing requirement as follows: "A manufacturing process for terminal sterilization of a large volume parenteral may employ steam, mixtures of air and steam, or superheated water as the sterilizing medium, provided the procedure has been shown to deliver an F_0 of 8 or more."

The examples cited above illustrate the specificity of many of the requirements in this proposal. Although many requirements are very specific, Section 212.5 provides flexibility by allowing manufacturers to use alternative facilities, equipment, processes, or control procedures. Thus, if a manufacturer has adequate data establishing that the alternative is equal or superior to that required in the proposal and provides assurance that the LVP meets the safety requirements of the Act and has the necessary quality and purity characteristics, the alternative may be used, provided it is documented and documentation is made available during an inspection. For those LVPs for which an NDA has been approved, use of any alternative shall be submitted in an NDA supplement. A total of 38 comments were received by the FDA on the proposed LVP regulations. Many of the comments were well reasoned, and some no doubt will be persuasive enough to produce changes in the final document,[19] although there are mounting indications that a final version may not emerge. The document has become a guidance document for industry and the FDA. The agency itself, in papers presented to industry symposia, backed off on some of the proposed requirements (e.g., the proposed mandatory F_0 of 8).

2. *Small Volume Parenterals*

Small volume parenterals or injectables, unlike LVPs, are a diverse and heterogenous group of drugs. They include not only terminally sterilized solutions but highly sophisticated suspensions, emulsions, and lyophilized products produced by specialized technologies. The FDA, in an addendum to its proposed CGMPs for LVPs, recognized these characteristics of injectables. Thus, in considering future regulations of these products, it requested comments and information for manufacturers of injectables on the sections of the proposed LVPs applicable to their products. The most comprehensive comments were submitted by the Parenteral Drug Association (PDA), a professional association of individuals and companies with the objective of fostering and advancing, in the interest of public health, the art and science of parenteral therapy, and to preserve and improve the integrity and stability of the parenteral drug industry.

The PDA comments[20] pointed out the many differences between LVPs and SVPs that would make it impractical to apply many sections of the proposed LVPs to the latter and ended with a proposal that CGMPs for SVPs not be proposed until yet unresolved problems for LVPs are addressed in final regulations. In the interim, the FDA has received a great deal of information on the processes and practices in the manufacture of diverse types of SVPs. With this information, much of it confidential, the FDA has a basis for determining current good manufacturing practices for different types of SVPs and can thus apply the umbrella CGMPs to these products. This may make it unnecessary for the FDA to promulgate regulations for SVPs, and the agency has issued draft guidelines on SVPs as an alternative.

IV. FDA ENFORCEMENT ACTIVITIES

The FDA is the agency in the Department of Health and Human Services responsible for the enforcement not only of the FD&C Act, but two other health regulatory statutes—the biologics licensing provisions of the Public Health Services Act (Sec. 351) and the Radiation Control for Health and Safety Act of 1968. Since biological products are legally defined as "drugs," they are also subject to the drug requirements of the FD&C Act. Thus, some biological parenterals are regulated under both statutes.

To administer these statutes, the FDA is organized at its Washington headquarters (Fig. 1) on a subject-oriented basis, and in the field, on a network of 10 regional offices, 22 district offices, and 124 resident inspection posts. FDA investigators are located in almost all cities of over 150,000 population. Total FDA personnel as of 1984 is approximately 7300, of which 4700 are located in headquarters and about 2600 are in the field. The headquarter's units are organized into four "centers" (formerly bureaus) on a subject matter basis, namely, the Center for Food Safety and Nutrition, the Center for Drugs and Biologics, the Center for Devices and Radiological Health, and the Center for Veterinary Medicine. The Center for Drugs and Biologics exercises major control of parenterals (Fig. 2). Two other headquarter units, the Office of Regulatory Affairs and the National Center for Toxicological Research, have a status equivalent to the centers. Two officers of the commissioner's staff, the Associate Commissioner for Regulatory Affairs and the Associate Commissioner for Health Affairs, have major impacts on decisions affecting parenteral drugs. The Office of the General Counsel, Department of Health and Human Services, Drug Division, located at FDA headquarters, exercises control over all regulation and major regulatory decisions as legal advisor to the Commissioner of Food and Drugs.

Because of the broad scope of FDA regulatory and other responsibilities and the necessity for coordination of the activities of the headquarters and field staffs, as well as with other agencies, a program management system (PMS) was adopted in 1970. The PMS is administered by the Associate Commisssioner for Planning and Evaluation and is an umbrella system, encompassing planning, budgeting, reporting, and evaluation of all FDA program activities. The program management system divides FDA activities into seven major program areas, such as food safety, human drugs and biologics, medical devices, and radiological health. These program areas are divided into projects. Human drugs and biologics includes 12 projects, such as bioresearch monitoring and drug quality assurance. Of interest to the regulated industries is the allocation of resources each fiscal year for the various projects. These allocations are published in the PMS annual Blue Book.[21] For fiscal year 1984, the allocation for the drug quality assurance project is 29% of the $112,832,000 for the human drugs and biologics program. This includes 586 equivalent positions for the field and 201 for headquarters. Work plans for the use of field resources for each project are determined by compliance programs, statutory requirements to inspect each drug firm once every 2 years, and by emergencies, such as the recent tampering with Tylenol. Of these obligations, the largest are compliance programs.

A. Compliance Programs

The field's resources are used mainly for inspections and the collection and analysis of samples and administrative follow-up, in accordance with directions

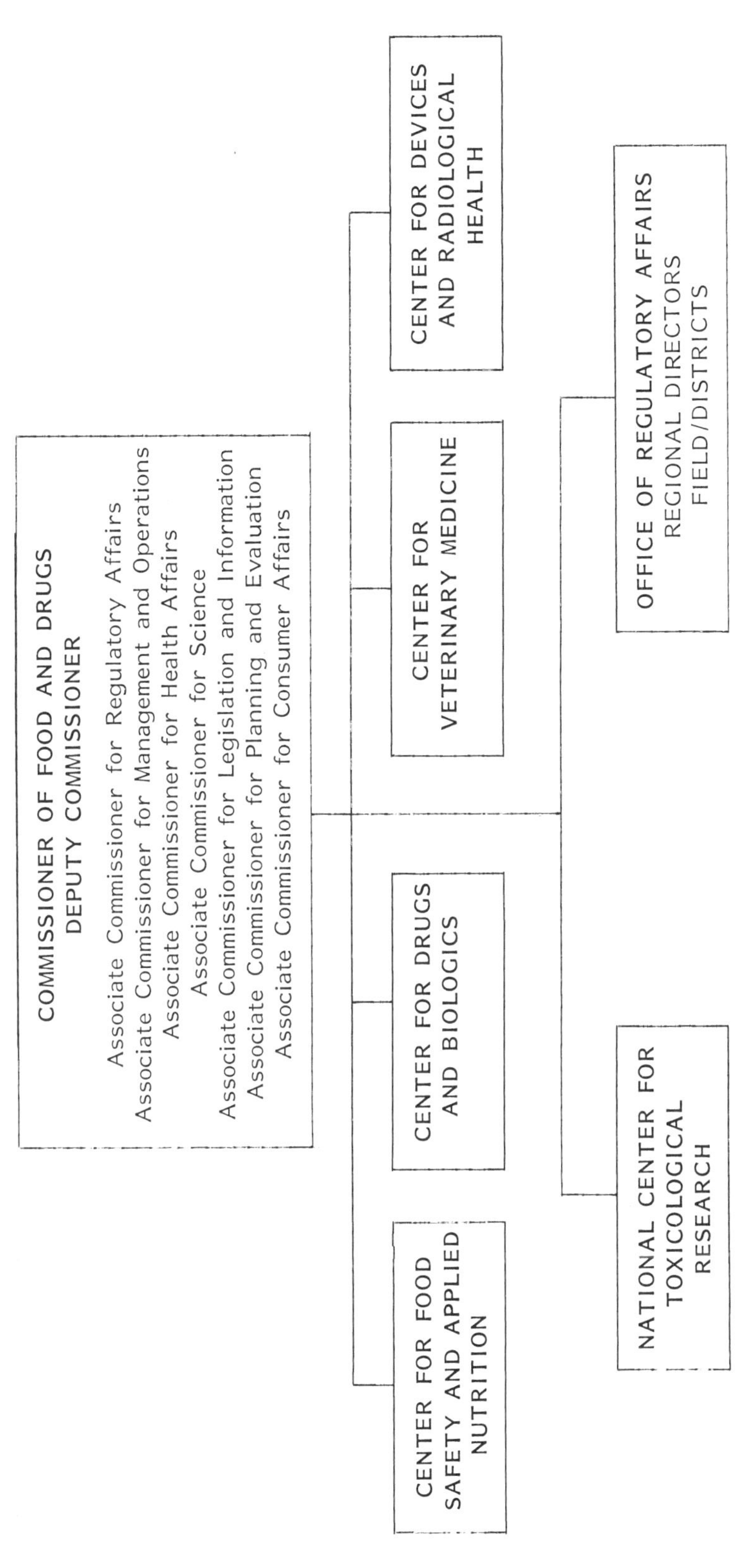

Figure 1 Organization and delegations, FDA 1260.1.

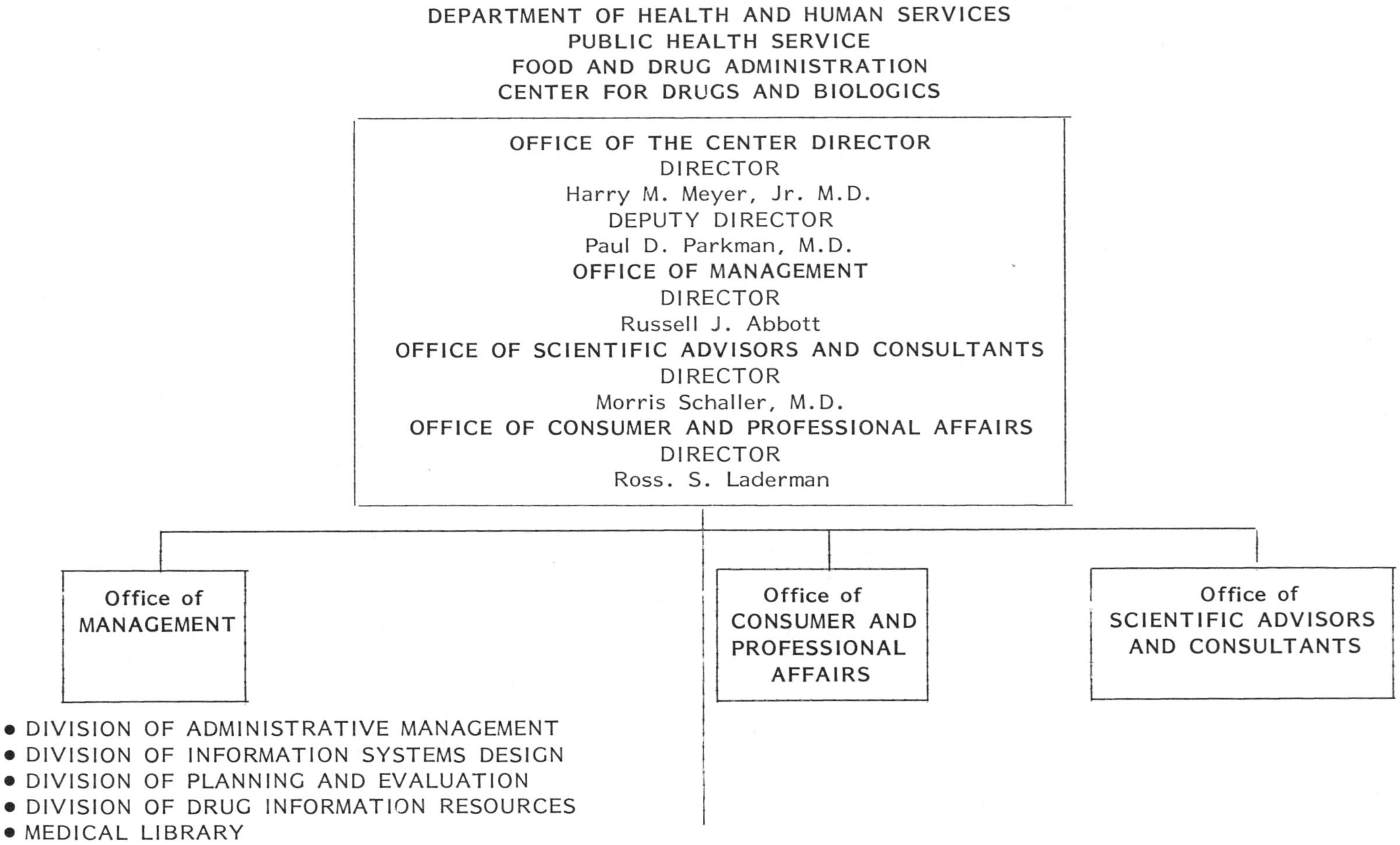

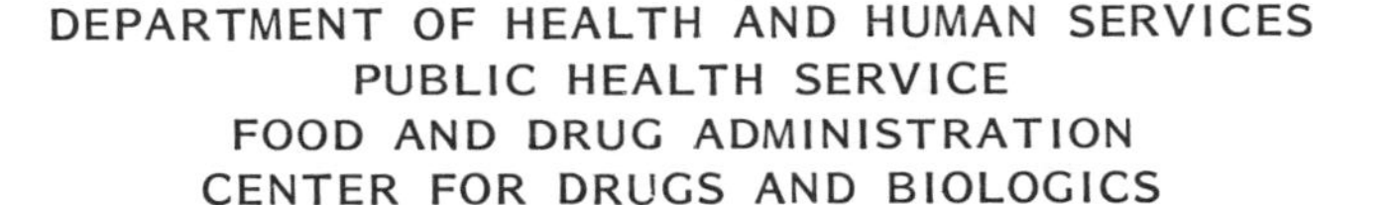
DEPARTMENT OF HEALTH AND HUMAN SERVICES
PUBLIC HEALTH SERVICE
FOOD AND DRUG ADMINISTRATION
CENTER FOR DRUGS AND BIOLOGICS
OFFICE OF THE CENTER DIRECTOR
DIRECTOR
Harry M. Meyer, Jr. M.D.
DEPUTY DIRECTOR
Paul D. Parkman, M.D.
OFFICE OF MANAGEMENT
DIRECTOR
Russell J. Abbott
OFFICE OF SCIENTIFIC ADVISORS AND CONSULTANTS
DIRECTOR
Morris Schaller, M.D.
OFFICE OF CONSUMER AND PROFESSIONAL AFFAIRS
DIRECTOR
Ross. S. Laderman
Office of MANAGEMENT
Office of CONSUMER AND PROFESSIONAL AFFAIRS
Office of SCIENTIFIC ADVISORS AND CONSULTANTS
• DIVISION OF ADMINISTRATIVE MANAGEMENT
• DIVISION OF INFORMATION SYSTEMS DESIGN
• DIVISION OF PLANNING AND EVALUATION
• DIVISION OF DRUG INFORMATION RESOURCES
• MEDICAL LIBRARY

(A)

Office of COMPLIANCE

- DIVISION OF DRUG LABELING COMPLIANCE
- DIVISION OF DRUG QUALITY EVALUATION
- DIVISION OF DRUG QUALITY COMPLIANCE
- DIVISION OF SCIENTIFIC INVESTIGATIONS
- DIVISION OF BIOLOGICAL PRODUCT COMPLIANCE
- DIVISION OF REGULATORY AFFAIRS

Office of DRUG RESEARCH AND REVIEW

- DIVISION OF CARDIO-RENAL DRUG PRODUCTS
- DIVISION OF NEUROPHARMACOLOGICAL DRUG PRODUCTS
- DIVISION OF ONCOLOGY AND RADIOPHARMACEUTICAL DRUG PRODUCTS
- DIVISION OF SURGICAL-DENTAL DRUG PRODUCTS
- DIVISION OF DRUG BIOLOGY
- DIVISION OF DRUG CHEMISTRY
- CENTER FOR DRUG ANALYSIS

Office of BIOLOGICS RESEARCH AND REVIEW

- DIVISION OF BIOCHEMISTRY AND BIOPHYSICS
- DIVISION OF BIOLOGICAL PRODUCT QUALITY CONTROL
- DIVISION OF BLOOD AND BLOOD PRODUCTS
- DIVISION OF VIROLOGY
- DIVISION OF BACTERIAL PRODUCTS
- DIVISION OF METABOLISM AND ENDOCRINE DRUG PRODUCTS
- DIVISION OF ANTI-INFECTIVE DRUG PRODUCTS
- DIVISION OF BIOLOGICAL PRODUCT CERTIFICATION
- DIVISION OF BIOLOGICAL INVESTIGATIONAL NEW DRUGS

Office of DRUG STANDARDS

- DIVISION OF OTC DRUG EVALUATION
- DIVISION OF GENERIC DRUGS
- DIVISION OF BIOPHARMACEUTICS
- DIVISION OF DRUG ADVERTISING AND LABELING

Office of EPIDEMIOLOGY AND BIOSTATISTICS

- DIVISION OF DRUG AND BIOLOGICAL PRODUCT EXPERIENCE
- DIVISION OF BIOMETRICS

(B)

Figure 2 (A) Office of the Center Director. (B) Offices and divisions—Center for Drugs and Biologics.

in compliance programs. Drug compliance programs are prepared by the Center for Drugs and Biologics, with input and concurrence of the staff of the Associate Commissioner for Regulatory Affairs. These programs represent the center's identification of program needs and priorities for a particular project, such as drug quality assurance. Of the 11 compliance programs under this project as of October 1983, all involved parenteral drugs to a greater or lesser degree. One current (1984) program concerned with small volume parenterals provides the field with guidelines on inspecting parenteral manufacturers and in recommending regulatory action when noncompliance is found. Programs change from year to year. An earlier program, on large volume parenterals, issued after publication of the proposed CGMP regulations for large volume parenterals, offered very specific guidance to the field, as well as to those in industry who obtained copies of the program. Although this program is no longer officially in effect and is not available, it contains some basic information of value in considering compliance for large volume parenteral operations. Thus, we have summarized this program below. Compliance programs provide FDA headquarters staff with information on the existence or extent of a problem and data on current industry practices. In addition to broad programs, such as on parenterals, others focus on specific problems, such as testing for endotoxins using the *Limulus* amebocyte lysate (LAL) test in USP XXI.

Upon completion, compliance programs may be evaluated. Several sampling and testing programs[22] for particulate matter in large volume parenterals were evaluated and it was shown that all samples were well within the limits in USP. Since current compliance programs are available,[23] they can be valuable as guides in setting up indistry self-inspection programs.

B. Large Volume Parenteral Compliance Program

1. *Background*

This section describes problems that led to the program. This included several massive recalls of large volume parenterals in 1971, leading to an FDA in-depth study of conditions and practices of the industry that affected their safety, particularly avenues of microbial contamination. This study led to an FDA-industry exchange on what the FDA considered important changes that were needed to assure current good manufacturing practice. These changes were subsequently incorporated in the proposed CGMP regulation for LVPs.

2. *Program*

Objective

The primary objective was to determine whether the practices of individual LVP manufacturers conform to CGMP. The program notes that the CGMP regulations are only proposals and hence should not be used as compliance criteria but to determine their feasibility if incorporated in final regulations. The program definition of LVP incorporated irrigating fluids.

Field Responsibilities

Inspectional. This program requires annual inspections of LVP manufacturers and that CGMP inspections be done only by qualified investigators, usually those who have completed a training course on parenterals.

When inspectional evidence indicates there may be an imminent hazard to health, special procedures to speed up corrective action, known as the "Alert system for hazard assessment—parenteral drugs" (ASHA), are to be followed.

3. Inspectional

In addition to the routine coverage under the CGMP drug regulations, investigators are to report in detail on specific aspects of LVP production under the following elements:

a. Raw materials
b. Manufacturing procedures
   1. Water-handling practices
   2. Controlled environment area: evaluation
   3. Sterilization procedures
   4. In-process sampling
   5. Pyrogens
   6. Particulate matter
   7. Packaging
   8. Finished product analytic testing
c. Sampling

4. Analytical

Part IV identifies the laboratories assigned to do specific tests, such as potency, sterility, particulate matter, pyrogen testing, and bioassays.

5. Regulatory/Administrative Follow-up

Part V includes guidelines to follow in recommending legal action based on adulteration or misbranding and sterility and potency for official and non-official drugs.

This introduces a new regulatory approach for LVPs, where an imminent hazard is indicated, namely, the ASHA. The procedures under ASHA are designed to speed up corrective action for CGMP deviations that are considered likely to result in an "imminent health" hazard. When immediate voluntary corrective action is not forthcoming, then the FDA is prepared to invoke legal sanctions, FDA-initiated recall, seizure, or injunction. In the absence of an "imminent hazard," a "regulatory letter" is the action of choice.

One problem with the ASHA is that the judgment about the existence of an imminent hazard may be subjective, and there is little recourse for the firm that believes such a hazard is not involved. Section 2.5 of 21 CFR defines "imminent hazard" and specifies that the declaration of imminent hazard can only be decided by the commissioner. ASHA does not address this regulation.

C. Inspections

All drug establishments are required to register annually with the FDA. Independent laboratories that engage in control activities for a registered establishment are considered extensions of the registered firm and must register themselves. The FDA is obligated to inspect each establishment at least once every 2 years. Inspections are conducted under the provisions of Section 704 of the Act. This section authorizes accredited FDA employees to enter drug establishments during business hours after furnishing the owner or operator with a notice of inspection. Inspections are unannounced, with a few exceptions. The statute requires that inspections be conducted in a reasonable manner and within reasonable limits. Manufacturers of prescription drugs are required to permit inspection of all things, including records, processes, and controls bearing on whether such drugs are adulterated or misbranded. However, inspectional authority does not include financial or sales data, personnel data (other than data as to qualifications of personnel under the CGMP and GLP regulations), and research data (other than that related to NDAs or other premarketing submissions). Refusal to permit inspection may cause the investigator to obtain a "warrant for inspection" from a U.S. District Court. Any further refusal after the warrant is served may result in a contempt of court action.

Inspections are the primary tool used by the FDA in gathering information on violations, as a basis for enforcement. There are many reasons for initiating inspections, in addition to those planned under specific compliance programs. FDA policy[24] requires the investigator to explain the purpose of the inspection if asked, except when such disclosure would thwart a pending investigation of fraud or similar activity.

At the completion of an inspection, if the investigator has noted what he or she believes to be violative conditions, an FDA form FD-483 will be left with the responsible official, listing all observations that in the investigator's judgment may lead to violations of the Act. Form FD-483 also serves as a basis for the prescribed discussion with management designed to give the official(s) an opportunity to indicate what if any corrective action they plan or, when they disagree with an observation, to explain the reasons for their disagreement. In addition to management's oral response to the observations listed in form FD-483, many firms have a policy of voluntarily responding in writing to form FD-483. They send their response to the district director as soon as possible after an inspection. The advantage of responding is that it provides the FDA official file with a written record in the firm's own words to complement the investigator's report. One advantage of a written response is that if the FDA district office considers the response adequate, it may ward off any regulatory follow-up. Since the firm's response may contain commitments for specific corrective actions, there is an obligation to carry them out, and in timely fashion. The FDA usually schedules a reinspection to check on the status of promised corrective actions.

D. Enforcement Policies and Procedures

FDA enforcement policies and procedures have changed slowly over the past years. Prior to 1965, formal legal actions—seizures, prosecutions, and injunctions—were the only enforcement tools used in achieving compliance. With the establishment of a Bureau of Voluntary Compliance in 1965 as a result of a recommendation of a Citizens Committee Report, the FDA slowly adopted some new enforcement approaches. Thus, in 1968, the agency instituted a procedure of supplying drug firms with written reports of inspectional observations even though there was no such statutory requirement that they do so.

Beginning in 1972, the FDA, upon advice of its general counsel, initiated two types of warning letters—regulatory letters, and information letters or notice of adverse findings, which notified top officials of drug firms of any potential or actual violations observed during the course of an inspection. "Regulatory letters" are so titled conspicuously, and are sent by certified mail to the top official(s) of a company. These letters cite specific sections of the Act or two other health statutes enforced by FDA and give brief descriptions of the violation. They usually issue from the office of the director in the district in which the establishment is located. Before such a letter is issued it must have the approval of compliance officials of the centers. The letter states in effect that the FDA is prepared to apply legal sanctions or administrative action unless the violative conditions are promptly corrected. A response must be made by the firm within 10 days of receipt of the letter, specifying the steps taken to ensure that the violations have been or will be corrected. If the firm's response is deemed inadequate, the district office is committed to initiate legal or administrative action. If the response appears adequate, the district office will promptly initiate a reinspection or other check to verify that the commitments have been fulfilled. The nature of some "administrative actions" are described in regulatory letters where appropriate as follows:

> No pending NDA's, ANDA's or requests for procurement by government agencies will be approved until adequate corrective action has been taken with respect to the above violations.

Regulatory letters are public information and are on display at the FDA's FOI office at headquarters. Such threatened administrative actions are powerful stimuli for immediate corrective action.

A "notice of adverse findings" letter is a warning letter sent following an inspection where violations are noted but their nature does not require immediate corrective action by the firm. A response time of 30 days usually is granted. Normally follow-up by the FDA is by reinspection to verify what if any corrective action has been taken.

The FDA has described its policy on regulatory letters and other types of compliance correspondence in its *Regulatory Procedures Manual.*[25] The FDA states that corrective action as a result of a regulatory letter does not preclude initiating legal action where the circumstances warrant. The agency has acknowledged that voluntary corrective actions very often benefit the consumer more than formal legal actions by accomplishing correction quickly, with less expenditure of FDA resources and with no burden on the federal courts. In its annual reports,[26] the FDA always includes statistics on the number of seizures, prosecutions, and injunctions of foods, drugs, cosmetics, and devices. Only since 1978 has it included statistics on regulatory letters in its annual reports. Of all the programs, the human drug program contained the largest number of regulatory letters.

V. VOLUNTARY COMPLIANCE

A. Industry FDA Cooperation

Efforts to promote voluntary compliance, begun in 1965 by the then Bureau of Voluntary Compliance, emphasized planned FDA-industry workshops and conferences to explain new complex regulations, such as the drug CGMP regulations, and to reduce the number of drug recalls by improving industry understanding of CGMP. Although parenterals were covered in these general workshops, a survey by the FDA of hospital stocks of large volume parenterals in 1964–1965 revealed a significant number of defective containers. This stimulated the FDA to hold a symposium in 1966 devoted exclusively to the safety of large volume parenterals. Because problems associated with parenterals involved not only their manufacture, but storage, handling, and use, experts from the fields of medicine, hospital pharmacy, nursing, military procurement, the FDA, and the USP were invited to participate. The proceedings of this symposium[27] contained research papers and recommendations that set the stage for FDA sponsorship in 1971, under a contract with the USP, of the formation of the National Coordinating Committee on Large Volume Parenterals (NCCLVP). Several large-scale recalls of parenterals in 1971 with reports of deaths and injuries associated with microbial contamination of two manufacturers' solutions hastened the organization of the NCCLVP.

Ten professional organizations representing medicine, pharmacy, nursing, hospitals, scientists in parenteral production and control, the FDA, the Centers for Disease Control (CDC), the USP, and the four major LVP manufacturers constituted this committee. This committee, considering its varied constituencies, accomplished many of its objectives in tackling many problems associated with parenterals. The final report of 11/30/79[28] at the conclusion of the contract, lists 21 accomplishments, such as the adoption by the USP of a test method and a standard limiting particulate matter; development of guidelines for selection, processing, and use of containers and closures for both manufacturers and hospitals; development and recommendation to hospitals of a system for surveillance and reporting of problems with LVPs; and recommendations for labeling of LVPs from the user's standpoint.

The contributions of voluntary corrective actions by industry in achieving compliance may be underestimated by the FDA because the agency has not included until recently any statistics on such actions in its compliance statistics. Undoubtedly, a majority of the drug firms receiving an FD-483 following an inspection have voluntarily corrected the deficiencies; otherwise there would be many more regulatory letters issued than are listed in the annual reports. However, until 1979, the FDA did not acknowledge a firm's voluntary corrective action response to an FD-483. An EDRO directive to its field offices issued in 1979 required districts to reply to all correspondence from firms regarding an FD-483.[29] In 1981, the FDA began a voluntary corrective action reporting system to recognize industry's efforts in raising the level of compliance.

B. Freedom of Information

Several references have been made in this text on the availability of various types of information in FDA files, such as summary basis of approval of

NDAs; establishment inspection reports (EIR); and compliance programs. These became generally available with the passage of the 1974 Amendments to the Freedom of Information Act (FOIA) and publication of FDA's implementing regulations in the FR 12/24/74 (pp. 44604–44657). This document contains an extensive preamble explaining and justifying the liberal approach of the FDA in opening up most of its files to the public. The final regulations are now codified in part 20 of 21 CFR. The Freedom of Information Act contains nine categories of information that are exempted, such as national security documents; trade secrets; other statutes that require certain documents to be held in confidence; and others. Usually only four categories are applicable to FDA documents, namely, IND, NDA, PMA, (premarket submissions requiring FDA approval); trade secrets and commercial (financial) information; personnel and medical files, and investigatory files compiled for law enforcement purposes.

Examples of information available on parenterals include the "Summary basis of approval" of NDA's for specific parenterals; results of FDA surveys of particulate matter in small and large volume parenterals; and compliance programs and establishment inspections reports (EIR) of facilities of registered manufacturers. Some of the above items are available from the National Technical Information Service (NTIS) on a subscription basis, whereas others are only available from the FDA FOI staff. A description of the various types of technical and compliance information available with sources and costs will be found in a recent journal article.[31]

Requests for information from the FDA FOI staff should preferably be limited to a single topic and be as specific as possible. The FDA is required to respond to requests within 10 working days of receipt by either furnishing the document or advising the requestor by a "letter of determination" whether it will be furnished. The FDA maintains a public log of all requests, which lists the name of the requestor and the information requested. If the FDA denies a request, the requestor may appeal to the Assistant Secretary for Health, and if this appeal is denied, the requestor may institute a suit in a U.S. District Court. Charges for documents are based on copying costs, postage, and, in some cases, search time. Current fee schedules will be found in Section 20.42 of 21 CFR. There is a provision for waiver of fees under certain circumstances as set forth in Section 20.43.

C. Drug Product Problem Reporting

The FDA initiated a voluntary surveillance program in 1971 on the quality of marketed drugs in cooperation with the American Society of Hospital Pharmacists (ASHP) and the United States Pharmacopeial Convention (USP). The drug product problem reporting (DPPR) system, was based on the concept that the expertise of hospital pharmacists and their concern over the quality of drugs could be used to report voluntarily apparent and actual defects and other problems with the drugs they dispense. Thus, this program would supplement the FDA drug surveillance program[32] in which samples of selected marketed drugs are collected and analyzed. The excellent cooperation and results from hospital pharmacists led the FDA to expand the program to include other health professionals through their professional organizations. The DPPR now includes not only hospital pharmacists but community pharmacists, nurses, dentists, and physicians. Participation in the DPPR system became a requirement in 1978 for hospitals under the standards of the Joint Commission for Accreditation of Hospitals.

The USP operates the DPPR system under a contract with the FDA. It furnishes reporting forms to health professionals. All DPPR reports are then distributed to the manufacturer or distributor of the drug involved and to the FDA. A brochure describing USP procedures and how health professionals can become involved is available from the USP.[33]

The growth in the annual volume of DPPR reports has been impressive, from 2000 in 1972 to 5631 in 1982. As of 1982, the number of reports by participating groups were as follows: hospital pharmacists, 3082 or 55%; community pharmacists, 1850 or 33%; and other health professionals, 699 or 12%.

A significant percentage of the reports emanates from hospital pharmacists, since the inception of the program deals with small and large volume parenterals and prefilled cartridges or syringes. For example, in 1982, of the 3082 reports from hospital pharmacists, 56% dealt with these parenterals. Shroff,[34] commenting on these figures, points out that the nature of the hospital pharmacy work would tend to encourage reporting problems with parenterals routinely. The large volume of historical data from reports on parenterals has enabled the FDA Product Surveillance Branch to prepare a quality trend report on these products.[35] The DPPR system supplements drug manufacturers' quality assurance programs by calling to their attention actual or potential defects that may have escaped their quality control. Thus most drug manufacturers, upon receipt of a DPPR, will initiate a prompt investigation. If the investigation discloses that the reported defect causes the product to be in violation of the FD&C Act, most manufacturers will initiate a voluntary recall of the particular lot and will also check to see if any associated lots may be involved. Also it gives manufacturers the opportunity to close any gaps in their manufacturing or quality control operations to prevent a recurrence of the violation. Frequently, when the investigation reveals no violation, it may suggest needed improvements in product packaging or other product characteristics. Undoubtedly, voluntary corrective actions are stimulated by the knowledge that the FDA is aware of the DPPR and may follow up by sending an investigator to check on the firm's action on most reports. But then voluntary compliance is posited on the existence of its alternative, regulatory compliance.

D. Recalls

1. *FDA Recall Guidelines*

FDA recall policy is contained in two documents. The first is Part 7 of Title 21, Code of Federal Regulations.[36] The second is Part 5 of Chapter 5-00 of the FDA *Regulatory Procedures Manual*.[37] Those sections of Part 7 of Title 21 concerned with recalls are intended to provide guidelines for manufacturers and distributors to follow with respect to their voluntary removal from the market, or correction of marketed products that are violative of the laws that the FDA administers. The recall guidelines are intended to explain the regulatory practices and procedures of the FDA, enhance public understanding, improve consumer protection, and assure uniform and consistent application of practices and procedures throughout the FDA itself. Part 5 of Chapter 5-00 of the FDA *Regulatory Procedures Manual* is directed to the FDA itself.

To better understand FDA recall policy and procedures, one should be aware that FDA thinking and practices with respect to recalls have been in a continuous state of evolution. The policy and procedures have been improved upon as the agency gained experience, usually by mistakes, with the recall process. For a history of the development of FDA recall policy, the reader is referred to the *Federal Register* of June 30, 1976, in which the FDA proposed regulations describing the policies and procedures the FDA follows, and that regulated firms should follow, in the conduct of product recalls.[38] The proposed regulations were finalized as (what the FDA called) regulations intended as guidelines in a *Federal Register* announcement of June 16, 1978.[39] It is these "regulations intended as guidelines" that are found in Part 7 of Title 21, Code of Federal Regulations.

Pharmaceutical manufacturers had been recalling portions of their products from the market for as long as there had been an industry, and for many reasons, some involving serious problems and some involving little more than pharmaceutical elegance. The FDA had also for many years been requesting firms to initiate recalls because recall was a more effective and more efficient means of removing objectionable products from the market. But, it was not until the 1960s that the FDA developed any kind of coordinated recall program, and not until 1971 that the agency published for the first time a formal statement concerning recalls. The reason for the long and tortuous path to formulating a recall policy was that the FDA had no legal authority under the FD&C Act to direct any firm to recall any product from the market. With the exception of certain limited recall authority with respect to medical devices, which was written into the Act in the Device Amendments of 1976, the FDA still, as of this writing, has no legal authority to order recalls.

The only enforceable legal tool the FDA has to remove violative products from the market (with the sole exception of medical devices discussed above) is the formal seizure process initiated through the U.S. District Courts. Frequently, when the FDA initiates injunction actions alleging violations of the FD&C Act, the FDA will ask a U.S. District Court to order a recall of violative products from the market; in doing so, the FDA relies on the court's equity powers, not on any authority contained in the FD&C Act. Often, the courts have acquiesced to such requests and ordered the recalls, but sometimes the courts have refused.

The FDA acknowledges it does not have recall power (except with regard to devices), but it insists it has the right to promulgate regulations telling how recalls should be conducted and monitored. The agency has chosen to label its recall regulations as guidelines, however, and this necessarily means that the firms involved are legally free to not follow them. When a recalling firm does not follow FDA guidelines, the agency can always initiate voluntary recalls at lower levels of distribution, and it can also initiate seizures.

FDA policy defines a recall as a firm's removal or correction of a marketed product that the FDA considers to be in violation of the laws it administers and against which the agency would initiate legal action (e.g., seizure). Under the policy, recall does not include a "market withdrawal" or a "stock recovery." A "correction" means a repair, modification, adjustment, relabeling, destruction, or inspection (including patient monitoring) of a product without its physical removal to some other location.

A market withdrawal is defined by the FDA as a firm's removal or correction of a distributed product, which involves a minor violation that would not be subject to legal action under existing FDA policies, or which involves no violation at all (e.g., normal stock rotation practices). A stock recovery is defined by the FDA as a firm's removal or correction of a product that has not been marketed, or that has not left the direct control of the firm (e.g., the product is located on premises owned by, or under the control of, the firm and no portion of the lot being recovered has been released for sale or use).

Under FDA guidelines, a "recalling firm" is the firm that initiates a recall. In the case of an FDA-requested recall, the firm that has the primary responsibility for the manufacture and marketing of the product to be recalled is the recalling firm. A "firm-initiated recall" is a recall initiated by a firm on its own volition, without a formal request from the FDA. An FDA-initiated recall is a recall initiated by a firm in response to a formal request for such action by the FDA. From a legal point of view, recalls (except of devices) are all voluntary. As a matter of fact, many firm-initiated recalls and all FDA-initiated recalls result from prodding by the FDA.

The guidelines direct that for every recall there be a "recall strategy," which is a planned specific course of action to be taken in conducting a specific recall, and which addresses the depth of the recall, the need for public warnings, and the extent of effectiveness checks planned for the recall. A recall strategy must take into account the following factors: (a) results of health hazard evaluation; (b) ease in identifying the product; (c) degree to which the product's deficiency is obvious to the consumer or user; (d) degree to which the product remains unused in the marketplace; and (e) continued availability of essential products.

When the FDA learns of a recall that has been initiated by a firm or when the FDA is the initiator of the recall, the agency assigns a "recall classification" to the recall. There are three classes. Class I is a situation in which there is a reasonable probability that the use of, or exposure to, a violative product will cause serious adverse health consequences or death. Class II is a situation in which use of, or exposure to, a violative product may cause temporary or medically reversible adverse health consequences or where the probability of serious adverse health consequences is remote. Class III is a situation in which use of, or exposure to, a violative product is not likely to cause adverse health consequences.

The depth of the recall will depend upon the product's degree of hazard and extent of distribution. FDA guidelines say that the recall strategy will specify the level in the distribution chain to which the recall is to extend, as follows.

Consumer or user level. Including any intermediate wholesale or retail level. The consumer or user may include the individual consumer or patient, the physician, or a hospital.

Retail level. Recall to the level immediately preceding the consumer or user level. It includes pharmacies, hospital pharmacies, dispensing physicians, institutions, such as clinics and nursing homes, and any intermediate levels.

Wholesale level. All distribution levels between the manufacturer and the retailers. This level may not be encountered in every recall situation (e.g., the manufacturer may sell directly to the retailer).

FDA guidelines state that the recall strategy should consider whether there is need of the issuance of a public warning. The purpose of a public warning is to alert the public that a product being recalled presents a serious hazard to health. It is reserved for urgent situations. When a recalling firm decides to issue its own public warning, the FDA requests that the firm submit its content and proposed distribution to the agency for review and comment. FDA public warnings are issued in consultation with the recalling firm. Public warnings may issue through the general news media. They may be national or local, as appropriate. Or, they may issue through specialized news media, such as professional or trade press or specific segments of the population, such as physicians and hospitals. The FDA has learned through experience that there must be a degree of fluidity in determining who, if anyone, should receive a public warning, lest more harm be done than good.

Regardless of whether there is a public warning, the FDA publicizes all recalls in its weekly FDA Enforcement Report,[40] including firm-initiated recalls. Sometimes, when in its judgment the FDA decides that publicity may cause unnecessary and harmful anxiety to patients when initial consultation between patients and their physicians is essential, the FDA may intentionally delay publication of some recalls.

FDA guidelines request the recalling firm to submit periodic reports to the appropriate FDA district office. The frequency of such reports is determined by the urgency of the recall and is specified by the FDA in each recall case. Generally, the reporting interval is between 2 and 4 weeks until the recall is terminated.

Effectiveness checks are an important part of the recall strategy. The purpose of effectiveness checks is to verify that all consignees at the recall depth specified by the recall strategy have received notification about the recall and have taken appropriate action. Consignees may be contacted by personal visits, telephone calls, and/or letters. There is available from the FDA a guide document entitled "Methods for conducting recall effectiveness checks"[41] that describes the use of these different methods. The guidelines place the responsibility for conducting effectiveness checks on the recalling firm but state that the FDA will assist in the task when necessary and appropriate. The guidelines provide five levels of effectiveness checks. Level A is 100% of the total number of consignees to be contacted. Level C is 10%. Level B is some percentage of the total number of consignees to be contacted, to be determined on a case-by-case basis, but greater than 10% and less than 100%. Level D is 2% effectiveness checks. Level E requires no effectiveness checks.

FDA recall guidelines suggest that all firms prepare and maintain a current written contingency plan for use in initiating and effecting a recall, that they use sufficient coding of regulated products (other than what is otherwise required by other regulations) to make possible positive lot identification and to facilitate effective recall of all violative lots, and that they maintain such product distribution records as are necessary to facilitate location of products that are to be recalled. The guidelines suggest that such records should be maintained for a period of time that exceeds the shelf life and expected use of the product and is at least the length of time specified in other applicable regulations concerning records retention.

Finally, the guidelines provide for FDA audits of recalls. Such audits may or may not be aided by state and local officials. The level of FDA audit checks shall be in accordance with the effectiveness checks level discussed above. The FDA considers a recall terminated when all reasonable efforts have been made to remove or correct the violative product in accordance with the recall strategy and proper disposition has been made according to the degree of hazard. For monitoring purposes, the FDA classifies a recall action "completed" at the point at which the firm has actually retrieved and impounded all outstanding product that could reasonably be expected to be recovered or has completed all product corrections.

2. Recall of Parenterals

There are many reasons an injectable product might be recalled. Like other drug products, injectables sometimes have label mix-ups, and sometimes batch numbers and expiration dates do not appear clearly on the labels. This is a particularly troublesome problem with ampuls when label information is printed directly on the glass. There may be problems with the closure system, low volume of contents, or even leaking of some vials or ampuls. There may have been complaints of pharmacological inactivity of the drug in patients. Laboratory testing subsequent to a manufacturer's release of the batch may disclose that the product does not comply with one or more of its specifications. Postmarketing experience may demonstrate that a tentatively established expiration date was too long; the product is breaking down. These are problems associated with all kinds of drug products.

There are other problems associated with injectable drugs that are not ordinarily associated with other dosage forms. These are the problems of sterility and pyrogenicity, and these problems have resulted in hundreds of recalls involving literally millions of doses since the latter part of 1969, during and after which time both the FDA and the industry advanced tremendously in their knowledge of how to achieve sterility during the manufacture of injectable drugs.

Between July 1, 1965, and November 10, 1975, there were recalls of 608 large volume parenteral products involving over 43 million individual containers that had been distributed to the market. Between January 1, 1970, and November 10, 1975, there were 17 recalls of biological LVP products. Most of these recalls were due to microbiological contamination or suspected microbiological contamination associated, in most cases, with manufacturing problems. At the request of U.S. Senator Gaylord Nelson, the Comptroller General of the United States through its General Accounting Office (GAO) conducted an investigation of these circumstances. The GAO report of that investigation is contained in a comprehensive report to Senator Nelson dated March 12, 1976, entitled "Recalls of large volume parenterals (Liquid drugs administered intravenously or by other non-oral means)"[42].

The incidents that led to those recalls involved injury and death associated with manufacturing problems in the LVP industry. The intensive investigations conducted at the time by the Food and Drug Administration and the Centers for Disease Control—as well as by the industry—resulted in greatly increased knowledge of potential problems in the manufacture of LVPs that might cause the products to lack the assurance that they were sterile and nonpyrogenic. This knowledge resulted in a closer liaison between the FDA and the CDC and in far more intensive inspectional regulation of the entire injectable drugs industry than ever before. This extended regulatory coverage, in turn, resulted in permanent shutdowns of some manufacturing plants, temporary shutdowns of others, technological updating and improvements in all injectable-manufacturing plants, and product recalls and destructions in the range of many millions of dollars.

The FDA had promised Senator Nelson that it would develop separate current good manufacturing practice regulations to cover large volume parenterals because it believed that the general CGMP regulations then in effect for drug products (actually, at the time the term "drug products" was not yet in use; the regulations used the undefined term "finished pharmaceuticals"). The FDA also told the industry at the time that the development and promulgation of separate regulations to cover small volume parenterals would also be given high priority. The FDA did develop and did publish in the *Federal Register* of June 1, 1976, proposed current good manufacturing practice regulations for LVPs, and those proposed regulations played a large part in the updating of not only the LVP industry but also the SVP industry as well. Curiously, as of this writing, the LVP regulations have not yet been published as final enforceable regulations (although they may yet be) and the plans to publish separate CGMP regulations for SVPs have been abandoned. This does not represent any diminution of FDA regulatory efforts with respect to injectable drugs but rather a reaction to a political trend that, except when absolutely necessary, government agencies issue "guidelines" rather than regulations. The FDA has given the industry much guidance through its sponsorship of and participation in industry and academia symposia and conventions and through the presentation of many speeches and the publication of many papers on the subject.

In initiating recalls of injectable drug products, the FDA has often been in the position where it had to carefully weigh whether the recall might cause more harm than good. If the product being considered for recall is a lifesaving drug and there is only one manufacturer, or there is more than one manufacturer but the lots being considered for recall consist of the bulk of what is available in the market, then a careful benefit-versus-risk decision must be made. To that end, the Center for Drugs and Biologics works closely with the Associate Commissioner for Health Affairs in weighing all the facts. Sometimes, drug products that had been recalled because of a lack of assurance of sterility have been released by the FDA for emergency use in surgery. Sometimes, recalls of batches of injectable drugs have been postponed pending the availability of replacement stocks. Ordinarily—and almost always—when injectable drug products have been recalled because inspectional evidence indicates a lack of assurance of sterility, those recalled injectable drugs have been destroyed.

Wherever, in the recall of injectable drugs, there is evidence of nonsterility or pyrogenicity, or if there is evidence of lack of assurance of sterility, the FDA has always classified the recalls in class I or class II.

VI. JUDICIAL REVIEW

A. Impact of Court Review

Whereas the meaning of a law often seems obvious to the casual reader, it is not until the courts have ruled on its meaning that the law can be regarded as "settled." The interpretations put upon laws by the courts are sometimes radically different from what people thought the laws meant when the Congress passed them in the first place. So it has been with the Federal Food, Drug, and Cosmetic Act. Although it would be far beyond the scope of this chapter to explain in detail how case law develops, some discussion is necessary so that the person who manufactures, tests, or dispenses injectable drug products may have a general understanding of how case law develops and of its significance.

Article III of the Constitution of the United States provides that the judicial power of the United States shall be vested in a Supreme Court and in such inferior courts as the Congress may from time to time establish. It provides that the judicial power shall extend to all court cases, in law and equity, arising under the constitution and the laws of the United States, and to controversies to which the United States is a party. It says the Supreme Court shall have appellate jurisdiction, both as to law and fact, with such exceptions and under such regulations as the Congress shall make.

All litigation under the FD&C Act is initiated in the name of the United States. Thus, a criminal indictment or information, or a complaint for injunction, might be entitled: "United States of America vs ABC Injectables Corporation." A complaint for forfeiture (seizure) might be entitled: "United States of America vs 66 Cases of ABC Injectables."

The Congress has established circuit courts of appeals and U.S. District Courts. There is at least one U.S. District Court in every state. Appeals from the decisions of the district courts are taken to the circuit courts of appeals in their respective circuits. The decisions of the circuit courts of appeals are binding in the courts within their own respective circuits, and they may be considered persuasive in other circuits, but they are not binding in other circuits. This sometimes causes situations of inequity wherein one circuit court will rule one way on an issue and another circuit (or a district court within another circuit) will rule another way. Then, if the law is to be settled, the matter must be brought before the Supreme Court.

Most FD&C Act cases that find their way to the Supreme Court reach it through a legal process called "certiorari," wherein a petitioner asks the Supreme Court to issue a writ of certiorari to one or more lower courts ordering that the records of the case be forwarded to the Supreme Court for review. Decisions of the Supreme Court settle the points of law or fact in question (unless, of course, the Congress changes the law).

With some exceptions, cases filed under the FD&C Act are filed in the U.S. District Courts. Venue (i.e., the particular U.S. District Court in which a case shall be filed) is generally determined by the geographical location where the alleged violations took place. Under some circumstances, venue can be changed.

Some of the provisions of the FD&C Act were regarded by some, from the beginning, as being vague and indefinite, and even unconstitutional. Many of those issues were settled early in the life of the Act. As time goes on, though, other parts continue to be interpreted in different ways, and the amendments to the Act have required judicial interpretation. So, the court opinions seem to be unending. It has been necessary, for example, that the courts settle what is meant by terms used in the Act (even though the terms might be defined in the Act itself). Thus, court opinions have settled what is meant in the Act by such generally used terms as "interstate commerce," "drug," "new drug," "prescription drug," and "over-the-counter drug."

Although an in-depth discussion of the case law under the Act would be beyond the scope of this chapter, some comments on the most important cases should be helpful. For those wishing to explore case law further, there is extensive literature. The Food and Drug Law Institute sponsors the publication of a series of texts on the Act itself and on cases under the Act.[43,44]

Section 301 of the Act cites the acts that are prohibited. The opening clause of Section 301 states that those acts, *and the causing thereof* are prohibited. Many cases have upheld the concept that one who causes a violation is just as much a principal in the crime as the perpetrator. Another section of federal law (18 U.S.C. 2) states that whoever commits an offense against the United States or aids, abets, counsels, commands, induces, or procures its commission is punishable as a principal. The lead case in this area is the Dotterweich case,[45] a drug case. The legal principles were affirmed, and even made clearer, in the Park case,[46] a food case, but equally applicable to drugs, in 1975. Dotterweich was on a fishing trip when his violation took place. Park had delegated to a subordinate the responsibility to correct a filth problem. Each was president of his company, but it was not specifically because of his corporate title that either man was convicted. In each case, the Supreme Court held that the defendant had stood in a responsible relation to the violation and was in a position to have prevented it, whereas the consumer could not.

It is important to people who are concerned with the manufacture, including testing and holding, of injectable drug products to understand that anyone who stands in a responsible position from which, for example, the sterility of injectable drug products might be assured and does not do so, can be held criminally responsible for any violation of the Act that might ensue. This is an awesome position for anyone to be in, but it is part of the role of those who produce drugs for the American people.

B. Specific Cases Affecting Parenterals

One case that involved a number of issues, and that (though it did not involve injectable drug products) explored at some length the concepts of sterility and sampling and testing for sterility, deserves particular mention here. It is a 1978 decision of the U.S. District Court for the Northern District of New York, U.S. vs Morton-Norwich Products, Inc.[47] The product involved was individually packaged gauze pads impregnated with nitrofurazone, an antibacterial dressing. Each count in the indictment alleged adulteration in two separate and distinct senses: one was violation of Section 501(c) of the Act in that the purity involved differed from that purported (the samples examined by FDA were found to be nonsterile), and the other alleged violations of Section 501(a)(2)(B), the current good manufacturing practice section, in which the government contended that the drugs were not manufactured, processed, packaged, or held in conformity with CGMP to assure that they would conform to the Act's requirements as to safety, and would have the strength and identity and meet the quality and purity characteristics they purported to possess. The court did not base its decision at all on the CGMP evidence presented by the government. We will here not treat of the CGMP issues, but will confine our comments to what the court had to say about sterility and sterility testing, concepts that are eminently important in the injectable drugs field.

The FDA analysts had not used the official *U.S. Pharmacopeia* method for sterility testing. The court held it was not necessary to do so. The products involved were not articles that were the subject of an official USP monograph. Had they been USP drugs, the charges based on the results of finished product examination would have been brought under Section 501(b) of the Act, which says that a drug is deemed to be adulterated if it purports to be or is represented as a drug, the name of which is recognized in an official compendium, and its strength differs from, or its quality or purity falls below, the standards set forth in the compendium, and the FDA would have been required to use the USP sterility test as its referee test in order to prove its case in court.

Persons concerned with the manufacture of injectable drugs should be aware that USP or NF tests and assays are never specifically required to be used by anyone except by the FDA when it analyzes samples of "official drugs" (i.e., drugs that are the subject of a compendial monograph) for law enforcement purposes, or by persons who because of contractual requirements must use tests specified in the contracts.

If one is manufacturing a USP or NF drug product, that product must conform to all the requirements of the monograph that governs it. Whatever tests and assays are performed must therefore be validated to prove that they are as good as, or better than, the official monograph tests and assays. If the product is a new drug, the FDA will insist on auditing the validation data during the new drug application review process, or if the test methodology is developed subsequent to FDA approval of the new drug application, the firm involved is required to submit the data to the FDA. The same is true with regard to certifiable drugs. Whether the product is a new drug or a certifiable drug, the validation data are always subject to FDA audit during its regular inspections of the manufacturer.

Another important finding of the court in this case was that sterility is an absolute concept. The court cited the standard of absolute liability established in both the Dotterweich and Park Supreme Court cases. In a footnote, the court indicated that the courts have somewhat ameliorated the hardships resulting from such a literal application of the Act by utilizing a *de minimis* doctrine to forgive minor, technical violations shown to be unavoidable even through the use of good manufacturing practice. The FDA has, in the food area, established certain "tolerances," for example, for mold in certain foods or for rat pellets in bulk wheat. But in this case, the court said it could not regard the contamination found (nonsterility) as *de minimis*. Clearly, no tolerances can be established permitting a certain number of units in a lot of injectable drugs to be nonsterile. On the other hand, there seems to remain a disparity between what can be demonstrated as scientifically probable and what this case says is legally necessary.

The defendants, according to the court's opinion, had taken the position that sterility is not an absolute concept, rather that it depends upon the results of probabilistic testing performed upon random samples of the product in accordance with USP testing methods. Thus, an article would be properly labeled "sterile" if it had passed preshipment sterility tests performed pursuant to the USP method, notwithstanding that some untested product units were in fact contaminated. The court did not agree.

The importance of the court's finding to persons involved in the manufacturing and testing of injectable drug products is immense. The court, knowing that an absolute cannot be measured, insisted that the absolute situation must prevail. Every single unit in every single manufacturing batch is required by the Act to be sterile if the product purports to be sterile or is represented in its labeling to be sterile. The law remains to be settled on this issue of fact. The Morton-Norwich case is binding only in the Northern District of New York.

In this case, the court rejected the defense's argument that the government had examined its samples after they had been in interstate commerce, whereas the indictment had alleged a violation of Section 501(c), nonsterility, when the products were shipped (introduced) into interstate commerce. Had there been evidence that something adverse might have happened to the packages while they were in interstate commerce (e.g., leaks or tears), or had the FDA failed to concomitantly test negative controls along with their test samples, the court might have rejected the government's findings. But the packages were intact, and the government's analyses did include controls.

With regard to the government's having not used official USP test methodology, the court cited a 1952 case, Woodard Laboratories, Inc., vs United States.[48] In Woodard, a court of appeals decision, the drug product involved had been admitted to the USP, but it was admitted after the date of the alleged violation and prior to the date the government filed its case with the court. In Woodard, the court found that the government was not required to use the official USP methodology because at the time of the alleged adulteration the USP test was not yet official.

The case law in the area of particulate matter in and clarity of solutions is also far from settled. Indeed, the state of the art is still far from where the FDA and the industry would like it to be. The USP, in its chapter on general tests and assays, says with regard to products intended for injection that every container whose contents show evidence of contamination with visible foreign material shall be rejected. The FDA, in its CGMP enforcement activities, also uses this "no visible particulate matter" requirement as its own standard for injectable solutions. Beyond this requirement, there are no other USP or FDA requirements with regard to particulate matter in small volume parenterals. There are USP particulate matter tests for large and small volume parenterals, which are discussed elsewhere in this text.

In his 1966 paper, The History of the Clarity Test,[49] Miller of the USP discussed the scientific and regulatory problems associated with particulate testing. His paper contains an account of a U.S. District Court seizure case, the Bristol Laboratories case, tried in 1949 at Syracuse, New York. The FDA witness who had examined the samples for the government and upon whose adverse findings the case was based was required to examine a number of test ampuls in court. When the code was broken, it was revealed that he had "passed" (in his court examination) as acceptable 36 of 38 ampuls from the government's own samples. Bristol promptly motioned for dismissal on the grounds that the USP test was arbitrary and unreliable. The court granted the motion.

The USP test that the court rejected was (and necessarily so, given the state of the art) subjective. It involved a visual examination against both a white and a black background. The general chapter on injections (USP XII, p. 666) said that medicaments intended for parenteral administration must be substantially free of any turbidity or undissolved material that can be detected readily. Miller said that the outcome of the case confirmed what was generally conceded by those familiar with the test, namely, that it was too subjective to be used as the basis for legal enforcement of a statute such as the Federal Food, Drug and Cosmetic Act.

There have been a number of cases dismissed by the courts in which the government had failed to establish that it followed compendial procedures in the analysis of samples of compendial drugs. Those in the industry responsible for the analysis of drugs must be scrupulously careful that they follow specifications, whether they be public (USP or NF) or private (NDA) specifications, during their laboratory testing of samples in order that their results might always be regarded as credible.

NOTES

1. United States v. Sullivan, 332 U.S. 689, 1948.
2. United States v. Dotterweich, 320 U.S. 277, 1943.
3. Section 707 of the Federal Food, Drug, and Cosmetic Act, 21 U.S.C. 377.
4. Section 502(d), Federal Food, Drug, and Cosmetic Act, 21 U.S.C. 352(d).
5. Administrative Procedures Act of 1946, 5 U.S.C. 551 et seq. For a detailed description of this Act, see *A Guide to Federal Agency Rule-making*, GPO, 1984. Stock #436-0661-796.
6. Title 21, Code of Federal Regulations, Sec. 201.51(d) (21 CFR 201.51(d)).
7. Federal Register (FR), Friday, September 29, 1978, Part II (Pages 45021–45026).
8. Federal Register Act of 1935. The FR is published daily, Monday through Friday, and can be ordered from the Superintendent of Documents, U.S. Government Printing Office, Washington, D.C., 20402.
9. Title 21, Code of Federal Regulations (21 CFR) contains all regulations promulgated by FDA for foods, drugs, cosmetics, colors and devices. It also includes regulations covering articles regulated under the Radiation Control For Health and Safety Act of 1968, as well as regulations covering controlled substances; these latter regulations are administered by the Drug Enforcement Administration, U.S. Department of Justice.
10. 21 CFR 210.1(b).
11. 21 CRF 25.
12. 21 CFR 58.
13. Executive Orders Nos. 12044, FR 3/24/78, p. 1220; and 12291, FR 2/19/81, p. 13193.
14. Bureau of Drugs, Investigational and New Drug Regulations Revisions. Concept Document. Food and Drug Administration, October 1979, pp. 1–193.
15. FDA Bureau of Drugs Clinical Guidelines, General Considerations for the Clinical Evaluation of Drugs. HEW(FDA) 77-3040, September 1977. Additional guidelines have been published periodically, and their titles are available from the Center for Drugs and Biologics.
16. Bureau of Drugs Staff Manual Guides, BD 4820.3, Drug Classification and BD 4850.7, End of Phase II Conference. Available under the Freedom of Information Act (FOI).
17. Copies of Summary Bases of Approval for individual approved new drugs are available under FOI.
18. Bassen, J. L., Ten years of GMP. *Drug Cosmetic Ind.*, December, 1973.
19. All comments are referenced under Docket 76 N-0099 and are available for public inspection or copying from Docket Management Branch (HFA-305) FDA, 5600 Fishers Lane, Rockville, MD 20857.
20. Comment by Parenteral Drugs Association, Docket 76 N-0100.
21. PMS Bluebook is published annually by the FDA Office of Planning and Evaluation.
22. Drug Product Survey Evaluation Reports are available from the FDA Center for Drugs and Biologies, Division of Drug Quality Compliance (HFD-334), FDA, 5600 Fishers Lane, Rockville, MD 20857.

23. Drug Compliance Programs may be obtained on a subscription basis from National Technical Information Service (NTIS), Springfield, VA 22161.
24. FDA Inspection Operations Manual (IOM), Section 511, Notice of Inspection. The IOM is available from NTIS on a subscription basis.
25. Regulatory Procedures Manual, Chapter 8-10. Available under FOI from the FDA FOI staff.
26. FDA Annual Reports, 1950-1974. For sale by Superintendent of Documents, U.S. Government Printing Office, Washington, D.C. Stock No. 017-012-002358. Later Annual Reports available from Consumer Communications Staff, FDA (HFE 88).
27. National Symposium Proceedings Safety of Large Volume Parenteral Solutions, July 28–29, 1966 (out of print).
28. Final Report of the National Coordinating Committee on Large Volume Parenterals, 11/30/79, by Dr. Kenneth N. Barker, Project Director and Chairperson NCCLVP and Chairman of the Division of Pharmacy Administration, School of Pharmacy, Auburn University, Auburn, Alabama 36830.
29. EDRO Field Management Directive No. 120. Available from FOI Staff.
30. FOI requests for information should be addressed to Freedom of Information Staff HFW-30, Food and Drug Administration, 5600 Fishers Lane, Rockville, MD 20857.
31. Bassen, J. L., FDA Manuals: A Source of Technical and Compliance Information. Pharmaceutical Manufacturing. August, 1984, p. 39.
32. Compliance Programs: Drug Product Problem Reporting, 7356.006, and Drug Product Surveillance, 7356.008.
33. The United States Pharmacopeia, 12601 Twinbrook Parkway, Rockville, MD 20852.
34. Shroff, A. P., Drug Quality Surveillance of Rx and OTC Drug Products. Pharmaceutical Technology, December, 1979, p. 28.
35. Available from FDA Freedom of Information Staff.
36. Part 7, Title 21, Code of Federal Regulations, 21 CFR 7.
37. FDA Regulatory Procedures Manual, Part 5 (Revised January 4, 1980), Chapter 5-00. Available under FOI from the FDA FOI staff.
38. Federal Register (FR), Wednesday, June 30, 1976 (pp. 26924–26930).
39. Federal Register (FR), Friday, June 16, 1978 (pp. 26202–26221).
40. FDA Weekly Enforcement Report. Includes information about recalls and about regulatory actions (seizures, injunctions, criminal prosecutions) that were filed during that week. Available under NTIS on a subscription basis.
41. Guidance document entitled Methods for Conducting Recall Effectiveness Checks. Available from FDA from the Freedom of Information Staff.
42. Recalls of large volume parenterals (liquid drugs administered intravenously or by other non-oral means), Food and Drug Administration, Center for Disease Control, Department of Health, Education, and Welfare, March 12, 1976. Available from the U.S. General Accounting Office, Washington, D.C. 20548.
43. Cases and Materials on Food and Drug Law, Thomas W. Christopher, Food and Drug Law Institute Series, Commerce Clearing House, 1966. Available from the Food and Drug Law Institute, 1200 New Hampshire Ave. N.W., Washington, DC 20036.
44. Institute Series. Eight volumes covering food and drug law from 1938 through 1974. The authors have included Vincent A. Kleinfeld (all

volumes); Charles Wesley Dunn (Volumes I–IV, 1938–1957); Alan H. Kaplan (Volumes V–VIII, 1958–1974); and Stephen A. Weitzman (Volume VII, 1969 through 1974). These volumes are available from the Food and Drug Law Institute, as are other case materials on Food and Drug Law.

45. See Note 2.
46. United States v. John R. Park, 421 U.S. 658, 1975.
47. United States v. Morton-Norwich Products, Inc., U.S. District Court, Northern District of New York (75 Cr. 114, 1978).
48. Woodard Laboratories, Inc., v. United States, United States Court of Appeals For the Ninth Circuit, 1952. (198 F. 2nd 995).
49. Safety of Large Volume Parenterals Solutions, National Symposium Proceedings, July 28–29, 1966. Dr. Lloyd C. Miller's paper The History of the Clarity Test is on pages 6–9. This Food and Drug Administration publication is out of print. Copies made from the original can be obtained from co-author Jonas L. Bassen, 12205 Fleming Lane, Bowie, Maryland 20715.

10
Medical Devices
DESIGN, MANUFACTURE, AND QUALITY CONTROL

David H. Wayt
Abbott Laboratories, North Chicago, Illinois

I. INTRODUCTION

The technical aspect of medical practice has developed in recent years with notable advances in many areas, including the development of sets and devices. Sets range from relatively simple items, such as a transfer tubing set with a bottle spike on one end and a needle on the other, to complex tissue-implantable electronic devices, such as heart pacers. Hospitals are faced with making decisions concerning the selection of both sets and devices. These decisions involve not only the demonstrated quality of a supplier's particular devices but the degree of duplication of devices from different suppliers, the variety of devices to be utilized, and the degree of complexity of devices and their combination in sets. Further, with the increased concern for cost containment, a very large economic factor has been introduced into the decision-making process. This affects devices, particularly, since most devices are currently supplied as disposable items. The latter has greatly reduced the responsibility of the hospital in repairing or reprocessing sets and devices, but has placed the responsibility on the device manufacturer. The buying requirements and policies of hospitals, at times, dictate the purchase of large numbers of more universal or general-purpose sets (Fig. 1) rather than smaller numbers of the more specialized sets (Fig. 2). The industry has responded to this requirement by producing a large number of extension or auxiliary sets (Fig. 3), which allow general-purpose sets to be converted to specialized uses. The buyers are becoming increasingly aware of the requirements and the end use for which the sets and devices are destined. (The term "sets and devices" will be used interchangeably throughout the rest of this chapter.)

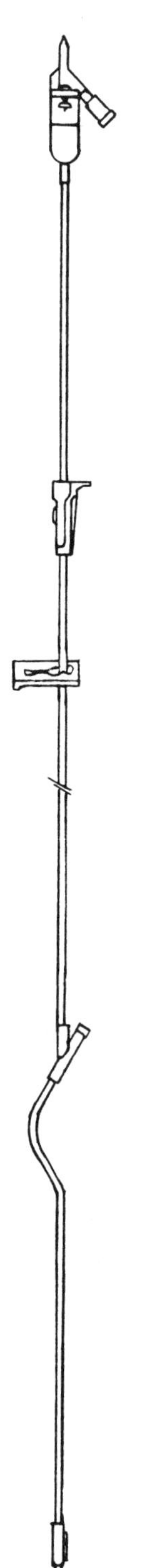

Figure 1 General purpose sets are characteristically simple in configuration and vary mostly in length.

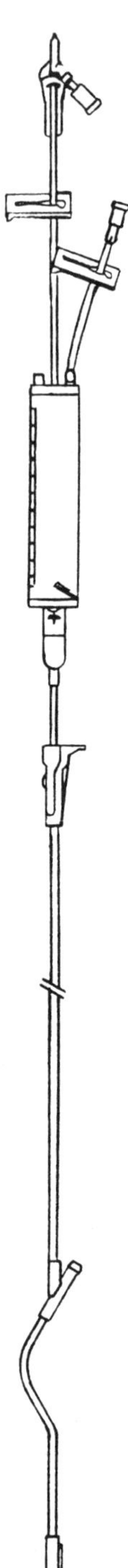

Figure 2 A specialty set such as the precision volume set is designed to meet specific needs.

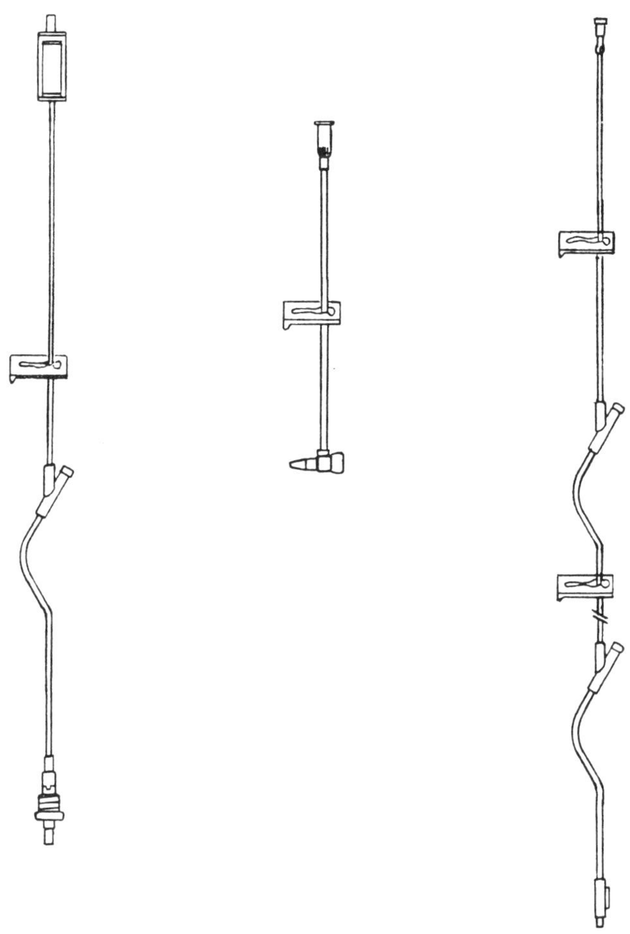

Figure 3 Extension sets are used to convert general purpose sets to specialized uses.

II. GENERAL CONSIDERATIONS

General-purpose devices, such as those illustrated in Figure 1, constitute the majority of those required in the hospital. They provide an inexpensive set with infusion control in the form of an adjustable clamp and a Y injection site providing a site for emergency procedures if required. However, consideration must be given to the specialized needs of the surgical and anesthesia departments in particular, as illustrated in Figure 4. The additional Y site is a specialized back-check valve assembly that allows the anesthesiologist to administer an anesthetic without having the drug diluted by the primary intravenous (IV) solution. The syringe is attached to the Y site. As the syringe plunger is depressed, the back-check valve closes, shutting off the primary flow from the IV bottle. Decisions must be made between single use versus multiple use, sterile set versus sterile fluid path only sets, and sterile versus nonsterile devices. Personal preference,

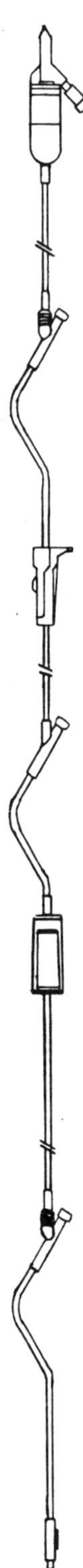

Figure 4 Anesthesia sets perform a specific purpose in the operating room environment.

special procedures and protocols used within the hospital, and bid or contract procurement requirements may all have an impact on the actual devices chosen for use by the hospital.

III. DESIGN OF DEVICES

Vendors in the health care industry are devoted to supplying products with very high product quality with respect to both design and conformance. The factors affecting the quality of design are that combination of physical principles in the design that meets the requirements of the user. The quality of conformance relates to how well the product complies with the specifications, formulations, and drawings of the design. In other words, these factors are concerned with quality assurance.

A. Function

The prime consideration in the design of any device is its functionality. Most devices are designed to provide a specific function, e.g., conveying medication from a bottle to the patient's veins (Fig. 1), providing a specialized service, such as allowing the introduction of an anesthetic to the patient through the IV fluid administration system (Fig. 4), or providing precision control of fluid administration, as with an electronic flow control device, such as a pump or controller.

The desired functionality of a set may be obtained when making only one of two models under laboratory or prototype conditions, but some degree of functionality may be lost when going to a large-scale operation. This is illustrated in the construction of a disposable needle valve in the pilot or prototype stage (Fig. 5). The threads in the stem can be very fine, resulting in precise control of the number of drops. However, in order to make the valve more manufacturable, a courser thread pattern may have to be used that will result in less precision. This trade-off is weighed during the design phase of a set or device and a choice made.

Whenever possible, the design is patient oriented, providing maximum comfort for the patient while still maintaining its functionality. This can be achieved by removing protrusions and sharp corners from patient contact, as illustrated in Figure 6. The filter illustrated can be taped to the patient's arm without discomfort. Further, areas of manipulation affecting the functionality of the device can often be moved away from the patient to where accidental contact cannot occur. There is also an element of use-directed design in devices, allowing reliability of function for its intended use along with patient safety as the result of safeguards built into the intrinsic design of the set. This is illustrated by the set and pump in Figure 7. All areas for nurse manipulation are placed above the pump and well out of the area of accidental patient contact.

The final element of the design revolves around user orientation. A well-designed set or device will allow for easy setup and use with a minimum amount of instructions. Equally important is consideration of the possibility of user misuse or misapplication of the product being designed. Rightly or wrongly, all failures of the product in the field reflect on the vendor's reputation even if the problem was caused by the user.

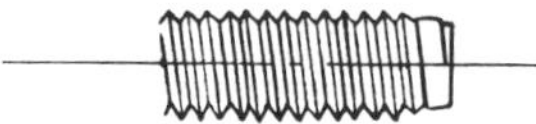

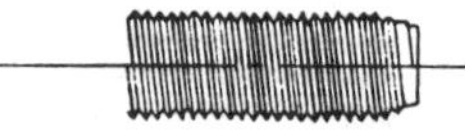

Figure 5 Prototyping allows designs to be tested before the final design is decided upon. The number of threads per inch will decide how fine the control of the valve may be. (a) Course thread, $\frac{1}{4}$ in. = 20 threads per in., (b) extra fine thread, $\frac{1}{4}$ in. = 32 threads per in.

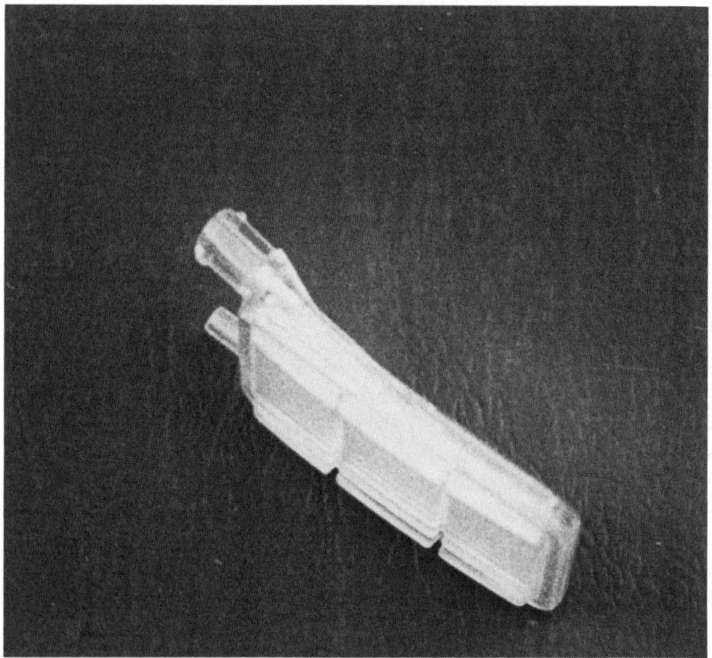

Figure 6 The experimental filter has been designed to give maximum comfort to the patient. The corners have been rounded and the bottom contoured to fit the curve of the patient's arm.

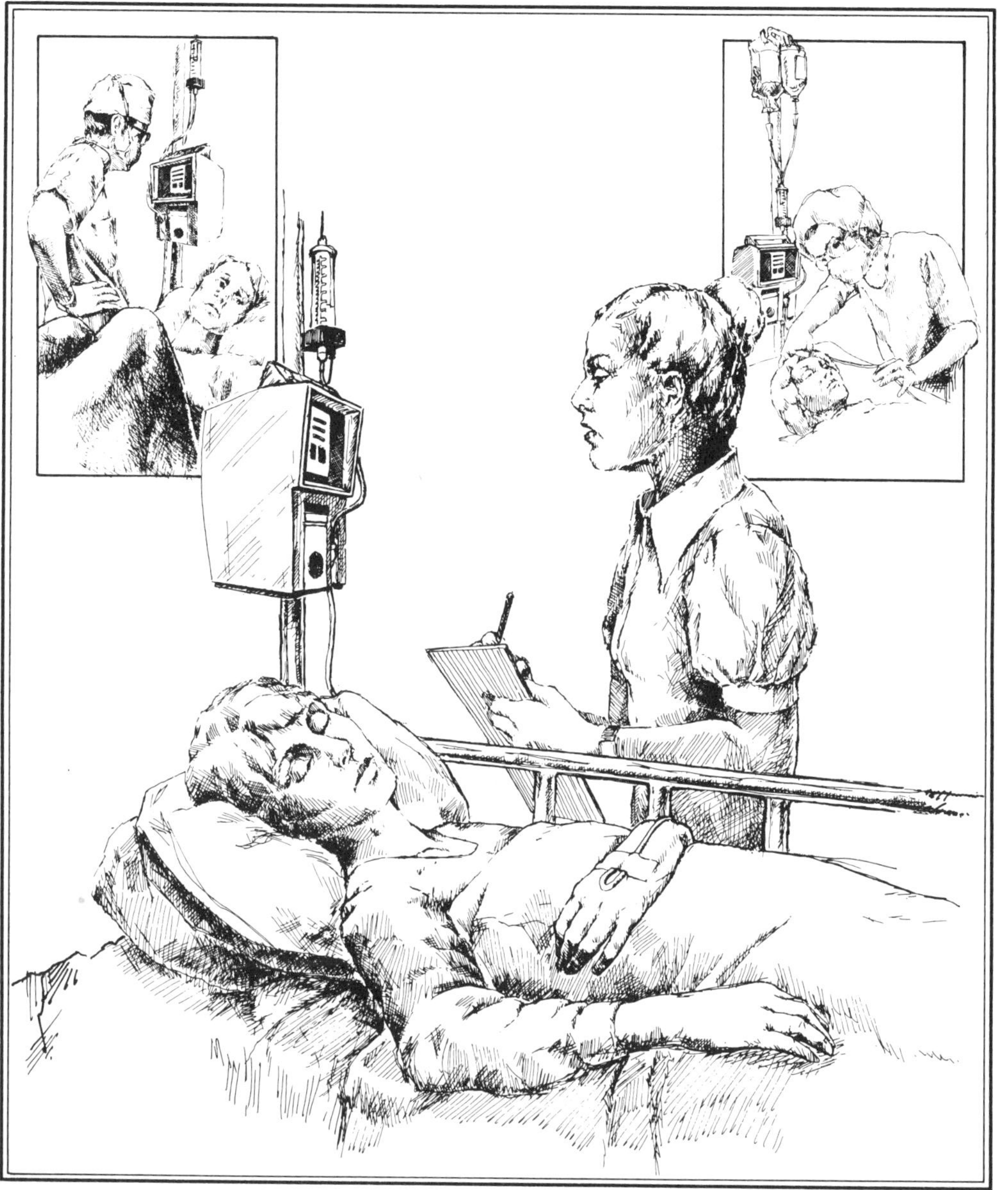

Figure 7 All bedside electronics, such as this IV pump, are designed to be placed in a convenient location for the operator but out of the way of the patient.

B. Materials

The selection of materials for a device plays a very important role. Since a large number of the devices in the current marketplace are disposable, there is a trade-off between permanence of the material and cost effectiveness. A product is no better than the parts, material, and processes required to produce it. Therefore, several factors are evaluated in material selection, including previous history of the material in similar products or design, flow characteristics of the material for molding complex parts, the manufacturing techniques to be used to assemble the device, and, if the device is to be sterilized, the sterilization mode once the device is assembled (ETO versus radiation or steam). All these must contribute to the intended use of the device. The list in Figure 8 gives common polymers used in many sets.

Once the device design has been finalized and the types and classification of materials to be used in the device determined, total characterization of the material is necessary. Usually this includes USP XXI testing (Fig. 9), as well as the characterization of the material by its physical attributes, such as tensile strength, tear resistance, and elongation.

C. Configuration

A design that can be easily used in more than one procedure or situation in the hospital is considered to be much more flexible and desirable than designs specifically targeted for a given procedure. Compare the sets in Figure 10. The general-purpose set on the left is considerably less complicated than the speciality set on the right and as a consequence is less expensive. Although a more general purpose set has great appeal, both the universal and targeted set have a place in most hospitals.

When the functionality and materials for a given design have been identified, the designer looks at the configuration of the actual device. Families of sets or devices can be characterized by placement of features in the same place within the set. In Figure 11, the piggyback sets are characterized by placement of the back-check valve the same distance below the drip chamber of the primary spike. In many sets the sequence of placement of features in the device is required to achieve device functionality. This is especially true in specialized sets, such as piggyback sets (Figs. 12 and 13). One of the paramount features in the configuration of the design is its manufacturability. Research and development must consider the manufacturing environment, process controls and equipment, and the technical limitations of the productive process in order to ensure compatibility and minimization of potential problems. Sets and devices that lend themselves to easier straight-line progressive assembly are more desirable. Compare the sets in Figure 10 again. The general-purpose set can be made either on a straight line or progressive assembly or in subassemblies that can be easily introduced into a simple assembly line. In contrast, the burette set requires more complicated subassemblies that do not readily fit into simple assembly procedures.

D. Processing and Handling

Generally, disposable sets and devices are relatively inexpensive items being produced in large number. As a given set or device gains in acceptance,

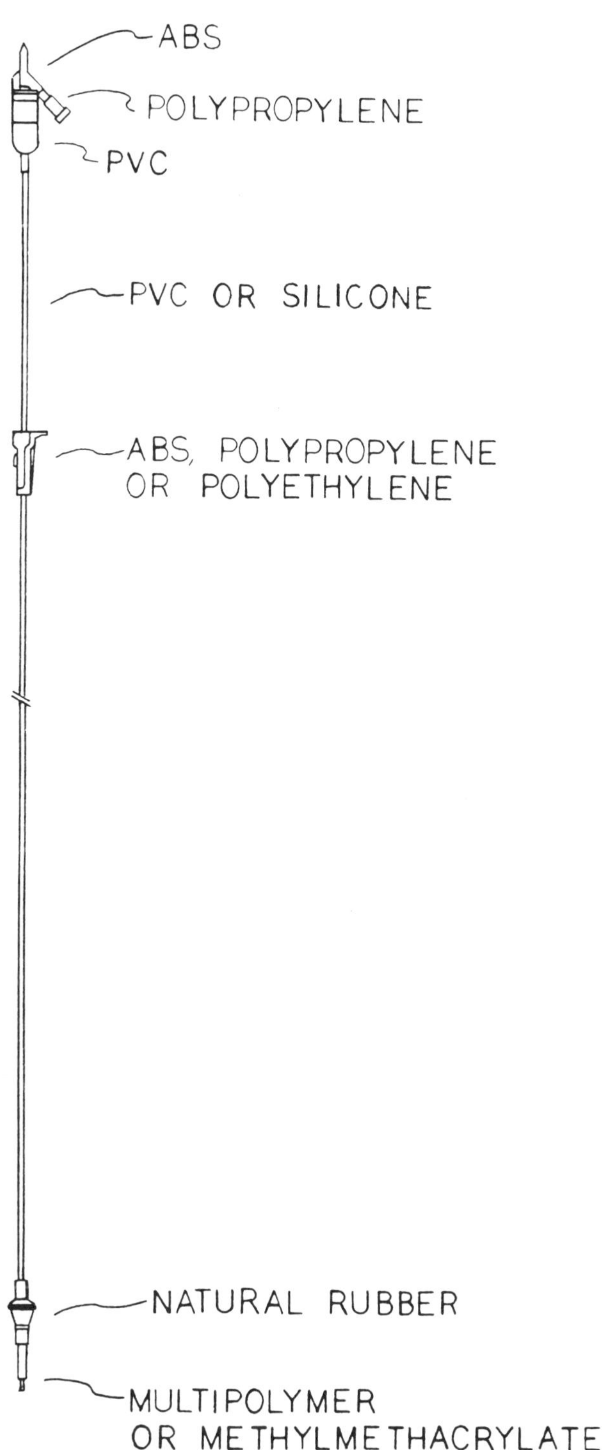

Figure 8 A large number of polymers are used in sets and are balanced against properties and cost.

I. MATERIAL REQUIREMENTS

All material shall be Class IV (to include saline, alcohol, vegetable oil extracts and implant) per USP test for plastics - USP XXI Page 1235.

Figure 9 Materials requirements can have requirements for specialized testing as illustrated by the above paragraph.

the number of units demanded by the market will increase considerably. In the design of sets expected to become high-volume sellers, considerable attention is given to producing uniformity within families and utilization of existing components. Components of a given class are handled within the plant environment in a manner to allow streamlining of the manufacturing operation.

Wherever possible the components are designed with automatic assembly as the goal. These parts should allow for manual assembly during the low-volume production phase (Fig. 14) but have the capability of being assembled automatically once the volume of sets increases (Fig. 15). The design should be such that the processing and handling do nothing to impair the functionality of the set or device.

The parts should be so designed that particulates are not generated during the manufacturing operation. This requires considerable coordination between the design group and the manufacturing group during the initial design phase of the device. Closely tied to this is the consideration of manufacturing processes to ensure there are no areas within the device that are hard to sterilize. The area circled in Figure 16 would have to have verification of its sterility under its normal sterilization cycle or be redesigned.

Paramount in the design is the requirement that the commodities and devices can be readily tested without undue increase in the cost of the product. Wherever possible the parts should be designed for in-line testing as well as final product testing. The subassembly in Figure 17 can be easily checked for functionality and completeness with a simple rotometer test that measures airflow through the subassembly. Too much airflow can indicate a hole in the filter membrane; too little flow can indicate blockage of some sort.

E. Voluntary Standards

A growing number of products require specific features in order to be both safe and efficacious. To address this issue a number of organizations, such as the Association for the Advancement of Medical Instrumentation (AAMI), the American National Standards Institute (ANSI), the Canadian Standards Association, and the International Standards Organization (ISO) are issuing voluntary standards for products.

These standards outline the *minimum* functional requirements and performance parameters considered necessary for safe and effective products. The voluntary standards are considered a consensus of expert opinion among manufacturers, users, and government agencies. Parts of sets produced to the voluntary standard, such as the ANSI luer taper standard, will mate with products from different vendors produced to the same standard (Fig. 18).

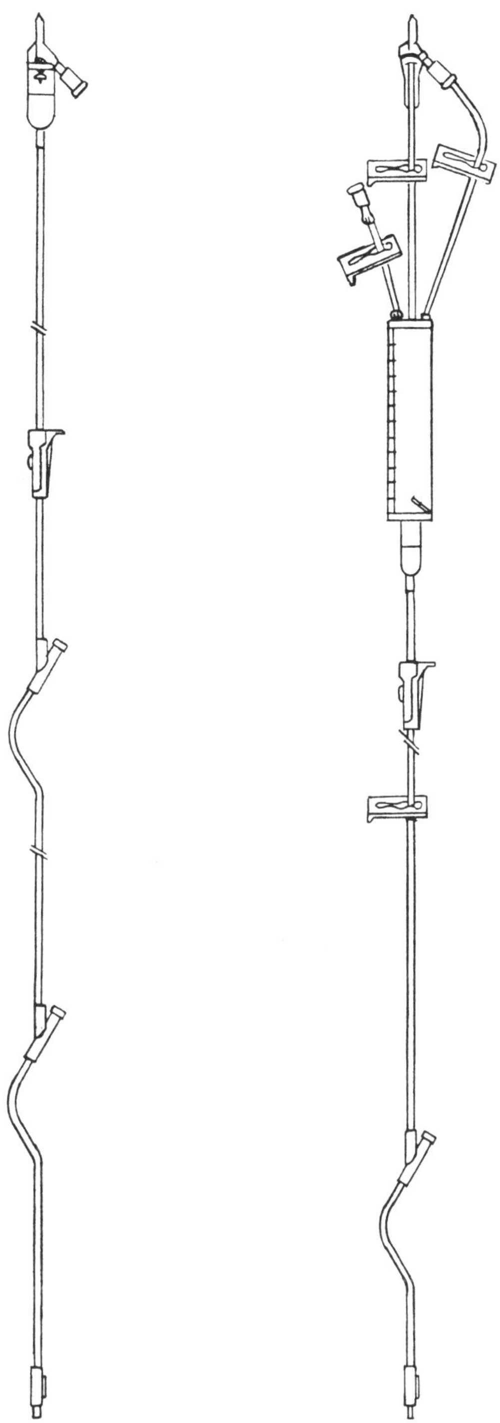

Figure 10 The complexity of a set has a direct bearing on the cost.

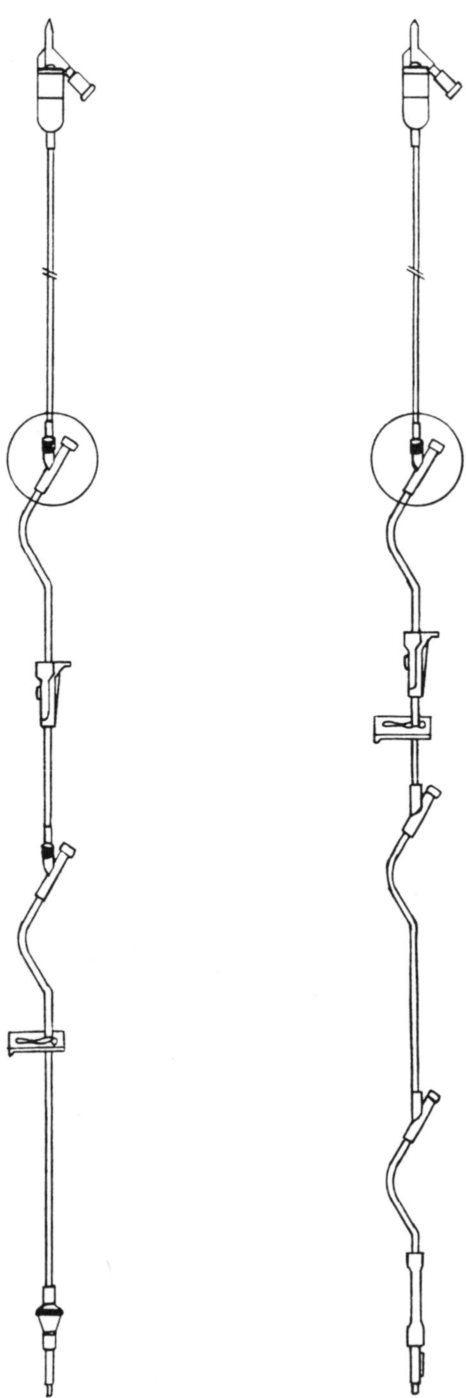

Figure 11 Families of sets are characterized by repeating elements found in each set, such as the backcheck valve in piggyback sets.

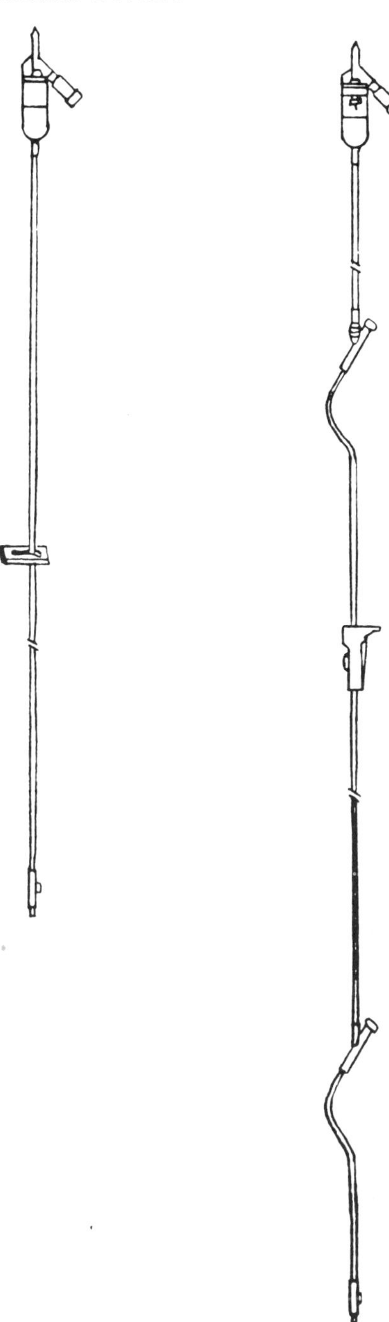

Figure 12 A piggyback "set" is usually composed of two sets and a needle to connect them.

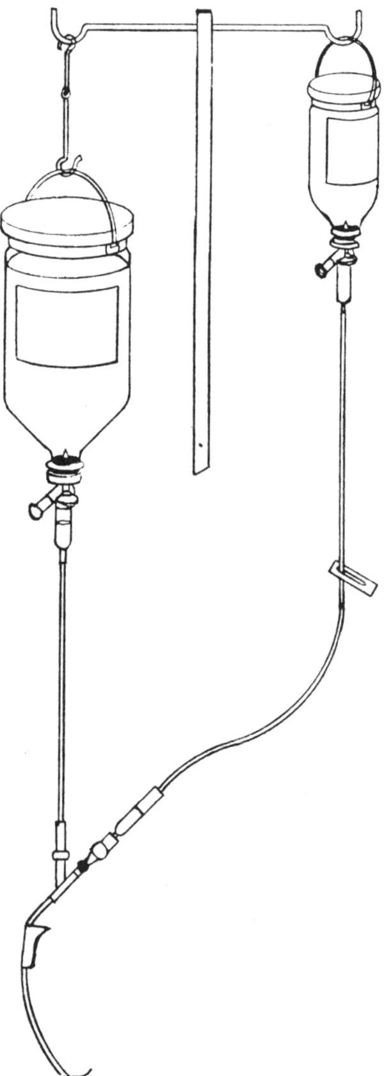

Figure 13 The pressure from the secondary set and bottle (the highest) will hold the valve closed, shutting off the flow from the primary bottle. Once the fluid in the secondary tubing falls to the level of the fluid in the drip chamber of the primary container the backcheck valve releases and flow from the primary container resumes.

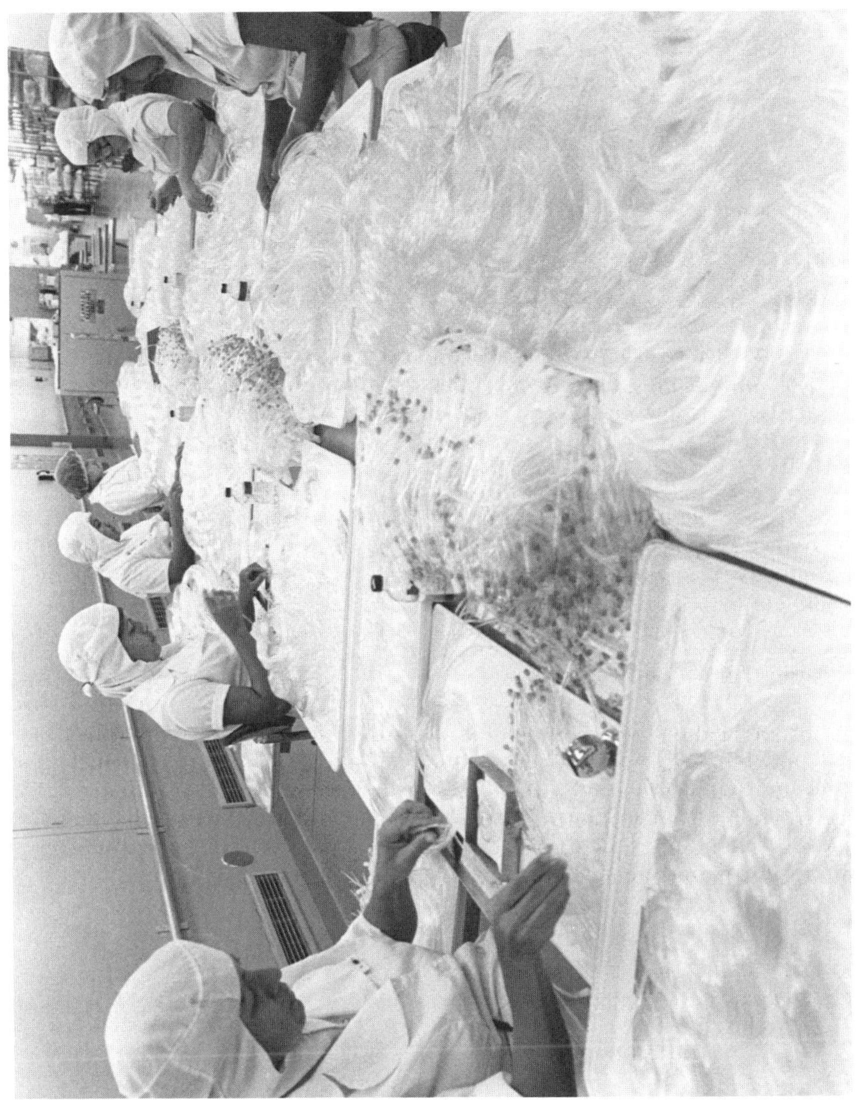

Figure 14 Since most low volume operations start as manual assembly operations the parts must be designed to make manual assembly easy.

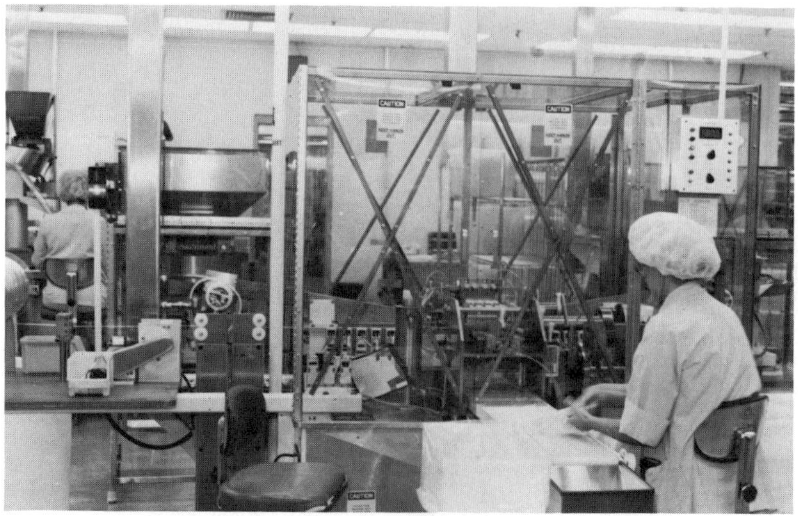

Figure 15 Once the demand increases to the point the assembly can be automated the parts should be easily assembled by the machine. This machine performs a task similar to that shown in Fig. 14.

The AAMI also issues publications called recommended practices, written primarily to provide guidelines for the use, care, and processing of medical devices, that cover a variety of subjects from sterilization to cleaning of reusable devices.

F. Disposable Versus Multiple Use

The designer of medical devices must take into consideration whether the device will be disposable or can be cleaned, resterilized, and reused. Some of the current disposable devices have multiuse capabilities but due to the complexity of design, manufacturers have chosen to retail them as disposable devices. They do this by permanently displaying the single-use requirement in the label claims (Fig. 19). This removes the liability of

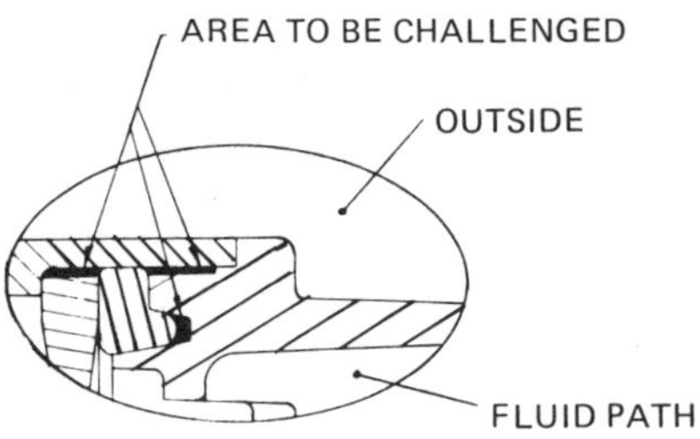

Figure 16 Blind areas must be addressed in selecting a sterilization process and cycle.

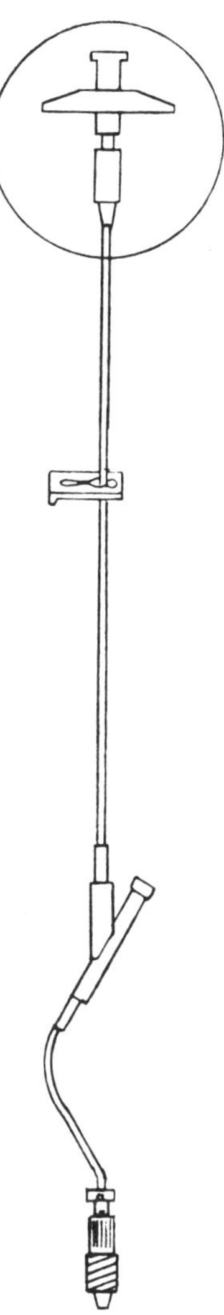

Figure 17 Ease of testing utilizing a simple test method is important in the design criteria for sets.

having a multiuse device with all its attendant procedures for cleaning and resterilization.

G. Packaging

Packaging within the medical device industry is almost as diverse as the number of devices themselves. But, as far as sterility is concerned, they can be divided into three main categories. One is the *sterile pack*, which delivers the entire device to an operating field in a sterile condition. The second is the *sterile pathway*, in which the container acts as a dust cover and general particulate eliminator until the time of use, but sterility is

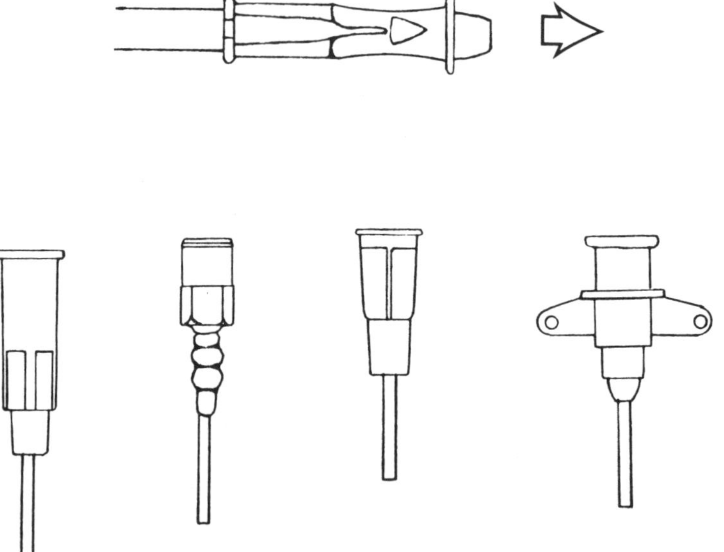

Figure 18 A plug made to the ANSI luer taper standard should fit any vendors' mating hub regardless of the external configuration.

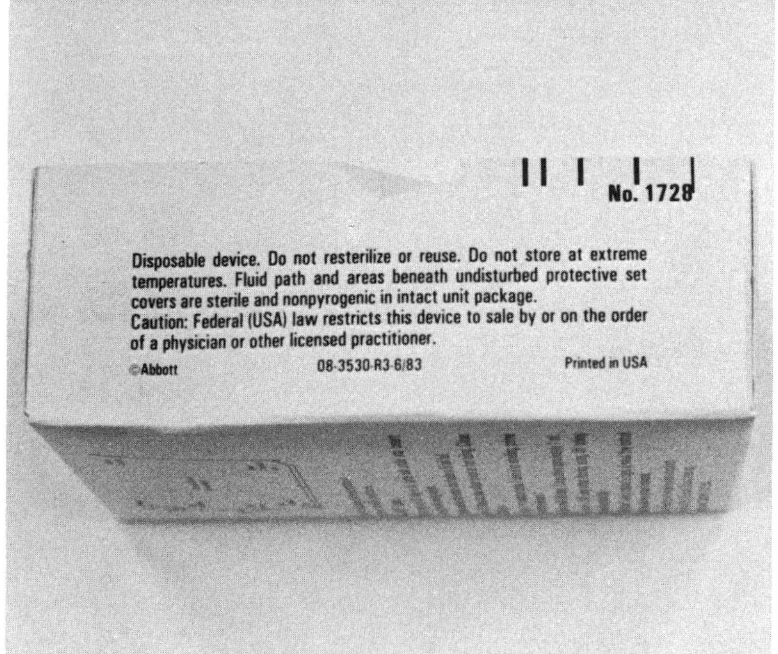

Figure 19 A typical device carton or box will have a legal statement limiting its use to one time and stating its use must be prescribed by a physician.

maintained only in the fluid pathway under the protective covers. The third category is the *nonsterile device*.

The package category is normally dictated by the label claims for sterile product or sterile pathway and decided upon by the manufacturer. When claiming sterile product, the package must be so designed to pass a number of maintenance of sterility tests that show that, under most normal and sometimes even abnormal conditions, the product within the package remains sterile. For devices maintaining a sterile pathway, the same type of testing is done to assure that the fluid path within the device and under the protective covers remains sterile during the testing programs. Whether the packaging is designed to make the actual product visible or depends upon a schematic on the package to show the product is left to the discretion of the vendor. Most packages are designed to provide security for the product. The sterile product package must show immediately if the package has been tampered with or opened. Most of the packages for devices with a sterile pathway also have some tamper-indicating feature. Choice of materials in packaging is usually determined by the type of presentation the vendor wishes to make. There are blisters with Tyvek covers, blisters with impregnated paper covers, peel pouches with breather patches, and paperboard boxes either with overwrap or glued end construction that allows a tamper-proof package.

IV. MANUFACTURING OF DEVICES

Manufacturing procedures are influenced by key regulations from the Food and Drug Administration (FDA), found in the FDA publication 21 CFR 820 entitled "Manufacture, packaging, storage and installation of medical devices" or, as more commonly known, "The device GMP's (good manufacturing practices)." These regulations not only affect the general layout of any given manufacturing area but also influence the selection of equipment and accessories used in the manufacturing process.

A. Plant Environmental Considerations

Components for a medical device are handled in the cleanest way possible. It is becoming common practice for the components to be manufactured in a Class 100,000 clean room before shipping to the device manufacturer. The components are packed in such a way that they can be transferred from one area to another or one plant to another without contamination.

The plant environment for most device manufacturing plants is Class 100,000 or better. This includes HEPA filtration or equivalent for the actual manufacturing areas, with balancing of the air pressures to restrict the introduction of particulates into the manufacturing areas as much as possible. Most plants also have stringent hand washing requirements for the operators to reduce the biological loading of the process area. Protective clothing is also an important part of controlling particulates and contamination in the plant environment. Specialized suppliers supply lint-free clothing and hair coverings for this purpose. Wherever possible the manufacturing areas are designed for one-way flow of materials; i.e., unfinished materials come in from one side of the room and finished materials exit from the other side of the room. Most manufacturing areas have restricted access, which allows strict control of both material and personnel coming into and going out of the area. Additionally, one of the functions of the plant quality assurance group includes continually monitoring the quality of the air and work surfaces in the manufacturing areas, including monitoring the work surfaces for bioburden.

The manufacturing processes should be designed to reduce the possibility of additional particulate generation or contamination of the material passing through the process. Therefore, the selection of the manufacturing process when making decisions concerning the initial design is very important. The manufacturing operation will routinely use solvent-sealing operations, siliconing operations, sonic sealing or welding operations, and a large variety of mechanical automatic operations using one or more of the above technologies. A typical set may be assembled with the technologies as shown in Figure 20.

Once the process has been selected, the marriage of the process to the equipment becomes an important consideration. Normally the equipment is validated for the operating parameters decided upon by the engineering or manufacturing functions to ensure the equipment or process will continue to make acceptable assemblies or subassemblies. In order to do this, one or more important measurable parameters are selected. An example would be the force necessary to separate tubing from an adjoining plastic part after being joined by a solvent-based adhesive. A typical validation worksheet may look like Figure 21. Detailed instructions on data entry and interpretation will accompany the worksheet. The bell-shaped curve generated on the validation sheet should fall within the accepted limits for the process, with a comfortable margin between the acceptance limits to allow for minor shifts of the process.

The design and use of equipment in the areas is also important from the standpoint of reducing particulate loading and allowing maximum ability to clean and service the equipment without jeopardizing the product being made in the area. Since most of the equipment used by device manufactureres is either custom-made or a highly modified version of commercial equipment, the necessary safeguards and modifications can be effected before the equipment is introduced to the manufacturing floor. This means that all moving machine parts should be essentially nonparticulate generating and easily cleaned. When air-operated equipment is used, the incoming and exhaust air should be carefully controlled to assure that no additional particulate contamination is introduced into the environment. If a "dirty" machine must be used, it is usually isolated or enclosed to minimize the impact on the process area. Cleanliness is one of the major concerns with the manufacturing area requiring frequent cleanups and frequent checks. The design of the equipment should be simplistic, so it can be cleaned easily since daily cleanups are a way of life within device-manufacturing processes.

In-process controls are extremely important during the manufacture of medical devices. The controls must cover both the subassemblies being made and the equipment and processes used to make the subassemblies. One way to maintain tight controls is to have an in-plant subassembly lot-numbering system tied either to a particular period of time or to a specific number of subassemblies being made. This allows frequent checks to make sure the process and the subassemblies being produced remain within the specifications necessary for the finished product.

Many products have characteristics that cannot be economically and effectively measured after the product has been completely assembled. Some of these characteristics can only be controlled by controlling the production

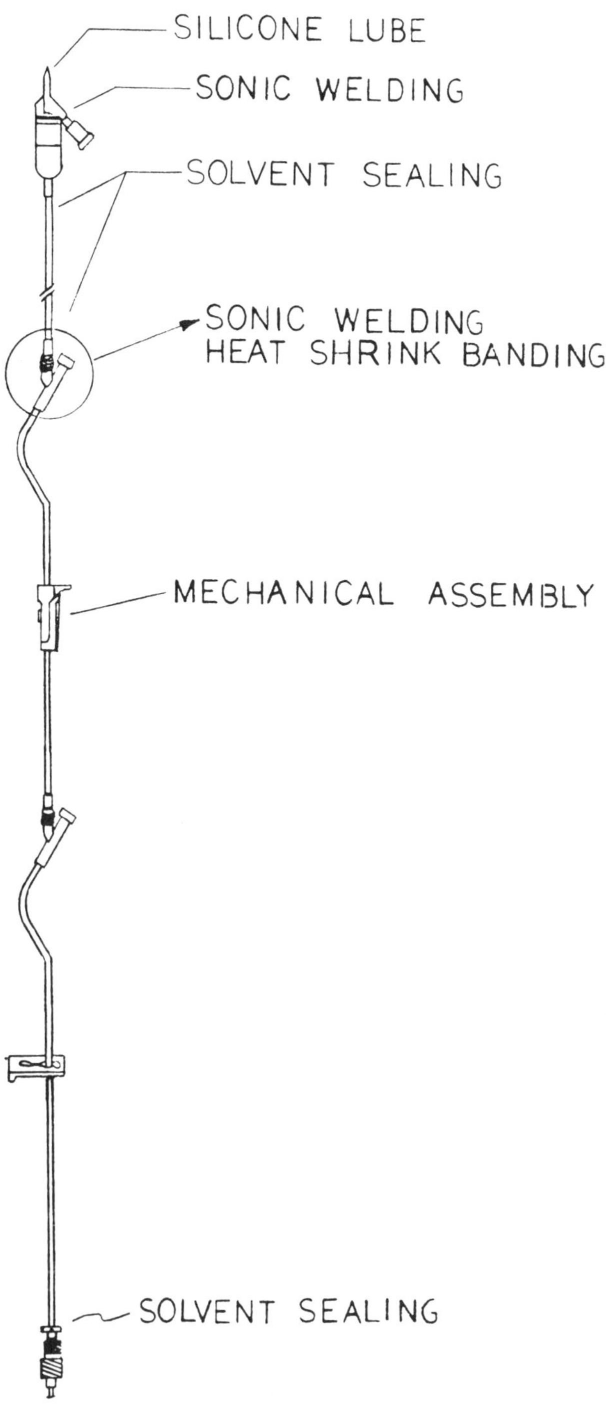

Figure 20 There are numerous technologies that can be used to assemble sets, with the above being only one such combination.

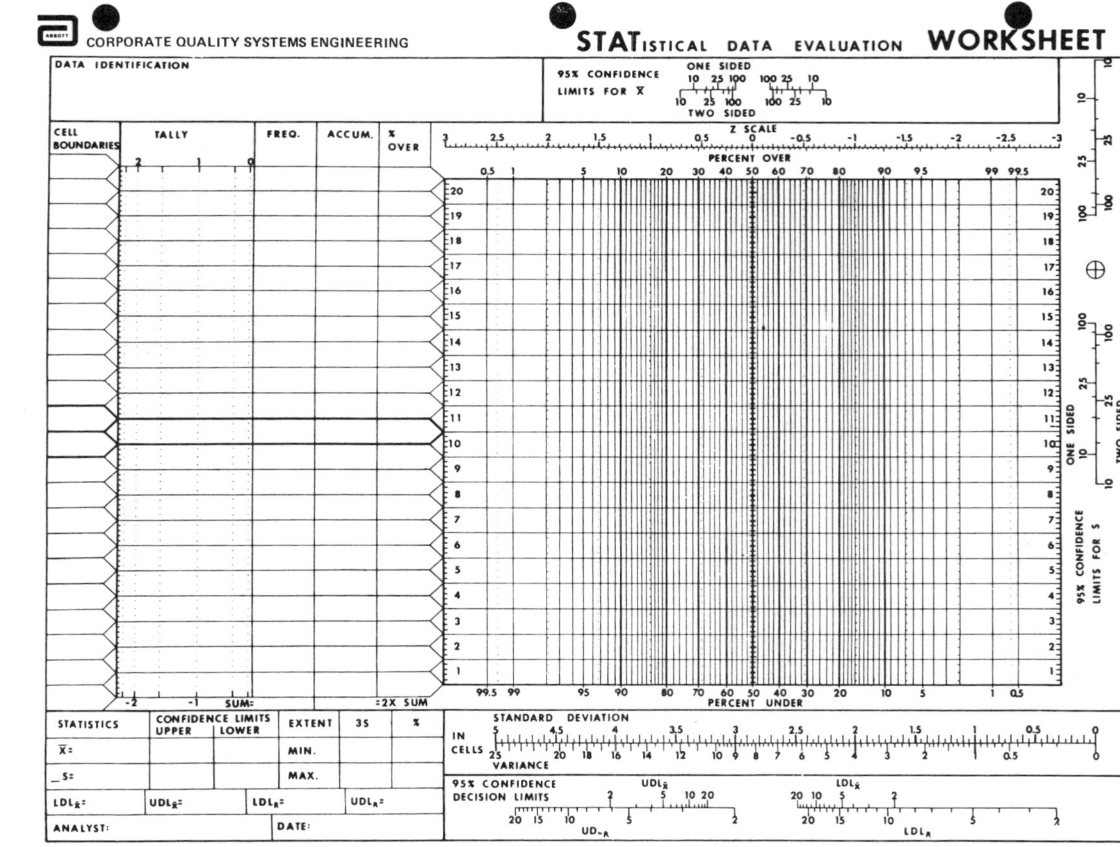

Figure 21 There are numerous statistical tools and forms available to the professional to allow quick evaluation of data from a process.

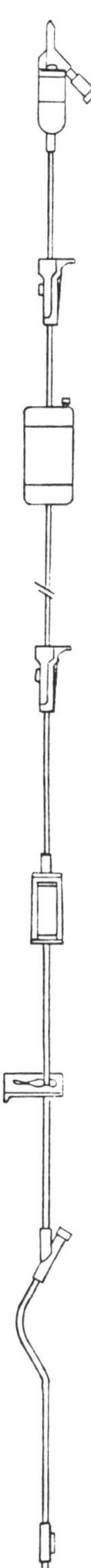

Figure 22 Increasing complexity of sets also adds increasing complexity to the testing methods. In some cases validation of the process becomes the easicr way to insure quality through a process.

process and the environment through which the product is passing during its manufacture. In the case of the membrane sets, for example (Fig. 22), flow testing becomes increasingly difficult as assembly progresses. Once the process and its equipment has been established, it is necessary to validate either the equipment and/or the process to ensure adequate quality of the subassemblies being produced. This is an activity usually coordinated between the manufacturing engineers and the quality engineers. Normally an attribute is chosen that can be readily measured and a specification set for the acceptable limits. A "window" is then established utilizing the best and worst cases of the parameters selected. Figure 23 illustrates a window that has been established for a sonic welding operation. This may be equipment settings or a time-related parameter. Once the window has been established, the parameters for the processing machine are posted or recorded in an accessible place and the process is considered satisfactory for production of the product. The in-process controls for machinery, equipment, and mechanical adjuncts to the manufacturing process are monitored by the quality assurance group but maintained by personnel with the plant engineering group. They have the responsibility of maintaining the equipment within the established parameters, performing preventive maintenance wherever necessary, and generally ensuring that the equipment functions correctly during the manufacturing process.

To tie the manufacturing cycle together in a controlled manner, detailed descriptions of each of the processes are written by the industrial engineering or manufacturing engineering department in the plant. Not only does this give a written record of how the product is being made but it gives a systematic means of "tollgating" the product from one step in the operation to the next. The process description describes a single process, or two

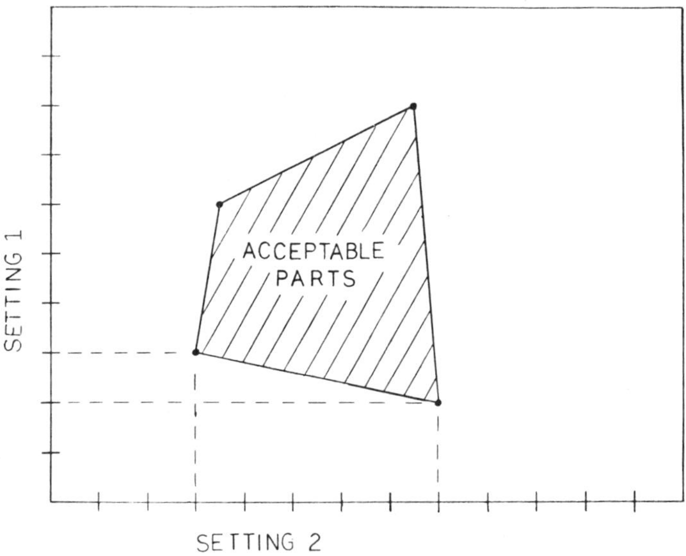

Figure 23 By establishing a "window" for given process parameters, a working grid of settings that will produce acceptable parts can be posted with the equipment or become part of the Quality Manual.

or more processes resulting in a single subassembly, which allows the parts or subassemblies to be collected in an area at the end of the assembly process. These "tollgates" give a natural point for the quality control group to sample and determine the quality of the product in production, as well as a point for collecting and counting the finished subassemblies. The entire manufacturing process requires the maintenance of cleanliness. This is generally achieved by the constant cleaning of the work surfaces and wiping down of the equipment on a daily and sometimes hourly basis using such disinfectants as alcohol or an activated dialdehyde. These activities reduce both the particulate and biological loading on the work surfaces. Major cleanups are performed between the manufacturing of different lots and sometimes between shift changes.

V. PACKAGING AND LABELING

The packaging and labeling of devices is very critical since this is the primary way of identifying the device. The plant must be fully aware of the importance of maintenance of complete control of the labeling material. To maintain the proper storage and labeling in a very controlled manner, the packaging area is isolated from other manufacturing areas. The type of packaging also is important since a sterile product requires slightly different handling than a product that is considered sterile in the fluid pathway only.

Packaging and labeling equipment is generally standard "off the shelf" equipment. It is controlled by some of the requirements outlined for equipment in the manufacturing area, although they will be less stringent than for the manufacturing equipment. The working area in the case of wrappers or cartoners may be isolated and considered less critical as far as particulate generation is concerned. However, in the case of blisters with Tyvek or paper lids for sterile sets, the area should be the same as the manufacturing area. The process for packaging equipment should be validated under the same program used for manufacturing equipment. Validating the packaging to be used for producing a product with sterile contents is much more stringent than a standard overwrap carton type of packaging since the contents must remain sterile. This requires additional quality control testing on the package itself during the manufacturing process.

VI. QUALITY ASSURANCE

The quality assurance unit in the plant has an extremely important function. The mass of record keeping required by the device GMP is within the responsibilities of this group. For this reason, quality assurance can represent from 5 to 15% of the total plant personnel in a device-manufacturing operation. A distinction should be made between quality assurance (QA) and quality control (QC). Quality assurance has the overall function of providing top management with the confidence that the quality function is performing adequately. This embraces formal reports, problem analysis, and trend evaluation as well as quality review of designs and processes. Quality control is defined in the more restricted sense as the actual inspection and inspection methods used in the plant. To ensure performance in a uniform manner throughout the plant, the quality assurance organization has a QA or QC manual for the plant operation. The QA manual will be more policy oriented than the QC manual, but both give sampling plans with the accept or reject levels for the operations within the plant. These plans are usually based on MIL-STD-105D, MIL-STD-414, or one of the generally recognized plans from Dodge and Romig. Most plant QA systems are geared to reduce the possibility of rejecting a final product finished lot. To achieve this objective, the tightest sampling plans are usually assigned to the beginning operations of any series. The product then goes through a normal tollgating from one assembly operation to the next with QA monitoring at each tollgate. The data collected at these tollgates not only provide an accurate record but also can be used as a basis of analysis and action in the resolution of manufacturing quality problems and the obtaining of corrective actions when needed (Fig. 24).

One of the major responsibilities is the receipt, control, and traceability of materials. To trace the material flow of incoming parts, one starts with the receipt from the vendor and continues through all the manufacturing operations to the finished product (Fig. 25). The material specifications will have the vendor identify the material used in making the parts, identify lot number, and mark the cases containing all materials according to corporate standards. Once this material is received, it is assigned a plant lot number and then is placed in quarantine until all incoming tests can be performed. Most device plants have a separate incoming quality assurance group that takes the specifications for each part and performs all the necessary tests. Since these specifications will give pre-established requirements that have been identified to the supplier, subjective decisions based on the inspector's judgment will be minimized. Figure 26 illustrates this by stating the attribute to be measured and the deviation that can be accepted. Once the tests are performed and the material is found to be acceptable, it is moved from the quarantine area into the general inventory. From general inventory it may go into one or more work orders, with strict records kept as to the number of parts placed in each work order. Materials are tracked and accounted for through the entire manufacturing process, including sterilization, to the completed finished goods work order. At outgoing, quality assurance again takes a specification that gives all the tests and requirements for the outgoing product and checks the product. If the product passes all these requirements, it is released to finished goods inventory for sale and distribution in the field.

With the completion of the manufacturing cycle, the product is presented by manufacturing to the quality assurance function in its batch or lot form for acceptance as the final marketable product. At this point, the quality assurance function takes the final marketable product specifications and performs the tests required by this document. Once the final test results are obtained, QA performs an in-depth review of the product, monitoring the process followed (with documented instructions), the use of properly approved raw materials, the various measurements of the environment of the process, and any deviations within the process or product during the manufacturing phase. At this time quality assurance function also concerns itself with ensuring that all necessary data have been collected and documented to meet both regulatory requirements and any requirement for future review of the data.

Once the product is finally accepted for distribution, it is introduced into the storage and distribution system. The QA function continues throughout these systems since it is imperative that the quality and integrity of the

ABBOTT

PROBLEM ANALYSIS AND CORRECTIVE ACTION REPORT

TO: (ACTION)	W.O./P.O.	LIST/COMM/CODE	LC	SC
VIA:				

You are requested to furnish a PROBLEM ANALYSIS AND CORRECTIVE ACTION REPORT for the following discrepancy(s) stating the cause for the discrepancy, the action taken by you to prevent recurrence, and the effective point of corrective action by ____________________ date. Retain one (1) copy of the report for your file and return one (1) copy to ____. If an extension is required for answering, direct your request to the (Plant Q.A. Manager) (Div. Q.A. Manager) giving the date that you expect an answer to be completed. Use additional sheets if required.

DISCREPANCY:

ESTIMATED COST OF DISCREPANCY (PER YEAR):

ORIGINATOR:	DIV. PLANT	DEPT:	DATE:

REPLY

CAUSE OF DISCREPANCY(S):

CORRECTIVE ACTION (State Effectivity Date and/or Lot Number):

SIGNATURE:	TITLE:	DATE:

FOLLOW-UP

CORRECTIVE ACTION VERIFIED AS FOLLOWS:

SAVINGS (PER YEAR):

SIGNATURE:	TITLE:	DEPT:	DATE:

4353-5-R2

Figure 24 Formalized corrective action forms are used as tools to help identify and correct problems. Records should show what actions have been initiated when a problem has been found and what resulted from the activity.

II. MATERIALS

Material shall be Polymer XYZ grade 2, manufactured by Polymer Manufacturing, Inc. A certificate must be sent with each lot of parts stating polymer and lot number. All parts must be boxed and marked according to Corporate Standard 1234 dated 10 Oct 1983.

Figure 25 The specification is a tool that can be utilized to control the materials coming into a device plant. As illustrated, the material identification can be quite specific and include instructions that make tracing the material easy.

product be maintained through controlled storage under proper environmental conditions to assure that they reach the customer in an undamaged state. At this point there must be adequate history and documentation for the product to allow review of the manufacturing process as well as the ability to trace and retrieve the product once it gets into the field.

Quality assurance systems will address both design and conformance requirements. Portions of the system are active in the designs and preproduction state; others follow the product during production and out into the field. All these activities are addressed to assure the product that results is in accordance with the written specifications and will reach the customer in such a state as to satisfy the user requirements. The systems are record and data oriented because of regulatory requirements and have the capability of tracing the product from the receipt of the raw material from the original vendors through its use by a customer in the field.

II. Functional Evaluation - Sample per MIL STD 105D, Level S-3, single sample plan.

The following are cumulative: 1.0%

A. On/Off switch functions appropriately.

B. Light box lights when "Light" control button is depressed.

C. Timer, when set at 10 minutes, shuts off unit in 10 minutes, ±30 seconds.

See Test Procedure

D. Speed, when set at 100RPM, will be 100RPM, ±3RPM.

See Test Procedure

Figure 26 Specifications should be written in such a way as to minimize subjective decisions by the inspector.

VII. SELECTED DEVICE CONSIDERATIONS

Because of the large variety of devices space does not permit a detailed discussion of each, but examples have been selected to illustrate how devices are handled in the areas of design, manufacture, and quality control.

A. Catheters or Needles

Venipuncture devices are the means of connecting sets to the patient's vein. The major devices in this area are the winged infusion set and the catheter-over-needle (Fig. 27), with the catheter-over-needle the preferred device.

1. Design

The most important part of this device is the catheter itself. As can be seen in Figure 28, the catheter is only a small part of the assembly. In the initial design consideration, the tip configuration was found to be critical to the smooth functioning of the device in the user's hands. Different manufacturers have approached the design from different directions (Fig. 29). In the design phase considerable thought had to be given to the tip configuration and the manufacturing process required to give the designed tip. Although some of the basic technology used by each manufacturer is similar, the actual process varies considerably among individual manufacturers. The rest of the design of the unit is one of esthetic or ergometric consideration.

Ideally the design should result in a smooth progression from the needle point past the bevel of the catheter tip. The tip of the catheter itself should be straight with no ragged edges or thin spots to curl back during tissue penetration. The angle of the bevel of the tip is of prime importance since it is a major factor influencing the penetration force required for a successful venipuncture. Each manufacturer has approached the design of the bevel slightly differently (Fig. 30), and each has its users in the marketplace. The catheter should never protrude over the heel of the needle but should come as close as possible to the heel, which makes for smoother insertion through tissue.

The type of material selected for the catheter is of great importance to the well-being of the patient. Currently the majority of manufacturers use fluoroethylenepropylene (FEP) as the material of choice, although over the years polyethylene (PE), polyvinyl chloride (PVC), and tetrafluoroethylene (TFE) have been used with some success. Newer materials that have been considered include several varieties of the polyurethanes. The materials selected have gone through numerous screening tests as well as clinical studies to show the absence of venous complications.

2. Manufacture

A large number of diverse technologies are used in producing catheter-over-needle assemblies. The technologies can be broken down into three general areas. The needle requires metallurgical and metal-working skills, the first general area of technology. The needle in the assembly is usually purchased from an outside vendor since the technique needed to produce an acceptable needle from the blank cannula stock is specialized and requires experience to consistently produce the specialized bevels and grinds required for an intravenous needle. Once the point has been ground, specialized packaging and handling is required to preserve the sharp point. On

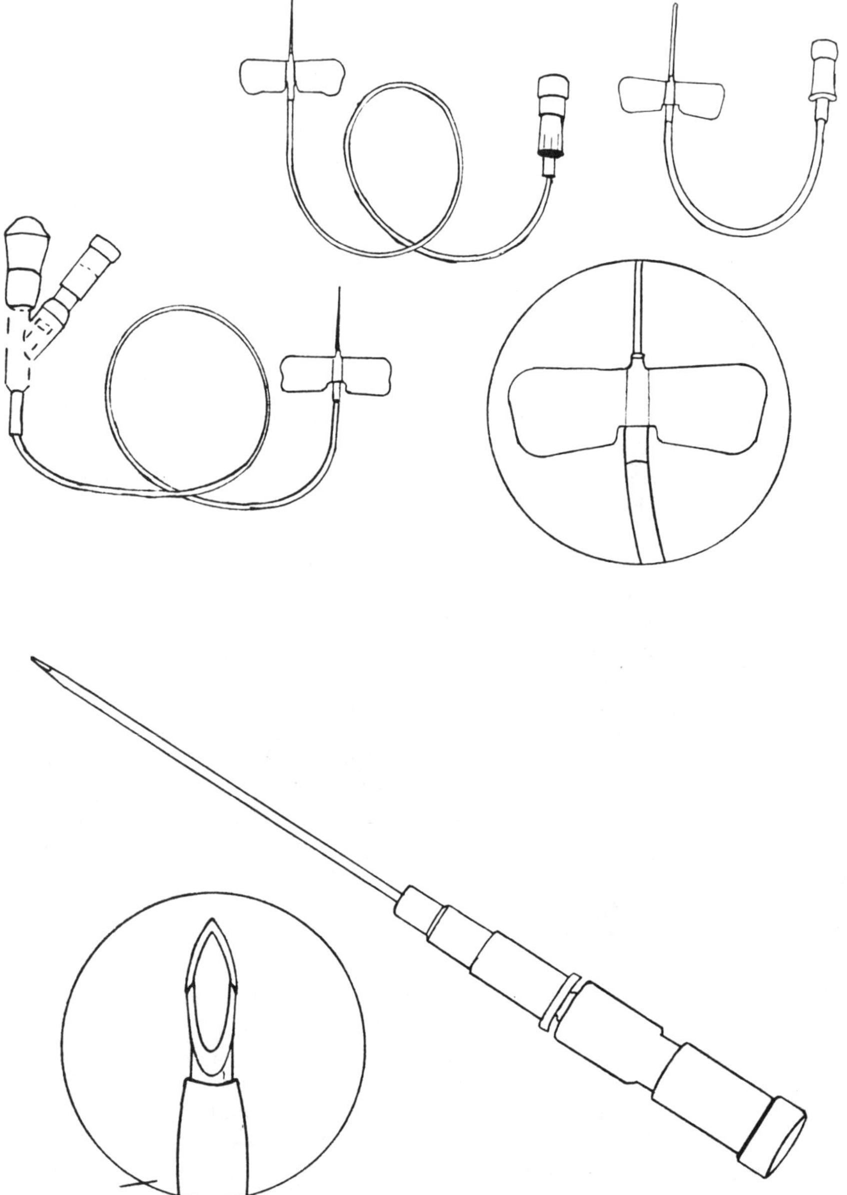

Figure 27 Over the past few years the winged infusion set has been slowly replaced by the catheter-over-needle.

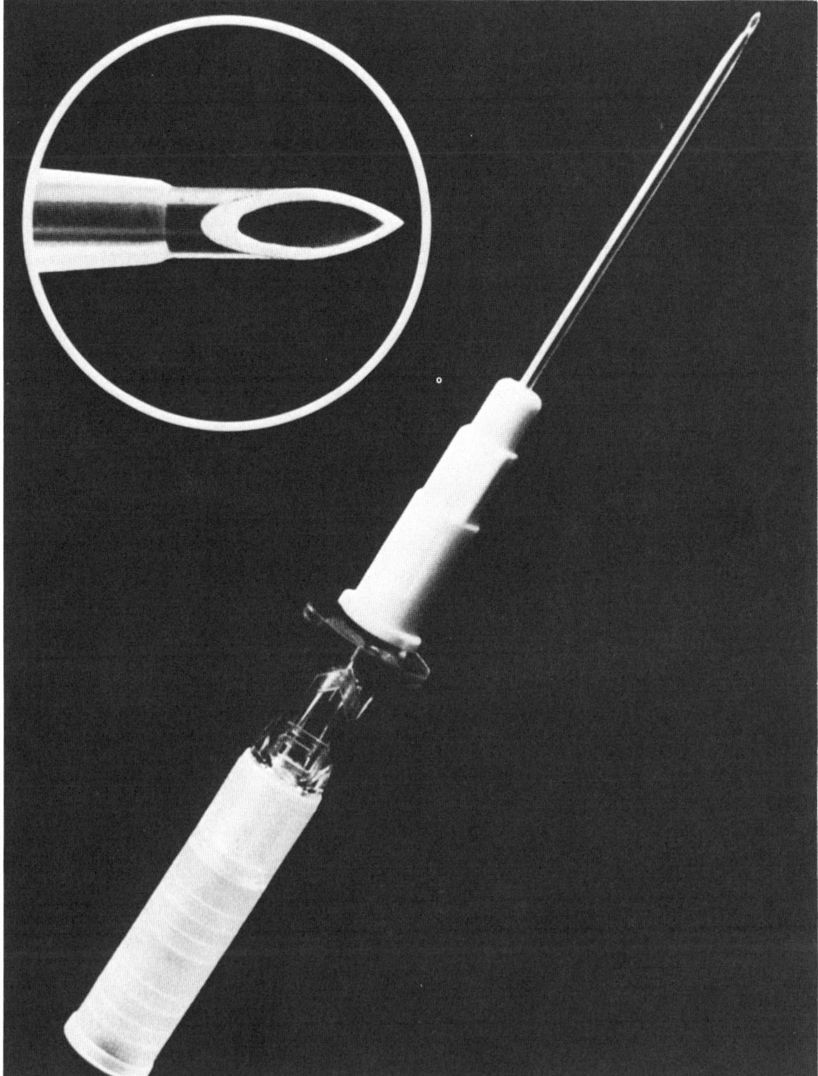

Figure 28 The actual catheter is only a small part of the device delivered to the customer.

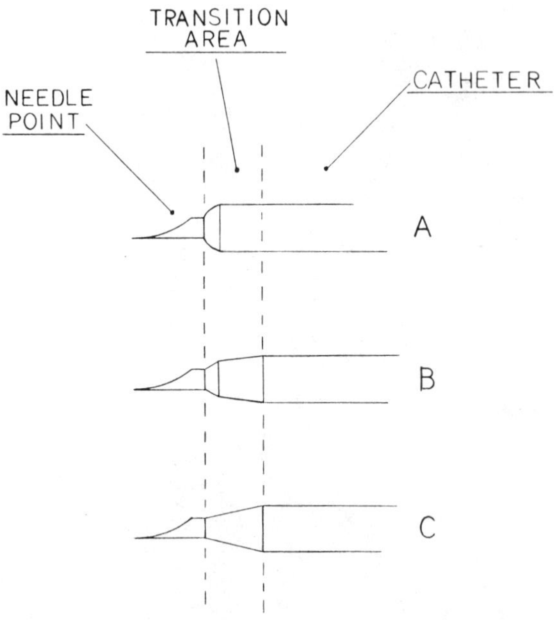

Figure 29 The three designs of the transition area shown above represent the major designs in the market today. Catheter A has a blunt transition area while C has a long feathered edge. Catheter B utilizes the best features of each.

receipt, the pointed cannulae are handled in bundles until they reach the first assembly operation, which is insert molding. There the cannulae are inserted in molds or "tools," as they are referred to in the trade, and have the hub molded to the blunt end of the cannula. The assembly is referred to as a needle assembly from that point.

They are then placed in a protective carrier and moved to the next operation. Meanwhile, the plastic catheter material has been checked for the correct length and also sent to a subassembly area to receive its hub. This is the second area of technology. The technology to put the hub on the catheter varies from insert molding through mechanical wedging with a separate piece, as can be seen in Figure 31. Once the hub is in place, the subassembly is moved into the main assembly area. The bevel on the catheter can be put on the catheter either before or after the catheter subassembly is matched with the needle assembly. The finished needle-catheter assembly is then placed in a sheath and sent to the packaging area (the third area of technology). The finished assembly is then placed in a sterile blister or pouch, boxed, and placed in a carton for sterilization and shipment.

3. *Control*

Control begins with the cannula or needle vendor who must provide analytical identification of the stainless steel used in the cannula as part of the package sent to the device manufacturer. Upon receipt of the needles at the plant, the incoming QC group tests the material according to the

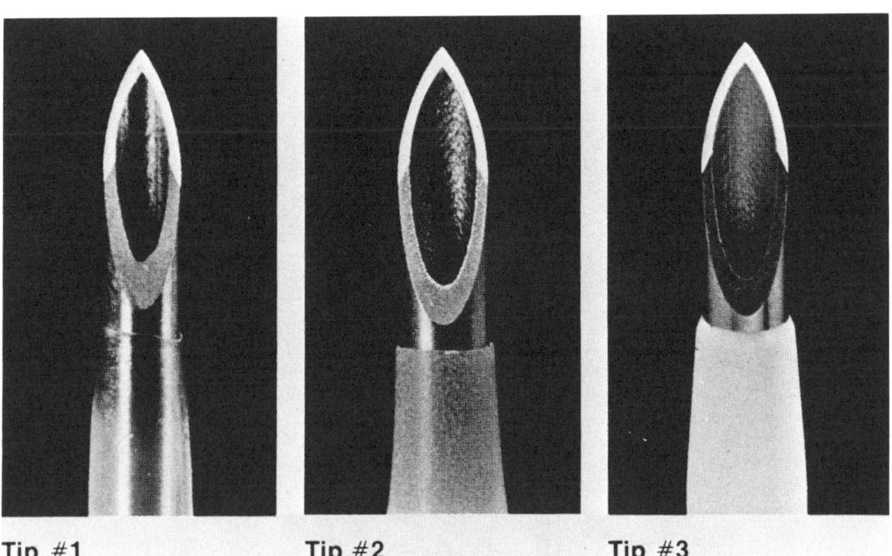

Figure 30 The bevel on the catheter tip is important and will vary according to the vendor's preference.

specification requirements. Sharpness of the point is usually checked according to MIL-STD-414, which allows for points that are too sharp as well as not sharp enough. The plastic used in the parts is identified both generically and by trade name by the parts vendor. If the parts meet all dimensional and chemical requirements, they are moved into the acceptable stock for manufacturing use. During the assembly process the subassemblies are checked after each operation against the requirements in the QA or QC manual before passing to the next operation. The final assembly is placed in the sheath, packaged, and sterilized. After sterilization, a statistical sample is pulled from the finished lot and checked. The catheter-needle assembly is checked for penetration values of the needle, catheter needle interface (the bevel), and value for the insertion of the shaft. The needle-catheter separation force is also checked. If the value is too low, the assembly can separate in transit. If it is too high, it will be hard to separate at the time of use.

B. Procedural Kits and Trays

1. *Design*

Kits and trays offer a unique challenge to the designer. The first challenge is in the selection of the procedure for which the tray is designed. Selection is based on the number of such procedures done through the year and

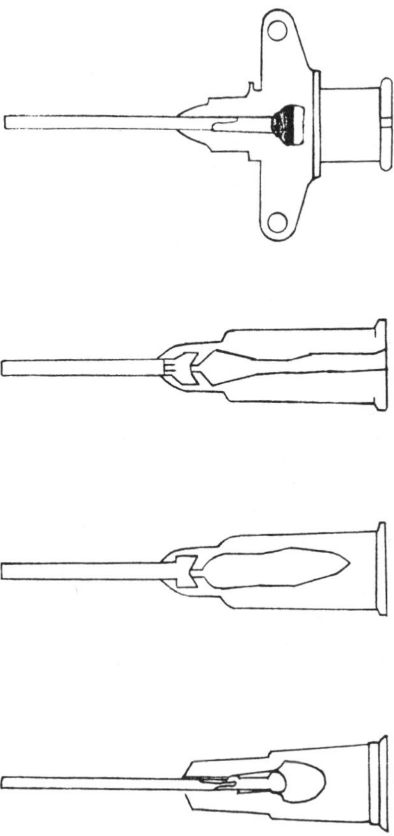

Figure 31 The method of attaching the catheter to the hub varies from mechanical wedging through insert molding.

how much time can be saved by having a preassembled kit or tray for the practitioner's use. The complexity of kits vary from the simple (Fig. 32) to the very complex multilayered unit, such as a spinal anesthesia tray (Fig. 33). The selection of the materials and their suppliers offers an interesting challenge. In the more complex kits there are considerations of dating the contents since some items, such as drugs (as in the anesthesia kit), have expiration dates. Whenever possible the most expensive of the dated items should be the limiting factor in dating the kit.

The tray is laid out to promote efficiency as well as provide the hospital personnel or physician with a complete array of the necessary components to perform the procedure so the hospital does not have to take the time and effort to assemble a sterile tray from their own stock. The contents are laid out in order of use, usually left to right. In case of procedures with a preparation procedure, the two major procedures are enclosed in the same package but are separated in trays or subpackages. In Figure 34 the preparation deck fits over the drug deck, providing protection of the drug deck while the patient is being prepared. When the preparation deck is removed, the drug deck is exposed. Color-coded ampuls can be used to allow the user to confirm the ampul selection at a glance, and the tray

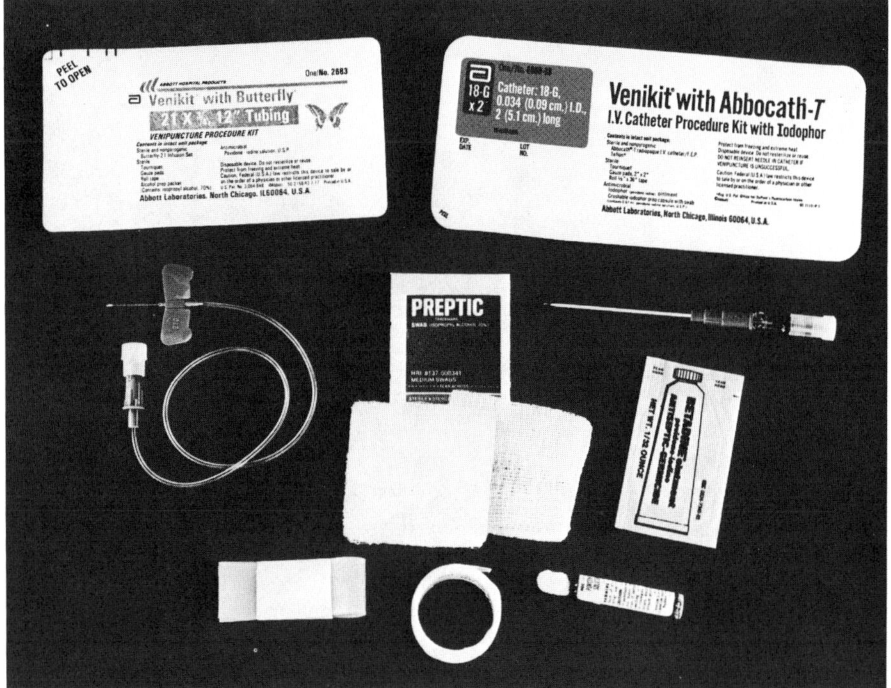

Figure 32 A simple venipuncture kit contains all the supplies necessary to place a catheter or needle in the patient's vein.

should have adequate finger room to allow easy grasp of the ampul. The ampul wells can be designed to allow the opened ampul to stand upright with the trough serving as a handy compartment in which to lay the filled syringe. Because of the layout, the user can proceed, step by step, without passing his or her hands over the opened ampuls.

2. *Manufacture*

Most tray suppliers are the manufacturer of one or more of the drugs, but the majority of the components in a kit or tray will be purchased from an outside vendor. The assembly operation for a kit or tray is primarily a packaging operation. However, it still goes through the previously described tollgate assembly.

3. *Control*

The generic manufacturing control system shown in Figure 35 holds true for the manufacture of kits and trays. In kits and trays another element has been introduced, expiration dating. Most sets and devices do not have expiration dates, but since trays contain drugs that do have expiration dates, the QA or QC function must pay special attention to the dating of the components used. If two or more drugs are used, the component with the nearest expiration date sets the expiration date for the tray assembly. Beyond this added requirement, the kit or tray is controlled like any other set or device.

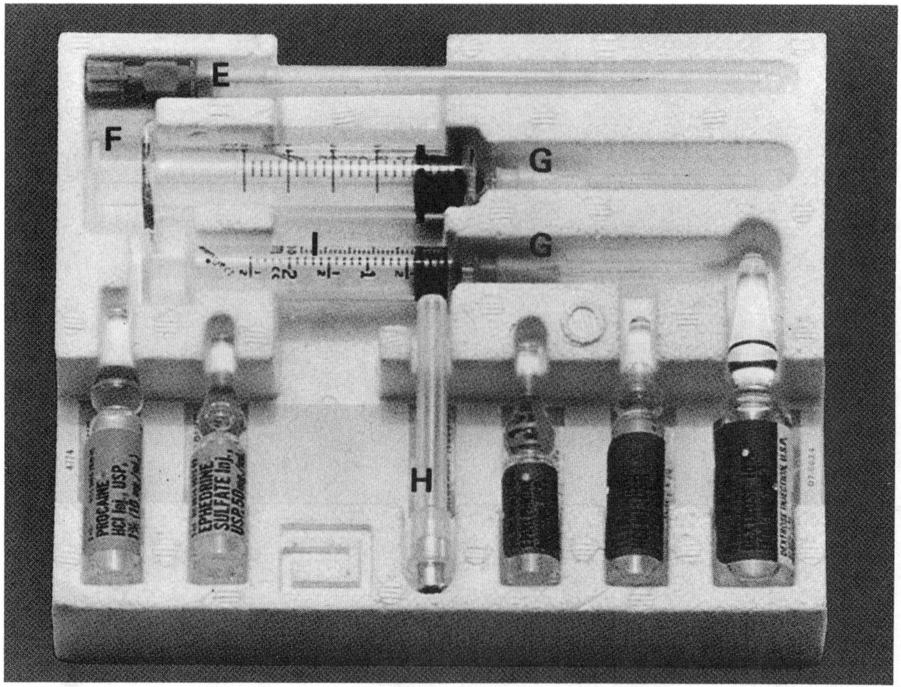

Figure 33 The upper or Prep Deck will contain drapes and sponges while the lower Drug Deck illustrated will contain the necessary drugs and accessories for the procedure. E is the spinal needle, F is the drug administration syringe, G are detachable needles on each syringe, and H is an introducer needle. The drugs for the procedure are placed in the order of use in the tray.

C. Intravenous Sets

1. *General Purpose*

Design

The designer of general-purpose sets, such as those in Figure 36, must consider such basic matters as dimensions. What length is most acceptable for general floor use in the hospital? Most manufacturers have standardized on-set lengths between 75 and 79 in. What are the minimum features the set must have to gain acceptance for general floor use? The more basic sets are found to contain a bottle or bag piercing pin, a sight chamber to allow the counting of drops, tubing somewhere in the neighborhood of 0.100 in. internal diameter, a flow control clamp, a Y reseal to allow emergency entry, and a male needle adapter to connect to the venipuncture device. With minor variations in tubing length and the possible inclusion of an extra Y site, all general-purpose administration sets will fit this description (Fig. 37).

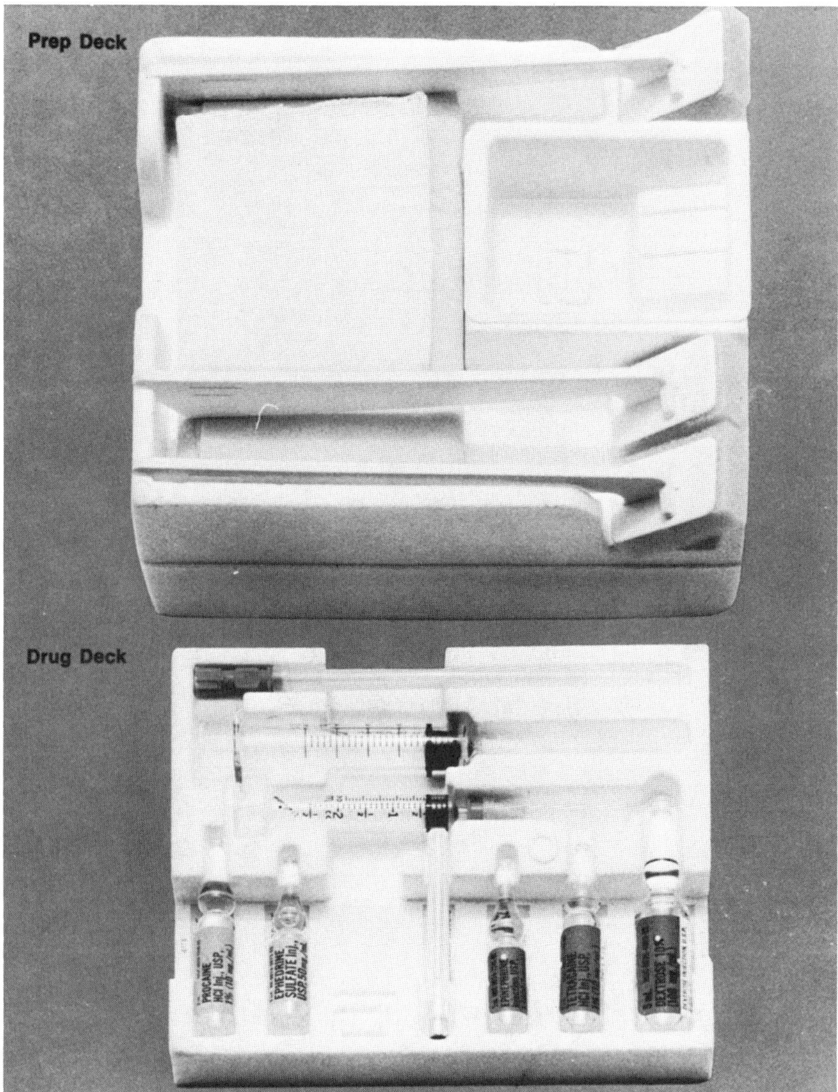

Figure 34 Packaging and presentation are important in a kit.

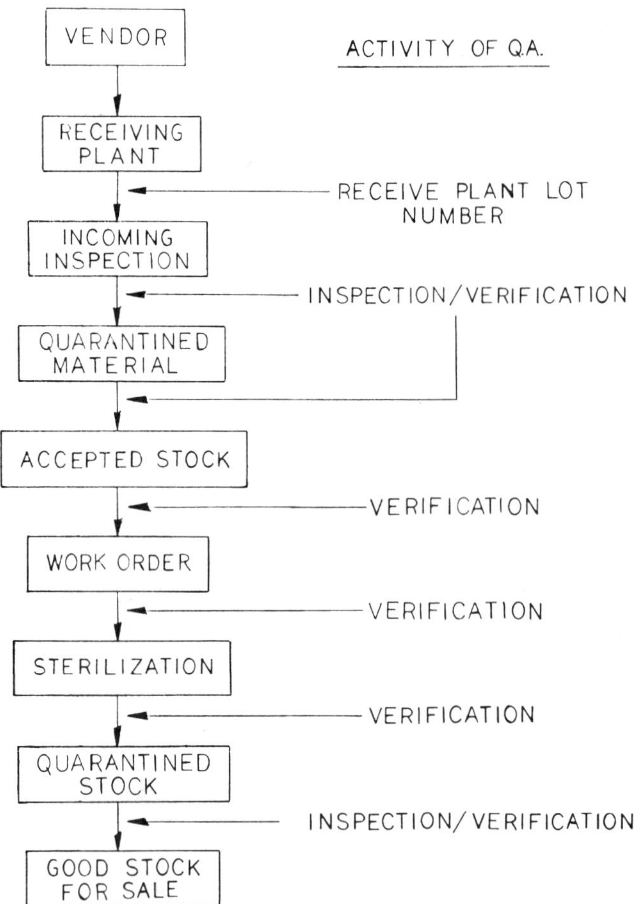

Figure 35 Kits and trays are subject to the same controls as the sets and devices during manufacturing.

Manufacture

The general-purpose administration set is one of the simpler sets to manufacture, with the possible exception of the extension set (Fig. 38). It lends itself well to straight-line assembly. The tubing can be cut to the required lengths and introduced directly into the assembly operation. The piercing pin assembly can be made as a subassembly or assembled directly on the line.

Control

The generic QA-QC flow diagram (Fig. 39) is an example of this type of operation. The actual test procedure and equipment required for control of the process can be minimal, requiring only a pull tester for tubing-to-component solvent seals and flow test equipment to assure there is no blockage or leakage in the set. Beyond the ability to do sterility testing, little more is required.

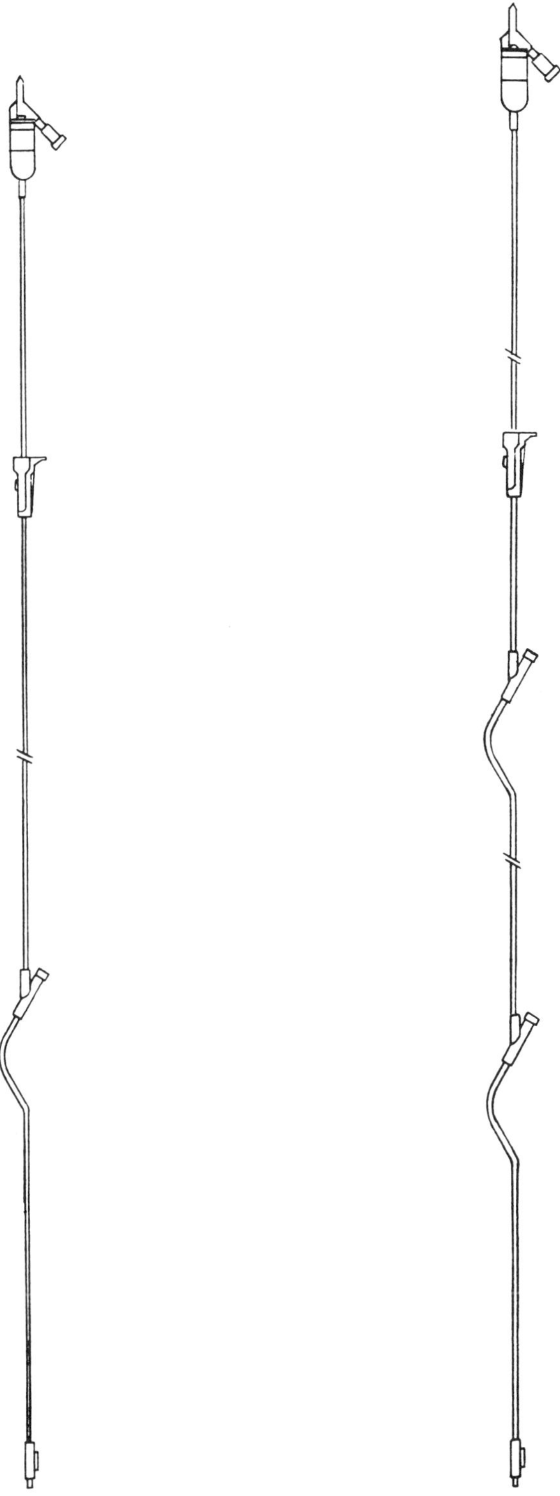

Figure 36 The utilization of a general-purpose set is in many cases determined by where the user wants to hang the IV fluid container.

Figure 37 General-purpose set configurations vary within narrow limits which allows minimum changes in an assembly line operation between sets.

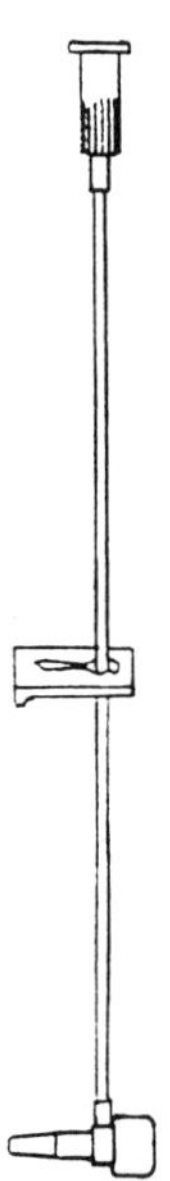

Figure 38 Simple sets such as extension sets can be manufactured on short uncomplicated assembly lines.

2. Controlled Volume Sets

Design

In the administration of IV fluids, there are times when the control of the amount of fluid administered is critical, as in the case of some of the more potent drugs and in intermittent additive therapy. Since the market needs are diverse, the designer is forced to address a specific need. Over the years the controlled-volume burette set has evolved in a variety of sizes, ranging from a 50-ml to a 250-ml burette, with the most common sizes the 100- and 150-ml burette sets. Despite the large number of configurations available, they have a number of common features (Fig. 40). Primary among these is the safety feature of the automatic shutoff. After the desired amount of fluid has been administered, the automatic shutoff prevents air from entering the lower fluid pathway and minimizes any chance for air embolism.

Manufacture

The critical part of the manufacturing process for these sets is the assembly of the calibrated burette. In most cases the automatic shutoff is assembled to the lower lid before the sight chamber or cylinder is added. The assembly of the cylinder to the lid is done in two steps, with time in between to allow the solvent adhesive to dry.

Control

All the normal checks and controls explained in the assembly control of the general-purpose set apply, as well as some specialized testing, such as functionality of the automatic shutoff. After final assembly the automatic shutoff feature must be tested. This is a destructive test, since only IV fluid will give an accurate test of the shutoff feature.

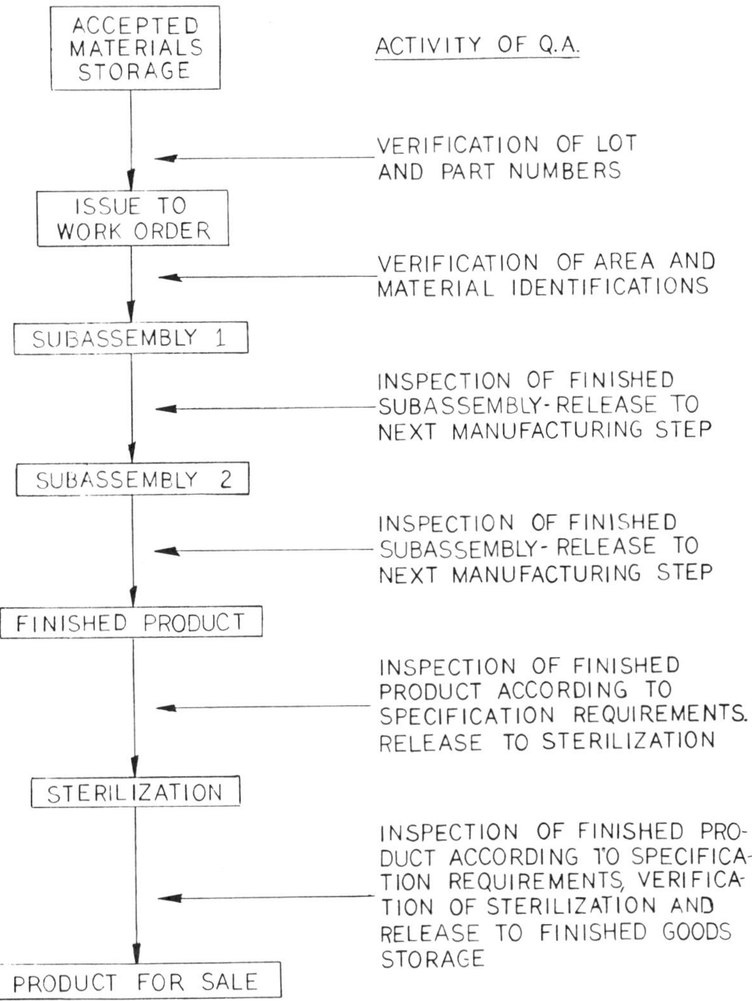

Figure 39 Again the QA organization plays an important role in the manufacturing operation.

3. *Blood Administration Sets*

Design

Blood sets present another set of design problems due to the characteristics of the fluid administered through them. The blood can vary from fresh whole blood to packed red cells. The temperature can vary from ambient room temperature to cold (just out of the cooler in emergency situations). Because of the presence of the red blood cells and protein in the plasma, the fluid reacts as a non-Newtonian fluid (Fig. 41). The blood cells themselves are also fragile and should be traumatized as little as possible. The longer cells or whole blood is stored before use, the more aggregation is possible. For this reason blood sets are required to have a gross filter as part of the design. Filter porosities used for this application

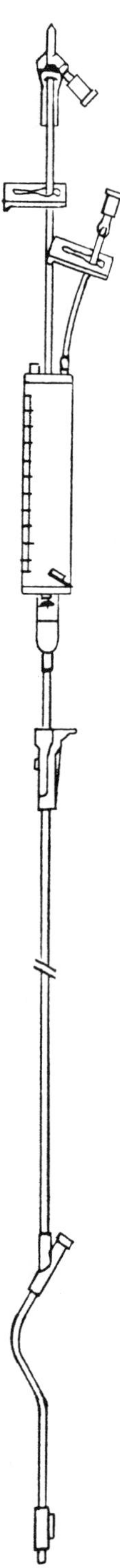

Figure 40 The burette set above displays the features usually found in this type of set. It has a calibrated cylinder, a controlled vent to the cylinder, and an automatic shut-off feature.

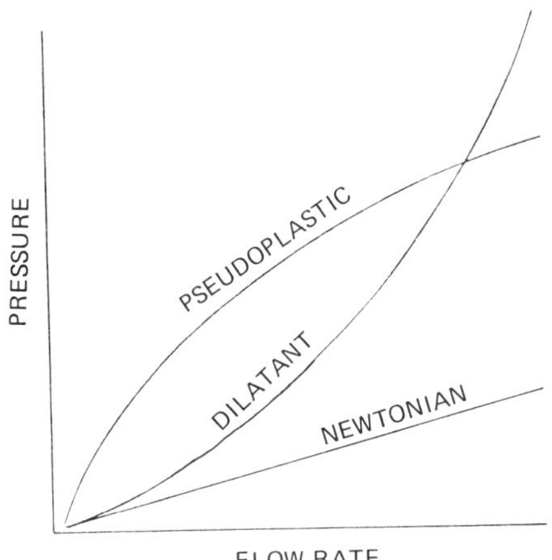

Figure 41 The fluids administered through a set can vary from a Newtonian fluid, such as saline, to a non-Newtonian fluid, such as blood. Designers must take this into consideration during the initial design phase.

range from 170 to 210 μm. The sight chamber can be a rigid cylinder (Fig. 42a) or flexible (Fig. 42b). Both designs reduce the likelihood of cell damage when priming and running. The bag-piercing pin is specifically designed to fit blood bags, not IV bags. Some sets are made to have the added capability of use with parenteral fluids as well as blood. In those cases the blood pins are further identified by a colored protective cover.

Manufacture

These sets are manufactured for the most part like any other set in the plant. Special consideration must be given to the assembly of the filter assembly. In most cases the filter goes through a 100% visual inspection for rips, tears, or missing threads in the woven filter material. The 100% inspection process is more frequently associated with the more complex sets since in many cases defects are easily seen but hard to pick up without a complicated test fixture or procedure. As an added step, the process is qualified as well.

Control

Quality control for these sets is similar to the general-purpose set since, unlike the membrane filter-containing sets, there is no easy way to check the integrity of the blood filter in the final product other than visually and by total destruction of the sight chamber in order to get at the filter. For this reason, the primary control rests with the process validation and testing procedures associated with the incoming filters.

D. Electronic Flow Control Sets and Devices

1. *Design*

The infusion devices were first introduced into the critical care units but have gradually been introduced into the rest of the hospital. They have found use in areas requiring a more accurate and consistent flow control

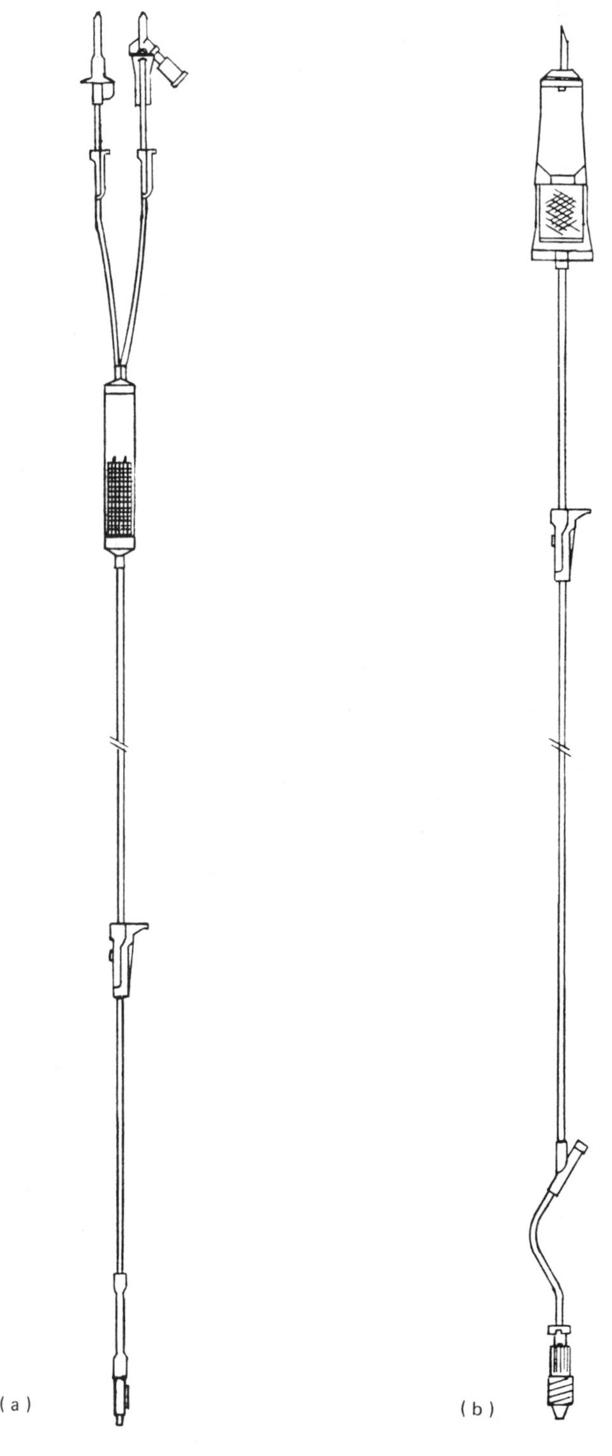

Figure 42 (a) The rigid cylinder has long been a feature with some blood sets and is similar to burette sets in that feature. (b) There are a growing number of users for the sets containing the flexible sight chambers.

than can be achieved with conventional sets. Sets required for electronic flow control must be matched with electromechanical equipment, which is part of this medical area. The electronic flow control devices cover drop counters, which, from their name, only count the number of drops going through a drip chamber, controllers, which act as electronic clamps, working by gravity but exerting no pressure, and volumetric pumps, which pump accurate amounts of fluid to the patient. The type of set used in each situation varies in minor but significant detail. Drop counters can be used on almost any set currently on the market. The only requirement is that the drop detector fit on the piercing pin flange and is in position to count the falling drops (Fig. 43). Controllers have the same drop detector requirement and have the added requirement of having tubing compatible with the clamping of the controller. The controller (Fig. 44) has two arms or pincers that close down on the tubing for flow control. The hardness of the tubing has a direct effect on the ease of maintaining the flow rate. The softer the tubing, the more the tubing "flows" after the clamp action has stopped, leading to inaccuracies. For this reason the manufacturers use the harder tubing if the set is being designed specifically to be used with a controller. Most sets can and are used with controllers with success. The most complex and specialized is the pump system. The electromechanical pump driver (Fig. 45) has a matched set that works only with a manufacturer's specific driver. For this reason, manufacturers have made available sets for nearly every fluid delivery procedure, and all are designed to operate in the gravity flow configuration as well. The systems are virtually all-fluid administration systems that can precisely deliver most parenteral fluids, including electrolytes, irrigation fluids, blood, drugs, and nutritionals. The pumps in the set operate in the same manner regardless of the actual design. The pump is filled from one side to a specific volume and

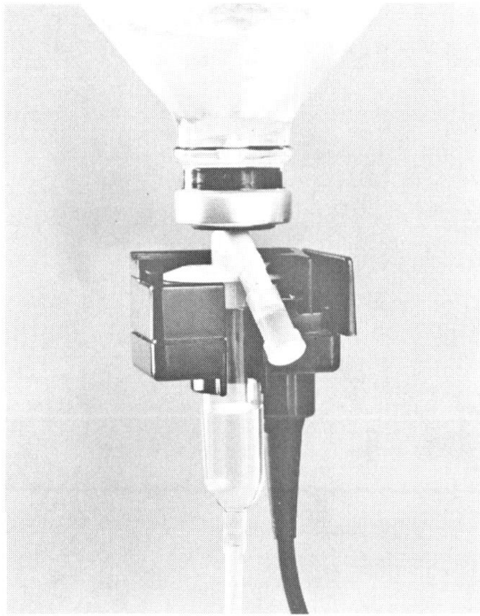

Figure 43 A drop counter takes over the laborious task of counting the individual drops and relaying the information to the electronics of the instrument where it is converted to rate and possibly volume.

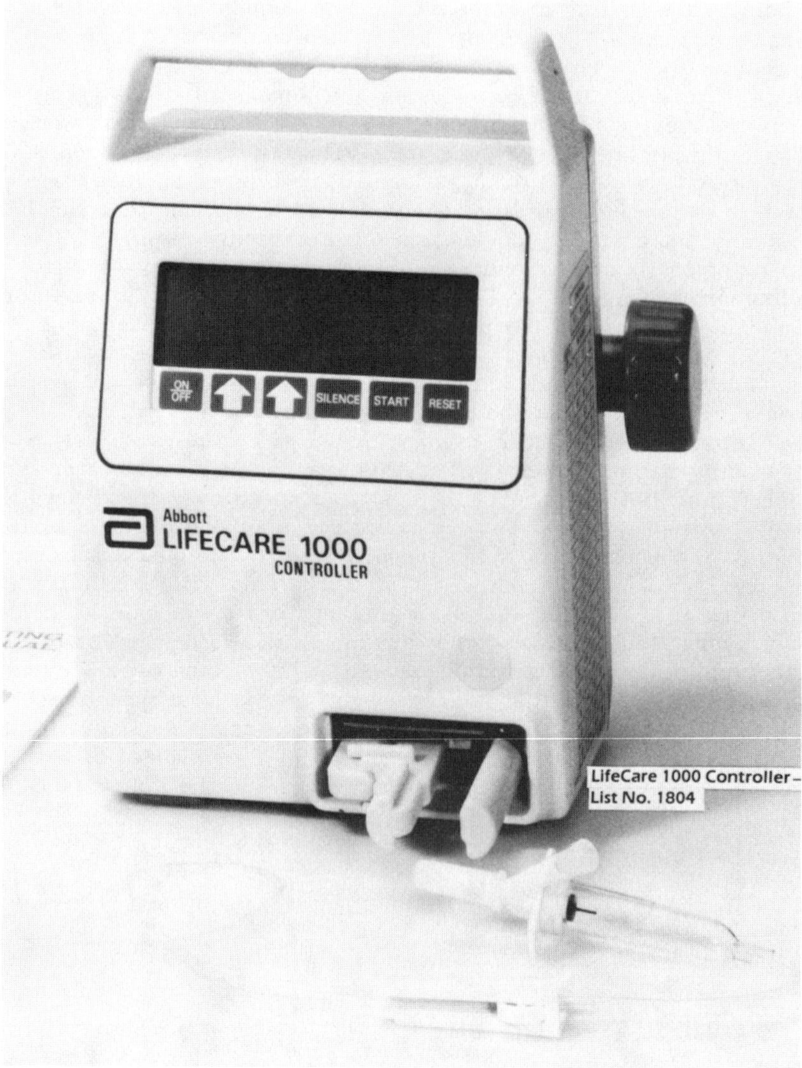

Figure 44 Controllers are among the least complicated of the electronic flow control devices in the market place. The two arms in the above illustration act as an electronic flow control clamp.

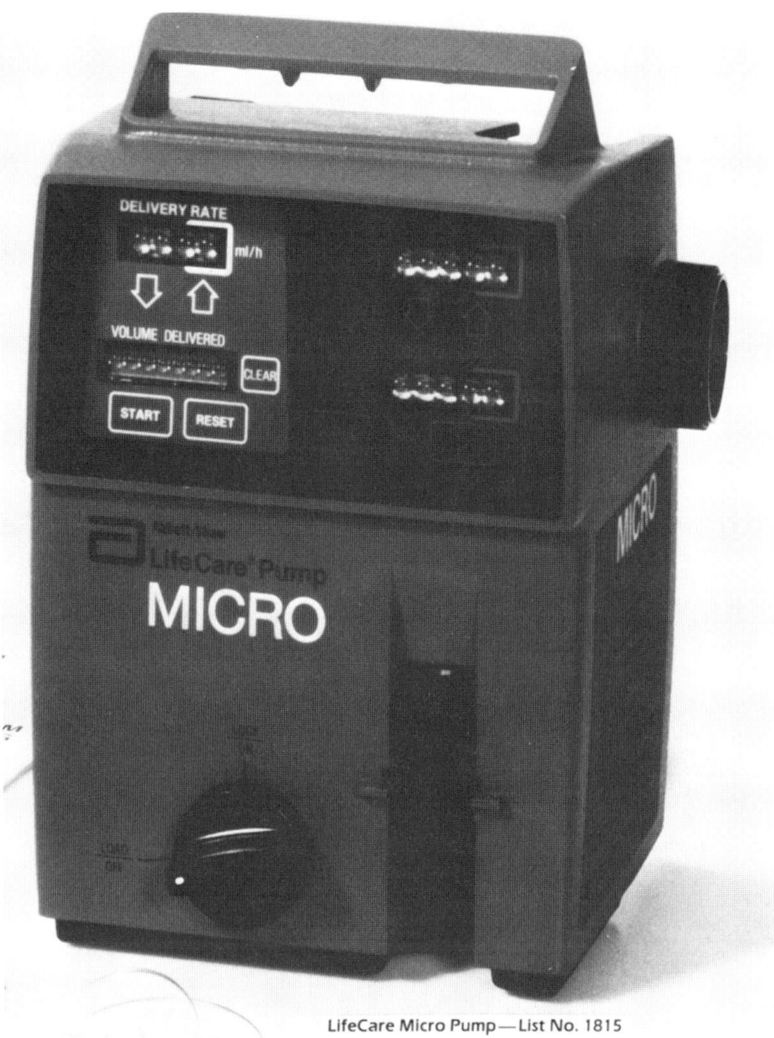

LifeCare Micro Pump—List No. 1815

Figure 45 The driver or pump for the system concept offers many features such as programable delivery rates and other information of interest to the user. It also requires a dedicated set for operation.

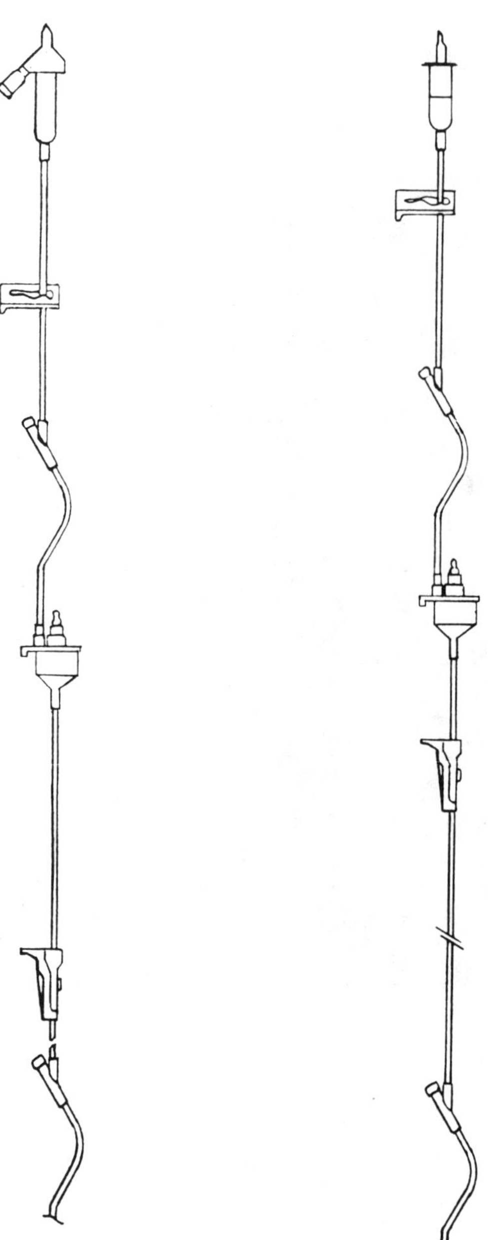

Figure 46 The pump sets differ from the other sets primarily through the inclusion of the pump itself.

expresses it out the other side. The chamber then refills. The number of strokes determines the actual volume to be delivered. The set configuration will be the same as a general IV set except it will contain the pump in the line (Fig. 46).

The "hardware" in the system is much more complicated. The electromechanical driver for a pump system, for instance, may have a large number of features. It can be run on AC or a battery or have the capability to use either. Some models will automatically switch to battery operation in the case of power interruption and can maintain a delivery rate of 125 ml/hr over an 8-hr period on battery power. Most models have adjustable delivery rates with a display of cumulative volume delivered. All drivers have some form of air infusion prevention. Some have detectors; others have been designed to pump fluid only and cannot pump air (air disabling). A variety of detector alarm indicators are available—audible, visual, or nursing station monitor. Some drivers automatically drop back into a keep vein open (KVO) status in the alarm condition.

Unlike many of the sets discussed earlier, the pump sets must be matched to the compatible driver from the manufacturer.

2. *Manufacture*

Manufacture of the sets for this segment of the market is similar to manufacture of the standard sets of similar configuration. In many cases they will be made on the same assembly lines. The drivers, on the other hand, present a completely different type of manufacturing. The regulations and requirements controlling the electronics industry are considerably different than those controlling the sets and devices industry. They overlap in the voluntary standard now being put together by AAMI entitled "Infusion devices." This standard covers both mechanical and electromechanical infusion devices intended for general hospital use.

The state of the art continues to advance, especially in the area of electronics. Couple this with the increasing number of biocompatible polymers, and potential future sets and devices become almost limitless. There is a move toward miniaturization of sets and devices to make the patient more comfortable. Trends also indicate a move to intermittent therapy (connecting the patient to bottles, bags, and pumps only when administering the therapy) as a means of making the patient mobile and leading to less nursing attention since the fluids or drugs are administered over a shorter period of time. These trends necessitate the design of new sets and devices to meet the new requirements, but the methods of designing, manufacturing, and control will not change drastically.

BIBLIOGRAPHY

1. A. L. Plumer, *Principles and Practice of Intravenous Therapy*. Little, Brown, Boston, 1982.
2. Nursing 80 Photobook Series, *Managing I.V. Therapy*. Intermed Communications, Inc., Horsham, Pennsylvania, 19044.
3. Military Standards. U.S. Government Printing Office. MIL-STD-105D, Sampling Procedures and Tables for Inspection by Attributes, April 29, 1963. MIL-STD-414.

4. Publications of the Association for the Advancement of Medical Instrumentation, 1901 N. Ft. Myer Drive, Suite 602, Arlington, VA 22209-1699.
   General-interest publications:

   a. Standard for Blood Transfusion Microfilters
   b. Standard for Autotransfusion Devices
   c. Standard for Hemodialysis Systems
   d. Water Requirements for Dialysis

   Technology assessment reports:

   a. Inhospital Ethylene Oxide Sterilization
   b. Hospital Electrical Safety
   c. Medical Technology for the Neonate

   Recommended practices:

   a. Reuse of Hemodialyzers
   b. Good Hospital Practice: Steam Sterilization and Sterility Assurance
   c. Process Control Guidelines for Gamma Radiation Sterilization of Medical Devices

5. Manufacture, Packaging, Storage and Installation of Medical Devices, Federal Register, Friday, July 21, 1978, Part II.

11
Quality Assurance for Parenteral Devices

Carl W. Bruch*

Skyland Scientific Services, Inc., Belgrade, Montana

I. CONTROL TESTS FOR THE MATERIALS USED IN PARENTERAL DEVICES

Significant advances have been made in the development of biocompatible materials for use in parenteral devices, i.e., those devices that have contact with parenteral fluids, blood, and/or internal tissues other than the alimentary canal or other mucosa. Currently, there are no officially promulgated rapid toxicity screening tests for materials used in parenteral devices. Although the development of tests for biological compatibility of device materials has progressed during the past decade, knowledge of the availability of these tests by manufacturers and their acceptance for regulatory purposes has not kept abreast of current biological assessment capability. Any material to be used as a part or whole of a parenteral device should function as intended without bringing about short- or long-term adverse effects. Neither the material itself nor any leachable constituents should cause adverse local or systemic responses. As a result of the Medical Device Amendments of 1976 to the Food, Drug and Cosmetic (FD&C) Act, most device manufacturers are aware that adequate biological tests and studies should be undertaken to demonstrate the suitability of any materials used in the manufacture of parenteral devices.

The tests most commonly employed for assessment of biocompatibility of materials are those for "Biological tests—plastics" [1] of the *U.S. Pharmacopeia* (USP). In general, these tests are intended for product contact surfaces, but used alone they are not entirely suitable for the thorough evaluation of the biocompatibility of an implant intended to be placed and left within the body for a period of time beyond 7 days.

The Food and Drug Administration (FDA) has been active over the past 10 years with academia and industry in the evolution of both in vitro and

---

**Current affiliation*: St. Jude Medical, Inc., St. Paul, Minnesota

Table 1 Suggested Toxicity Assays for Device Materials: Short-Term (<30 Days) Internal Devices

In vitro toxicity

- Cellular effects
- Organ culture
- White blood cells: count, function

In vivo toxicity: 90-day subchronic

Immune (sensitization): Dermal (guinea pig maximization)

Gene toxicity

- Gene mutation
- In vitro repair
- Cell transformation
- Dominant lethal (mouse) or recessive lethal (*Drosophila*)

in vivo tests (to be noted in the following section) that would more adequately characterize the long-term compatibility of plastics and other materials in the human body. Table 1 is indicative of the range of these tests and their application to short-term parenteral devices, i.e., devices within the parenterum for less than 30 days. Some of the more rapid tests may be used on a batch-by-batch basis to assure that supplies of plastics and other materials maintain suitable characteristics for the manufacture of parenteral devices. Sufficient routine biological testing of each batch of materials for parenteral devices is necessary to provide assurance that satisfactory quality (material safety) is maintained through every production lot.

A. Formulation Checks and Chemical Assays

Specifications must be developed for the raw materials and/or components used to fabricate subassemblies or the total parenteral device. If it is necessary to procure a raw material or a component from a vendor who will not or cannot provide batch control or identity, at least batch identification should be assigned on the basis of an order or shipment. Every effort should be made to obtain and document as much information from the vendor as possible regarding the ingredients and chemical assays for raw materials and components. When such vendor certifications cannot be obtained, it is essential that the parenteral device manufacturer develop a set of chemical test procedures to show that the basic raw materials and components meet the original requirements specified in the development of a particular plastic or other material for use in the parenteral device. Chemical profile screens, usually to include infrared or ultraviolet (UV) analyses, should be established so that the uniformity of raw materials and components going into the manufacture of a parenteral device can be properly controlled.

B. Assurance of Required Physical Properties

The manufacturer of a parenteral device should establish the nature of required physical properties and stability characteristics for that device. If the device is composed of different materials united as subassemblies to form the completed device, then the physical properties of the subassemblies should be measured by adequate physical and chemical tests. Examples of these properties are light transmission, tensile strength, flexibility, and rigidity. In addition, the USP [2] contains procedures for plastics, which assess the nonvolatile residue, residue on ignition, heavy metals, and buffering capacity. Most parenteral device manufacturers will have modified these USP procedures to assure that the final parenteral device will have immediate use characteristics and long-term stability to properly serve the function intended for that device.

C. Toxicological Safety Tests

1. Basic Toxicological Tests to Assure Safety of Device Material in the Development of a New Medical Device

Any new device material should undergo a battery of in vitro and in vivo tests to assess both the short-term and long-term biocompatibility of that material when in contact with body tissues. For parenteral devices that are used to deliver blood or blood derivatives or various types of parenteral solutions, the following types of in vitro investigations are recommended: cytotoxicity tests including either agar overlay, direct cell contact, minimum essential medium (MEM) elution, or inhibition of cell growth; blood compatibility, including tests for hemolysis; and mutagenic screening tests, such as the Ames test [3] or the mouse lymphoma assay [4]. The following types of in vivo investigations should be conducted on both the materials and the finished parenteral device: use of selected eluates (leachates) to assess acute systemic toxicity, intracutaneous toxicity, and sensitization; and implantation either subcutaneously or intramuscularly to assess short-term material compatibility. The details of such testing procedures are beyond the goals for this chapter, but such information can be obtained by writing the Center for Devices and Radiological Health (CDRH) of the FDA [5].

2. Routine Toxicity Tests for Batch-to-Batch Release of Devices

The section in the USP on transfusion and infusion assemblies [6] refers to the use of a "mouse safety test" to assess the batch-to-batch release of parenteral devices as nontoxic. However, this procedure is now outmoded as a demonstration of the basic safety of parenteral plastic materials. The following critical evaluation is presented to show parenteral device manufacturers and testing laboratories for materials used in such devices that the USP mouse safety test is unable to detect low levels of toxic leachables from plastic materials.

a. The test is similar to a mouse LD_{50} procedure, except that the number of mice required for the test is not adequate to assess the statistical significance.
b. Transfusion and infusion assemblies and similar types of medical devices usually consist of various lengths of plastic tubing and various molded plastic components (fitments) used primarily for making connections to other equipment. For purposes of this critique, it is assumed that the parenteral devices would have an approximate fluid path volume of 25 ml, i.e., the volume of rinse solution.

c. If this volume of extracting solution is diluted to 250 ml, a 10:1 (v/v) dilution of any leachable substance occurs.
d. Based on a required test dosage of 0.5 ml per mouse, this dose is equivalent to 25 ml/kg.
e. In my experience, most extractable substances from plastics have LD_{50} values in mice greater than 100 mg/kg. For a 20-g mouse, this would require 2 mg to be extracted and injected for an LD_{50} level to be achieved.
f. For 2 mg of extractant to be delivered to the mouse, the 250-ml extracting volume would have to remove 1000 mg of extractant from the device (4 mg/ml concentration). Thus, at least 1 g of material would have to be extracted into the extracting volume or 2% of the total weight of a 50-g plastic device.
g. Since our experience indicates the usual concentration of chemicals from plastic is in the parts per billion or in the very low parts per million range (<10 ppm), the insensitivity of the mouse safety test becomes apparent.
h. Based upon the historical ppm range of extraction concentration noted above, the concentration in the volume of solution used in the USP mouse safety test for extraction would be 10 μg/ml in the worse case stated (10 ppm). Dilution caused by the addition of 0.9% NaCl solution to bring the volume to 250 ml would further reduce the concentration to 1 μg/ml, thereby providing a dose to the mouse of 0.5 μg, or 25 μg/kg.
i. Based on these calculations and the known LD_{50} values for the ingredients of plastic formulations, it is highly improbable that a plastic constituent would be so toxic as to cause an LD_{50} response in a mouse. Conversely, modest amounts of moderately toxic materials can be extracted and never detected in a mouse LD_{50} assay.

Any material that has passed a leachable extraction test as described in Section I.C.1 would have a higher degree of safety than a material that has passed only the USP mouse safety test. If the manufacturer maintains controls over the plastic formulation through an eluate test or a cytoxicity test, there is no need to run the USP mouse safety test. Furthermore, it is recommended that manufacturers use in vitro cytoxicity tests (agar overlay or MEM elution are most common) or blood hemolysis to assess the batch-to-batch safety of the plastic materials. These in vitro tests can be used as a more rapid and sensitive toxicity screen for any possible changes in plastic formulations purchased from vendors. Thus, parenteral device manufacturers have the flexibility to use any of several methods to assess the lack of toxicity of the plastic materials purchased in bulk quantities for use with parenteral devices.

II. PROCEDURES FOR ASSURING STERILITY OF PARENTERAL DEVICES

Sterility is classically defined as an absolute condition, i.e., the complete destruction or removal of all forms of life. The sterility of parenteral devices should be assured to the extent that the probability of microbial contamination or survival is one in a million (10^{-6}) per item, or less. To estimate the state of sterility by USP finished product testing [7] as an absolute condition for all items in a lot is not reliable, if indeed it is possible. The following discussion will give several ways in which a more direct mechanism of assuring sterility on a batch-by-batch basis can be derived. Several satisfactory approaches exist, but manufacturers are encouraged to use and develop different and improved methodologies. The following discussion should be used, therefore, as a general guideline to the types of necessary data. A key thrust is that the manufacturer have some knowledge of the resistance of microbial contamination on parenteral devices to the sterilization process, either as D values or as the quantity of resistant survivors to subprocess doses of sterilant.

In this analysis, terminal sterilization of devices in their shipping packages will be approached as a probability function, which is susceptible to measurement in physical and chemical terms. A D value (time to kill 90% of the organisms) is defined on the basis that the death of microbes usually follows first-order reaction kinetics [8–10]. The use of the D value allows a theoretical calculation of the probability of survivors from a terminal sterilization process.

The term "sterile" has been compromised in that the term covers a wide range of probabilities of survivors on products, i.e., from 10^{-2} to 10^{-9} probability of a survivor per item (PSI). The suggestion by Campbell of the Canadian Health Protection Branch [11] that the word *sterile* be modified by the addition of a microbiological survivor index (MSI) has merit. The MSI is a positive term derived by taking the reciprocal of the logarithm for the probability of a survivor per item (PSI) from a sterilization process. The Association for Advancement of Medical Instrumentation (AAMI), in its "Guidelines for gamma radiation sterilization of medical devices," uses the term "sterility assurance level" (SAL) to similarly assess the probability of a survivor per item (PSI) from the sterilization process [12].

A. Sources of Biological Contamination (Bioburden) During Manufacture

The world of microorganisms is one of rapid reproduction leading to large populations. For example, a single bacterium that weighs 10^{-12} g and has a generation time of 20 min could produce in 48 hr of exponential growth, approximately 2.2×10^{43} cells, or some 2.4×10^{24} tons, a mass approximately 4000 times that of the Earth. Various factors, such as the limitation of available nutrients and space as well as the accumulation of toxic metabolic waste products, prevent the full reproductive potential of a microbial cell from ever being realized. Table 2 lists approximate numbers of microorganisms that can occur in various types of specific environments.

Medicine was one of the first disciplines to recognize the need for control of microbial contamination. A most dramatic push to restrain the numbers of microorganisms in the industrial environment came from the activites of the space program to limit the microbial contamination of planets during extraterrestrial exploration (exobiology). Studies sponsored by the National Aeronautics and Space Administration (NASA) since the 1960s have shown that significant numbers of microorganisms can exist on surfaces and in the air of intramural industrial environments. However, if proper control measures are continuously employed, the level of microbial contamination can be kept low, i.e., from 0 to 3 viable particles per ft^3 of air and less than

Table 2 Numbers of Microorganisms Occurring in Specific Environments

Environment	Microorganisms per unit of measurement	Unit of measurement
Soils	10^4-10^7	g
Water	$<1-10^4$	ml
Ocean sediment	10^5-10^7	g
"Clean" air	1–10	ft^3
"Dirty" air	10^3-10^5	ft^3
"Stratosphere"	$<1-10^{-3}$	ft^3
Human feces	10^8-10^{10}	g
Human skin	$1-10^4$	$in.^2$
Plant dust	10^3-10^6	g
Sewage	10^6-10^7	ml
Floors	$10-10^3$	$in.^2$

1000 microorganisms per ft^2 of surface area in the work environment. Where contamination control programs have been established and monitored, it has been shown that people are the primary source of microbial contamination of the products being produced.

1. Environmental Control Over Various Manufacturing Steps

Industry has recognized a need for the control of particulates (fine dust, fibers, and others). In the aerospace industry, particulate matter (including microorganisms) is generally controlled to very low levels by performing work in controlled environmental facilities (i.e., clean rooms, clean enclosures, and laminar-flow work stations). Conventionally, a clean room is characterized as class 100, 1000, 10,000, or 100,000 as defined in Federal Standard 209B [13]. Classification of clean rooms is done according to defined limits of tolerable particulate matter of specific sizes. Particulate contamination is not differentiated into viable (microorganisms) or nonviable matter.

Microbiological control procedures should be instituted in any facility manufacturing sterile parenteral devices. These control procedures are directed toward limiting the presterilization microbial load (bioburden) on the products to a level compatible with the sterilization cycle to be employed. Many sterilization cycles are established on the basis that the presence of less than a given number of microorganisms on each device can be used to predict the PSI. Such estimates of survivors can only be accomplished by a carefully planned and executed program of microbial contamination control combined with vigorous monitoring of the terminal sterilization cycle.

For adequate analysis and surveillance of biological contamination control systems, criteria or standards should be established. The usual goal will be to limit, control, or reduce the number and types of microorganisms occurring on specific components and subassemblies during the assembly of the finished parenteral device. For example, one specific criterion might specify the number of bacterial spores allowable per finished device immediately prior to sterilization. If the device is too large to be sampled, then a specification for the number of spores per unit area could be established. Sometimes, the criteria will also specify the allowable number of airborne microorganisms and frequently other particulates as well. It is usually necessary to specify the assay techniques and other tests and procedures to be used in these monitoring activities.

In any microbial contamination control system, one or more of the following techniques is usually employed to assess whether the proper level of microbiological control has been established.

a. Microbial air sampling: air impaction samplers, liquid impingers, and settling plates are used most frequently.
b. Particle size sampling: liquid impinger samplers with preimpingers offer some particle-size selectivity; the Anderson cascade sieve sampler is frequently used to discriminate the airborne viable particles in a microbiological aerosol into six particle-size ranges.
c. Surface sampling: cotton swabs or Rodac plates are usually used.
d. Surface contamination accumulation test: small sterile strips of stainless steel, glass, or plastic are placed in the environment; after various exposure periods, strips are collected and assayed for viable microorganisms.
e. Component surface testing: small components and systems under microbiological contamination control may be tested by complete immersion in an appropriate bacteriological culture broth or by washing the component in a sterile rinse solution that is then quantitatively assayed either by plate counting or membrane filtration (to be discussed later).

2. *Role of Processing Machinery and Fluids on Bioburden*

Contact with Water

Water treated to remove chemical impurities by distillation, ion exchange, or reverse osmosis is widely used in the preparation of pharmaceuticals and other medical products. Ion-exchange resins have been implicated as the sources of gram-negative bacterial contamination of water that was used to prepare cosmetic lotions or other types of topical drug products that were later recalled because of the presence of opportunistic pathogens in the product [14]. Even with water that has been produced by distillation, contamination with gram-negative bacteria capable of multiplying rapidly and reaching high population levels ($>10^5$ cells per ml) can constitute a hazard to the products that are processed with such water. Not only will *Pseudomonas aeruginosa* and *P. cepacia* grow in distilled water supplies, but other organisms, such as *Yersinia enterocolitica*, and acid-fast organisms, such as *Mycobacterium chelonei* and *M. gordonae*, have been found to grow to high cell count levels (up to 10^7 ml^{-1}) in various types of water supplies. Most of these organisms are not very resistant to air drying and are of little consequence to the bioburden when the product is to be sterilized by either ethylene oxide, radiation, or steam sterilization.

A greater hazard to the sterile product from gram-negative bacteria is that they are a potent source of bacterial endotoxin (pyrogen) and can result in failure of the devices to pass tests for nonpyrogenicity. It is strongly recommended that all sources of water used in the processing of parenteral devices be monitored either by the USP rabbit test or preferably by the *Limulus* amebocyte lysate (LAL) test (to be discussed later). Although bacterial endotoxin (pyrogen) is water soluble, the adherence of this type of lipopolysaccharide onto the charged surfaces of plastic materials can make the removal of that contamination difficult in later processing steps.

Contact with Lubricants, Oils, Cleaning Solutions, and Solvents

It is recommended that all forms of silicone used in the lubrication of sterile parenteral devices be presterilized. The sterilization of such silicone lubricants is best accomplished through the use of dry heat at temperatures from 140 to 160°C. Sterilization containers for lubricants should be as small as practicable, be easily cleaned, and should afford minimal contamination of the lubricant between sterilization and use. In addition, steps should be taken to clean and presterilize reservoirs, transfer containers, and feed lines.

An inadvertent source of microorganisms contributing to the bioburden can be the growth of various organisms in the lubricants or oils used on machinery. Careful control should be exercised over all machine-lubricating oils since a wide variety of microorganisms can grow in these products. In addition, gram-negative bacteria and fungi have been found to grow in some aqueous cleaning solutions that have been used to process some of the component parts or subassemblies. The growth of microorganisms in nonpolar solvents is uncommon, and usually these solvents serve as a means to free the product of contaminating organisms, thus reducing the bioburden.

3. *Control over Human Contact*

Shedding by Personnel

The bioburden control problem on parenteral devices in various stages of manufacture is primarily a personnel problem, either through inattention to basic control procedures or as an ecological source of microorganisms. Of the great spectrum of bacteria, fungi, yeast, and viruses that comprise the natural microflora, a few find the inner and outer surfaces of the human body to be hospitable for growth. As greater attention is paid to the cleanliness of a manufacturing area, a greater proportion of the environmental microbes constituting product bioburden will be contributed by these organisms from humans.

Particular attention should be paid to the cleaning of exposed skin areas since contact with or shedding from the human skin is frequently the largest source of bioburden on parenteral devices. Since sterilization of the skin is practically impossible, it is recommended that various types of antiseptic (skin-compatible disinfectant) cleaning solutions be provided to allow a significant reduction in the number of organisms carried on exposed skin areas. Other procedures that provide a significant means of control for bioburden shedding from personnel are the following.

a. Masks and hair caps can provide a reasonable barrier for the shedding of microorganisms from the nose and mouth area, the lower extremities of the face and neck, and the top and back of the head. Frequent changes of masks are recommended to prevent overloading with organisms.

b. Gowns should be prepared in laundering facilities that prevent the growth of microorganisms and reduce lint during various stages of the laundering process. Following laundering, the gowns should be wrapped in protective packages to prevent an accumulation of microorganisms or dirt on the laundered clothing.

c. Footwear is worn in many parenteral drug-manufacturing areas. Various forms of disposable coverings, often of plastic, are available to limit the introduction of microorganisms and dirt into parenteral device-processing areas.

Use of Clean Rooms and Laminar-Flow Hoods

Clean rooms, clean enclosures, and clean work stations, which have been briefly mentioned previously (Section II.A.1), are installations that reduce the bioburden as well as particulate contamination of the supplied air. By themselves these physical facilities will not provide hardware or devices with low bioburden levels. The goal of low bioburdens is accomplished through the use of this type of physical facility by trained people who are properly garbed and are following prescribed procedures that prevent unnecessary accumulation of organisms on the parenteral devices.

Laminar-flow clean rooms represent an ultimate approach to cleanliness based on the isotropic flow of filtered air. The incoming air is recirculated through a high-efficiency particulate air (HEPA) filter for extensive reductions of airborne particles. The direction of flow may be vertical (downflow area) or horizontal (crossflow area).

Clean work stations or benches are similar to laminar-flow facilities in the degree of microbiological contamination control that can be achieved. They are ideally suited for critical operations on small assemblies or small finished devices. The principles of laminar airflow are utilized to prevent and even remove particulate contamination on devices. Commercially available laminar-flow benches provide environments with fewer than one microorganism per cubic foot at normal working distances from the HEPA filter face.

4. Decontamination and Cleaning Steps During Manufacture

Clean water (i.e., low microbial count) that contacts surfaces in various stages of processing will affect the bioburden on components and assemblies. Various types of chlorofluorocarbon compounds are used to clean metal and plastic materials during various stages of fabrication. Cleaning solvents will, in general, lower the bioburden on the finished parenteral device.

Besides these chemical procedures, various physical procedures, such as exposure to high-velocity clean air, will remove particulate contamination. In addition, ultraviolet or microwave radiation, as well as other types of low-temperature heating processes, can effect a significant reduction in the bioburden. However, these latter processes still can result in a significant microbial filth load that can show up if the device must be tested for nonpyrogenicity.

B. Characterization of Bioburden (Types and Numbers)

The kinetics of a sterilization procedure and the degree of bioburden on the device determine the PSI. Industrial microbiologists interested in determining the bioburden on finished parenteral devices immediately prior to sterilization have necessarily borrowed and adapted techniques developed for other applications. During the past 50 years, microbiologists in other fields, particularly in the food and dairy industries and some medical care facilities, have developed suitable methods for microbiological sampling of various materials and/or items. These techniques can be grouped basically into four categories: swabbing, agar contact plates, direct surface agar plating, and fluid rinses. Most microbiologists working with medical devices are employing variations of rinse techniques to determine the bioburden on parenteral devices immediately prior to sterilization.

It should be noted that the spacecraft sterilization technology effort of NASA has investigated and adapted techniques from other microbiological applications for use with the quantitation of microorganisms on/in aerospace hardware. As part of the NASA policy of standardizing microbiological procedures, it was decided to utilize a single broad-spectrum recovery agar medium and a single incubation sequence for all bioburden determinations. It was recognized that no single growth medium or single incubation sequence could recover all viable microorganisms occurring on spacecraft. It was decided therefore that maximal counts from one broad recovery agar medium would be preferable to the use of multiple media and varied incubation sequences, which could well make the entire bioburden assessment effort unmanageable. Trypticase soy agar (TSA), also known as soybean casein digest agar, was chosen by NASA scientists as the optimum recovery medium and 32°C for 72 hr as the incubation sequence to be used. The emphasis of this approach was the recovery of spore-forming species.

1. *Total Aerobic Microorganisms on Subassemblies and Finished Devices Prior to Sterilization*

Most Probable Number (MPN) Assays per *U.S. Pharmacopeia* Procedure

The first opportunity for the CDRH of the FDA to use the characterization of bioburden in the definition of sterilization cycles came in 1977 with the document entitled "Guidelines for sterilization of intraocular lenses by manufacturer" [15]. Since the medical device industry has in the past looked to general information contained in the USP as a guide for its own activities, it was decided to use the procedures listed for the USP microbial limits test as a way to determine bioburden on intraocular lenses [16]. The main difficulty with the USP procedure is that it was designed to test a small subportion of lots of dry powders or liquid medications and is not fully applicable to the testing of all available surfaces on a parenteral device. Another limitation is that the estimate of total aerobic microbial count through serial dilution with growth/no growth end points in multiple broth tubes at each dilution is more difficult to manipulate and to extrapolate to a true bioburden determination on the device. In some situations, such MPN estimates can be satisfactory.

Total Aerobic Counts per NASA Standard Procedures

The applicability of the procedures developed by NASA for microbial counts on spacecraft surfaces to bioburden analyses for medical devices should be explored. The NASA method, which is excellent for bioburden determination on small parenteral devices or in the fluid path of larger devices, is outlined in Figure 1. It is an adaptation of the rinse technique employed in the dairy and food industry and is further described in a NASA report [17]. The finished devices (intact or broken up) are placed in individual bottles containing 50 ml of sterile 0.1% peptone water. The bottles are mechanically shaken to dislodge contaminants. Duplicate 5-ml aliquots of the peptone water (or serial dilutions thereof) are then plated in 20 ml of TSA agar (identical with SCD agar of the USP method) and incubated aerobically; two other 5-ml aliquots are incubated anaerobically. The remaining 30 ml of the diluent is transferred to a large test tube and heat shocked at 80°C for 15 min. The purpose of this step is to destroy all non-spore-forming species so that spore formers can be separately estimated. After heat shocking, duplicate 5-ml aliquots are plated in 20 ml of TSA agar and incubated both aerobically and anaerobically. In addition, the item itself after shaking can be removed from the diluent and plated directly in melted TSA agar. After the agar hardens, the plate is incubated aerobically at 32°C for 72 hr.

An adaptation of the NASA procedures was investigated and reported by West [18]. The modifications included the following: longer contact time with diluent on a shaker followed by brief insonation; diluent filtration through membrane filter; membrane filter plated directly or blended for serial dilution and plated in TSA medium; and no incubation under anaerobic conditions. West used these modified procedures with syringes, drape material, and catheters.

C. Development of Sterilization Cycle

The procedure that has been most in vogue to assure the sterility of pharmaceutical or medical items is a sterility test of a small sample of the treated products. In the past, the official drug compendia (USP and National Formulary, now combined) relied extensively on such tests as the way to judge the adequacy of a sterilization cycle. Some experts have characterized the USP finished product sterility test as legally acceptable but scientifically inadequate. The biological as well as statistical inadequacy of finished product sterility testing as the basis on which to assess terminal sterilization of medical products has been shown. Conventional sterility tests cannot provide sufficient confirmation of the sterility of a lot of treated items unless extremely large sample numbers are taken, and even then the analyst is confronted by the dilemma of extrinsic contamination from his or her own body or from the testing environment.

Recent experience has shown that two other approaches can be used either separately or together to bring about a much greater degree of assurance of sterility in processed items. The first approach centers on studies that establish the kinetic rates of kill that take place during the destruction of various types and quantities of microorganisms expected to be present on the product during a particular terminal sterilization process. Determination of the kinetics of microbial destruction by a given sterilization treatment yield D values from which the probabilities of survivors per item can be calculated. The basic mechanics of this approach will be briefly presented, but the nature of this chapter does not allow a generalized discussion of the kinetics of microbial destruction.

The second approach that has come into recent use is that of biological indicators (BI) placed in each batch of the product to be sterilized. Usually,

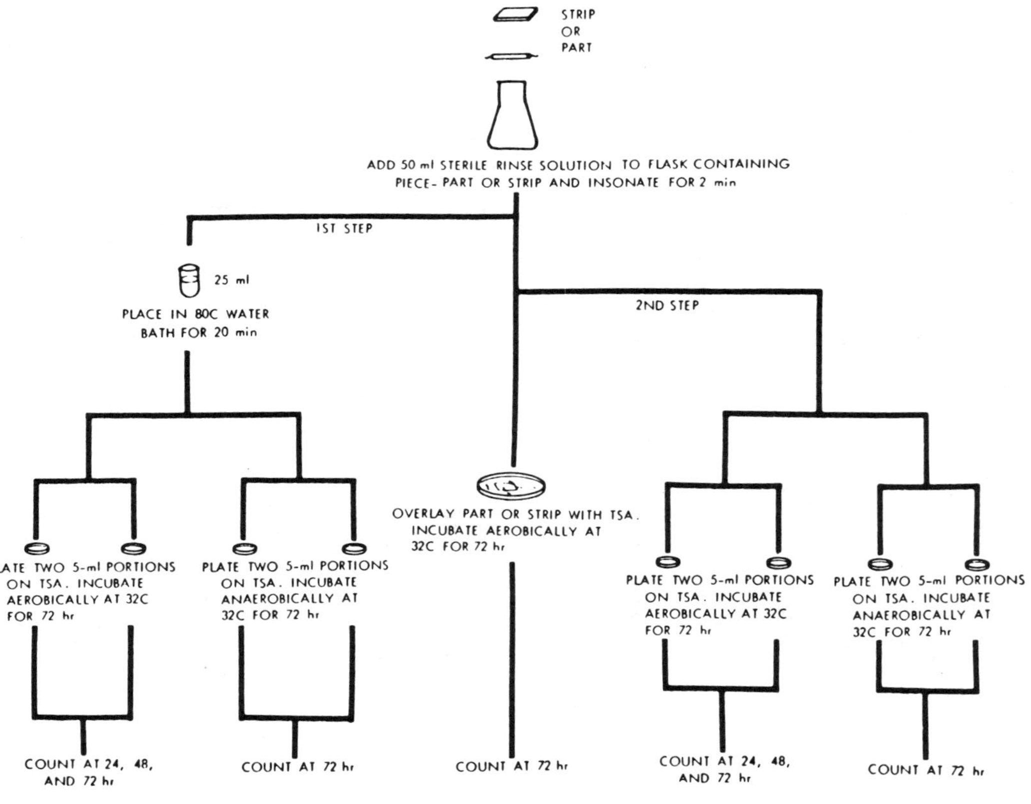

Figure 1 Schematic outline of NASA standard procedure for microbiological examination of spacecraft components. (From Ref. 17.)

the BI is a bacterial spore suspension that has been dried on a suitable carrier or placed directly on the sample items of the product to be sterilized. The destruction of these positive microbial controls provides excellent support that sterilization of a given batch of material has been achieved. Ideally, the organisms used in the BI should have their resistance characterized in terms of D values. The destruction of a known or graded series of populations of organisms of defined resistance (D value) when correlated with the resistance (D value) of the natural bioburden can allow a reasonable estimate of the probability of a survivor per item from a given sterilization process. The basic philosophy behind the use of BI is that this procedure provides a more rigorous control of a sterilization cycle then a sterility test of treated products that usually have only a low level of random contamination before entering the sterilizer.

When the physical variables of a given sterilization procedure can be rigorously controlled and monitored by physical means, then the concept of dosimetric release, i.e., no finished product sterility test, can be utilized. Dosimetric release assumes that the kinetics of microbial destruction for the bioburden has been defined and the associated probabilities of a survivor or sterility assurance level for a particular sterilization process have been calculated based on that bioburden. Interim challenges with BI can be utilized to assure that the monitoring of all physical variables has been held constant, but the continued use of BI in dosimetric release procedures is not necessary.

The order of death for a sterilizing process can be determined by plotting the number of organisms (bioburden) on the logarithmic (Y coordinate) against either the length of heating time, the length of exposure time at a given gaseous or chemical concentration, or the radiation dose on the linear scale (X coordinate). Such a curve is referred to as a death rate or survivor curve (Fig. 2). For most sterilizing agents and under most conditions, the death rate curve usually exhibits a straight-line exponential function or first-order reaction kinetics. The D value is the reciprocal of the rate function K of the first-order reaction equation. In more simple terms, the D value is the time for a 90% reduction in the microbial population exhibiting first-order reaction kinetics.

It should be understood that the plot in Figure 2 represents the idealized situation; i.e., destruction curves for pure cultures of microorganisms usually follow first-order reaction kinetics. The generalized straight-line plot graphically illustrates the effects of the terminal sterilization process on microbial contamination. Mathematically, the number of organisms decreases logarithmically to log 0 (one organism). Below log 0, the plot indicates that the population is now in a negative logarithmic function. Thus, at 10^{-1}, the exact phraseology is that there is 1 microbial survivor per 10 processed items. At 10^{-2}, the probability is of 1 survivor per 100 items. Therefore, considering that the reduction of organisms is never absolute but rather a probability function, then there exists a reasonable way to express the effect of further exposure times. It is now currently accepted that this expression is in terms of probability of a survivor per item (PSI) or sterility assurance level (SAL). It is easy to visualize in this context that absolute sterility is never achieved, but instead there will always remain a probability, no matter how small, that a survivor can be obtained.

The commonly accepted value of a probability of survivor for sterile parenteral devices is one in a million, or 10^{-6} per item. Those manufacturers who rely on the USP finished product sterility test [7] with a 20-item sample have a 95% confidence of detecting the probability of a survivor per item at

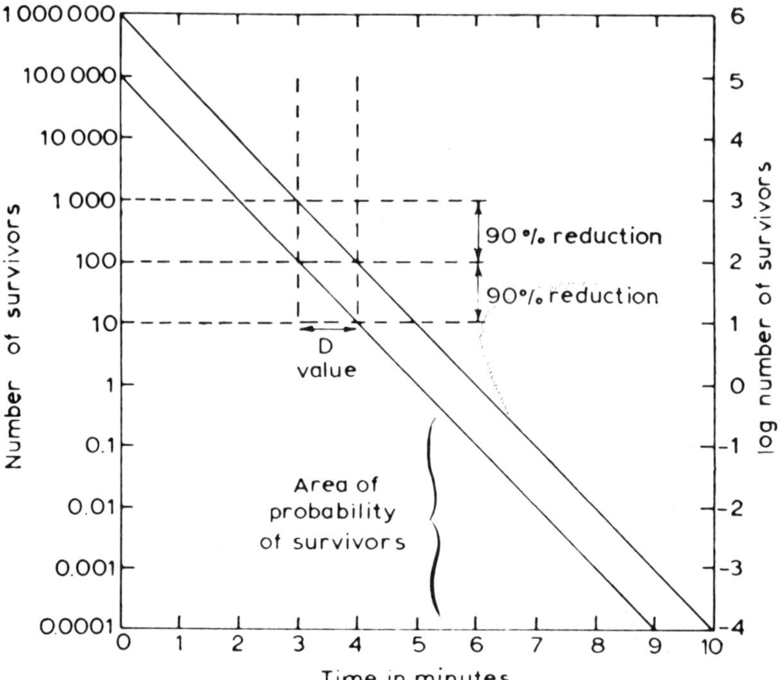

Figure 2 Microbial death rate curves that illustrate concept of decimal reduction (D values) and probability of survivors.

approximately the 10^{-1} level. It is obvious that one cannot test for PSI at levels much below 10^{-2}. Table 3 is a listing of PSI for various products contacting a hospital patient. It should be realized that there is a billion-fold difference in sterile quality when one analyzes the various processes used to produce the sterile products listed in Table 3. It is for this reason that the Health Protection Branch of the Canadian government has recently proposed [11] that the word *sterile* should be replaced by a microbiological survivor index, which is the reciprocal of the probability of a survivor that a device is contaminated with an organism. An MSI of 3 would mean that the PSI is 1 chance in 1000, or that only 1 device out of 1000 would contain one or more contaminants. The terminology of PSI, SAL, and MSI is equivalent.

1. Definition of Resistance of Bioburden to a Sterilization Procedure: Derivation of D-Values and Qualification of a Pre-existent Sterilization Cycle

Application of the Stumbo Equation

Most analyses of microbial destruction data from any sterilization procedure require that the data be in the dose-response format, i.e., temperature-time for heat, concentration-time for chemicals, and absorbed dose for radiation versus numbers of surviving organisms. If the semilogarithmic survivor curve (first-order inactivation reaction) is other than a straight line (Fig. 2), direct utilization of the data is difficult. Data utilization

Table 3 Estimates of Probability of Survivors for Sterilized Items

Item	Probability of survivor/unit
Canned chicken soup[a]	10^{-11}
Large volume parenteral fluid	10^{-9}
Intravenous catheter and delivery set[a]	10^{-6}
Syringe and needle[a]	10^{-6}
Urinary catheters[a]	10^{-3}
Surgical drape kit[a]	10^{-3}
Small volume parenteral drug (sterile fill)	10^{-3}
Laparoscopic instruments (processed with liquid chemical sterilants)[b]	10^{-2}

[a]Dosimetric release: no sterility test.
[b]Limits of USP sterility test: $10^{-1.3}$ (with 95% confidence).
Source: From C. W. Bruch, Process-control release of terminally sterilized medical devices. In *Sterilization of Medical Products*, Volume II (E. R. L. Gaughran and R. F. Morrissey, eds.). Johnson & Johnson, New Brunswick, N.J., 1981, p. 104.

limitations have encouraged researchers to (a) attempt to describe the survivor curve by a single straight line, regardless of shape, (b) use of end-point methods of analysis that develop a survivor curve directly without facing the actual problem of the slope of the intermediate points of that curve, or (c) use of fractional negative (FN) data from replicate unit exposures where original number of organisms per replicate is known so that a D value can be calculated that assumes the survivor curve is a straight line from the original population to whatever value of survivor is desired. This last approach is a refined version of b and is basically a two-point plot that is extrapolated to the desired level of probability of a survivor and the corresponding dose then read from the curve.

Data for which a fraction of the replicate units from subprocess (incremental) dosing are negative can be analyzed statistically using the most probable number (MPN) technique to yield the probable number of survivors at the respective dose point. Such methods of evaluation were originally developed for thermal destruction data. Stumbo [19] proposed that each positive tube in a multiple replicate unit thermal destruction testing program, where FN data existed, be considered to contain one viable organism. His formula for the calculation of the D value, which defines the slope of the destruction curve, is

$$D = \frac{T}{\log A - \log B}$$

where

A = total number of samples to be assayed at zero dose (zero time interval), multiplied by the presterilization microbial count (bioburden) per replicate sample
B = value calculated by assuming one surviving spore per replicate when less than the total number of replicates show survival
T = time of exposure (dose) at a given temperature

Subsequently, Stumbo et al. [20] suggested that the MPN equation of Halvorson and Ziegler [21] be utilized to evaluate more accurately the number of survivors when FN data were obtained using a multiple replicate testing program. The equation utilized by Halvorson and Ziegler turns out to be the first term of the Poisson distribution. The reader is referred to the following references [10,22,23] to gain more theory about this overall approach to the calculation of the D value.

West [18] has presented an analysis of how the Stumbo technique can be utilized for the derivation of D values from ethylene oxide (EtO) sterilization. Similarly, Berube [24] gives a demonstration of how the FN technique can be utilized in the derivation of D values for bioburden on product to be radiation sterilized. The CDRH of the FDA has accepted the FN technique as a simplified means to estimate D values for any sterilization procedure. The derivation of the D value then allows a rapid calculation of the total dose of sterilant needed to achieve a desired PSI.

The following brief outline gives a simplified way to determine D values using subprocess (incremental) treatments and FN data.

a. Determine the microbial load for at least 20 items per load for several loads (not less than three).
b. With EtO sterilization, expose loads to normal processing conditions at a fixed gaseous (EtO) concentration, temperature, and relative humidity.
c. Withdraw 20 samples at 1/4, 1/2, 3/4, and at normal process time and culture per USP finished product sterility test procedures [7].
d. With radiation sterilization, withdraw 20 samples at 0.2, 0.4, 0.6, 0.8, 1.0, 1.3, 1.6, and 2.0 Mrad doses and culture per USP finished product sterility test procedures [7].
e. Calculate the D value for the microbial load using the Stumbo equation given above.

Calculation of the D Value from the Stumbo Equation

The following example shows how the D value is actually calculated from raw data using the Stumbo equation.

Of 20 replicates, 18 gave a positive response (growth) at 0.4 Mrad; $\log_{10}$ of 18 = 1.255. Of 20 replicates, 2 gave a positive response at 0.6 Mrad; $\log_{10}$ of 2 = 0.301. The average bioburden per device was 50 organisms.

The D value at 0.4 Mrad:

$$D = \frac{0.4 \text{ Mrad}}{\log_{10} (20 \times 50) - \log_{10} 18}$$

$$= \frac{0.4}{\log 1000 - \log 18} = \frac{0.4}{3 - 1.255} = \frac{0.4}{1.745} = 0.229 \text{ Mrad}$$

The D value at 0.6 Mrad:

$$D = \frac{0.6 \text{ Mrad}}{\log 1000 - \log 2} = \frac{0.6}{3 - 0.301} = \frac{0.6}{2.699} = 0.222 \text{ Mrad}$$

The average D value is 0.226 Mrad for the bioburden of 50 organisms per device.

2. *Acceptable Estimates of Probabilities of Survivors for Both Parenteral and Nonparenteral Devices*

Calculation of Process Times to Show PSI $<10^{-6}$ for Parenteral Devices (Includes Implantable Devices)

The thrust of the discussion until now is that sterilization is defined as a probability function, which is susceptible to measurement in physical and chemical terms. The D value is defined on the basis that the death of microorganisms follows first-order reaction kinetics. The use of the D value allows a theoretical calculation of the probability of a survivor from a terminal sterilization process. Because of limits for the extent of this chapter, the theoretical background for this calculation has not been developed in depth. Other references have been given previously that adequately discuss the realities of these concepts.

For parenteral devices, the PSI is desired to be 10^{-6} or less. The following example is a simplified version of the use of the bioburden estimate combined with the D value to yield a desired dose level (time at a given EtO concentration at a specified temperature range) for EtO sterilization of parenteral devices.

> The $\log_{10}$ of N_{sd} plus the reciprocal of the $\log_{10}$ of PSI, multiplied by the mean D value, yields the desired process cycle.
>
> N_{sd} is the average bioburden count (N_o or organisms per total item or per fluid path of item) to which has been added three standard deviations of that mean value. In this example, N_{sd} is equal to 150 organisms per device; $\log_{10}$ of 150 = 2.17.
>
> The D value is equal to 13 min.
>
> The calculated process time at the temperature selected (112–128°F; approximately 120°F): $(2.17 + 6) \times 13$ min = 106 min.

Currently Accepted Probabilities of Survivors for Different Types of Devices

The concept of probabilities of survivors allows different magnitudes of this value to be placed on devices according to the hazard posed by the use of that device. This concept is relatively new to the medical products industry but has been accepted in the food-processing (canning) industry for the past 70 years. Table 3 gives a presentation of the sterile quality defined as PSI, which are currently accepted for various types of products containing a hospital patient. The first item, canned chicken soup, has the lowest PSI. This situation has come about because of the rigorous heat cycles developed by the food canning industry to alleviate the hazard from *Clostridium botulinum* in canned foods. The canned food industry has never relied on a USP-type finished product sterility test to assess the quality of its canned goods. The statistics of detecting survivors through that type of test are so poor that the public confidence in the safety of canned foods would be severely compromised through outbreaks of botulism.

You will note that the PSI established for parenteral devices in Table 3 are set at the basic level for all implantable devices, i.e., 10^{-6} or less. Some will question why this higher PSI is allowed in a parenteral device as opposed to the PSI in canned chicken soup of 10^{-11} or less. The basic answer is that parenteral devices do not provide a growth medium for the organisms as would a canned food and that the probabilities or removing the device from its packaging and placing it in sterile fashion into the parenterum of the patient do not justify a lower PSI for these types of devices. It should be noted that small-volume parenteral drugs are not terminally processed. The use of sterile filtration-aseptic filling techniques with these types of products does not allow an achievement of the PSI beyond 10^{-4} with the most modern equipment in a rigorously monitored laminar-flow clean room.

D. Validation of Effectiveness of Sterilization Procedure (Cycle)

Two basic approaches are utilized by the medical device industry in developing sterilization cycles. The more elegant approach is to establish cycle conditions based on the number of microorganisms in or on the product (bioburden) and the interior of the packaging and the resistance of those microorganisms to the sterilant being employed. The interplay of bioburden and its resistance to the sterilant will determine the conditions necessary for the cycle to achieve a certain level of PSI or SAL. This approach, which has been extensively discussed above, is referred to as the PSI approach through bioburden analysis. The AAMI guidelines for industrial sterilization of medical products with gamma radiation provides a broad description of this approach [12].

The second approach is more commonly found with steam sterilization under pressure and EtO sterilization and is characterized as an "overkill" sterilization approach [25,26]. It is normally applied when the device can withstand long exposure to high-temperature steam or any other sterilant without adverse effects. Any steam sterilization cycle that results in an F_O (to be defined in Section III.C.2) of greater than 8 can be characterized as an overkill approach [27]. When experience exists to use the overkill approach, it offers the manufacturer the advantage of less need for characterizing the bioburden and its resistance to the particular sterilant. However, the manufacturer must be aware that the sterilization of large populations of microorganisms can result in the presence of microbial filth, which in the case of parenteral devices can be a source of pyrogens.

It has never been the intention of the CDRH of the FDA to dictate the methods and validation approaches that must be followed by a manufacturer in sterilizing a device [28]. The manufacturer should design the sterilization process for a product in such a manner that the device is rendered sterile without adversely affecting the quality (safety) of the device or compromising its packaging. The validation of a sterilization process assures that the specified sterilization cycle can reproducibly achieve a safe product whose quality and efficacy can be evaluated against developed specifications. Validation of the sterilization process means that the total process can be translated to a routine production basis with assurance that the product bioburden is killed to the extent specified by the manufacturer in the design protocol. This approach allows industry to use technically equivalent methods in achieving the same end result. Every manufacturer must evaluate the advantages and disadvantages of any particular process to assure the sterility of the product on a routine manufacturing basis.

1. Validation Approaches for Sterilization Cycle Development

Subprocess (Incremental) Dosing With Characterized Bioburden

This approach has been described in "Guidelines for sterilization of intraocular lenses by manufacturer," which is available from the FDA [15]. Basically, the manufacturer withdraws a fixed number of samples, usually about 20, at 1/4, 1/3, 1/2, 2/3, and 3/4 of normally used process times known to be employed for the processing of a specific product by a particular sterilant. The withdrawn samples are cultured per the USP finished product sterility test procedures. The goal is to arrive at a point where fractional-negative (FN) data can be obtained as has been described under Section II.C. The presence of FN data allows the use of the Stumbo equation to calculate a D value (see Section II.C.1.a) for the resistance of the population normally expected to be present on the device from the routine manufacturing process. Once the D value can be estimated, then that value can be employed in the equation given in Section II.C.2.a to calculate the cycle (dose) necessary to achieve the desired levels of probability of a survivor.

Inoculation of Product with Biological Indicators (BI) When Bioburden Is Low or Is Not Known

In the sterilization of intraocular lenses, it was determined that many manufacturers had very low bioburdens, less than two organisms per lens, which would not allow the proper use of the Stumbo equation to arrive at a D value. Therefore, the lenses were directly inoculated with either an aqueous or an alcoholic suspension of spores of *Bacillus subtilis* var. *niger* to the 10^6 level and then employed in an incremental or subprocess dosing procedure. The D values derived for this inoculated population were then used to calculate a process cycle with a 10^{-6} PSI. This approach is feasible when one has a smaller scale model of the sterilizer in which to develop the cycle, which can then be transferred to the actual production sterilizer. However, if one is attempting to establish the cycle in a production-size vessel, then this approach may not be practical.

A modified approach, called "half-cycle validation," has been applied to those processes currently used in production but never previously qualified. The manufacturer continues production as normal but inoculates a minimum of 40 finished packaged samples with 10^6 spores per item (this is inoculum level for EtO sterilization) or places paper strip BI in the most difficult to sterilize portion of the packaged device. The regular loads are processed as before, but the sterilization cycle is interrupted at one-half of its normal time and 20 of the product with BI retrieved. The cycle is restarted and run to completion (normal time). The remaining 20 samples with BI are retrieved, and both sets of samples are assayed by USP finished product sterility tests.

If the level of 10^6 spores is not killed at the half-cycle, the inactivation of this level by the full cycle allows the load to be released. However, the total cycle must be increased on the next validation run. If this challenge level is killed by the half-cycle, the processor repeats this procedure two more times. The kill of the 10^6 level of spores per device by a half-cycle definitely assures that the PSI is less than 10^{-6} for the overall cycle. Actually, this "half-cycle validation" is really an example of the "overkill" approach to sterilization process verification.

Use of a Graded Series on Inoculated Product with a Fixed Sterilization Cycle

In the situation discussed immediately above, some preprogrammed (microprocessor controlled) production size vessels are not always amenable to subprocess (incremental) or half-cycle qualification treatments. A previously established cycle can be qualified if the product is inoculated with a graded series of a BI, either directly on the product or by filter paper strips placed in the most difficult to sterilizer portion of the packaged device. Thus, with an EtO sterilization cycle, the product could be serially inoculated with 20 units at the 10^3 spores per device, another 20 units with 10^4 spores per device, and so on up to a level of 10^8 spores per device. The fixed cycle is then run that would allow an estimate of the D value provided FN data are obtained for a series of 20 units at one of the inoculated levels. The FN data from that inoculum level are used in the Stumbo equation to obtain the D value. The D value is then used to calculate the dose (time of exposure) for a PSI of 10^{-6} or less per the procedure described in Section II.C.2.a.

2. *Implementation of Sterilization Cycle During Routine Manufacturing Operations*

The discussion in Section II.D.1 indicates that the use of smaller scale equipment to develop and qualify the sterilization cycle is not followed by all manufacturers of sterile disposable devices. Some operators prefer to develop the cycle using actual production equipment. When the cycle is developed in smaller scale equipment and then is transferred to the actual production equipment, extensive control of the chemical and physical variables specified in the smaller scale equipment must be monitored in the production sterilizer. Thus, a limited amount of qualification of the large-scale routine manufacturing unit will be required when the cycle has been previously developed in a pilot-scale unit.

Control of Physical and Chemical Variables Through Instrumentation

Any sterilization procedure used on a manufacturing basis will have equipment with process variables controlled by various types of gages and monitors. For example, any unit employing temperatures above ambient must have associated with it temperature gages to indicate temperature at specific points in the unit. In addition, for large sterilizers where the temperature of the load has been brought up to a particular value, the validation of the cycle will require the use of various types of temperature probes, such as thermocouples or resistance temperature detectors (RTD), to show that the desired temperature can be achieved in the most difficult to penetrate sections of the sterilizer load. Routine monitoring with such thermocouples or RTD is not necessary after the sterilizer, with a defined load, has gone through the performance qualification and validation phases. The other routine monitors used with the sterilizer for actual production runs must be calibrated against some standard or reference base that is acceptable to regulatory authorities. With radiation sterilization, the routine dosimeters must be calibrated against a primary dosimeter standard referenced back to the radiation dosimeter calibrations established by the National Bureau of Standards (NBS).

Use of Noninstrumented Chemical and Physical Monitors

The chemical or physical variables of a sterilizing process can be checked for minimal or maximal values through the use of simplified approaches. For example, various types of heat-sensitive tapes can be placed on the outside of pallets or on the actual packaging for individual units of devices to show that a certain minimal temperature was reached during the processing cycle. Similarly, relative humidity monitors of a simple chemical nature can be included in the process loads.

If the performance of the cycle is to be rigorously monitored through such noninstrumented monitors, then these monitors must be calibrated back against some primary source and be capable of reproducible results before they are employed in a particular sterilization process. This means that every time a new lot of these monitors is purchased, they are either bought with a vendor's certificate that states their performance or their performance is checked by the user against a primary standard that has been previously established.

Use of BI Whose Resistance Has Been Checked During Qualification Phases as Routine Production Monitors

With EtO sterilization cycles, many manufacturers prefer to utilize BI during the performance qualification approach, either in a pilot-scale equipment or in the actual production units. If the performance qualification phase has employed the use of product-inoculated BIs, these do not have to be continued during routine production cycles. Paper strip BIs, which are included during performance qualification, are acceptable for routine cycle monitoring. These commercial BIs must be purchased against a resistance specification (D value) for the particular sterilant being used. The processor can evaluate the efficiency of these purchased BI against the actual D values for the natural bioburden or against the D values obtained from the use of inoculated product in the performance qualification of the cycle.

E. Functional and Stability Tests for Product Packaging

1. *Role of Packaging in Development of Sterilization Cycle*

It has been assumed in the discussion under qualification and validation of effectiveness of the sterilization cycle that the manufacturer had established what type of packaging would be most suitable for the product, prior to the undertaking sterilization cycle development. Ideally, the packaging should provide a minimal barrier to the effectiveness of the sterilant being employed but a maximal barrier to the ingress of contaminants during shelf life. With physical sterilization procedures, the penetration by ionizing radiation or by dry heat is affected slightly by the characteristics of the packaging material. However, in steam sterilization, where penetration by the water molecules is a necessary adjunct to the kinetics of kill, and in EtO sterilization, where moisture must be present for the EtO molecules to alkylate the key moieties in the bacterial cell, then packaging can have a key role in the efficacy of the cycle to be employed. Alternatively, even if the packaging allows the penetration of the sterilant, but certain procedures are employed in the sterilization cycle, such as a vacuum to achieve a sufficient gaseous concentration of EtO, that vacuum itself may play a key role in the integrity of the packaging system. The key variables in the sterilization process, such as temperature, moisture, gas penetration, and ability of packaging seals to withstand various levels of negative pressure, should be determined prior to the initiation of the qualification of the effectiveness of the sterilization cycle itself.

2. *Effect of Packaging on Release or Generation of EtO Residues*

It should be appreciated that those types of packaging material that are more resistant to EtO permeation can be penetrated through the use of long cycles or cycles with high gas concentration. If the product is brought out of the sterilizer rather quickly, there can be significant concentrations of EtO remaining within the packaging and also within the device if the device materials can solubilize the EtO. Thus, packaging that tends to be restrictive to the rapid ingress or egress of EtO has the potential to result in higher levels of residue, depending on the degassing conditions being employed. This subject is rather complex, and it is not possible to go into an in-depth discussion. It is suggested that those readers who are new to the role of packaging in EtO sterilization should consult the papers by Ernst and associates [29] for a more complete discussion of the role of this factor.

3. *Resistance of Packaging to Shipping Abuse and Consumer Insults*

The manufacturer is responsible for the sterility of the product until it is deliberately opened by the user, whether doctor or patient. The packaging for a device must be developed using conditions that mimic the nature of shipment and storage during all phases of its delivery to a particular site of use. It cannot be assumed that because an item is going to be used in a hospital operating room that the people handling that product, prior to its actual use, will be considerate about the type of handling that the product should receive. If the packaging for the device cannot take specific kinds of abuse, that information should be included on the package labeling to properly caution the user.

4. *Stability (Shelf-Life) Testing for the Sterile Packaged Device*

At the present time, most sterile medical device manufacturers do not give an expiration date on the package. However, in some situations the FDA has required an expiration date. This has occurred with the packaging for intraocular lenses. In this situation, the intraocular lens manufacturers were required to come up with data to show that the lenses in the final sterile shipping package would have shelf lives for defined periods of time. Thus, if the manufacturer wanted to claim an expiration date of 12 months, data had to be provided to show that the sterile packaged items, after storage at 12 months, under normal shipping, vendor, and hospital storage conditions, would still be sterile and have their integrity maintained. The USP finished product sterility test is used to assess sterility in the tested items. Similarly, if an expiration date of 3 years were to be placed on the package, then data must be provided either by the intraocular lens manufacturer directly or from the packaging supplier to the intraocular lens manufacturer that the packaging had the capability under the use conditions for which the intraocular lenses would be shipped and stored of providing 3 years of shelf-life stability. Storage or stability data obtained for the same packaging (and seals) used with other types of devices are acceptable in this regard.

III. RELEASE CRITERIA FOR A STERILIZED PARENTERAL DEVICE

A. Legal Acceptability of the Scientifically Inadequate USP Finished Product Sterility Test

During the previous discussion in Section II.C on the development of a sterilization cycle, frequent mention was made of the USP finished product sterility test. It was noted that two major industries that employ sterilization processes (food canning versus pharmaceutical products) have taken widely divergent positions in establishing the safety of these cycles. It was discovered early in the canning of foods that the public would not accept the frequency of outbreaks of botulism that occurred from the processing of foods at flowing steam temperatures (212°F). As containers for food and better sterilizing equipment became available, allowing the use of steam under pressure, it was found that the incidence of botulism decreased. Still, the food canning industry could not rely on small numbers of cans taken from lots of canned goods as a way to assure the safety of the food from *C. botulinum*.

Therefore, in the period 1915–1921, the National Canners Association Laboratories determined the kinetics of kill in phosphate buffer for a large population of spores of *C. botulinum*. It was noted in laboratory tests that the destruction of the largest quantity of spores that could be suspended in 1 ml of phosphate buffer approximated 10^{11} spores. The destruction of this population of spores took 2.45 min at 250°F. The D value was calculated to be 0.21 min. This value later became the classic D value for heat resistance of *C. botulinum* in various canned goods.

At about the same time it was discovered that another organism, spores of *Bacillus stearothermophilus*, had greater resistance to moist heat at temperatures of 250°F than did the spores of *C. botulinum*. Therefore, the food canning industry put greater reliance on the destruction of spores of *B. stearothermophilus* strain 1518 as a biological indicator to show that a particular canning cycle, for a particular food, had an assured level of safety. The food canning industry could not live with the rates of botulinal outbreaks that would occur if it relied on the USP finished product sterility test, which has a 95% confidence level of detecting a PSI of $10^{-1.3}$ with a 20-item sample.

In contrast to the way the food canning industry developed safe and effective sterilization cycles, the medical products industry has tended to rely on sampling of a population of treated materials as indicative of the quality of the treated lot. Specifically, it was found that many medicaments of interest to pharmacists could not withstand rigorous heat treatment cycles. The procedure evolved early in the practice of pharmacy to use tyndallization to achieve PSI in the treated products at a level of 10^{-1} to 10^{-2}. Tyndallization refers to the practice of heating the product to flowing steam temperatures, cooling, followed by an incubation cycle, for at least three such cycles. It was assumed that those spores that survive the initial heating period would germinate following incubation and that the repetition of this type of cycle would eventually destroy a high proportion of the spores present in the product. With the newer techniques for steam sterilization at high temperature and pressure, the practice of tyndallization has fallen into disfavor, though it is still occasionally encountered in some long-established (grandfathered) drug products. Tyndallization is totally out of place in the modern practice of sterilization for medical products.

The previous discussion has cited briefly the biological inadequacy, as well as the statistical limitations, of the USP sterility test. This test is best applied and has its greatest utility in assessing the sterility of aseptically filled nonterminally sterilized products, where use of BI or dosimetric release is not possible. The many facets involved in sterility testing of aseptically filled products is adequately covered in the sterility test chapter of the USP [7]. It is suggested that terminally sterilized products will move away from any reliance on the USP sterility test and employ the use of BI initially to gain information on the probability of survivors from a developed cycle. Later, the cycle can be physically monitored and controlled so that the use of BI is not necessary. This is the situation for many products sterilized with steam under pressure or with radiation sterilization, which are released dosimetrically or on the basis of control of process variables alone.

B. Use of BI as a Batch Release Mechanism

The use of BI as a legally acceptable means to assure the microbiological safety of terminally sterilized lots of medical products occurred in USP XVIII (1970). The details for the use of BI in lieu of finished product tests was included in the sterility test chapter, which is legally enforceable by the authorities of the FDA under the FD&C Act. Some regulatory officials and industry lawyers became concerned that options were being allowed in this chapter to assess the sterility of a load of treated drug products. It was the legal position that there could be only one official test in an adversary proceeding in a court of law to assess legally the sterility status of a lot of material. Accordingly, in USP XIX (1975), the use of BI was removed from the sterility test chapter and placed in a nonlegally enforceable (informational) chapter on sterilization methods. However, this informational chapter in USP XIX contained a table that gave the suggested numbers of BI to use in lieu of finished product sterility test samples. As such, this chart could be used by industry to satisfy the questions of FDA investigators during periodic reviews of manufacturing and sterility assurance procedures.

The dialogue continues today, and in USP XX (1980) and XXI (1985), the table on the use of BI in lieu of finished product samples that was present in USP XVIII and USP XIX was dropped. Instead, there is a discussion of BI in the informational sterilization chapter and legally enforceable product monographs for dry heat, EtO, and steam BI. It was stated in Section III.A that the USP finished product sterility test is a legal test but cannot satisfy scientific concerns as to biological adequacy or statistical sufficiency of testing. The USP does allow the use of alternative procedures of equal sensitivity and reliability in place of any of the official methods listed in the compendium [30]. On this basis, a manufacturer of sterile products is free to use BI without any finished product testing to assure the sterility of a lot of sterilized goods. For those manufacturers who understand the kinetics of sterilization processes and the means to adequately monitor and control such processes, the concept of dosimetric or process release is applicable and is now being widely used.

1. *Use of Adventitious BI (Spore Strips) in Assuring Low Levels of Probabilities of Survivors*

Although BI in the form of paper strips, with spores contained in glassine envelopes or as spores in vials of liquid, have been available for approximately 30 years, their use has grown extensively since 1965. The many articles that have been published on the use and performance of BI have shown that the way the indicators are carried is not critical to their destruction by either moist heat or by ionizing radiation. However, this is not true for the spores carried on paper strips used in dry heat or EtO sterilization processes. With these latter two sterilants, the rate of kill of the microbial contamination is dependent on the amount of moisture associated with the product at the point where the microbial contamination is lodged [31,32]. West [18] has shown that spores of *B. subtilis* var. *niger* die much faster on paper strips than do the same spores placed on some plastic devices or than does the bioburden on those same devices. If manufacturers want to use spore strip BI, they should qualify the kill of these indicators vis-a-vis the natural bioburden through the use of subprocess (incremental) doses as described in Section II.D.1.a.

2. *Limitations for Inoculated Product BI*

The use of the product itself to carry the BI can result in artificial situations that are difficult to sterilize with gaseous chemicals, such as EtO. The spore contamination forms hard crusts on hydrophobic plastic surfaces through the piling up of spores. This crusting phenomenon is further encouraged if the spore preparation is not highly cleaned. Furthermore, these spores on inoculated product BI are not as easily assayable as they are from a paper strip. When it is desirable to locate spores in long lengths of tubing or in small complex devices, a syringe with a long needle can be used to place the spores at various sections of the lumen (bore) of the tubing or in intricate locations in the device, which can then be sectioned out or flushed during assays for viability of surviving spores. For bulky equipment, such as blood oxygenators and renal dialysis equipment, reject specimens of materials from which the various portions of the device are assembled may be used as carriers for the spores, which should then be placed in difficult to penetrate sections of the device. However, the use of plastics with hydrophobic surfaces must be evaluated with caution to prevent unrealistic situations of BI resistance to EtO.

C. Acceptability of Dosimetric Release (No Sterility Test)

1. Dosimetric Release for Products Sterilized by Ionizing Radiation

An examination of the kinetics of microbial kill by radiation sterilization will show that this sterilizing method is as efficient as moist or dry heat sterilization, and under usual operating condition is much easier to control than EtO gaseous sterilization. Because of the simplicity of this sterilization process, the number of variables that must be regulated is at a minimum. Only a brief analysis of several key factors associated with radiation sterilization of medical supplies will be discussed here. The two chief factors determining the level of sterility (probability of survivors) attained from radiation processing under usual manufacturing conditions are the average bioburden on the items and the radiation resistance of that bioburden.

The first step in developing a dosimetric program for radiation sterilized products should start with a program of environmental microbial monitoring. Through the use of various aerosol samplers, swab techniques, and Rodac contact plates, the sources of microbial shedding and buildup in the processing environment can be determined and suitable restrictive measures taken to limit the accumulation of microorganisms on the finished items (see Sec. II.A for further discussion). The average bioburden on each type of product, as manufactured, should be determined. The previous discussion in Section II.B describes the assay procedures currently in use.

Some manufacturers going into radiation sterilization initially employ a biological indicator, usually spores of *Bacillus pumilus*, to serve as an integrator of all factors that could be involved in the sterilization process. The sterilization of product inoculated with spores of *B. pumilus* can be correlated with the destruction of the natural bioburden on the product. It has been found that the inoculum level of 10^6 spores of *B. pumilus* on the product will not survive a dose beyond 1.2 Mrad. The manufacturer then places greater reliance on the use of primary and secondary chemical dosimeters to assure that the load has received the necessary amount of energy (dose) to achieve the desired level of a probability of a survivor.

The purpose of dosimetry is to measure the energy transferred by radiation to the treated material. As indicated, the use of a BI to measure dose is not that precise, and in commercial usage will not go beyond 1.2 Mrad. Physical and/or chemical dosimeters are available that are easy to use, relatively precise, and reliable. The qualities that a good physical and/or chemical dosimetric system should have are the following: (a) it should be independent of the dose rate and only record the total dose received; (b) it should be small in size, and (c) it should be reasonably precise, reliable, and reproducible.

In order to achieve these latter objectives, the sterile disposable device industry has utilized the concept of primary and secondary dosimeters. The primary dosimeters can be considered "the gold bar" type of standard and are employed during the initial phases of commissioning of a facility or the introduction of a new product line to be sterilized in a particular sterilization facility. Calorimeters, ionizing chambers, and chemical dosimeters, such as ferrous sulfate solution and ceric sulfate solution, are considered the techniques for primary standard reference dosimetry. In the day-to-day monitoring of radiation-sterilized medical products, secondary dosimeters that can be related back to the primary dosimeters are routinely employed. Liquid solutions of radiochromic dyes, ceric plus cerous sulfate, undyed plastics, such as clear Perspex (polymethyl methacrylate) and PVC, and dyed plastics, such as red Perspex, which can be read spectrophotometrically or potentiometrically, are the materials of choice. The absorbed dose levels currently being used in radiation dosimetric release programs range from approximately 1 Mrad for products desiring a PSI of 10^{-3} or less, to 1.6–1.8 Mrad for products having a PSI of 10^{-6} or less. As of 1984, radiation dosimetric release programs in the United States rarely employ dose levels as high as 2.5 Mrad.

2. *Process (Dosimetric) Release for Products Sterilized by Steam Under Pressure*

The approach to have steam-sterilized products released processwise is similar to that described for radiation dosimetric release. The bioburden on a sample of items from the load to be sterilized should be determined. However, it is not necessary to go through subprocess (incremental) dosing to obtain a D value for the steam resistance of the bioburden. Instead, the bioburden should be exposed to a heat shock of approximately 10 min at 80°C to kill vegetative forms, the survivors indicating the spore load in the bioburden. If the number of spores per item is less than 100, then the use of an F_0 of 8 or greater will provide a PSI of 10^{-6} or less [27]. The F_0 is equivalent to the amount of time that the hardest to penetrate portion of a load is at the temperature of 250°F. Thus, if an item can be shown through various techniques involving the integration of lethality [10,22] to be at a temperature equivalent to 250°F for 8 min, then it has an F_0 of 8. Similarly, if the rates of microbial destruction at a lower temperature can be related to the rates of microbial destruction at 250°F, i.e., the use of the z function [10,22], then a longer processing time at a lower temperature can have an F_0 of 8.

Unlike radiation dosimetric release, steam process release does not usually employ a steam dosimeter as such. If the use of thermocouples shows that the center of a load is at a temperature of 250°F for 8 min or more, or the integration of lethal rates through the come up, holding, and cool-down times will summate to an F_0 of 8, then the product can be released on a process basis alone. The routine use of thermocouples or RTD is not required after the initial validation of an F_0 of 8 has been established for a specific sterilizer with a particular load configuration. Some manufacturers do utilize heat and steam integrating chemical indicators as a form of steam sterilization dosimeter for lot-by-lot release of their products. These steam sterilization dosimeters are widely used by hospitals to monitor their autoclave cycles.

As an adjunct to the steam process release program, some manufacturers during the initial development phases of the program will use a BI challenge of sproes of *B. stearothermophilus*. It is not necessary to have these spores carried on the product, since there is an equivalence of resistance between spores carried on adventitious carriers, such as paper strips, and those carried directly on product for this sterilization method. Frequently, it is found that the number of spores on the BI must be decreased from the 10^6 level, since the D value for many lots of spores of *B. stearothermophilus* will exceed 2 min at 250°F. Ideally, the destruction time for the BI should not come closer than two D values to the total time desired for the steam sterilization cycle. The instrumentation used to follow the temperature, pressure, and time of a steam sterilization cycle should be properly calibrated and rechecked at periodic intervals (6 months) to assure that the steam process release variables are still within control.

D. Pyrogen Release Criteria

The only devices in the United States currently required to be tested for lack of pyrogenicity are transfusion and infusion assemblies. This requirement comes about through the listing of these two items in the USP [6], which outlines how the pyrogen test is to be performed on these devices. All other manufacturers of the various devices entering or contacting the parenterum, who label their products for lack of pyrogenicity, do so on the basis that the presence of pyrogen, if detected by the FDA, could be legally cited as a form of adulteration under the FD&C Act.

It is commonly assumed that the cause of the febrile reaction, characterized as a pyrogenic response to materials entering the parenterum, is a lipopolysaccharide derived from bacterial endotoxins. Pyrogens are of widespread occurrence as a result of microbial growth, although not all types of microorganisms produce them. The most potent pyrogens are obtained from gram-negative bacteria, although other microorganisms, such as yeast and mold, as well as a few viruses, can produce substances that are pyrogenic in nature. The amount of material required to produce a specified rise in temperature, to be classed as a pyrogenic response, varies from 0.1 ng up to approximately 1 μg/kg of rabbit body weight.

By definition, a pyrogenic substance is capable of producing fever, i.e., of significantly elevating the body temperature of a mammalian species. The test currently listed in the USP [33] sets the significant elevation of a rabbit at 0.6°C, which is equivalent to about 1.0°F. A second effect generally produced by pyrogen in the mammalian system is an alteration of the blood picture: there is a brief reduction followed by an increase in the white blood cell count. The release of endogenous pyrogen from the white blood cells leads to other physiological effects.

The previous and still legally acceptable procedure for assaying for the lack of pyrogens in parenteral devices was the USP rabbit test, which involves a presumptive procedure with three animals. If the test device passes, it is judged nonpyrogenic. If the test result is positive, however, the completed USP test with an additional five animals is to be performed [33].

USP XXI describes a bacterial endotoxin test employing the reagent derived from the aqueous extracts of the circulating amebocytes of the horseshoe crab, *Limulus polyphemus* and referred to as the *Limulus* amebocyte lysate (LAL) procedure. This test has been described in the literature as the most sensitive and convenient method currently available for detecting bacterial pyrogen. In the presence of picogram (0.001 ng) quantities of endotoxins, the LAL reagent exhibits a protein coagulation reaction (gel, turbidity, or precipitate) under prescribed in vitro test conditions and in the absence of interfering substances.

In the Federal Register (FR) of March 29, 1983 [34], the FDA issued a notice stating the conditions under which manufacturers can use the LAL test for determining that medical devices are nonpyrogenic. Basically, manufacturers must show that the LAL reaction is not inhibited by substances eluted from their devices and that the test in their hands is at least as sensitive as the USP rabbit pyrogen test. Guidelines cited in the above FR outline the types of data that the device manufacturer must develop before relying on the LAL test for release of product as nonpyrogenic. Prior to the publication of this FR in 1983, over 50 medical device manufacturers had submitted data packages to the FDA and had received approval to use the LAL test solely as the pyrogen release mechanism for their products. Submission of data on LAL use to the FDA is not now required.

E. Acceptable Levels of Residues from Gaseous EtO Sterilization Procedures

The use of EtO as a gaseous sterilant for parenteral devices results in residues of EtO itself, ethylene chlorohydrin, and ethylene glycol. In those plastics that can solubilize EtO, the residue of this gas can be contained within the plastic matrix. Usually, the other two residues, ethylene chlorohydrin and ethylene glycol, are formed on the surface of the device and can be easily eluted with solvents.

EtO is an alkylating agent and has been shown to be mutagenic to microorganisms, pollen, seeds, and insects. Recent studies indicate that EtO is teratogenic at high dose levels and gives a positive response in a dominant lethal assay for mutagenicity. Ethylene chlorohydrin is also mutagenic, but its activity on a molar basis is much less than that of EtO. The hazard from the chlorohydrin comes through its serious systemic toxic effects, which can occur through its being swallowed, inhaled, or absorbed through the intact skin. Ethylene glycol is much less toxic then the other two compounds and can be tolerated in low doses for a long period of time.

In the *Federal Register* of June 23, 1978 [35], the FDA proposed maximum residue limits and maximum levels of exposures for EtO, ethylene chlorohydrin, and ethylene glycol in drugs and medical devices. An extensive review of the toxicological hazards from each of these compounds was presented. Assay methodology for the detection of these residues with medical devices centered on the three procedures contained in the proposed standard for EtO sterilization [36] published by AAMI: (a) vacuum extraction, (b) acetone extraction, and (c) headspace gas analysis. All three procedures rely on the use of gas chromatography for the detection of these residues.

The AAMI proposed standard [36] contained a recommendation that the residue limit in implantable devices not exceed 250 ppm of EtO. In the June 23, 1978, proposal by the FDA, the residue limits for both EtO and ethylene chlorohydrin in parenteral devices is basically at a level of 25 ppm each, except that in small devices a level 250 ppm for each of these residues is suggested. The residue level for ethylene glycol ranges from 500 ppm in implantable devices up to 5000 ppm on topical devices.

F. Resterilization of Parenteral Devices by User

One of the current concerns in the United States is the rapidly rising cost of hospital and medical care. One of the factors that could contribute to a decrease in such medical care costs is the limited reuse of many disposable or single-use items. The difficulty with encouraging such reuse lies in identifying which disposable devices can be safely reused and what specific precautions should be observed in reprocessing any particular device. In the absence of assurance from manufacturers that such disposable products can safely be reused, medical practitioners or patients often have no practical alternative way, aside from testing, of verifying that such products can be reprocessed without adverse effects.

If a manufacturer gives instructions in the labeling for the product that states the conditions under which the device can be resterilized, then the FDA has no objections to such reuse. Basically, the FDA has not ruled out the reuse of disposable devices by health care institutions, provided those institutions are able to ensure that such reuse is safe when not specified by the device manufacturer. Any group that engages in the resterilization of disposable or single-use devices bears legal responsibility if the manufacturer has not given indications that the device can be resterilized or has not provided instructions on such resterilization.

G. Adequate Record Keeping for Every Lot of Sterilized Parenteral Devices

It is the responsibility of either the plant production manager or the chief quality control official, at each production location, to assure that an adequate number of reference samples are retained to allow for analyses in the event of legal challenges over the sterility, nontoxicity, or nonpyrogenicity of each lot of parenteral devices. The actual number of such samples is not defined in the good manufacturing procedures (GMP) for medical devices promulgated by the FDA [37]. Usually, a manufacturer will hold as a reserve sample approximately twice the number of samples that would have been tested if a finished product sterility test had been performed. All such stored samples must be reasonably protected from dust and crushing and held under storage conditions approximating room temperature and relative humidity. A master reference sample book indicating all reference samples in storage should be maintained by the responsible designated person for each plant location.

Every lot of sterile parenteral devices produced by a manufacturer should have extensive record keeping and documentation of the history of that lot. Among the items that should be considered for such record keeping include preconditioning room records and recording charts, all sterilizer logs, the recording chart for each sterilizer run, any animal test records associated with the materials for each lot, the lot numbers for the biological indicators, sterility test records, if performed, for each lot of product, and the dates when the product was released for shipment. A more complete grasp of what is required in a device history record can be obtained by consulting the GMP regulations for medical devices [37].

REFERENCES

1. U.S. Pharmacopeia XXI, Biological Tests—Plastics, U.S.P. Convention, Inc., Rockville, MD, 1985, pp. 1235–1237.
2. U.S. Pharmacopeia XXI, Physico-Chemical Tests—Plastics, U.S.P. Convention, Inc., Rockville, MD, 1985, pp. 1237–1238.
3. B. N. Ames, J. McCann, and E. Yamasaki, *Mutation Res.*, 31:347–364 (1975); also *Proc. Natl. Acad. Sci.*, 70:1181–2285 (1973).
4. D. E. Amacher, S. C. Paillet, G. N. Turner, V. A. Ray, and D. S. Salsberg, *Mutation Res.*, 72:447–474 (1980); also *Mutation Res.*, 64:391–406 (1979).

5. Toxicological Guidelines for Medical Device Materials, Division of Small Manufacturers Assistance, Center for Devices and Radiological Health, FDA, Rockville, MD 20857.
6. U.S. Pharmacopeia XXI, Transfusion and Infusion Assemblies, U.S.P. Convention, Inc., Rockville, MD, 1985, p. 1183.
7. U.S. Pharmacopeia XXI, Sterility Tests, U.S.P. Convention, Inc., Rockville, MD, 1985, pp. 1156–1160.
8. C. W. Bruch and M. K. Bruch, Sterilization. In: *Dispensing of Medication* (E. W. Martin, ed.), 7th Edition. Mack Publishing Co., Easton, Pennsylvania, 1971, pp. 592–623.
9. C. W. Bruch, *Dev. Ind. Microbiol.*, 14:3–16 (1973); also *Bull. Parent. Drug Assoc.*, 18:105–121 (1974).
10. I. J. Pflug and R. G. Holcomb, Principles of thermal destruction of microorganisms. In *Disinfection, Sterilization, and Preservation* (S. S. Blcok, ed.). Lea & Febiger, Philadelphia, 1983, pp. 751–810.
11. R. W. Campbell, Microbiological Safety Index. In Information Letter No. 563, Health Protection Branch, Health and Welfare Canada, Ottawa, 1979; also see *Med. Instrument.*, 14:232–233 (1980).
12. Process Control Guidelines for Gamma Radiation Sterilization of Medical Devices, Association for Advancement of Medical Instrumentation (AAMI), Arlington, Virginia, 1984.
13. Federal Standard 209B, Clean Room and Work Station Requirements for a Controlled Environment. General Services Administration, Washington, D.C., 1973.
14. C. W. Bruch, *Drug Cosmet. Ind.*, 111(4):51–54; 150–156 (1972).
15. C. W. Bruch, Proc. Amer. Soc. Quality Control, February 28, 1977, pp. 173–176, ASQC, Cherry Hill, NJ; also Sterile Medical Devices: A GMP Workshop Manual, pp. 165–168, Center for Devices and Radiological Health, FDA, Rockville, MD, 1984.
16. U.S. Pharmacopeia XXI, Microbial Limit Tests, U.S.P. Convention, Inc., Rockville, MD, 1985, pp. 1151–1156.
17. NASA Standard Procedure for Microbiological Examination of Space Hardware, NHB 5340.1A, National Aeronautics and Space Administration, Washington, D.C., 1968.
18. K. L. West, Ethylene oxide sterilization: A study of resistance relationships. In *Sterilization of Medical Products* (E. R. L. Gaughran and K. Kereluk, eds.). Johnson & Johnson, New Brunswick, N.J., 1977, pp. 109–168.
19. C. R. Stumbo, *Food Technol.*, 2:228–240 (1948).
20. C. R. Stumbo, J. R. Murphy, and J. Cochran, *Food Technol.*, 4:321–326 (1950).
21. H. O. Halverson and N. R. Ziegler, *J. Bacteriol.*, 25:101–121 (1933).
22. L. J. Joslyn, Sterilization by heat. In *Disinfection, Sterilization, and Preservation* (S. S. Block, ed.). Lea & Febiger, Philadelphia, 1983, pp. 3–46.
23. I. J. Pflug, Heat sterilization. In *Industrial Sterilization* (G. B. Phillips and W. S. Miller, eds.). Duke University Press, Durham, N.C., 1973, pp. 239–282.
24. R. Berube, Resistance levels for biological indicators for use in sterilization by ionizing radiation. In *Sterilization of Medical Products* (E. R. L. Gaughran and K. Kereluk, eds.). Johnson & Johnson, New Brunswick, N.J., 1977, pp. 169–192.

25. Guideline for Industrial Steam Sterilization of Medical Products, Association for Advancement of Medical Instrumentation (AAMI), Arlington, VA, 1985.
26. Guideline for Industrial Ethylene Oxide Sterilization of Medical Devices, Association for Advancement of Medical Instrumentation (AAMI), Arlington, VA, 1981.
27. U.S. Pharmacopeia XX, Steam Sterilization, U.S.P. Convention, Inc., Rockville, MD, 1980, p. 1037 (footnote 2).
28. Guideline on General Principles of Process Validation, FDA, Rockville, MD, 1984.
29. J. E. Doyle, A. W. McDaniel, K. L. West, J. G. Whitbourne, and R. R. Ernst, *Appl. Microbiol.*, 20:793–797 (1970).
30. U.S. Pharmacopeia XXI, Tests and Assays—Procedures, U.S.P. Convention, Inc., Rockville, MD, 1985, p. 5.
31. W. G. Murrell and W. J. Scott, *J. Gen. Microbiol.*, 43:411–425 (1966).
32. G. L. Gilbert, V. M. Gambrill, D. R. Spiner, R. K. Hoffman, and C. R. Phillips, *App. Microbiol.*, 12:496–503 (1964).
33. U.S. Pharmacopeia XXI, Pyrogen Test, U.S.P. Convention, Inc., Rockville, MD, 1985, pp. 1181–1182.
34. Draft Guideline for Validation of the Limulus Amebocyte Lysate Test as an End-Product Endotoxin Test for Human and Animal Parenteral Drugs, Biologic Products, and Medical Devices, Federal Register 48: 13096 (1983); also published in Pharmacopeial Forum, May–June 1983.
35. Ethylene Oxide, Ethylene Chlorohydrin, and Ethylene Glycol: Proposed Maximum Residue Limits and Maximum Levels of Exposure, Federal Register 43:27482 (1978).
36. Standard for Ethylene Oxide Sterilization (Proposed). Association for Advancement of Medical Instrumentation (AAMI EOS-P 11/77), Arlington, VA, 1977.
37. Good Manufacturing Practice for Medical Devices, Code of Federal Regulations, Title 21, Part 820; available from U. S. Government Printing Office, Washington, D.C., 1984.

12

Regulatory and GMP Considerations for Medical Devices

Larry R. Pilot

McKenna, Conner & Cuneo, Washington, D.C.

I. INTRODUCTION

In 1906, the first Food and Drug Act, known as the Wiley Act, was enacted into law [1]. The needs of society were relatively simple, and the procedures for implementing this law were far from complex. Since that time the needs of the public have changed, there have been dramatic technological advances and federal laws applicable to foods, drugs, cosmetics, and devices have been modified by Congress and judicially applied and interpreted through thousands of court cases.

Today, the Food and Drug Administration (FDA) has the responsibility to administer this complex of laws and the manufacturer has the basic responsibility to assure that what it manufactures is safe and/or effective. Violations of the Federal Food, Drug, and Cosmetic Act [2] can lead to the destruction of a business or a criminal penalty for an individual. Consequently, it is important to know something about the law, the function of the FDA, and the intent and significance of FDA regulations on good manufacturing practices (GMP).

II. HISTORY OF DRUGS AND DEVICES

The Food and Drug Act of 1906 was designed to prevent the manufacture, sale, or transportation of adulterated or misbranded drugs. There was no provision to require a premarket demonstration of safety or effectiveness, and devices, as distinguished from drugs, were not considered. Difficulties in enforcing the 1906 law led to the obvious conclusion that amendments to the law were necessary. In 1912, the Act was amended to prohibit the appearance of a false statement of curative or therapeutic effect on labeling of drugs. During the 1930s, Congress considered various amendments to the Act, but it was not until a number of fatalities occurred after patients consumed a toxic suspension of sulfanilamide that Congress passed the Federal Food, Drug, and Cosmetic Act of 1938 (the Act). This new Act enabled the FDA to regulate cosmetics and devices for the first time and, more importantly, to require that new drugs be approved for safety by the FDA before such drugs could be generally made available to the public.

In 1962, largely because of serious incidents relating to the teratogenic effect of the drug thalidomide, the 1938 Act was amended to require that any new drug be approved by the FDA for effectiveness as well as safety before a new drug could be made available to the public. However, no changes in the law were made with respect to devices, and the FDA was limited to applying the 1938 provisions of the Act against devices. Thus, the FDA had the burden to establish that a device was adulterated or misbranded.

The device nomenclature in 1938 was intended to cover things like trusses, ultraviolet lights, orthopedic shoes, surgical instruments, contraceptives, prosthetic devices, and the like; and the concern over these and other items considered to be devices related to the truthfulness of their labeling claims. Most of the legal actions taken over the years were based on the misbranding provisions of the Act. These involved actions against such devices as colonic irrigators, spechtochromes, generators liberating chlorine gas, galvanometers, and products that delivered ultrasonic waves or electrical energy. Although drug discovery and development was proceeding at a rapid rate and legislation, regulations, and court decisions were filling in the void to provide a sound, often controversial, body of law relating to drugs, scientific and regulatory activity in the device industry occurred at a slower pace. Device discovery, development, and innovation was somewhat less noticeable, and the technological advances that occurred far outdistanced the formulation of an adequate basis in law. In the 1950s, concern was expressed over the lack of authority to properly control problems arising from the use of devices. This concern intensified during the early 1960s, when the device nomenclature began to fill out with such respectable terms as cardiac pacemakers; ceramic and plastic surgical implants; kidney dialysis units; defibrillators; cardiac, renal, and other catheters; artificial veins, arteries, and heart valves; and other devices equally descriptive of the types of products that have enriched medical science.

It was not until 1967, however, that the first comprehensive legislative proposal affecting devices was introduced into Congress.

Shortly thereafter, the Supreme Court of the United States reviewed two different cases involving the application of the new drug provision of the Act to products that were covered by the definition of the term "device." In 1968, the Supreme Court denied certiorari in *AMP Incorporated vs. John W. Gardner, HEW Secretary, et al.* and thus left standing the decision of the Second Circuit Court of Appeals [3]. The circuit court held that two products consisting of a disposable applicator (a hemostat in one product and a long slender tube in the other), a nylon ligature loop, and a nylon locking device used for tying off blood vessels during surgical procedures were essentially products that were sutures. Because sutures were identified in the *U.S. Pharmacopeia*, the court reasoned that these products were drugs, and not devices. That a suture was listed in the *U.S. Pharmacopeia* was some evidence that the product was a drug. Inasmuch as the suture was capable of coming within the definition of either a "drug" or a "device," a liberal construction of the Act warranted classifying the product as a drug to protect the public health. Because there was a difference of medical opinion among the experts concerning the safety of the product, it was construed to be a "new drug."

In the other case, *United States vs. An Article of Drug . . . Bacto-Unidisk*, the Supreme Court decided in 1969 that antibiotic sensitivity disks were drugs and reversed the Sixth Circuit Court of Appeals [4]. The Sixth Circuit had affirmed the District Court's finding that these disks, which were used for in vitro identification of antibiotic effectiveness against organisms, were not drugs. The District Court had further suggested that these disks would be more appropriately identified as "devices" under the Act. The Supreme Court held that Congress did not intend to limit a drug to the medical concept of articles that were administered to humans either internally or externally. The definition of drug* should be read literally and, thus, include antibiotic sensitivity disks. In rejecting the suggestion that these disks were devices, the Court held that the Federal Food, Drug, and Cosmetic Act is a form of remedial legislation that must be given a liberal construction consistent with the Act's overriding purpose to protect the public health.

These court decisions created some confusion and a new sense of awareness on the need to modify the Act to provide the FDA with appropriate authority to regulate the device industry. In particular, the device industry was concerned about the confusion these court cases would generate because of the uncertainty as to whether the definition for drug or device applied to a particular product. If a product could be covered by the definition of the term "drug," then such product would be subject to all the provisions of the law applicable to drugs. If the product was new, then preclearance for safety and effectiveness as a new drug was required. For example, in the early 1970s, new contact lenses that were distinguishable from hard contact lenses because they were soft or hydrophilic were regulated by the FDA as new drugs. Likewise, all accessories to these products, including heat disinfection units, were regulated as drugs. Application of these court cases to products like contact lenses stimulated renewed public interest in a new law to solve the problems that were being created.

During October 1969, President Richard M. Nixon became the third President to request legislation for devices. As a result, the Secretary of HEW appointed a committee chaired by Dr. Theodore Cooper, Director of the Heart and Lung Institute. This group was to thoroughly review this matter and prepare a suitable report [5]. This report, which was released in late 1970, lead to the introduction of various legislative proposals, and after years of careful, deliberate discussion of these proposals by representatives

---

*Drug is defined as "(a) articles recognized in the official *United States Pharmacopeia*, official Homeopathic Pharmacopeia of the United States, or official National Formulary, or any supplement to any of them; and (b) articles intended for use in the diagnosis, cure, mitigation, treatment, or prevention of disease in man or other animals; and (c) articles (other than food) intended to affect the structure or any function of the body of man or other animals; and (d) articles intended for use as a component of any articles specified in clause (a), (b), or (c); but does not include devices or their components, parts, or accessories."

of industry, the health professions, Congress, government, and consumers, the Medical Device Amendments of 1976 became law on May 28, 1976.

III. MEDICAL DEVICE AMENDMENTS OF 1976

A. Legislative History and Intent

The development of the Medical Device Amendments of 1976 (the Amendments) took several years, and during this time, Congress reviewed the input provided by consumers, industry, the health professions, and the government. The experience of the FDA in regulating drugs represented a constant reminder to the Congress of the need to avoid creating a statutory scheme that would complicate or confound the invention, manufacture, and availability of new devices. In general, the various interest groups agreed on the need for a new law, and these interest groups worked well with the Congress and one another to develop an approach that was workable and reflected the major differences between drugs and devices. There was a sense of urgency but no panic or calamity of the type that accompanied passage of the 1938 and 1962 drug amendments. As a result, the congressional hearings, debates, and committee reports represent a clear and deliberate attempt to justify and explain the many new provisions in the Amendments.

These Amendments provided the FDA with more direct authority to regulate a product subject to its jurisdiction than it had for any other product. The provisions of the Act applicable to drugs are not nearly as broad, complicated, or flexible. Congress recognized the need to develop a statutory mechanism that would be responsive to the concerns of the Cooper Committee and the public. In large measure as a result of this continuing concern, the Medical Device Amendments of 1976 conferred upon the FDA certain immediate authorities and a mechanism whereby certain other authorities could be exercised after completion of administrative procedures and/or the final publication of appropriate regulations.

B. Unique Provisions

Under the Amendments, Congress redefined the definition of device to avoid overlap with the drug definition and provided for different levels of control to apply to devices depending on the characterization of the device and intended use.

The revised definition of *device* appears in the Act as follows:

> The term 'device' (except when used in paragraph (n) of this section and in sections 301(i), 403(f), 502(c), and 602(c)) means an instrument, apparatus, implement, machine, contrivance, implant, in vitro reagent, or other similar or related article, including any component, part, or accessory, which is—
>
> (1) recognized in the official National Formulary, or the United States Pharmacopeia, or any supplement to them,
> (2) intended for use in the diagnosis of disease or other conditions, or in the cure, mitigation, treatment, or prevention of disease, in man or other animals, or

(3) intended to affect the structure or any function of the body of man or other animals, and which does not achieve any of its principal intended purposes through chemical action within or on the body of man or other animals and which is not dependent upon being metabolized for the achievement of any of its principal intended purposes.

The amendments provide that the FDA, with the assistance of outside expert advisory committees, must review and classify all devices into a category for which distinguishable controls are applicable. In theory, this approach would apply controls that are in reasonable proportion to the nature of the device. Thus a simple device would be subject to certain general controls, whereas a device intended to support or sustain human life would be subject to more stringent controls, including premarket approval by the FDA. The classification categories and regulatory requirements that apply to the manufacturer of a device in the class are as follows [6]:

Class I, General controls. General provisions of the Act relating to adulteration; misbranding; registration; banning; repair, replacement or refund; record keeping and reporting; and good manufacturing practices, among others, are sufficient to provide a reasonable assurance of the safety and effectiveness of a device.

Class II, Performance standards. In addition to the controls applicable for class I devices, it is necessary to establish a performance standard in order to provide a reasonable assurance of the safety and effectiveness of the device.

Class III, Premarket approval. In addition to the controls applicable for class I devices, it is necessary to require premarket approval by the FDA in order to provide a reasonable assurance of the safety and effectiveness of the device. Such premarket approval could also require compliance with an applicable performance standard.

The Food and Drug Administration began the process of classifying devices prior to the enactment of the Amendments and continues the process [7]. The composition of the advisory committees is described in the Amendments. The voting members, are physicians, engineers, and other qualified scientists with expertise in the specialty of the committee (e.g., orthopedics, dentistry, circulatory system, and neurology). In addition, each committee consists of two nonvoting members, one representing the interests of consumers and the other representing the interests of industry. The committees meet in open session, and the product of their efforts to classify devices is published in the *Federal Register* for public comment. After the FDA has reviewed the comments of the public, a final classification order, with an appropriate preamble, is published in the *Federal Register*.

Final classification determines whether a device is in class I, II, or III. A manufacturer of a device subject to class III, premarket approval, would not be required to submit an application until 30 months have elapsed from the date of final classification. This assumes that the device was in commercial distribution prior to May 28, 1976, or is substantially equivalent to such device. Whether any submission for these "pre-Amendment" type of devices will be required is left to the FDA.

Devices that are new because they are not substantially equivalent to "pre-Amendment" devices are automatically classified into class III. This automatic classification applies irrespective of the intended use or simplicity of the new device. The manufacturer must either obtain FDA premarket approval (PMA) for the device or successfully petition the FDA for reclassification of the device into the general control (I) or performance (II) category. Any device in class I may be exempted by the FDA from requirements applicable to registration, records or reports, or good manufacturing practices. Finally any device for which a PMA is required may be marketed without such approval if the FDA has approved a product development protocol (PDP). The PDP enables the manufacturer of a device for which changes are certain to occur (e.g., a complicated electronic device) to market the device and make necessary improvements consistent with advances in technology. Apart from premarket approval by the FDA, devices can be made available to the public through a premarket notification procedure or as an investigational device.

C. Premarket Notification

Under the Amendments, manufacturers and certain distributors must register with the FDA and list their devices with the FDA. This enables the FDA to maintain an inventory of registered establishments and classified devices. Whenever a registered manufacturer or distributor is about to market a device for the first time or a new manufacturer or distributor wants to market a device for the first time, the FDA must be notified at least 90 days in advance of the commercial distribution of the device. This premarket notification procedure is authorized under Section 510(k) of the Act (21 U.S.C. 360) and is often referred to as a 510(k) notification.

The FDA promulgated regulations to implement this authority. These regulations are found in the Code of Federal Regulations at Title 21, Part 807 (21 CFR Part 807). Under these regulations, the manufacturer must submit a notification if

a. A device is to be marketed for the first time
b. A device being marketed by someone else is to be marketed by the registrant for the first time
c. An existing device is to be significantly changed or modified to effect its safety, effectiveness, or intended use

The manufacturer must submit certain information describing the device and its equivalence to classified devices not requiring premarket approval or devices marketed before the effective date of the Amendments and for which premarket approval is not required.

In general, the FDA recommends that a premarket notification contain the following information:

a. Product name (include the proprietary and the common or usual or classification names).
b. Registration number assigned by the Bureau of Medical Devices to the notifying establishment (where applicable).
c. Present class of the device, if any, and the appropriate classification panel that considered the device. If the device has not yet been classified by the FDA, include a statement to that effect.
d. Action taken to meet performance standards (where applicable).

e. Samples of proposed labels, labeling, and advertisements that describe the device and identify its intended use and directions for use.
f. A statement of how the device is similar to and/or different from others on the market. Include copies of labeling, studies, or other material that supports the statement.
g. For changed or modified devices, include data showing how the change or modification affects the safety or effectiveness of the device.

The FDA will evaluate the information submitted by the manufacturer. If the FDA determines on the basis of the information reviewed that the device described in the notification is substantially equivalent to a device for which premarket approval is not necessary, the manufacturer will be notified. The device can then be marketed subject to applicable provisions of the Act even though the 90 days have not elapsed. If for some reason the FDA determines that a device is not substantially equivalent and the manufacturer cannot provide additional evidence to support a change of the FDA position, the device can be marketed in the United States only after a premarket approval (PMA) by the FDA has been obtained or the manufacturer has successfully petitioned the FDA to reclassify the device into class I or class II.

If the manufacturer elects to pursue FDA review of a PMA submission, it must limit use of the device to investigation by qualified practitioners in accordance with FDA regulations. However, the manufacturer may export the investigational device to other countries provided the laws of the foreign country are followed, the government of the foreign country has no objection, and the FDA agrees to the export of the device.

D. Investigational Devices

Whenever clinical studies are undertaken in an effort to demonstrate the safety and effectiveness of a device prior to FDA consideration of a PMA, the sponsor of the investigation must comply with regulations applicable to investigational devices. These investigational device exemption (IDE) regulations are found in 21 CFR Part 812 and, depending on the nature of the device, the sponsor may have to obtain FDA approval prior to the commencement of the investigation. The FDA distinguishes two types of devices, namely, significant risk or nonsignificant risk devices. Only the term "significant risk device" is defined, and this definition includes a device that presents a potential for serious risk to the health, safety, or welfare of a subject and (a) an implant; (b) used in supporting or sustaining human life; or (c) substantially important in diagnosing, curing, mitigating, or treating disease or in preventing impairment of human health.

The sponsor must determine whether the device is a significant risk device. If the device falls into this category, then the sponsor must submit an application to the FDA with a comprehensive description of the investigational program. It is essential that this submission, among other things, describe the investigational plan, provide for patient informed consent, identify qualified investigators who have obtained institutional review board approval of the investigational plan to be conducted at the facilities identified, and the labeling for the device. The FDA will review the IDE application and advise the sponsor within 30 days whether the IDE is approved, approved with modifications, or disapproved. If the IDE application is disapproved, the sponsor has the opportunity to request a hearing in order to pursue administrative remedies.

If the device is regarded by the sponsor to be a "nonsignificant risk device," there is no requirement to submit the IDE to the FDA for review and approval. However, it is necessary that the Institutional Review Board approve the investigation before any clinical studies are undertaken. Likewise, it is the responsibility of the sponsor to comply with all other provisions of the regulation because there is no functional distinction between significant risk and nonsignificant risk devices. Thus the only practical, but important, difference between an investigation for a significant risk device as opposed to a nonsignificant risk device is the need for the sponsor to obtain FDA review and approval of an investigation for a significant risk device.

E. Premarket Approval

Any postamendment "new" device or device that has been classified into the premarket approval, class III, category must undergo premarket review by the FDA for safety and effectiveness before commercial distribution of the device can take place or continue. The manufacturer or other party who submits a premarket approval application (PMAA) has the responsibility to provide adequate evidence to satisfy the FDA that there is a reasonable assurance of device safety and effectiveness in relation to the intended use of the device.

Under Section 515 of the Act (21 U.S.C. 360e), the applicant must submit the following information:

a. Full reports of all information, published or known to or which should reasonably be known to the applicant, concerning investigations that have been made to show whether such device is safe and effective
b. A full statement of the components, ingredients, and properties and of the principle or principles of operation, of such device
c. A full description of the methods used in, and the facilities and controls used for the manufacture, processing, and, when relevant, packing and installation of, such device
d. An identifying reference to any performance standard under Section 514 that would be applicable to any aspect of such device if it were a class II device, and either adequate information to show that such aspect of such device fully meets such performance standard or adequate information to justify any deviation from such standard
e. Such samples of such device and of components thereof as the Secretary may reasonably require, except that where the submission of such samples is impracticable or unduly burdensome, the requirement of this subparagraph may be met by the submission of complete information concerning the location of one or more such devices readily available for examination and testing
f. Specimens of the labeling proposed to be used for such device
g. Such other information relevant to the subject matter of the application as the Secretary, with the concurrence of the appropriate panel under Section 513, may require

If the required information is present, the FDA must approve or disapprove the PMAA within 180 days of the submission. Unlike new drugs, the Amendments require that the PMAA be reviewed by an advisory panel of experts who are not employees of the FDA. The expert panel is charged with the responsibility to review the PMAA during a meeting that is open to the public and to recommend approval or disapproval of the PMAA.

The FDA is not required to accept the findings of an expert panel, but if it rejects the panel recommendation, it carries a burden to demonstrate support for its position. If the FDA disapproves the PMAA for a device, the applicant has the opportunity to petition the Commissioner of the FDA for a hearing on the disapproval prior to initiating any proceedings in the Federal Courts. If the FDA approves the PMAA, it will notify the applicant by letter and publish a notice to this effect in the *Federal Register*. This notice will provide a summary of the data on safety and effectiveness and provide the public with an opportunity to comment on the approval. Moreover, after the PMAA is approved, any member of the public has the opportunity to formally challenge the approval by the FDA in accordance with procedures outlined in the Act.

There are many other provisions of the Amendments that are unique and permit the use of custom devices, export of devices not available in U.S. markets, and use and distribution of restricted devices and provide the FDA with other authorities.

IV. OTHER LAWS

In addition to the Federal Food, Drug, and Cosmetic Act, the FDA administers the Radiation Control for Health and Safety Act, which was enacted into law in 1968. Under this law, any device that emits ionizing or nonionizing radiation is subject to the provisions of the law, and a performance standard for such product could be established by regulation. Many products that fall under the definition of the term "device," as defined in the Federal Food, Drug, and Cosmetic Act, are included in this definition, and standards for devices, such as dental x-ray equipment, have been established. Manufacturers of such devices are subject to the provisions of both laws.

Other regulatory agencies possess authority to regulate the activities of device manufacturers. These include the Environmental Protection Agency, the Occupational Safety and Health Administration, and the Consumer Product Safety Commission, to mention a few. In 1978, these government agencies formed a working group to coordinate activities of mutual interest and reduce unnecessary overlap. The Interagency Regulatory Liasion Group coordinated various efforts and implemented a basic program to assist one another in making observations during inspections of plant facilities. Although this group no longer exists, it did provide a mechanism whereby duplication of effort was minimized.

In general, when there is a possibility of overlapping regulatory requirements by government agencies, the respective agencies will often prepare and agree to a memorandum of understanding. For example, the Federal Trade Commission (FTC) has the responsibility to regulate the activities of those who advertise over-the-counter drugs and medical devices. The

FTC is concerned about the truthfulness of advertising representations that are made about devices that are available to the public and for which the FDA has not identified these as restricted devices.* A number of years ago, the FDA and the FTC entered into an agreement that established procedures whereby they could coordinate their programs and exchange information and evidence. In theory, this would avoid overlap and enable the FDA its expertise with respect to liability and the FTC to apply its expertise in matters relating to advertising [8].

Another example of agency cooperation relates to federal government purchase of medical devices. The Department of Defense (DOD), as well as other agencies of the government (e.g., the Veterans Administration and the General Services Administration) have a need to inspect manufacturers prior to purchase of devices. At one time, the DOD conducted its own inspections of device manufacturers even though the FDA had this responsibility for the public under provisions of the Act. In an effort to avoid needless duplication of effort, the DOD and the FDA agreed that the FDA would conduct all future investigations of device manufacturers seeking to do business with the DOD [9].

Irrespective of the application of laws applied by other federal government agencies, anyone involved in activities relating to the development, manufacture, and marketing of products subject to the Federal Food, Drug, and Cosmetic Act should be familiar with the basic provisions of the Act relating to drugs and devices and the process the FDA utilizes to accomplish its objectives. This is particularly important for manufacturers responsible for compliance with FDA regulation on device good manufacturing practices.

V. THE FEDERAL FOOD, DRUG, AND COSMETIC ACT: GENERAL PROVISIONS

A. Basic Provisions

The purpose of the Federal Food, Drug, and Cosmetic Act is to provide direction to manufacturers of drugs and devices and enable the FDA to take certain steps to prevent violations from occurring, detect the presence of violations, and take corrective measures when violative conditions are observed. The objective of this process is to provide the general public with a reasonable assurance that drugs and devices are safe and effective.

The Act describes in general what is expected of those who develop, manufacture, or market drugs and devices. Pertinent terms relating to label, labeling, and other aspects are defined, and general provisions relating to the responsibilities of manufacturers are discussed. The FDA has the authority to develop and enforce certain regulations, conduct inspections of certain facilities to acquire various kinds of information, and take other necessary steps designed to assure that drugs and devices are safe and effective. Some provisions of the Act are self-explanatory and do not require

---

*Under Section 520(e) of the Act [21 U.S.C. 360i(e)], the FDA can, by regulation or through premarket approval, restrict the use and distribution of devices. For example, if the FDA had reason to believe that a cardiac implant should be limited only to surgeons who have a particular type of training, it could order this restriction by regulation.

the development of regulations. Other provisions of the Act can become operational only after the FDA has promulgated a regulation. In addition, the FDA has the authority to promulgate regulations that are necessary for the efficient enforcement of the Act.

B. Substantive and Interpretive Regulations

The distinction between a provision of the Act and a regulation is important. Congress defines in the Act what is required and what constitutes a violation of the Act. In some areas, Congress has explicitly authorized the FDA to develop regulations that will have the force and effect of law. These regulations are referred to as "substantive" regulations and must be developed in accordance with procedures outlined in the Act or under the Administrative Procedure Act. This requires publication of a proposal in the *Federal Register* in order to provide the public with an opportunity to comment on the proposal. A period of time, usually at least 60 days, is allowed for interested parties to develop comments and transmit them to the FDA. After the time period for comment has elapsed and the FDA has reviewed all comments, it will publish a final regulation in the *Federal Register*. This final regulation is preceded by a preamble that describes the FDA position in response to the comments received. The final order in the *Federal Register* will identify the effective date, and the regulation, without the preamble, will be published in Title 21 of the Code of Federal Regulations.

The FDA often publishes other regulations intended to result in the efficient enforcement of the Act. These regulations are generally viewed as being "interpretive" as opposed to substantive. These interpretive regulations, which often carry force equivalent to substantive regulation, also appear in Title 21 of the Code of Federal Regulations after the public has had an opportunity to comment on the proposal and the FDA has issued a final order. For example, the general administrative procedures of the agency relating to citizens petitions, Freedom of Information requests, and so on, are codified in Title 21 of the Code of Federal Regulations. The FDA also publishes in the *Federal Register* from time to time general notices that announce an agency position on a particular matter, the scheduling of a meeting, or a general policy of interest to the public. In addition, the FDA maintains a number of manuals (e.g., Regulatory Procedures Manual and Inspector Operations Manual) that provide instructions to employees. These manuals are available to the public on request under provisions of the Freedom of Information Act.

C. Prohibited Acts

If a drug or device is in violation of the Act, including applicable regulations, the article is subject to seizure by the FDA or the FDA may proceed to enjoin the further distribution of the violative product. These actions against the device must be pursued in U.S. District Court, and a claimant has the opportunity to contest the position of the FDA. In addition, to actions taken against the device (in rem), actions for criminal prosecution can be taken against those persons (in personem) who violate the Act and regulations promulgated under explicit authority of the Act. However, prior to initiating any criminal proceeding against a person suspected of violating the Act, the FDA must give that person an appropriate notice and an opportunity to present his or her views, either orally or in writing. If the opportunity for a hearing has been accepted, no recommendation to the U.S. Attorney can be transmitted until the hearing is completed.

D. Adulteration

Under the Act, a drug or device is deemed to be adulterated if there is a failure to comply with any of the applicable provisions outlined in Section 501 (21 U.S.C. 351). These violations generally relate to the quality or purity of the finished product. A device, for example, would be adulterated if any one of the following conditions exist.

a. If it consists in whole or in part of any filthy, putrid, or decomposed substance; if it has been prepared, packed or held under insanitary conditions which could result in contamination with filth or render the device injurious to health; if the container is composed of an unsafe color additive [21 U.S.C. 351(a)]
b. If the purity or quality of the device falls below that which it purports or is represented to possess [21 U.S.C. 351(c)]
c. If the device is subject to a performance standard as a class II device and it fails to meet the standard in any respect [21 U.S.C. 351(e)]
d. If premarket approval is required for a class III device and the device is marketed without such approval or is not otherwise exempted from such approval [21 U.S.C. 351(f)]
e. If it has been banned by the FDA [21 U.S.C. 351(g)]
f. If it fails to comply with requirements on good manufacturing practices [21 U.S.C. 351(h)]
g. If it is an investigational device and it is not in compliance with the requirements for investigational devices [21 U.S.C. 351(i)]

Since 1938, a number of actions have been brought by the FDA against devices it considered to be adulterated. For the most part these actions were undertaken on the basis that the device contained improper substances, was manufactured under improper circumstances, or did not possess the level of quality or purity claimed for the device. For example, these cases often involved devices that were labeled as sterile but that were nonsterile. There have been few actions brought against devices as adulterated under new provisions of the Medical Device Amendments of 1976. Most of those that have been brought involve violations of the regulations on good manufacturing practices.

E. Misbranding

A drug or device is deemed to be misbranded for a variety of reasons identified in Section 502 of the Act (21 U.S.C. 352). These violations generally relate to matters involving the labeling or advertising of a device or the failure of the responsible party to comply with some required general provision of the law. A device, for example, would be misbranded if any one of the following conditions exist:

a. If the labeling is false or misleading in any particular [21 U.S.C. 351(a)]

b. If certain information necessary for the proper identification of a device is absent [21 U.S.C. 351(b)]
c. If a required statement is not prominently and clearly conveyed in the label or labeling [21 U.S.C. 352(c)]
d. If the established name does not appear prominently on the label [21 U.S.C. 352(e)]
e. If the labeling does not bear adequate directions for use and essential warnings [21 U.S.C. 352(f)]
f. If it is dangerous to health when used in the dosage or manner, or with the frequency or duration prescribed, recommended or suggested in the labeling [21 U.S.C. 352(j)]
g. If it fails to comply with general provisions of the law relating to mandatory filings with the FDA of information relating to establishment registration, product listing, or premarket notification [21 U.S.C. 352(o)]
h. If it is identified as a restricted device and the advertising is false or misleading in any particular or it is marketed in violation of other provisions of the Act relating to restricted devices [21 U.S.C. 352(g)]
i. If it is a restricted device and the advertising or labeling fails to provide certain information [21 U.S.C. 352(r)]
j. If it is subject to a performance standard and this labeling fails to comply with a requirement in the standard [21 U.S.C. 352(s)]
k. If there was a failure or refusal on the part of a responsible party to comply with other provisions of the Act relating to submission of reports, maintenance of records, or public notification on a repair, replacement, or refund of the purchase price of a violative device [21 U.S.C. 352(t)]

The provisions of Section 502 relating to labeling and hazard to health have been involved in numerous cases since 1938. However, there have been few cases litigated where the provisions of the law relating to the Medical Device Amendment of 1976 have been involved.

F. Other Provisions of the Act

The general provisions of the Act relating to adulteration and misbranding form the basis for most of the violations that exist under the Act. Thus, if a device is deemed to be adulterated or misbranded, the FDA can attempt, through the courts or by an administrative proceeding, to take an action against the device to correct the violative condition. Likewise, any person who is responsible for having adulterated or misbranded a device is subject to citation and possible prosecution.

There are other provisions of the Act not relating to adulteration or misbranding that could expose the individual who does not comply with these provisions to citation and possible criminal prosecution. These are outlined in Section 301 of the Act (21 U.S.C. 331) and include the refusal to permit inspection under Section 704 of the Act (21 U.S.C. 374) or make certain information available to the FDA; giving a false guaranty or undertaking; use of any statement in the labeling or advertising of a device that a premarket or investigational device exemption approval has been obtained; or the failure to comply with certain other FDA requirements or orders.

Finally, there is a provision in the Act [21 U.S.C. 331(j)] that makes it unlawful for any person, including a government employee, to use for his or her own advantage any information lawfully required under various provisions of the Act that concerns any method or process that as a trade secret is entitled to protection.

VI. AGENCY PROCEDURES

The overall direction of the FDA program in a particular product area is generally provided by an appropriate organizational unit. Consequently, the Center for Devices and Radiological Health is responsible for the development of policies and regulations necessary to implement FDA authority under law and, in particular, under the new authority provided under the Medical Device Amendments of 1976. The Center for Devices and Radiological Health has the functional responsibility to administer the law and work in cooperation with various FDA field offices to secure compliance with the law.

The Center is allocated resources in the field in order to gather information to verify whether violations of the law exist. Assignments from the Center are issued in one of two basic formats. One is to issue a special assignment to a particular district office or offices in order to investigate whether a problem exists or verify information previously received by the Center. These assignments are generally not planned and occur on a case-by-case basis as needs dictate. The other method that the Center uses is to develop a program that is subsequently distributed to all district offices. The "program" represents a planned activity to be conducted over time or during a period of time in order to gather information as part of a "surveillance activity" or determine whether the regulated industry is in "compliance" with the Act or regulations issued under the Act. These "surveillance" and "compliance" programs are available to the public on request and provide useful information to manufacturers about FDA interest and expectations.

A. Inspections

The field personnel consist of individuals who are trained as "investigators"* and whose function it is to conduct inspections. The investigators are authorized by law to conduct inspections under Section 704 of the Act (21 U.S.C. 374) and generally attempt to gather information pursuant to an assignment or a Center-initiated program. The investigator's instructions are provided in the Inspector Operations Manual mentioned previously. The investigator will usually appear at a facility unannounced and will present credentials and a notice of inspection (FD Form 482) to the responsible official in the facility. The investigator is entitled by law to certain information. Some information on this is outlined in Section 704 of the Act. The investigator may ask for more information than he or she is entitled to under law, and the person subject to the inspection has the option as to whether to provide this information. As a result, it is essential that management be aware of its rights and develop a company position prior to the inspection.

---

*In addition to the investigators, the FDA also employs inspectors who function in a similar capacity but who are not qualified by experience and education to become investigators.

Only experienced individuals who are familiar with company policy should accompany an FDA investigator.

During an investigation, the investigator may request to be provided with a sample of the device. The investigator will offer to pay and, if he or she obtains a sample, will provide the company representative with a document (FD Form 484) to verify receipt of the sample.

B. Communications with Plant Management

Upon completion of an investigation, which could take a few hours to several weeks, the investigator will review findings with management and provide a list of any observations noted that in his or her opinion suggest a violation of the law. This "Notice of Observation" (FD Form 483) is available to the public and may form the basis for a subsequent action by the FDA. Management should carefully review any Form 483 and decide whether and how to respond.

The investigator will prepare a written report of findings for his or her supervisors. This will not be available to the public under the Freedom of Information Act until the FDA has made a decision not to pursue regulatory action or the regulatory action has been legally completed. As a general principle, if a Form 483 is issued and the observations justify some further comment by FDA officials in the district office, one of several types of letters will be issued. The FDA district director could issue a letter referred to as a "notice of adverse findings" (NAFL), which is intended to bring to management's attention the concern of the district about the observations. However, the FDA is not prepared on the basis of these observations to pursue any regulatory action involving seizure, injunction, or prosecution.

The other letter the FDA district director could issue is referred to as a "regulatory letter." This type of letter is transmitted only when the FDA believes that a device is misbranded and it is prepared to take legal action. If correction of the violation is not undertaken by the firm, the FDA will proceed to seize the device and/or enjoin the firm from shipping the device in interstate commerce. The company receiving a "regulatory letter" will have 10 days in which to respond. If a satisfactory response is not obtained by the FDA, then it will proceed to take appropriate regulatory action.

In some cases, the FDA will not issue a regulatory letter, but will proceed to seize the device or obtain an injunction. This will occur if the device is adulterated, represents a hazard to health, or involves a situation where the firm has been warned previously about similar violations.

In addition, the FDA has other procedures under the Medical Device Amendments of 1976 that it could apply to correct violations. These involve the banning of a device; detention of a device; or the repair, replacement, or refund of the purchase price of a violative device.

VII. REMEDIAL ACTIONS AND PROCEDURES

A. General

Irrespective of whether a violation of the law or regulations is discovered upon inspection or through some other method (e.g., analysis of a device purchased in the marketplace), the FDA is authorized to pursue a remedial action against the device or the person through the courts or apply an administrative procedure sanctioned by law to ban a device or correct a violation.

In addition, the FDA can apply an administrative procedure not found in the Act and referred to as a "recall" [10]. This latter procedure is used to describe any situation in which the person responsible for possible adulteration or misbranding of a product undertakes, on a voluntary basis, an effort to correct the alleged violation. When the FDA applies the designation "recall" to a remedial action taken by a responsible party, it represents a statement by the FDA that a device is adulterated and/or misbranded and, therefore, in violation of the Act. It is not necessary that the device be removed from the marketplace because the correction of the violation can occur through field modification of the device, revision of the labeling, or a suitable communication of information to users or likely users. The FDA will monitor the progress of the "recall" and provide assistance if indicated. The FDA will also assign a category of recall to reflect the seriousness of the recall, and it will publish pertinent information in its weekly enforcement report. A class I recall applies to a device where death is a possibility in the absence of the recall, whereas the class II and class III recalls are less serious.

If the FDA is satisfied with the progress of the recall, it will generally pursue no further action because the public need will be satisfied. However, if the recall is unsatisfactory, the FDA may proceed to invoke other penalties under the Act, including seizure or injunction.

B. Seizures and Injunctions

Whenever seizure or injunction are considered to be appropriate remedies to correct a violation, the FDA will transmit its recommendation to the FDA Office of the General Counsel. If this office agrees, the recommendation is transmitted to the Justice Department, which, if there is agreement, will pursue the matter in an appropriate U.S. District Court. In matters relating to seizure, if the district court agrees, then the U.S. Marshall, pursuant to a court order, will seize the device. A person who has a claim to the device may file such a claim and dispute the position of the government through appropriate court procedures. A claimant can also decline to claim the seized device or enter into a consent order with the FDA that will resolve the status of the devices. Likewise, in matters relating to injunction, the accused may contest this action in the federal courts.

Apart from seizure or injunction, the FDA can pursue other procedures sanctioned by the Medical Device Amendments of 1976.

C. Banning

Under Section 516 of the Act [21 U.S.C. 360(f)], the FDA can set in motion a process to ban a device in order to prevent its shipment in interstate commerce.

If a device for human use presents substantial deception or an unreasonable and substantial risk of illness or injury, the FDA may initiate a proceeding to promulgate a regulation that would ultimately identify the device as a banned device. In general, the public will have an opportunity to comment on the proposed regulation before a final regulation becomes effective.

If a request is made for an informal hearing on the proposed regulation, the FDA will provide for such a hearing, and the final regulation will not become effective until such procedures have been completed. Under certain circumstances, the FDA can make the proposed regulation effective upon publication of a proposal and prior to the publication of a final order.

After a device has been declared to be banned, its shipment in interstate commerce or for export is prohibited and the banned device is subject to seizure or injunction. Anyone who violates any provision of the law relating to a banned device is subject to possible criminal prosecution [11].

D. Detention

Under Section 304(g) of the Act [21 U.S.C. 334(g)], if, during an inspection of a facility, it is determined that there is reason to believe that a device may be adulterated or misbranded, the FDA can proceed to detain the device for up to 30 days. The procedures that apply to the detention of a device provide an opportunity for an informal hearing. During the period of time that a device is under detention, it cannot be moved in any way that would result in the possible distribution of the device in interstate commerce.

Upon expiration of the 30-day time period, if the matter has not been resolved, the device may be shipped in interstate commerce unless the FDA has obtained a court order to seize the device or enjoin shipment in interstate commerce [12].

E. Notification and Other Remedies

Under certain circumstances, if the FDA determines that a device presents an unreasonable risk of substantial harm to the public health, it may order that a firm or other responsible person give adequate notice to the public if such notice would eliminate the unreasonable risk. Before issuing a notification under this section, the FDA must consult with the persons who are to give notice under this order. The FDA could require that a notice be directed to all health professionals who prescribe or use the device and any other person, including manufacturers, importers, distributors, retailers, and device users. If necessary, the FDA could require that the notice go directly to a patient.

The FDA could also order the manufacturer, importer, or any distributor of a device it determines meets certain statutory criteria to take one of the following actions:

a. To repair the device so that it does not present the unreasonable risk of substantial harm with respect to which the order was issued
b. To replace the device with a like or equivalent device in conformity with all applicable requirements of the Act
c. To refund the purchase price of the device (less a reasonable allowance for use of the device under certain conditions)

Before issuing a repair, replacement, or refund order, the FDA would be required to afford an opportunity for an informal hearing. After the hearing opportunity has been provided, the FDA can issue its order if certain facts can be established. These include, among others, that the device "presents an unreasonable risk of substantial harm to the public health," and "reasonable grounds to believe that the device was not properly designed and manufactured with reference to the state of the art as it existed at the time of its design and manufacture."

Failure to comply with any of these provisions of the Act, which are described in Section 518 [21 U.S.C. 306(h)], result in the device becoming misbranded under Section 502(t) of the Act [21 U.S.C. 352(t)], and any person who fails to respond to such order may be subject to criminal prosecution.

F. Prosecution

Any person who commits a prohibited act as described in Section 301 of the Act (21 U.S.C. 331) is in violation of the Act. Before any violation of the Act is reported by the FDA to any U.S. Attorney for institution of a criminal proceeding, the person accused of committing the violation is given an opportunity to present his or her views, either orally or in writing. This is provided for in Section 305 of the Act (21 U.S.C. 335). If the FDA decides to prosecute, the matter is referred to the U.S. Attorney. If an indictment is delivered by the grand jury, the defendant will have the opportunity to be tried by a jury because any violation of the Act is considered to be a violation of a criminal law.

Any person found guilty of violating a prohibited act is subject to imprisonment for up to a year and/or fine of up to $1000. If a person commits a violation with the intent to defraud or mislead or after having had been previously convicted, then such person can be imprisoned up to 3 years and/or fined up to $10,000. There have been numerous convictions over the years, and some individuals have been jailed for committing violations of the Act.

Unlike most statutes describing criminal conduct, it is not necessary in food and drug law to establish intent to violate the Act. The mere existence of a violation provides sufficient cause for the FDA to proceed with a criminal prosecution. There are two individual Supreme Court cases that strengthen the position of the FDA and create understandable anxiety among executives responsible for complying with the Act.

In 1943, the Supreme Court upheld the conviction of a Mr. Dotterweich, who was president and general manager of Buffalo Pharmaceutical Company. The firm repacked under its own label drugs manufactured by someone else, and Dotterweich claimed that he should not be prosecuted because he was not aware of any wrongdoing. The court disagreed and clearly stated that any person in a position of responsibility to a corporation that adulterates or misbrands a drug must suffer the consequences of a criminal prosecution even though such person was not aware of the violation [*United States vs. Dotterweich*, 230 U.S. 277 (1943)].

In 1975, the Supreme Court had an opportunity to reconsider the strict liability established in *Dotterweich* when John R. Park, chief executive of Acme Markets, Inc., appealed a conviction that involved the holding of adulterated food products. Acme operated hundreds of retail food stores and numerous warehouses at the time of the violation. Over the course of several FDA inspections of warehouses in Philadelphia and Baltimore, it was demonstrated by the FDA that there was a continuing problem involving rat infestation. Mr. Park delegated responsibility for correction of these problems to subordinates and claimed this, in part, as a defense in order to avoid prosecution. He was found guilty after trial and appealed to the Court of Appeals, which reversed his conviction. The government appealed, and the stage was set for a review of the strict standard imposed by *Dotterweich*. In a 6-3 decision, the Supreme Court reversed the Court of Appeals, affirmed the *Park* conviction, and relied heavily on the decision in the *Dotterweich* case [*United States vs. Park*, 421 U.S. 658 (1975)].

It is largely because of these court decisions that executives of device companies are concerned about their liabilities under the Federal Food, Drug, and Cosmetic Act. This is particularly true with respect to the responsibility of an individual to comply with FDA requirements on good manufacturing practices.

VIII. GOOD MANUFACTURING PRACTICES

Prior to the enactment of the Medical Device Amendments of 1976, it became apparent to the FDA that many of the problems covered with respect to adulterated or misbranded devices related to the conditions under which the devices were being manufactured. As a result, the FDA undertook to develop regulations on good manufacturing practices (GMP) in an effort to reduce the frequency of recalls that occurred because of problems relating to manufacturing practices. GMP regulations for foods and pharmaceuticals had previously been implemented by the FDA.

The Medical Device Amendments of 1976, however, provided the FDA with explicit authority to prescribe good manufacturing requirements [13].

The FDA was instructed by Congress as part of the law to form an advisory committee of experts and to consult with the committee prior to promulgating GMP regulations. Further, once the GMP regulation became effective, any person subject to the GMP requirements had a right to petition the FDA for exemption or variance from any requirement. The FDA must also consider the advice and recommendation of the advisory committee when deciding whether to approve or disapprove a petition.

The FDA proposed a GMP regulation on March 1, 1977, and published a final order on July 21, 1978 [14]. The final order became effective on December 18, 1978. The preamble to the proposal and the final order set forth in great detail the process followed by the FDA in developing this regulation. The final regulation applies to manufacturers of all finished devices but does not apply to manufacturers of components or parts.

A. The GMP Regulation

The regulation attempts to avoid describing in any detail how a particular function is to be performed. The responsibility is on the manufacturer to develop and implement a system appropriate for the device, which is compatible with the intent of the regulation. The regulation itself consists of 10 major subparts. These are as follows.

Subpart A. General provisions
- 820.1 Scope
- 920.3 Definition
- 820.5 Quality assurance program

Subpart B. Organization and personnel
- 820.20 Organization
- 820.25 Personnel

Subpart C.	Buildings
820.40	Buildings
820.46	Environmental control
820.56	Cleaning and sanitation
Subpart D.	Equipment
820.60	Equipment
820.61	Measurement equipment
Subpart E.	Control of components
820.80	Components
820.81	Critical devices, components
Subpart F.	Production and process controls
820.100	Manufacturing specifications and processes
820.101	Critical devices, manufacturing specifications, and processes
820.115	Reprocessing of devices or components
820.116	Critical devices, reprocessing of devices or components
Subpart G.	Packaging and labeling control
820.120	Device labeling
820.121	Critical devices, device labeling
820.130	Device packaging
Subpart H.	Holding, distribution, and installation
820.150	Distribution
820.151	Critical devices, distribution, records
820.152	Installation
Subpart I.	Device evaluation
820.160	Finished device inspection
820.161	Critical devices, finished device inspection
820.162	Failure investigation
Subpart J.	Records
820.180	General requirements
820.181	Device master record
820.182	Critical devices, device master record
820.184	Device history record
820.185	Critical devices, device history record
820.195	Critical devices, automated data processing
820.198	Complaint files

The regulation provides general guidance and places great emphasis on the need to develop a good system, maintain adequate records to verify that the system is functioning properly, and implement an audit procedure to assure on a continuing basis the effectiveness of the manufacturing process and quality control procedures. The following subparts contain procedures worthy of special consideration.

Subpart A: General Provisions

Manufacturers of components are urged to use the regulation as a guide, and directions are provided for those who wish to seek an exemption or variance. Every finished device manufacturer is instructed to prepare and implement an appropriate quality assurance program.

Subpart B: Organization and Personnel

The basic requirements of a quality assurance program are identified, and manufacturers are instructed to implement plan and periodic audits of the quality assurance program to verify compliance with the quality assurance program.

Subpart E: Control of Components

Procedures relating to selection and control of components are emphasized, and additional procedures relating to the selection and handling of critical components for critical devices are described.

Subpart J: Records

Manufacturers are required to maintain a master record for the device and implement stringent procedures relating to any change in the master record. Manufacturers must also maintain a complaint file, investigate certain kinds of complaints, and allow the FDA access to these files.

Prior to the effective date of the GMP regulation, the FDA evaluated all recalls involving devices for a 10-year period of time when it was suspected that the reason for the recall was related to a GMP deficiency. The FDA is using this information, in part, to provide baseline data on the impact of these regulations over time. During 1979, the FDA in cooperation with the Biomedical Division of the American Society for Quality Control conducted two day meetings in each of the FDA regional offices and several additional district offices to educate industry on the requirements of the regulation.

B. Critical Device Designation

The regulation recognizes that there are significant differences between various kinds of devices and distinguishes a critical device from all other types of devices. The term "critical device" is defined as follows:

> A device that is intended for surgical implant into the body or to support or sustain life and whose failure to perform when properly used in accordance with instructions for use provided in the labeling can be reasonably expected to result in a significant injury to the user. Critical devices will be identified by the Commissioner after consultation with the Device Good Manufacturing Practice Advisory Committee authorized under section 520(f) of the act, and an illustrative list of critical devices will be available from the Bureau of Medical Devices, Food and Drug Administration.

Thus, all provisions of the regulation apply to critical devices, whereas all other devices are only subject to general provisions of the regulation.

C. Compliance Program

In February 1979, a compliance program was distributed to the field and the FDA began investigations of device firms to determine compliance with the GMP regulation. The FDA Center for Devices and Radiological Health [formerly Bureau of Medical Devices (BMD)] continues to provide industry with useful information designed to promote compliance with the GMP regulation. These included "Text of the GMP regulation with pertinent cross-references," June 1979; "A quality audit program for industry," September 1979; and "GMP questions and answers," Fall 1979.

In March 1980, the FDA issued its first evaluation of the device GMP compliance program for fiscal year 1979. The "executive summary" of this evaluation is as follows:

> This evaluation report summarizes the findings of 807 device Good Manufacturing Practice (GMP) inspections accomplished from February 1, 1979 to September 30, 1979.
>
> The inspectional findings show that as firm size increases, compliance with the GMP regulation increases. Additionally, the inspectional findings show that manufacturers of critical, non-critical, and in vitro diagnostic devices have approximately the same level of compliance; that is, there are no significant differences in the extent of GMP compliance attributable to the type of device produced. Fifty-nine percent of the firms inspected are complying with ninety-one percent or more of the applicable requirements. Seven percent of the firms inspected are complying with sixty or less percent of the requirements.
>
> Failure to meet audit requirements appears in the listing of the ten GMP requirements with the lowest level of compliance. This is true regardless of whether a manufacturer is producing critical, non-critical or in vitro diagnostic devices.
>
> As a result of the 807 inspections, 168 Notice of Adverse Findings Letters and 10 Regulatory Letters have been issued to device manufacturers. Firms receiving regulatory correspondence have been scheduled for reinspection within six months. In those cases where reinspection has taken place, firms, on the average, had corrected approximately seventy-five percent of the deficiencies noted at the time of the initial inspection.
>
> Based on a comprehensive review of each inspection report, BMD concludes that the field applied the GMP regulation in a uniform and consistent manner. Also, field investigators followed the directions contained in the compliance program.

In fiscal year 1982, the FDA issued another report on its evaluation of the device GMP inspection program. This confirmed many of the findings of previous years. The executive summary of this evaluation states, in part:

> This evaluation report summarizes the findings of the FY'82 Device Good Manufacturing Practice (GMP) Compliance Program and compares these to those findings of the three previous fiscal years. In FY'82, inspections were conducted at 1,116 establishments. The field spent 29,708 hours conducting these inspections.
>
> Four hundred and seventy-seven of these 1,116 establishments had never received a GMP inspection prior to FY'82. The most frequent deficiencies found in these firms were in the areas of auditing, calibrating of equipment, and maintaining the device master record. These are the same kinds of problems found in firms receiving an initial GMP inspection during the period FY'79–81. Noncritical device manufacturers which received their initial GMP inspection in FY'82 appear to have a significantly higher compliance with the GMP than firms which received their initial inspection in FY'79–81.
>
> During the four fiscal years that the GMP Compliance Program was in effect, a total of 1,185 firms received two comprehensive GMP inspections. These firms had, at the time of their initial inspection, a mean Compliance Index of 86 with a standard deviation of 16; while at the time of the second biennial inspection, the mean Compliance

Index had increased to 94 while the standard deviation had decreased to 10. Thus at the time of the second biennial inspection, firms were in a better state of compliance and there was less variability in compliance with the GMP. However, while there has been a considerable increase in compliance with the GMP, 56 firms (5% of the 1,116 firms) had Compliance Indices of less than 74. In addition, 135 medium and large sized firms (17% of the 1,116 firms) were still not auditing their quality assurance program after receiving their second biennial GMP inspection.

FY'82 represents the fourth year the GMP Compliance Program has been in effect. Those manufacturers of Class II and III devices receiving an initial inspection in FY'79 and 80 should have received a second biennial inspection during FY'81 and 82 if they had not gone out of business. In fact, only 74% of firms that manufacture Class II and III devices that were inspected in FY'79 and 80 were still in business in FY'81 and 82 did receive a second biennial inspection within the two year period as required by the Medical Device Amendments of 1976.

The date of this report suggests that FDA's voluntary compliance strategy of issuing a written warning to top management either in the form of an FD-483 or a NAFL* is an effective way to achieve significant compliance with GMP requirements.

The development and implementation of regulations on device good manufacturing practices represent a major initiative of the FDA since enactment of the Medical Device Amendments of 1976. Significant agency resources have been devoted to this activity in the expectation that conscientious adherence by industry to these regulations and to the system designed and implemented by the manufacturer will result in continuous manufacture of the device in compliance with the original design. It is essential to the continuing success of a device manufacturer that it faithfully manufacture a device for distribution that complies in every respect to design specifications. Failure to do this could result in recall of the device, exposure to civil actions for product liability, criminal or civil sanctions under the federal Food, Drug, and Cosmetic Act, or loss of sales. Any one of these consequences flowing from the manufacturer's inability to properly manufacture a device could result in loss of business and personal loss to those who are responsible. Representatives of the FDA have stated on numerous occasions that compliance with good manufacturing practices also represents good business practices.

D. Access to Records Disputes

Relatively few disputes have arisen between the FDA and the industry over application of this regulation. The notable exception to date involved a refusal by a heart pacemaker manufacturer to allow FDA investigators access to certain records relating to complaints about pacemakers. The FDA obtained a warrant for inspection from the U.S. District Court Magistrate for the purpose of inspecting and copying the following records:

---

*Notice of adverse finding letter.

a. Complete failure investigation reports
b. Computerized printout of failures, including all code or legend information needed to interpret the data
c. Complete complaint files
d. Complete file-handling procedures, failure analysis procedures, and return product-handling procedures

The manufacturer filed an appeal with the district court from the order of the U.S. Magistrate and argued that the warrant exceeded FDA statutory authority and violated the Fourth Amendment of the U.S. Constitution. The Court found that Congress expanded FDA inspectional authorities over device manufacturers and access to manufacturer records upon enactment of the Medical Device Amendments of 1976. The court further concluded that the GMP regulation requires production of the total written record of failure investigation and complete complaint files. The court struck the warrant request for complaint procedures and the computer printout because these were not explicitly required by the regulation [*In the Matter of Establishment Inspection of Medtronic*, 500 F. Supp. 536 (1980)].

IX. MANUFACTURER, INSTITUTION, AND HEALTH PROFESSIONAL RESPONSIBILITIES

In the device industry, as a general proposition, it is the responsibility of the manufacturer to assure that a device is properly designed and manufactured. Health professionals and health care institutions are usually not expected to further manipulate a device other than to follow instructions for maintaining and properly using a device. In this respect it is particularly important for health professionals to be aware of their responsibility to follow the instructions of the manufacturer. Proper transportation, storage, maintenance, and adherence to instructions are essential to the successful application of a device for the benefit of a patient. Failure to maintain the integrity of a device could expose the health professional and institutional or private enterprise employees to severe penalties under the Federal Food, Drug, and Cosmetic Act or in a civil action. This is a particular concern for devices that are disposable or reusable and devices that require regular maintenance or use by specifically trained or qualified individuals.

A. Disposable or Reusable Devices

Some devices are intended to be discarded after use on a patient. For example, devices used for the intravenous feeding or medication of a patient are often labeled explicitly for "single use" and with such admonitions as "discard after use," "do not reuse," or "do not resterilize." Any practitioner or institution undertaking to reuse or resterilize a device against these warnings does so at great risk. Certainly the reuse of a device that is clearly labeled as single use or disposable is not advisable.

If it is necessary to resterilize a device or sterilize a device that is reusable, the practitioner or institution must exercise great care to assure that the device is suitable for use and that the method of sterilization that is used is appropriate and implemented properly. Failure to take adequate precautionary and subsequent control measures could expose an individual and the institution to civil or criminal liability.

B. Device Maintenance

Devices used in medical care often require regular maintenance or calibration in order to operate effectively and as designed by the manufacturer. The manufacturer or other person responsible for the commercial distribution of the device has the responsibility to provide adequate information. This may include instructions on assembly, disassembly, schematic diagrams, maintenance, calibration, or other special instructions necessary for the proper functioning of the device. It is incumbent on the user to follow these instructions carefully and avoid any deviations from these instructions.

For devices that operate on principles of electricity, where electronic components are used or fail-safe systems are designed to prevent improper use, the user must avoid the temptation to alter the device or repair it without clear guidance from the manufacturer. If the user undertakes such an effort and this results in a modification of the device that compromises the quality of the device, under Food and Drug law the user may be liable for having committed a prohibited act. The possible violation relates to the performance of an act that could result in the device being adulterated or misbranded.

X. SUMMARY

The decision to develop, manufacture, and/or market a medical device requires a basic understanding of the application of the Federal Food, Drug, and Cosmetic Act and the responsibility of the Food and Drug Administration. In particular, individuals who are responsible for the manufacture of devices, whether as part of a production or quality control function, must recognize their potential exposure to criminal penalties if their actions result in the adulteration or misbranding of a device. This section is intended to describe basic provisions of the Act including the Medical Device Amendments of 1976, the general operation of the Food and Drug Administration as it relates to the manufacture of devices, and the development and current status of FDA regulations on device good manufacturing practices.

REFERENCES

1. Food and Drugs Act, 34 Statutes at Large, 768 June 30, 1906.
2. Federal Food, Drug, and Cosmetic Act as Amended, 21 U.S.C. 321 et seq.
3. AMP Incorporated vs. John W. Gardner, 389 F. 2d 825 (1968).
4. United States vs. An Article of Drug . . . Bacto- unidisk, 394 U.S. 784 (1969).
5. T. Cooper, HEW Study Group on Medical Devices, Medical Devices: A Legislative Plan (1970).
6. Section 513, Federal Food, Drug, and Cosmetic Act, 21 U.S.C. 360c.
7. 21 C.F.R. Part 860 (1984).
8. FDA Compliance Policy Guide No. 7155X .01, October 1, 1980.

9. FDA Compliance Policy Guide No. 7155d .08, July 15, 1982.
10. 21 C.F.R. Part 7, Subpart C (1984).
11. 21 C.F.R. Part 895 (1984).
12. 21 C.F.R. Part 800, Subpart C (1984).
13. Section 520(f), Federal Food, Drug, and Cosmetic Act, 21 U.S.C. 360j(f).
14. 21 C.F.R. Part 820 (1984).

BIBLIOGRAPHY

Federal Food, Drug, and Cosmetic Act, as Amended, Title 21, United States Code, Section 301 et seq.

Medical Device Amendments of 1976, Public Law 94-295, 94th Congress, S. 510, May 28, 1976.

Medical Device Amendments of 1976, Report by the Committee on Interstate and Foreign Commerce, 94th Congress 2d Session, House of Representatives, Report No. 94-853, February 29, 1976.

An Analytical Legislative History of the Medical Device Amendments of 1976, The Food and Drug Law Institute, Inc., Washington, D.C. 20036, 1976.

Medical Devices Reporter, Commerce Clearing House, Inc., Publishers of Topical Law Reports, 4025 W. Peterson Ave., Chicago, Illinois 60646.

Regulatory Requirements for Marketing a Device, U.S. Department of Health and Human Services, Public Health Service, Food and Drug Administration, Bureau of Medical Devices, Government Printing Office: 1982-0-374-900/1036.

Device Good Manufacturing Practices, A Workshop Manual, October 1982, U.S. Department of Health and Human Services, Public Health Service, Food and Drug Administration, Bureau of Medical Devices, U.S. Government Printing Office: 1982-0-386-960/8573.

Premarket Notification: 510(k) Regulatory Requirements for Medical Devices, U.S. Department of Health and Human Services, Public Health Service, Food and Drug Administration, National Center for Devices and Radiological Health, U.S. Government Printing Office: 1983 381-177/307.

13

Parenteral Products in Hospital Practice

John W. Levchuk

The University of Tennessee, Memphis, The Health Science Center, Memphis, Tennessee

I. INTRODUCTION

Professional personnel in the pharmaceutical industry may have little awareness of the pharmacist's responsibilities concerning sterile dosage forms in the hospital. This chapter is intended, in part, to help bridge that gap. The chapter is also for hospital pharmacists as an aid in the design of quality services and in the evaluation of program or operational performance. Those in industry may recognize in this material a common bond of interest with the practice of hospital pharmacy and see ways to apply their knowledge and experience to the hospital setting. As hospital pharmacists refer to preceding chapters of this collected work, they will recognize that industry indeed has much to offer them.

II. FACTORS AFFECTING THE USE OF STERILE DOSAGE FORMS IN THE HOSPITAL

A. Growing Usage

The concept of what constitutes good pharmacy services in a hospital is continually changing. Two dramatic advances during the past 20 years were the establishment of centralized parenteral admixture services (a parenteral admixture is the mixing of two or more parenteral products in the hospital to meet a patient's specific therapeutic requirements; one of the products is usually an infusion solution) and the pharmacist's direct involvement in assuring the quality of parenteral therapy. The number of hospitals providing admixture services has risen from a handful in the early 1960s to approximately 80% in 1983 [1]. During the growth period, many patient care benefits resulting from admixture programs have been documented, including greater dosing accuracy, reduction in dosing errors and in infusion-associated complications, such as sepsis and phlebitis, better monitoring of patient response to infusion therapy, and the prevention of deteriorated, incompatible, or precipitated products from being administered. Economically and administratively, the purposeful organization of centralized parenteral admixture services and functions brings together many previously scattered activities. This provides for benefits, such as the centralization of responsibility and accountability, better utilization of personnel, improved charge control, establishment of cost accounting and charge centers, comprehensive planning and quality assurance, and economies of scale.

There are no composite statistics available that can adequately portray the importance of parenteral therapy in the care of the hospitalized patient, but the 1669 respondents (of approximately 7000 hospital pharmacy directors) to the 1983 Lilly hospital pharmacy survey [1] provide a glimpse of the intensity of parenteral usage in U.S. hospitals. For example, the average U.S. hospital (a general hospital with 200 to 299-bed capacity) dispenses weekly approximately 1400 large volume solutions with and without additives. Larger institutions dispense more. Specialized facilities dispense more than general hospitals, probably because they treat more serious illnesses. Furthermore, parenteral prescription activity will continue to increase, according to the trend data. Trends also indicate that pharmacists are spending more time manipulating parenterals prior to dispensing. Augmented demands for unit-dose packaging of parenterals to support the increase in unit-dose systems can be expected. (A unit-dose system is, in brief, where no more than a 24-hr supply of drug is available on the nursing unit; where medications are packaged as to the number of units, volume, or quantity needed by a specific patient at a specific dosage time; and where each unit-dose amount is identifiable as to specific patient and administration time.)

B. Types of Products

Institutional markets use virtually every commercially available sterile pharmaceutical dosage form. However, the scope of inventory and usage rates vary among individual facilities, depending upon such factors as degree of specialization, intensity of care, census, and formulary policies. These dosage forms may be grouped operatively for the hospital into the five general categories now discussed.

1. *Infusions*

Infusions are parenteral products intended for injection into a vein by intravenous (IV) drip. They are packaged in plastic or glass large volume parenteral (LVP) containers to which is attached a suitable IV set (Fig. 1) at the time of infusion. Venous entry is by a metal needle or a plastic catheter. An infusion system provides continuous, regulated, fluid flow at a preset rate. Once a prescribed flow rate (e.g., 125 ml/hr) has been established, the fluid should continue to flow accurately from the unattended system until the container has emptied.

Flow is maintained by gravity or positive pressure. With gravity flow, the rate is usually established with a tube-constricting flow control device (e.g., roller clamp or screw clamp). The following steps are normally required clinically to establish a flow rate. First, the number of drops per minute must be calculated from a medication order often expressed metrically (e.g., mg or ml) or chemically (e.g., mEq or mM) per unit time (e.g., min, hr, 8-hr period). The nurse, for example, must refer to the manufacturer-

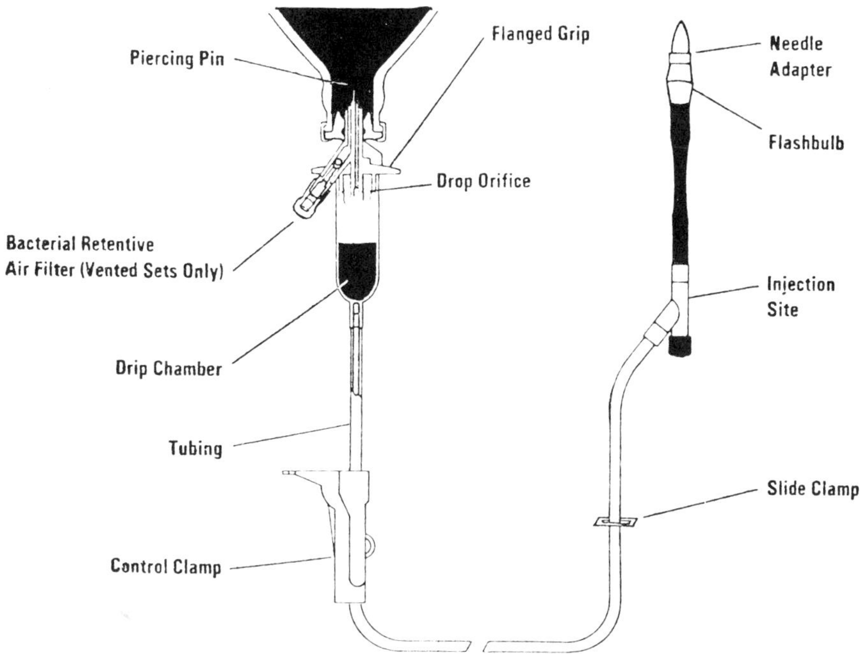

Figure 1 A standard intravenous infusion set. (From A. Rodrique and E. A. Parker, *Hosp. Pharm.*, *16*:332, 1981. Courtesy of J. B. Lippincott Co.)

supplied approximate drip chamber calibration value (e.g., 10, 15, 20, or 60 drops/ml) printed on the IV set package. The nurse then visually observes the number of drops per minute falling in the drip chamber, manually adjusting the flow control device as needed. Free-falling drops also may be counted electronically with an IV controller, a device having a continuous feedback system linking a drop sensor with a tube-constricting mechanism. Thus, a predetermined drip rate can be maintained electronically.

Positive pressure flow is produced by use of an IV pump, a device that propels fluid through an IV line at a constant controllable rate (the "peristaltic" pumps) or in conjunction with a constant volume (the "volumetric" pumps). Volumetric pumps operate on the principles of piston-chamber constant stroke volume displacement or of peristalticlike progressive occlusion of constant-length sections of IV tubing. Only those sets specified by the pump manufacturer may be used with the volumetric pumps.

Fluids are infused according to a continuous or an intermittent dose schedule. A continuous schedule involves the nonstop infusion of a relatively large volume of fluid (e.g., 1 liter per 8-hr period for adults) over a period of several hours or even days. Continuous therapy usually provides fluid, electrolytes, agents to adjust acid-base balance, nutrients, and some drugs by slow IV drip. The total fluid intake must not exceed the patient's requirements, approximately 2400 ml for an adult.

An intermittent schedule usually involves the dilution of a drug in 50–100 ml of a standard LVP solution (e.g., dextrose injection 5%, sodium chloride injection 0.9%) for infusion over a 15 to 30-min period, repeated at regular intervals, such as every 6 hr. The so-called piggyback IV administration system (Fig. 2) accommodates the periodic intermittent infusion of a secondary fluid during the continuous administration of a primary fluid. A back-flow check valve in the primary IV line stops primary fluid flow while the intermittent fluid is running.

Infusions are administered with or without additives. The preparation of IV admixtures constitutes by far the predominant involvement of the hospital pharmacist in sterile pharmaceutical compounding.

2. *Injections*

Injections are precisely measured volumes, usually less than 10 ml, of small volume parenterals (SVPs) for parenteral administration. A needle and syringe are commonly used to inject SVPs intravenously, intramuscularly, subcutaneously, and by virtually every other parenteral route discussed by Duma and Akers (Chap. 2, Vol. 1). The hospital pharmacist's usual involvement with SVPs is the supply, distribution, and control of commercially available products throughout the hospital and their use as additives in the compounding of IV admixtures. Hospital pharmacists may be requested occasionally to mix and dispense two or more commercially available SVPs in the same syringe, a common nursing activity. Repackaging in unit-dose syringes is a growing trend. Compounding SVPs from raw ingredients is not common practice.

3. *Ophthalmics*

Ophthalmics include sterile solutions or suspensions intended for topical dropwise instillation in the eye or ointments for topical application to the eye area. The hospital pharmacist's involvement with ophthalmics is similar to injections. Ophthalmics must be sterile and particulate free but are not required to be apyrogenic, so the same supplies, equipment, and facilities used for compounding injectables may also be used for ophthalmics. However, presterilized, ready-to-use polyethylene dropping bottles are apparently not as readily available commercially as are disposable syringes for repackaging SVPs, thus inhibiting the pharmacist's ability in packaging and hence activity in ophthalmics compounding.

4. *Dialysis and Irrigation Solutions*

These products should meet all the standards for infusions. The hospital pharmacist's involvement with these products is normally the supply, distribution, and control of commercially available products. Even these functions have been relegated in some hospitals to other departments, such as general stores or central sterile supply.

5. *Solutions for Inhalation Therapy*

Commercially available products are normally used in hospitals by respiratory therapists in conjunction with respirators and other respiratory therapy equipment to humidify the respiratory tract, help mobilize bronchial secretions for easy removal, and provide relief from bronchospasm and respiratory mucosal edema. These solutions should be sterile and free from pyrogens and particulate matter. Inhalation of microorganisms or particulate matter can be serious for the patient with a compromised respiratory tract. General

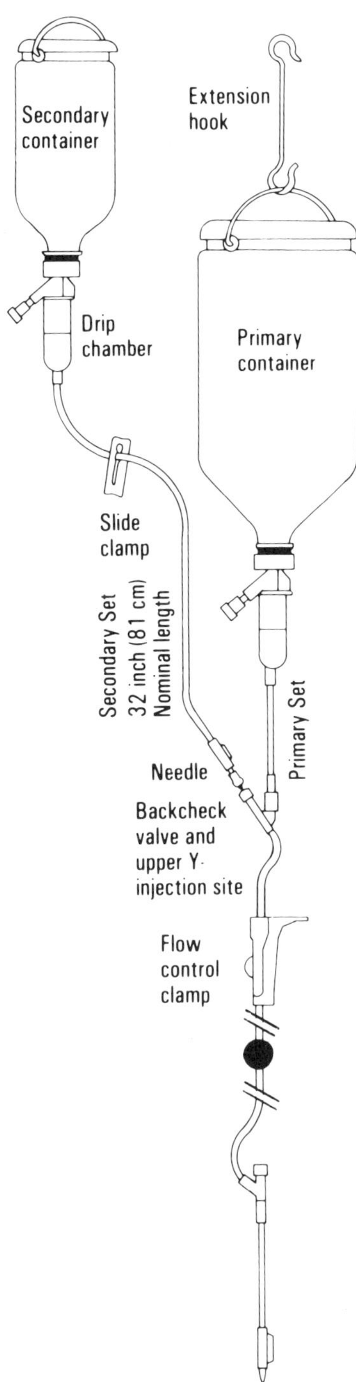

Figure 2 An intermittent ("piggyback") infusion system. (Courtesy of Abbott Laboratories.)

contamination of an entire respiratory therapy system can occur within hours from the addition of a single microbiologically contaminated solution. Thus, a patient receiving continuous therapy for several hours from a system with increasing levels of microbial contamination is subjected to a heavy cumulative microbial challenge deep into the lungs.

The pharmacy department has not normally been involved in respiratory therapy, leaving even the supply, distribution, and control of respiratory therapy solutions up to the respiratory therapists. The need for pharmacy involvement in this area has been recognized and met in at least one hospital through inclusion of respiratory therapy products in the pharmacy's unit-dose program [2].

C. The Functional Medication Cycle

An overview of the hospital use of parenteral products is presented to help industrial professionals distinguish between the industrial and the hospital perspective regarding the sterile product. Thus, a model depicting a functional cycle of parenteral products in a hospital with a centralized IV admixture program in the pharmacy department is presented (Fig. 3). The model illustrates the normal flow and relationships of activities involving parenterals in hospitals in general. In Figure 3, a sequence of activities and events is initiated when a patient's diagnosis prompts a treatment plan that includes parenteral therapy. The resulting sequence involves compounding, dispensing, drug distribution, and clinical functions in response to a patient-specific medication order. The functions associated with pharmaceutical supply are also depicted in Figure 3 but sequenced separately from and supportive to the order response sequence. The supply sequence is initiated on the basis of inventory levels rather than an individual patient treatment plan. Supply functions include IV admixtures, reconstitutions, repackaging, and other activities conducted as a batch process. The reader should note that the main topic headings used in this chapter closely parallel the activities and events sequenced in Figure 3.

No single department or staff has consolidated authority over, or responsibility for, deciding upon or fulfilling everything depicted by the functional medication cycle. Functional fragmentation does occur, generally following the traditional lines of professional responsibility. For example, physicians usually assess patient status and make therapeutic decisions. Pharmacists and their immediate appointees are responsible for product procurement, preparation, packaging, distribution, and control. Drug administration is normally the responsibility of the nursing staff. Interprofessional involvement and interaction usually occur in regard to patient monitoring, assessing patient response to therapy, and therapeutic decision making.

Figure 3 also reflects the floor stock (see Storage in Patient Care Areas) and nonpharmacy compounding that exist in some hospitals. Nonpharmacy personnel sometimes perform functions that are basically pharmaceutical. For example, the central stores or central sterile supplies departments are responsible, independent of the pharmacy department, for the procurement, storage, distribution, and control of LVP solutions in some hospitals, a practice that is strongly discouraged. Nurses sometimes prepare parenteral admixtures in patient care areas. Although IV solutions should be prepared by a pharmacist or under the direct supervision of a pharmacist [3], allowances may be made for others to compound [4] under special circumstances, such as emergencies, new admissions after hours, or when the pharmacist

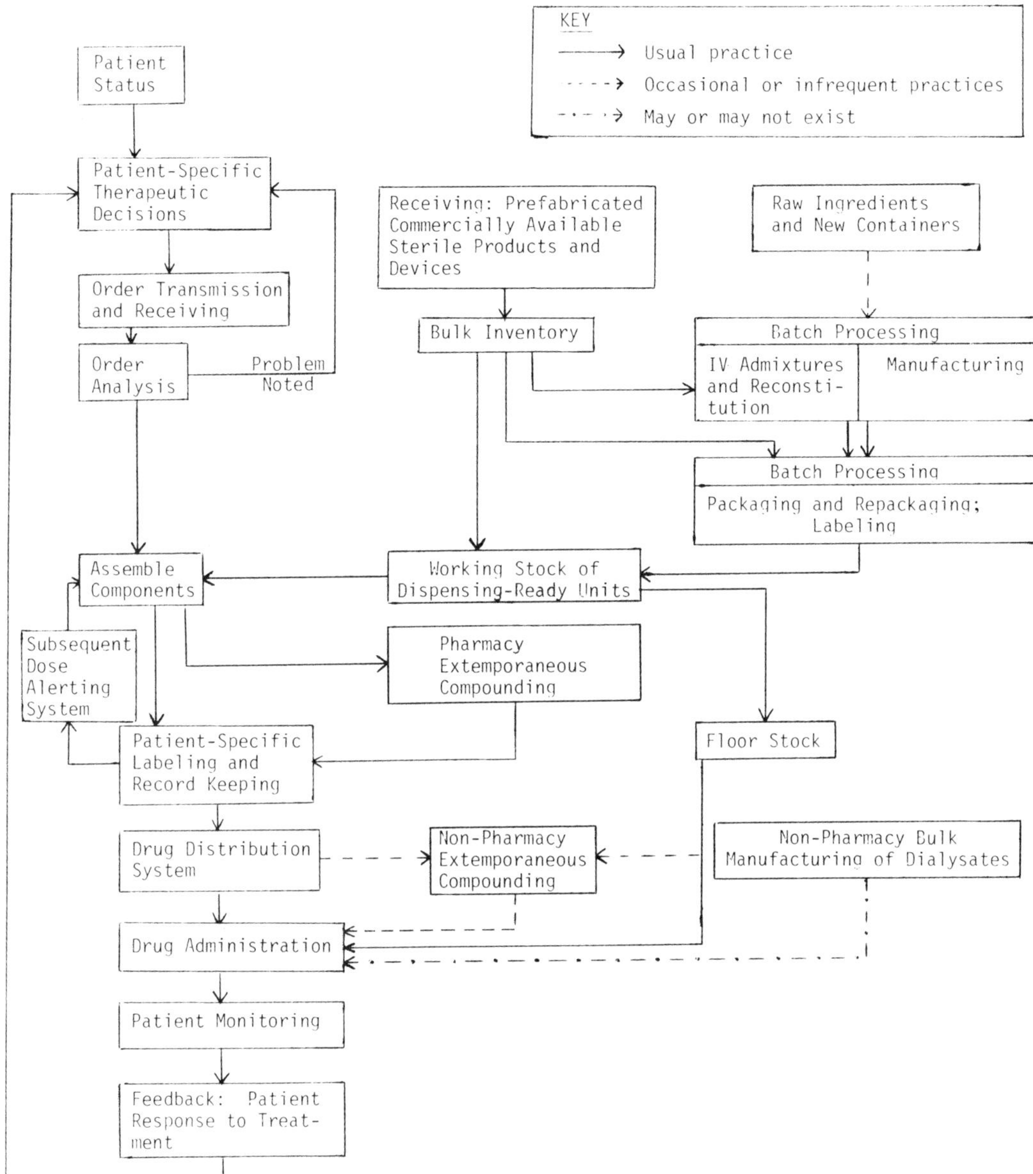

Figure 3 The functional medication cycle of parenteral products in a hospital with a centralized intravenous admixture program.

is not on duty. However, the pharmacist should be contacted whenever questions, such as potential adverse effects, dosing matters, or incompatibilities, arise [3]. Furthermore, the pharmacy department is responsible at least for preparing policies and procedures for extemporaneous compounding in patient care areas to assure that all pharmaceutical requirements are met [5].

All aspects of the parenteral medication cycle should be included in a comprehensive quality assurance program administered by the pharmacy department. Furthermore, comprehensive policies and procedures or operational protocols should be in writing. Interdepartmental coordination is essential to minimize gaps in coverage, needless overlap, and conflicting statements. Quality assurance responsibilities of the pharmacy department are discussed near the end of this chapter.

D. Organizational Control

The hospital's administrative structure, medical staff committees, and economics influence the goals and the means for providing parenteral products and services within the institution. Regarding administrative structure, responsibilities for most functions within the parenteral products medication cycle are spread among the pharmacy and nursing departments and the medical staff. The directors of pharmacy and nursing report independently to the hospital administrator (directly in a small hospital or through an assistant administrator in a larger hospital), who in turn is responsible to the hospital's governing board. All responsibilities of the pharmacy and nursing departments are subject to the usual administrative controls typically associated with the organizational hierarchy. Mutual interests between pharmacy and nursing are officially resolved through the chain of command. However, interdepartmental committees may be formed for good communication and mutual problem resolution.

A medical director oversees the entire medical staff and reports directly to the governing board, independently of the hospital's administrator-departmental structure. A pharmacy and therapeutics (P&T) committee and an infections committee are among the several standing advisory committees of the medical staff in an accredited hospital. The P&T committee may recommend institutional policies and procedures about any aspect of parenteral product use or parenteral therapy in the institution. They may also, pending approval of their recommendations, delegate authority to designated departments for procedural implementation and enforcement. The infections committee, operating under the same basic premises, is concerned primarily with any matter relating to infection control in the hospital, including nosocomial infections associated with parenteral products. The accreditation standards for these committees [5], because they are stated in general rather than specific terms, are subject to different interpretations as committees define their duties and responsibilities.

A pharmacist is normally a member of the P&T committee and should be a member of the infections committee. As a member, the pharmacist has the opportunity to help shape policy. Furthermore, a capable and interested pharmacist is likely to earn readily from these committees considerable authority to develop, implement, and enforce meaningful procedures consistent with committee policy.

E. Standard of Care

A hospital has a duty to provide reasonable care based on a standard consistent with prevailing, accepted practices and with the recommendations and guidelines published by professional, scientific, or scholarly bodies and accrediting agencies. Groups relevant to parenteral products in this regard include the Joint Commission on Accreditation of Hospitals (JCAH), the American Society of Hospital Pharmacists (ASHP), the National Coordinating Committee on Large Volume Parenterals (NCCLVP), the Centers for Disease Control (CDC), and the *U.S. Pharmacopeia* (USP). JCAH standards have been termed quasilegal standards, which must be consulted in hospital pharmacy practice. However, accreditation is voluntary. A hospital becomes accredited upon successful completion of an inspection by a JCAH survey team. Although the accreditation process has been a major impetus in upgrading and maintaining the quality of care in U.S. hospitals, JCAH falls far short of accomplishing in the hospital what the FDA does in the pharmaceutical industry with respect to the sterile pharmaceutical product.

A standard of care is not a list of regulations to which compliance is determined by inspection. Rather, it is cumulatively established in the courts through past judgments made in civil suits. These are brought against a hospital by an injured party when a suspected breach of duty is the alleged cause of the injury. The court hears expert testimony and consults past court cases to help determine the expected standard and the defendent's duty to follow that standard. The standard of care, especially as interpreted through the recommendations of the above-named organizations, is probably the most useful guide available in helping hospitals understand their duties with respect to the pharmaceutical aspects in the preparation and use of parenteral products.

State boards of pharmacy are the duly constituted bodies to enforce state laws pertaining to the practice of pharmacy. However, their regulations relevant to the preparation of defect-free sterile products are usually either vague or nonexistent. Although the FDA does not exercise jurisdiction over the practice of pharmacy in a hospital, the ASHP suggests that all manufacturing procedures in a hospital pharmacy should be consistent with the current good manufacturing practices (CGMPs) [6].

A significant form of economical control, especially when financial resources are limited, may occur when the priorities of the pharmacy department differ from the priorities of the institution as a whole. For example, hospital pharmacists are expected, as are their industrial counterparts, to give the highest of priorities to those compounding and quality assurance activities that lead to quality products. However, when these activities are competing with more dramatic and seemingly more influential ways for fulfilling the hospital's overall goals, they may be deemed relatively unimportant by the hospital's higher level financial decision makers.

As a licensed health professional, the individual practitioner is expected to fulfill the responsibilities of his or her profession in a manner consistent with all applicable federal and state laws, professional standards of conduct, and the current standard of care. Even so, the practitioner has considerable leeway for using professional judgment in matters ranging from establishing scope of services to moment-by-moment decisions about, for example, compounding details. Demands of the hospital as an organization are sometimes in conflict with professional duties and responsibilities as seen by the individual licensed pharmacist. However, the resulting apparent undermining of professional autonomy does not abrogate the hospital pharmacist from the responsibility of making individual professional decisions in accordance with the public trust bestowed upon him or her.

III. DISPENSING AND COMPOUNDING PROCESSES

A. Order Initiation and Transmission

The medication order that initiates the sequence of events depicted in Figure 3 must originate from a legally recognized prescriber (e.g., a physician). Many factors influence the prescriber's decisions in creating an order for parenteral medication, including consultation with the pharmacist, policies of the P&T committee, scope of the hospital's formulary, and established protocols, such as the standardized orders for total parenteral nutritional (TPN) solutions and priorities for allocating infusion pumps.

The order may be transmitted to the pharmacy verbally or in writing. An efficient transmission system for IV admixture orders is necessary for workload scheduling in the pharmacy department. For example, nurses in some hospitals must notify the pharmacy by telephone as soon as a new or changed IV admixture is prescribed. The pharmacy eventually must receive a direct copy of the order written by the prescriber in the patient's medical chart. Some hospitals use special order sheets for infusions or TPN solutions.

B. Order Analysis

The pharmacist should review all IV admixture orders upon receipt to detect any problems, such as an incompatibility, inappropriate dosing, or a therapeutic drug-drug interaction, before the order is prepared. The pharmacist should contact the prescriber as soon as possible about any problems requiring, in the pharmacist's judgment, a change in the order. Of special interest for this chapter is the prediction of incompatibilities during this review.

An incompatibility is a preventable, undesired physical or chemical phenomenon occurring when two or more pharmaceutical systems are combined. It may be visually detectable, such as a precipitate, haze, immiscible layering, turbidity, effervescence, or color change, or only instrumentally detectable, such as a change in pH or viscosity. An accelerated degradation of one or more of the mixed ingredients may remain undetected by the observational means normally available to the hospital pharmacist. A drug-container incompatibility also may occur, for example, sorption of the active drug in a SVP product to the wall of the LVP container to which it was added. Occasionally, poor patient response to drug therapy may prompt a suspicion of an incompatibility. Ideally, the observation should be followed up with planned research and confirmation. The now well-known sorption of diazepam and nitroglycerin to PVC infusion containers are examples where this has occurred.

When reviewing an order, the pharmacist must predict the likelihood that the compounded IV admixture will remain free from adverse chemical or physical changes until its administration has been completed, anticipating that up to 24 hr may transpire between mixing and initiation of administration

[4], plus up to another 24 hr [4], or even 48 hr in some hospitals [7], until the container is removed from the patient. The label on all IV admixtures should display a beyond-use time and date [4] that is not likely to exceed the time for any significant degradation or altered appearance to develop, as determined from information in the literature, other evidence, or professional judgment. Trissel's and King's incompatibility guides [8,9] and other references are available to help the pharmacist in this determination. The package insert and labeling for the additives may provide helpful information. The pharmacist should also keep abreast of current research on incompatibilities and the stability of IV admixtures as published in, for example, the *American Journal of Hospital Pharmacy*. Furthermore, the pharmacist should maintain for future reference experience profiles for admixtures not adequately described in the guides or for which the pharmacist's observations are unique or differ from those in the literature.

If the compatibility or stability of a particular combination of ingredients is not explicit, the pharmacist must make a prediction from general knowledge using any limited information that may be available. For example, the magnitude of the problem is reduced considerably from the infinite by the pharmacist's general understanding that most incompatibilities or hastened degradation are associated with accelerated hydrolysis or reduced solubility in a new environment (e.g., new pH or dilution of a cosolvent system), salting out, formation of an insoluble molecule (e.g., cation-anion reaction involving Mg^{2+} or Ca^{2+}), or hasten the oxidation of oxygen-sensitive agents upon dilution of an antioxidant system. The pharmacist should also recognize that phosphates, carbonates, and lactates, weak acids or bases or their salts, relatively nonpolar organic molecules, and dry products for injection may be especially problematic. When the outcome of an admixture is conjectural, two units should be prepared near the scheduled administration time, retaining one to observe for at least 24 hr for any visible changes. A change may require discontinuance of the unit being infused. Results from the observation should be documented in the pharmacist's experience profile. Newsletters or other prescriber awareness programs may help promote prudent prescribing practices as a way to reduce questionable combinations.

C. Dispensing

Dispensing is a legislatively defined activity limited to duly licensed pharmacists and their legally recognized and supervised appointees. The dispensing process for injectables usually involves selecting the correct product, labeling it according to the hospital's policies and procedures, and consigning the completed unit to the hospital's drug distribution system. The unit must be available at the patient's bedside in time for the scheduled administration.

Injectables should be dispensed in as ready to use form as possible. Many prefabricated commercially available parenterals are ready for use and therefore can be dispensed without manipulation of the contents or the container.

D. Compounding

Many occasions arise where the pharmacist must compound (i.e., mix two or more substances to achieve prescribed amounts in the final dispensed unit), subdivide, or repackage specific volumes of injectables to achieve dosage individualization, a combination of products in a single injection, a dilution, or a reconstitution.

1. *Extemporaneous Compounding*

The IV admixture is the most frequently encountered and perhaps the only type of parenteral that is extemporaneously compounded in U.S. hospitals. A typical IV admixture problem involves the transfer of required volumes of one or more SVPs into a LVP container using an appropriate transfer device, such as a syringe and needle. Each order is handled as a separate entity. A processing system accommodating a stream of separate orders should be a planned and controlled operation guided by written policies and procedures.

An IV admixture worksheet should be completed and filed for every compounded IV admixture. Information that should be recorded includes complete identification of all products used, including concentration(s) of active ingredient(s), volume, lot numbers, and expiration dates; preparation notes; dosage, infusion rate, and administration times; special handling or storage requirements; and other details. The worksheet is a transcription by a pharmacist from a physician's written order or from a nurse's verbal transmission of a physician's order. The accuracy of every transcription should be verified from the prescriber's written order as a part of a quality control check. The original order should be attached to or at least cross-referenced with the worksheet. Computerized label production allows the ready generation of a duplicate label for attachment to the worksheet. The worksheet should also provide space for noting such information as the name of the compounder and the time and date of compounding for each instance that the admixture was compounded (e.g., when the prescriber's order requires the preparation of multiple identical units). Quality checkpoints for each compounding instance should also be accommodated on the form. In general, the worksheet should be designed to serve as a source document containing adequate information for the exact duplication of any subsequent units. All worksheets should be filed as historical quality control documentation of processing. A master batch formula is irrelevant to extemporaneously compounded IV admixtures. Thus, all necessary guidance and standardization of practices must be provided through the written policies and procedures.

A central IV admixture service must have a reliable self-alerting system to know when subsequent admixtures must be prepared in fulfillment of an order. Time-specific alerting may be achieved by placing all worksheets in time-labeled pigeonholes corresponding to the first (for new orders) or next scheduled preparation or dose times. Computerized updating and alerting is used in some hospital pharmacies.

2. *Batch Processing*

Batch processing is the preparation of multiple identical units of product as a unified operation. The preparation of routinely encountered IV admixture orders, TPN solutions, reconstitutions, and unit-dose syringe filling by batch processing may result in improved efficiency, economy, or quality control. Batch processing in a central IV admixture program may be in anticipation of future demand (e.g., freezing a 30-day supply of a reconstituted antibiotic diluted in an IV fluid in plastic bags) or known orders (e.g., preparing a 24-hr supply of an IV admixture in response to amassed identical orders).

A written master batch formula with procedures should be available for all batch processing. An appropriate batch-processing report should be completed and filed for every batch prepared. The design of batch-processing records and reports in hospital pharmacy [10] are similar in principle but not in detail to batch documentation used in the pharmaceutical industry [11].

Criteria that may help in determining the feasibility of preparing a particular product as a batch operation include (a) usage rate, that is, number of required units per reference period; (b) stability and predictability of the usage rate; and (c) ability to schedule personnel and the compounding facility to batch operations. A threshold usage rate is required before the invested effort (e.g., time to plan, write master formulas, validate procedures, and maintain adequate quality control) provides sufficient benefits. Stability and predictability of usage is needed to avoid wastage from overproduction or inefficiencies caused by underproduction.

Conditions favorable to batch processing probably exist in many hospital pharmacies for the following preparations.

a. The addition of equal volume(s) of one or more additives to several LVP containers (same fluid and same size), for example, antibiotics in piggyback-size (50 or 100 ml) containers.
b. The reconstitution of several vials of a product for injection, obtaining the diluent from a common LVP container.
c. Repackaging an injection from multiple-dose vials into unit-dose syringes.
d. Premixing a specified volume of crystalline amino acids injection with a specified volume of dextrose injection 50% to make a standardized TPN solution. Constant amounts of selected additives, such as electrolytes, could also be included in the process. (Later, each standardized solution may be tailored to the individual patient with subsequent additives.)

Regarding scheduling, the sterile products compounding area should not be tied up with batch production during peak demand periods for extemporaneously prepared units. However, batches may be scheduled during low prescribing periods, such as evenings and nights. An additional compounding area could be considered if warranted by adequate anticipated workloads for both extemporaneously and batch-prepared IV admixtures.

A batching procedure is normally no more complex than the aseptic transfer of equal aliquots of fluid from an LVP container into several identical receiving containers using a specialized manual or electronic volumetric transfer device. A manual device would be a syringe-type, spring-return sterile disposable pipet. The electronic devices usually used by the hospital pharmacist are operationally similar to the IV pumps already described. However, some units, unlike IV pumps, have multiple transfer lines and pumping stations. The accuracy, dependability, simplicity and ease of use, speed, cost, and other factors relative to anticipated workload have been the subjects of research by hospital pharmacists.

Limitations on batch size include the work surface area in the hospital pharmacy's laminar-airflow workbench(es), the container size of commercially available products, and the beyond-use time limitation. Concerning the latter, the NCCLVP recommendation that an IV admixture should be administered promptly or, if refrigerated, within 24 hr after preparation [4] will continue to influence the hospital pharmacist in determining how many units to prepare as a batch. Hospital pharmacies normally do not have the means to perform studies for establishing product-specific beyond-use times before which insignificant degradation or no growth of accidentally introduced microbes can be assured.

Batches of parenteral solutions are frozen after dilution or reconstitution in some hospital pharmacies, for example, IV admixtures of antibiotics in flexible plastic LVP containers. A frozen unit is taken from the freezer as needed, ready for use upon thawing. The stability and activity of each product subjected to this process should be evaluated after freezing and after thawing. Some research of this nature has been reported in the literature. Freezing maintains the stability of several otherwise unstable drugs in solution for prolonged periods, such as 30 days [12]. Stability may not be maintained by freezing the solutions of some agents, for example, ampicillin [13]. Solutes may not redissolve upon thawing, for example, cimetidine [14]. Thawing methods have included ambient thawing (sitting out at room temperature), warm water baths, and microwave radiation. Ambient thawing may require up to 5 hr; microwaving may produce full thawing usually in 2–20 min, depending upon such factors as power used, container size, number of units in the chamber, a unit's chamber location, and shaking intervals. Uneven defrosting is more likely to occur during multiple-unit rather than single-unit microwave defrosting.

Prolonged ambient thawing of rapidly degrading products may be disadvantageous. Overheating, potentially adverse to product stability, may occur upon microwave thawing from haphazard control of the radiation period and irregularities in radiation intensity. Overheating may also result from prolonged immersion in water baths above room temperature. Stability or activity of several antibiotics, TPN solutions, and cimetidine has been shown not to be adversely affected by proper microwave thawing [14].

Microbially contaminated water baths, freezer compartments, and refrigerators place an undesirable contaminant challenge on the admixture container, as the integrity of the rubber closure had been violated during the admixture process. Situations to avoid include immersion of the medication ports in the water bath and contact between the ports and ice or water in a freezer or refrigerator. Defrosting of a freezer presents a serious problem in this regard, because melted freezer ice may remain in contact with container components for prolonged periods. Routine sanitization of water baths, freezer compartments, and refrigerators with a validated procedure and schedule is urged.

3. *Manufacturing*

Manufacturing of sterile products from raw ingredients in a hospital pharmacy has been encouraged as a means to meet patient care needs of a hospital when a suitable product is not commercially available. Hospital pharmacists are not likely to manufacture an item if it is commercially available, as purchasing is usually more cost effective and convenient than in-house manufacturing. Although not frequently encountered, manufacturing of special items can be very professionally stimulating, according to the testimony of hospital pharmacists who have manufactured. Involvement is usually dependent upon the personal initiative of a knowledgeable and concerned pharmacist who is perceptive to the often unrequested needs of the medical staff. Pharmacists' arguments justifying lack of involvement have included inability to provide adequate quality assurance or documentation of clinical efficacy, lack of knowledge and training, inadequate space or personnel, and lack of demand. Perhaps demand is low because prescribers are not accustomed to customized manufacturing by pharmacy personnel. Perhaps the pharmacist desirous of having such a service needs to take the initiative and actively promote it. Examples where hospital pharmacists have manufactured parenteral products for special needs include antibiotics in high concentrations for orthopedic total hip replacement surgery; intraocular injections for corneal replacement procedures; injections free from added substances for intrathecal or pediatric use; certain sterile powders, ointments, and solutions for use in surgery or isolation units; and trace minerals injections for IV admixture before their commercial availability. Hospital pharmacists are urged to consult Chapter 6 (Vol. 1) for insights in establishing small volume parenterals manufacturing or for evaluating existing procedures.

IV. TECHNOLOGY OF STERILE COMPOUNDING IN THE HOSPITAL PHARMACY

The maintenance of product integrity in the compounding of IV admixtures depends primarily on the control of environmental quality, the pharmacist's aseptic technique, and the use of filtration to control microorganisms and particulate matter. The maintenance of postcompounding container integrity is also important. In addition, special policies and procedures for the protection of the operator and the compounding environment are required when compounding involves the use of biohazardous agents, such as some anticancer drugs.

A. Environmental Control

Hospital pharmacy departments usually must compete with other departments for the space and the funding required to support a capital project such as a new or substantially upgraded IV admixture program. Space, physical renovations, and equipment needed for adequate environmental control normally comprise a major share of the total capital costs. With a limited ability to procure additional space, the astute hospital pharmacist must maintain a constant awareness of the hospital's long-range planning and should be vigilant for poorly utilized space to ask for. Obtaining capital and space for a new venture may depend upon the hospital pharmacist's ability to get the proposed program included as a part of a hospitalwide capital expansion program. Even so, the final level of funding for a new or expanded IV admixture program may be inadequate to fulfill all objectives. Thus, many IV admixture programs operate with marginal levels of space, facilities, and environmental control. Ironically, a major program justification has often been the claim that centralization in the pharmacy would provide better environmental control for the preparation of IV admixtures than would be achievable by nurses in patient care areas. Through centralization, focused resources and planning should result in quality compounding facilities and written policies and procedures for the proper maintenance and use of those facilities.

1. *The Laminar-Airflow Workbench (LAFW)*

The LAFW is the central component of an environmental control facility in an IV admixture program because (a) all critical activities should be done in it;

(b) it is the predominant workflow focal point; (c) most IV admixture procedures relate to it in some way. The LAFW is usually the first, and sometimes the only, environmental control device obtained by a pharmacy department. All critical activities, that is, any procedure that could directly or indirectly lead to contamination of a parenteral product, a fluid pathway for that product, or any surface of potential future product contact, should be conducted under Class 100 conditions (see Chap 9, Vol. I, for a comprehensive discussion on designing a parenteral production facility for environmental control).

A LAFW is capable of providing Class 100 conditions in its work space, although its achievement depends upon the device's design and configuration, adherence to proper procedures during use, understanding its limitations, and reliable performance in accordance with the unit's specifications. The hospital pharmacist must be able to select the right unit, write policies and procedures for its proper use, train and supervise personnel, and adhere to an acceptable monitoring and testing program to assure that Class 100 conditions are met.

Both horizontal and vertical flow workbenches are used in hospital pharmacy. The same basic principles apply to working in either one, for example, (a) no object or activity should intervene in the direct airstream between the HEPA-filtered, laminarized airflow source and the critical activity; (b) turbulence generation in or near the work space should be kept to a minimum; and (c) the existing flow of work space air should not be impeded. However, the difference in airflow direction requires modifications in technique [15]. For example, several critical objects usually may be positioned anywhere (except within a few inches of the perimeter) on the work surface in a vertical LAFW at the same time and still remain fully bathed in the unobstructed airstream. However, in a horizontal LAFW, an object should not create a barrier between the airflow source and any other object, objects should be placed close to the airflow source to minimize the risk of an intervening barrier relative to the airflow source, and objects should be adequately spaced so as not to impede the general airflow in the work space. To avoid obstruction of airflow between the source and critical objects, operators must learn to work essentially behind objects in horizontal flow units and under objects in the vertical flow configuration.

Particles entrained in the downward-flowing airstream in a vertical LAFW impact on the work surface and may be resuspended if airflow is disrupted. Thus, critical activities should not occur close to the work surface. An inch or more from the work surface should be allowed, depending upon the design of the vertical flow unit [16].

Vertically flowing air offers virtually no resistance to cross-stream gusts of room air, a factor to be considered where turbulence-generating work activity is unavoidable adjacent to the work space opening.

Vertical LAFWs are designed to be used with a front protective panel and a limited (e.g., 10–15 in.) work space opening. Matters such as these should be considered in conjunction with expected work arrangements, room design, and operator preferences when selecting a LAFW for purchase.

2. *The Buffer Area*

The quality of the air immediately surrounding a LAFW affects the air quality in its work space. Air quality in an active hospital pharmacy falls far below that required by the Class 100 standard. Thus, a LAFW should be located in a buffer area, that is, a dedicated room separated from the other activities of the department. This area should be maintained in a cleaner state than in the main pharmacy and should be protected from contaminant-generating sources, such as shipping cartons, the traffic of nongowned personnel, dirty ventilating air, and activities not associated with the preparation of sterile products. Furthermore, the facility should provide for adequate separation between preparatory activities and aseptic work. Probably because of the demand for IV admixtures, their compounding frequency, and the occasional rush order, some hospital pharmacists have tended to put LAFWs in busy readily accessible locations, even next to a hallway door, as observed in one pharmacy. Hospital pharmacists must locate LAFWs in accordance with the current state of knowledge about effective environmental controls.

The application of the following principles of facility design should result in air quality improvement for the buffer area. The buffer area may be conceptualized as a long tunnel (figuratively, not literally) with the LAFW located at the far end. Clean air for this tunnel would flow in at the far end, thus providing a general outward movement of air through the tunnel. The in-flowing air should be treated to remove particulates, preferably by HEPA filtration. The airflow rate should be high enough through the tunnel to minimize the ingress of airborne contaminants on wild air currents at the exit end. The direction of the airflow from the LAFW should be the same as the general room air flowing through the tunnel. Objects, including the LAFW, should be arranged for the minimization of dead areas or eddy currents.

The buffer area should have the construction characteristics of a clean room, that is, walls, ceiling, floors, and fixtures should be composed of nonshedding, smooth, impervious, readily cleanable surfaces. Examples of suitable ceilings include epoxy-painted plaster and epoxy-impregnated clean room ceiling panels. The porous, fibrous acoustical ceiling tiles found in many hospitals should not be used in the buffer area. Smooth-textured, solid sheet vinyl is useful as a flooring material. Seams can be heat welded and the flooring coved to the wall to eliminate crevices at the baseboard. Where new wall construction is not feasible, a buffer area can be created by isolating an area within a larger room with clear heavy-ply, polyethylene sheeting. The plastic surrounding the LAFW and associated activities would hang from ceiling to floor, except at the end opposite the LAFW, where the sheeting would stop a few inches above the floor. As another approach, prefabricated solid-walled modular areas are commercially available from clean room equipment suppliers.

Fixtures should be readily cleanable and should not be dust catchers. Preferably, wall cabinets should reach the ceiling; otherwise, their tops would require frequent cleaning. Open bins for such supplies as syringes and SVPs probably cannot be avoided, but they should be readily cleanable. Stainless steel is normally the best (and most expensive) material for fixtures and cabinetry. Good quality baked enamel or plastic laminated wood are usually suitable materials for countertops and cabinetry. Wood cabinetry should be avoided in the buffer room, because wood is porous and sheds particulate matter. Wet wood can harbor viable microbial colonies.

Some hospital pharmacists use wire utility carts in preference to fixed storage cabinets for their buffer room supplies. Carts offer the advantages of movability, storage flexibility, and cleanability. They may be wheeled to the buffer room doorway for restocking with a daily supply of sanitized LVP and SVP containers, transfer sets, syringes, and other items needed for a day's work. Supplies remaining on the cart from the previous day would be removed and the cart would be wiped down prior to restocking with sanitized items.

Work flow must be considered in the design of the buffer area. The procedures outlined in the Appendix would be carried out in the buffer area as a linear sequence. Only the compounding step must be carried out in a LAFW, because it is the only step involving critical activities or exposure of critical sites. Assembly, staging, finishing, and postcompounding inspection would be performed adjacent to the LAFW for efficiency. The consignment step and contaminant-generating support activities, such as bulk inventory storage, unboxing, scrubbing, gowning, sanitization of supplies, label preparation, and writing on work sheets, should be performed outside the buffer area. Sinks normally are not needed for buffer room activities. However, if sinks must be built into the buffer area, they should be at the exit end because of the contamination potential. With thoughtful planning, the layout of the buffer area can accommodate work efficiency and a smooth flow of personnel and material while adhering to principles of environmental control. A schematic floor plan consistent with the preceding discussion is provided in Figure 4.

3. *Procedural Controls*

A hospital pharmacy should have detailed written operating procedures directed toward (a) preventing contaminants from entering the buffer area and the LAFW, (b) reducing and containing contaminants generated within the buffer area and the LAFW, and (c) isolating critical sites and critical activities from any environmental contamination that may be present.

Controlling access of personnel and supplies is crucial for the prevention of contaminant ingress to an environmentally controlled area. Controlled access means that neither people nor supplies are permitted into the controlled area without a specific purpose relevant to processing or area maintenance and not before the person or object has undergone prescribed gowning, sanitization, or other preparatory activity. Contamination can also be controlled by maintaining a low population density in the buffer area and by designing operations to minimize movement. Arranging objects in the LAFW to best utilize laminar flow of HEPA-filtered air aids in isolating critical sites from contamination. The article by Frieben [17] should be consulted for more details on specific contamination control procedures. Because people and their activity contribute much of the contamination found in clean rooms, considerable attention should be focused on personnel when writing procedural controls for a hospital pharmacy's IV admixture area (Chap. 10, Vol. 1 offers guidance in this regard). Written procedures should also encompass the activities of maintenance and housekeeping personnel in the buffer area.

Procedural breakdown may occur from conflicting demands upon a pharmacist. For example, a pharmacist involved in compounding IV admixtures may be called away by a pressing demand elsewhere. Or the pharmacist may need to hustle into the buffer area just to prepare one rush order. Procedural breakdowns, especially adherence to proper gowning procedures, can be expected to increase as interruptions with conflicting demands increase. Reduction of interruptions, augmented staffing, and/or revised work schedules may offset the problem. Writing compromised procedures to compensate for interruptions is not appropriate.

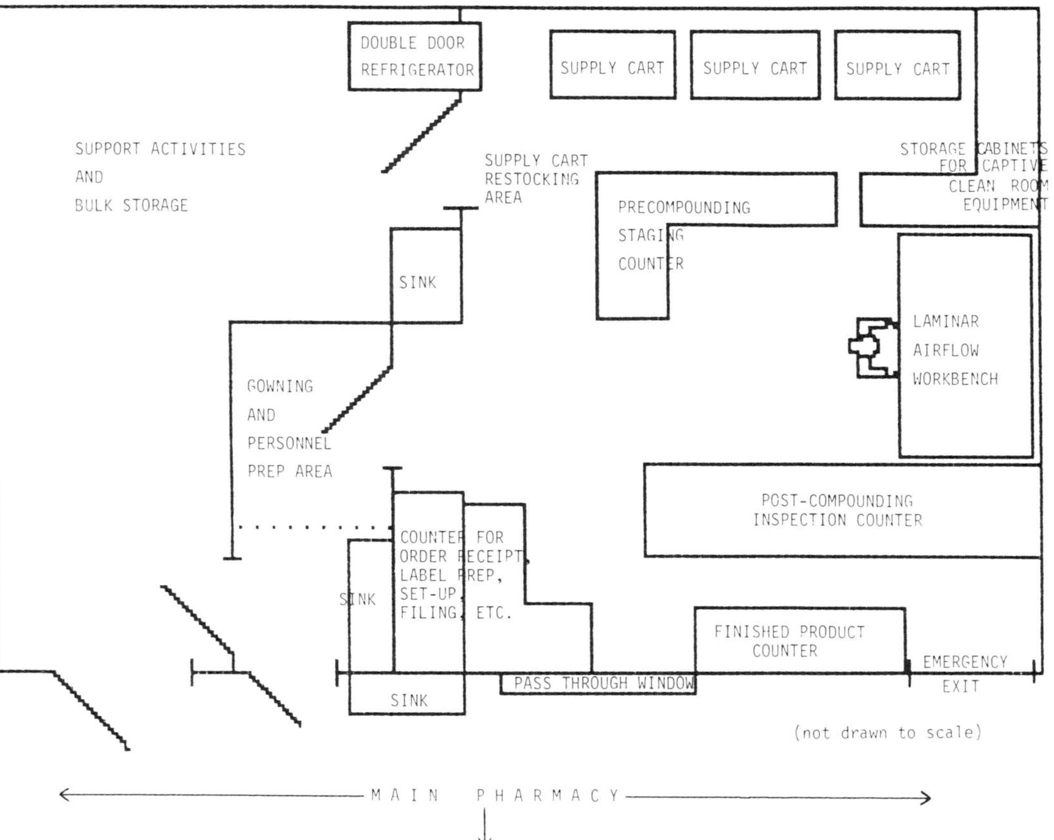

Figure 4 A schematic floor plan for a facility to prepare intravenous admixtures in a hospital pharmacy. (The floor plan is designed to facilitate a work flow consistent with the sequence of admixture procedures depicted in the Appendix.)

4. *Gowning*

Gowning for the buffer area should include preparatory scrubbing of hands and arms to the elbow with a germicidal detergent (such as povidone-iodine surgical scrub), donning a clean hair cover, beard cover for operators with facial hair, and a clean but not necessarily sterile nonlinting, low fiber-shedding laboratory coat. The coat should be knee-length, constricted at the wrists, neck high for the full circumference, and made from a high-barrier, low particulating material such as Tyvek. Clean shoe covers also should be worn. A face mask to deflect the breath is recommended for operators working at a horizontal LAFW. Masks should be changed frequently to prevent microbial overloading.

Wearing gloves in the buffer area reduces the transfer of contaminants from the hand to objects and provides a barrier to particulate transmission into the atmosphere from skin shedding. Gloves, however, are not effective for preventing the touch contamination of critical sites, because objects previously handled are not likely to have been sterile. Thus, wearing gloves may promote a false sense of security. Some believe that strictly controlled movement with clean, sanitized hands is preferable to routine gloving. Operators should wear gloves under certain special circumstances, for example, when handling hazardous substances or for conditions such as eczema on the hand where unusually high amounts of particles and microbes could be shed.

5. *Patient Care Areas*

The best conditions for preparing sterile products in patient care areas probably would be in areas having low traffic, low population density, and low activity. The nurse should at least wash the hands immediately prior to compounding.

B. Technique

The compounding of IV admixtures requires an array of manipulative skills in handling a variety of sterile, ready-to-use devices and containers in many different configurations under controlled environmental conditions. Most IV admixture orders involve a transfer procedure, mainly the withdrawal of the contents of a vial or an ampul using a needle and syringe; the transfer of the contents of a syringe with filtration to a LVP container; the reconstitution of the dry contents of a vial; the vacuum transfer of a solution from a SVP or LVP container to an evacuated bottle or a vacuumized bag; and the transfer of multiple increments of the contents of a LVP container into several receiving containers. A variety of devices are used, for example, transfer tubing, vented and/or filter needles, hydrophobic and hydrophilic membrane filters, evacuated LVP bottles and empty LVP bags, multiple additive syringes with spring-return plungers, volume control IV sets, and the standard needle and syringe.

Aseptic technique is any procedure or processing condition designed to keep materials as free as possible from viable contamination. Operators must use it during compounding to keep sterile items sterile. Complete reliance must be placed on the proper and consistent use of aseptic technique for the prevention of contamination, because IV admixtures do not include a sterilization step in their preparation. Training and experience are required for the pharmacist to develop consistently effective and aseptic manipulations.

The Avis and Akers illustrated manual of detailed, step-by-step procedures [18] is suggested as a training aid.

The procedural prevention of fluid pathway contamination, or anything that may come in direct or indirect contact with fluid pathways, focuses on (a) touch avoidance of critical sites; (b) bathing critical items and sites continuously in the unobstructed, direct flow of HEPA-filtered, laminarized air; and (c) minimizing duration of critical site exposure. Examples of specific procedures for operators include (a) keeping fingers and hands away from critical sites; (b) avoiding the same work surface location for placing critical and noncritical objects; (c) placing noncritical activities and objects toward the periphery of the work space; (d) performing critical activities close to the airflow source; and (e) not performing or not placing critical work or objects downstream from airflow barriers or at the work space periphery. Examples of critical sites or activities include any connection of fluid lines, an opened ampul, an unsheathed needle, and uncapped syringe tips or IV set spikes.

An open pathway for airborne contamination may exist during venting or with poor connections. Venting may be needed to allow fluid transfer to or from a rigid, nonvacuumized or nonpressurized container. A hydrophobic, bacterially retentive filter should be used when possible for venting airways. Devices creating open airways, such as venting needles without air path filters, are to be avoided.

Poor connections, often difficult to detect, augment the chances for contaminant ingress during vacuum transfers, which are very common in hospital pharmacy. Although a pressure transfer system would probably provide less chance for contaminant ingress, existing technology is geared more to the vacuum transfer. However, the hospital pharmacist can create pressure transfer systems by applying low-pressure, bacterially filtered compressed air or nitrogen to a LVP container via the airway on a vented IV spike (Fig. 1). Portable compressed gas tanks are available in a wide range of sizes. A hand-operated syringe pump also can provide pressure through the airway. Flexible plastic LVP containers can be pressurized with a standard blood pressure cuff. An infusion pump on the transfer line provides pressure distally, but the proximal part of the system would be under a vacuum. All connections should be maintained under unobstructed controlled airflow because of the continuing risk of contaminant ingress.

Several procedures, such as those that follow, establish an appropriate environment for aseptic technique.

a. All paper wrapping, dust covers, and the like should be removed at the outer edge of the LAFW as their sterile contents are introduced into the work space.
b. Items not directly from a sterile overwrap should be cleaned with a nonlinting wipe dampened with a liquid disinfectant, such as isopropanol 70% or ethanol 70%, immediately prior to their introduction into the work space.
c. Although previously scrubbed, the hands should be wiped occasionally during work with a hand disinfectant, such as alcohol foam or complexed iodine.
d. The side walls and work surface of the work space should be sanitized with a nonlinting wipe soaked with a surface disinfectant, such as isopropanol 70% or ethanol 70%, at the beginning of each shift, at appropriate intervals during a shift, and whenever spillage occurs. Wiping

should proceed progressively outward, that is, from the cleanest to the dirtiest part of the walls and work surface.

e. Movement in and out of the work space should be minimized. For example, all supplies needed for an order are introduced prior to beginning aseptic manipulations. Discards are placed near the outer side edge of the work space, to be removed upon completion of the manipulation. Unnecessary items should not be brought into the work space.

"Assembly line" procedures involving electronic transfer pumps, some with programmable multiple input and output channels, are also used in hospital pharmacy for multiple filling operations. As systems become more complex, the chances of breaches in aseptic technique increase. The hazard to patients increases, too, because contamination from a procedural breach may affect many units in a multiunit process. An operator must be trained and certified in aseptic technique at the required level of procedural complexity.

C. Biohazardous Agents

In addition to proper environmental control procedures and aseptic technique to protect the product, special procedures are needed to protect operators from any biohazardous materials, such as anticancer drugs, that they may be working with. Anticancer drugs may be carcinogenic, mutogenic, cytotoxic, or cause skin lesions, all justifiable concerns to the immediate operator and to those working in the immediate environment. Special procedures for handling these agents involve containment of the agent (e.g., using a biological safety cabinet and biohazard disposal methods), protection of the immediate operator (e.g., wearing proper gowns and gloves), and avoidance of splash, spills, spray-back, and aerosolization, and certifying the operator's technique.

Biological safety cabinets (BSCs) include vertical laminar airflow devices with a second HEPA filter to remove particles from the downflow air prior to exhaust or recirculation. Standards for the design and construction of BSCs, published by the National Sanitation Foundation [19], are for the express purpose of minimizing hazards inherent in working with biological agents. In purchasing a BSC, the hospital pharmacist must carefully assess whether Class 100 conditions are achievable by the unit(s) under consideration. For example, some units produce an unobstructed downflow air velocity significantly less than 90 ft/min ± 20%, the velocity that has been required for the entire history of LAFW devices for pharmaceutical application. While working in a BSC, operators are urged to perform their manipulations in the inner half of the work space because the air from that location would be exhausted away from the operator [20]. Some hospitals have a BSC to be used exclusively for the preparation of antineoplastics.

An appropriate garment for working with cytotoxic agents should be made of a material providing a good barrier. The garment should have long sleeves with closed cuffs and a closed front [2]. Although gloves should be worn, glove materials seem to offer only limited protection. Although latex may be generally less permeable to antineoplastic drugs then other glove material, such as polyvinyl chloride, some antineoplastic agents do permeate through latex [21].

Special compounding procedures include the use of Luer-lock fittings whenever possible, elimination of internal pressure or vacuum in containers by venting with a hydrophobic filter, opening ampuls only after all liquid is out of the neck and with a pad around the neck, and by using a closed vessel to contain discarded solution. Special procedures are also required for handling emergency exposure [20], spills [22], and waste disposal [23].

The hospital has a responsibility to minimize the occupational exposure of its employees to biohazardous materials. Regular medical surveillance, including laboratory tests [20], training programs, and written policies and procedures, are helpful in fulfilling this responsibility.

D. Filtration

Filtration should be employed to prevent process-related particulate contamination in IV admixtures. Sources of particulate matter include glass slivers from ampul breaking, sheared-off plastic particles from line connections, rubber cores from stopper punctures, and residual particulate matter intrinsic in certain devices. Furthermore, certain SVP injectable products, notably penicillin, other antibiotics, and powdered drugs for reconstitution, have been associated with higher levels of particulate matter. In general, the particulate load in an IV admixture increases as the number of added SVP drugs increases.

All fluids added to the final LVP container normally should be passed through a filter of 5-μm porosity or smaller. The filtration device should be placed in line as close to the point of final container entry as possible. A variety of sterile, ready-to-use filter units are commercially available, for example, membrane filters in plastic housings, sintered stainless steel filters affixed inside needle hubs ("filter needles"), and various transfer sets with inline membrane filters. Virtually every routine IV admixture transfer can incorporate filtration through the use of a convenient, sterile, commercially available filter unit. However, for some applications, certain devices are more efficient or are more appropriately designed than others. For efficiency, an adequate flow rate should be maintained. Flow rate through a membrane filter is directly proportional to pore size, membrane surface area, and pressure and indirectly proportional to fluid viscosity. Flat disk membranes with a diameter of 25 mm are commonly used. At a porosity of 5 μm, the membrane offers little resistance to the gravity flow of a mobile solution. Although a 0.45-μm membrane offers more resistance, it still permits reasonable flow rates for the gravity transfer of a liter of a mobile solution. Although more rapid flow rates would be expected by increasing the surface area or the porosity, the lumen diameter of an in-line delivery needle or Luer connector may be the rate-limiting factor for the system.

The application of pressure normally will provide a proportionate increase in the flow rate of a fluid through a membrane of a given porosity. In some instances, for example, with viscous solutions or when using 0.22-μm membranes with small diameters, a pressure greater than that provided by gravity flow may be required to establish and sustain an adequate flow rate. However, the application of pressure above the capacity of the system may cause system leakage. Furthermore, there should be concern for operator safety whenever pressure systems are employed. Regulated pressure at 6–8 psi normally is satisfactory. Higher pressures should be used with caution, extremely so with glass systems. Safety pressure vent valves should be used whenever there is the possibility that excessive pressure may cause injury or significant damage to personnel or equipment.

Sterile, ready-to-use disposable membrane filter units, IV filter sets, and various commercially available fluid transfer sets with inline membrane filter units are commonly used in hospital pharmacies. The filter units themselves normally can be expected to withstand pressures at least up to their bubble points (e.g., 55 psi for a 0.22-μm membrane). However, when a filter unit is an integral part of a commercially available set, the maximum allowable pressure is usually considerably lower (e.g., 10–25 psi, depending upon the set). The hospital pharmacist should compare the maximum allowable pressure for a set with the maximum pressure that would be applied to it, for example, when the set is to be used with an automatic pipeting device. This information is usually printed on the set's package or available in the product literature.

Some filter units may lack adequate filter support, making the membranes they contain vulnerable to breakage from forward or reverse pressure surges. Surges may occur with quick application or release of pressure on the system. Stronger membranes, such as those composed of a nylon-supported filter material or adequate support in the filter housing, should be used when higher pressure or surges are anticipated. Even excessive forceful syringe plunger depression may create excessive pressure.

Filter integrity should be checked when possible. A rapid, qualitative approach based on the bubble point principle can be included as a step in the compounding process. For example, after the required amount of fluid has been expelled, the filter unit is detached from the syringe. Air is drawn into the syringe, the filter unit is reattached, and the plunger is depressed until significant resistance is felt. The plunger is then released abruptly; it should spring back to its original position. Lack of resistance and rebounding would indicate a defective unit. The amount of resistance and the forcefulness of rebound decrease with increasing pore size until perceived resistance becomes too low to be reliable. The perceived resistance is a function of the bubble point rating of a membrane, that is, the amount of pressure required to force air through a wet membrane (e.g., 55 and 33 psi for 0.22 and 0.45 μm, respectively, for cellulose acetate membranes). The required pressure decreases as pore size increases. Quantitative bubble point testing is unrealistic in an IV admixture program because of the high pressures involved.

Air locking is the shutdown of a fluid line resulting from trapped air in the upstream side of the filter housing. Its occurrence can be explained by the bubble point principle. Trapped air usually can be avoided procedurally [18]. Air venting filters, such as the Millipore IVEX-2 (Millipore Corporation, Bedford, MA 01730) and the IMED Filterset (IMED Corporation, San Diego, CA 92131) (Fig. 5) may be used when air elimination through manipulative procedures is unreliable or inefficient.

IV admixtures normally are compounded using sterile components and aseptic technique under controlled environmental conditions, and it is expected that they would remain sterile. Thus, filters removing nonviable particles but not necessarily bacteria are normally adequate. However, a bacterially retentive membrane (0.22 μm) should be used to minimize the chances of bacteremia occurring in immunocompromised, debilitated, or other high-risk patients who may not be able to cope with the infusion of any bacteria.

The use of inline filters during infusion is not a substitute for filtration during compounding. The pharmacist is responsible for providing defect-free products to the user. Unnecessary reliance upon the user to carry out a step that can and should be done in the pharmacy is inappropriate. Because all infusions may not be administered through an inline filter (the

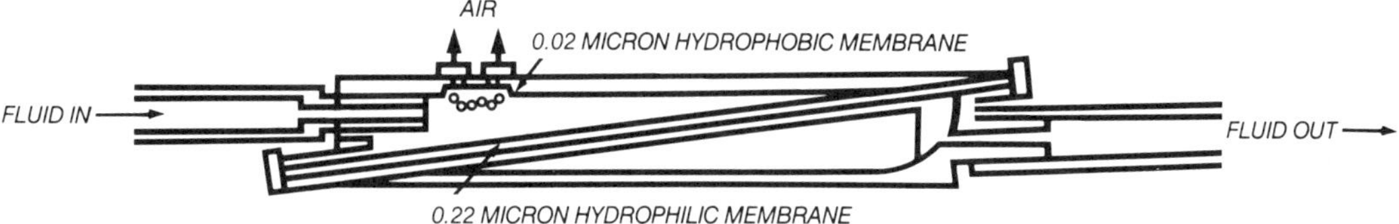

(a)

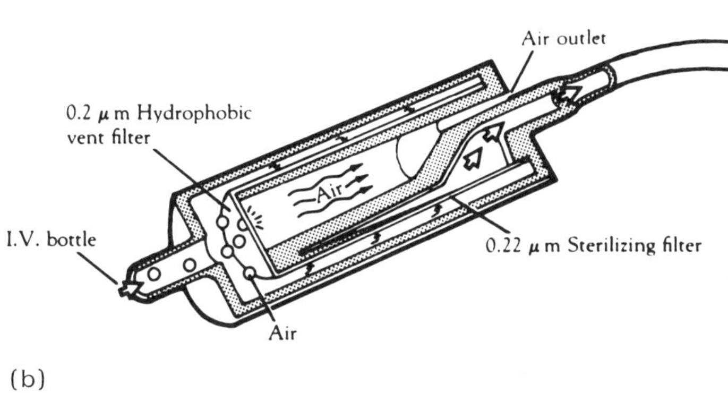

(b)

Figure 5 Air venting filters for the infusion of intravenous solutions. (a) The IMED Filterset. (Courtesy of The IMED Corporation.) (b) The Millipore IVEX-2 Filterset. (Courtesy of The Millipore Corporation.)

decision may be beyond the pharmacist's control), consistency in the quality of products actually administered may be questionable. Furthermore, IV admixtures not filtered in the pharmacy may lead to a high rate of clogged inline filters, and higher levels of contaminant challenge on a filter increase the probability of contaminant passage.

E. Packaging

Processing of container components is rarely encountered in the hospital pharmacy. IV admixtures are normally dispensed in the manufacturer's original container for the LVP solution to which the components were added, the original container of a powdered drug to which a diluent had been added, or commercially available sterile, pyrogen-free evacuated glass bottles or empty plastic containers to which the solution had been transferred. Hospital pharmacists also subdivide parenterals into ready-to-use unit-dose glass or plastic syringes. Because seal integrity may be compromised as a result of compounding activities, the hospital pharmacist must provide for adequate postcompounding protection of container contents. All products leaving the pharmacy must bear proper labeling.

1. Containers

Hospital pharmacists should assess the container-contents compatibility for every injectable product repackaged in the pharmacy. Concerns include the loss of drug due to sorption into plastic or adherence to glass walls of containers. Clinically significant decreases in drug concentration from binding to plastic containers have been reported for several drugs used in IV admixtures, including nitroglycerin, insulin, diazepam, carmustine, bleomycin, and vitamin A. Significant adherence of insulin to glass has also been reported. Sorption to IV sets may also occur. For example, considerable loss of nitroglycerin can be expected during infusion through a polyvinyl chloride infusion set. This loss can be greatly diminished by using polyethylene infusion tubing.

Loss of active ingredient to IV admixture containers and infusion administration sets should be ascertained for new drugs. Where loss is significant, temperature, surface area of contact, container materials, solution pH, drug concentration, contact time, and other parameters that may affect rate and extent of loss should be evaluated and the results published by the manufacturer. Manufacturer-provided product fact sheets containing data similar to that published by Mason et al. about diazepam binding [24] would be beneficial to the hospital pharmacist.

The hospital pharmacist is responsible for labeling unit-dose syringes repackaged in the pharmacy with an appropriate expiration date. A national survey disclosed that a wide variety of arbitrarily assigned expiration dates on injections are being used by hospital pharmacists [25]. Assigned expiration dates have been 24 hr, 1 week, one-quarter of the manufacturer's expiration, 6 months, the manufacturer's expiration, or other fixed interval general formulas [25]. When a single fixed arbitrary expiration dating interval is used in the absence of analytic data, it should be conservative enough to ensure the stability of the least stable repackaged drug product. Product-specific expiration dating based on data would be preferred. To illustrate the inappropriateness of fixed interval expiration dating, the average potency loss of gentamycin injection was experimentally determined to be 16% and 7% in 30 days after hospital pharmacy repackaging in plastic and glass syringes, respectively [26].

Stability loss upon unit-dose repackaging is likely to occur with light-sensitive drugs and agents prone to oxidation. Both problems are usually predictable from the manufacturer's original packaging or labeling. For example, the manufacturer's amber vials or ampuls inhibiting transmission of ultraviolet wavelengths may indicate a product's light sensitivity. An antioxidant in a labeled list of ingredients may be a cue that a product is prone to oxidation. Prolonged storage in clear or plastic syringes may result in hastened degradation of light- or oxygen-sensitive products. A box or an ultraviolet-absorbing plastic pouch may be used to enclose a clear container for reducing light transmission. (An IV admixture of sodium nitroprusside is so light sensitive that the container must stay protected from light until administration is complete.) Glass syringes prevent the permeation of oxygen encountered with plastic syringes. However, substituting glass for plastic may not fully protect oxygen-sensitive products, because rubber syringe plunger tips or syringe tip caps may be permeable to oxygen. Furthermore, the product may be exposed to oxygen during repackaging.

The pharmacy department should have written, detailed procedures for a precompounding integrity inspection of all LVP containers to be used in IV admixture compounding. For example, glass LVP bottles should be inspected for cracks, fractures, evidence of damage, and presence of vacuum. Areas prone to damage are the bottoms, the cap area, and the necks. The plastic overwraps of LVP plastic bags should be inspected for tears or other evidence of damage or breach of integrity. The overwrap provides a vapor barrier and thereby reduces water loss from the product. After the overwrap is removed, a systematic series of firm pressing of the bag should reveal any pinhole leaks. Glass and plastic containers should be scrutinized for evidence of leakage, such as dried residue or wetness. The written procedure also should provide guidance for the disposition of products in which defects have been noted. For example, intrinsic defects should be reported as requested by the USP-FDA drug products defects reporting program. The NCCLVP has recommended a detection-response protocol for isolating and dealing with both intrinsic (manufacturer source) and extrinsic (hospital-induced) contamination of parenterals [27].

2. *Sealing*

Intact stoppers on LVP containers are pierced by needles or IV spikes during the preparation of an IV admixture. The resiliency of elastomeric stoppers should provide adequate resealing upon withdrawal of the piercing device, unless too many punctures were made or the diameter of the piercing device was too large. Various commercially available overseal devices, such as additive caps and adhesive-backed foil, provide protection against post-compounding contamination. Overseals also provide tamper-evident sealing and a means to alert clinicians that additives are present. LVP containers to which IV sets have been attached in the pharmacy should be individually enveloped in protective plastic bags during transport and holding.

Filled unit-dose syringes are sealed at the syringe tips with a Luer-locked sheathed needle or a pressure-attached plastic or rubber syringe tip cap. Held on by friction, the latter are prone to detachment during handling. Pressure-slip attachment is dangerous because a detached tip can be readily reattached by untrained or unmotivated personnel instead of returning the defective unit to the pharmacy for replacement. This type of problem can be circumvented by using an adhesive-backed foil seal (commercially available) to retain the cap and by dispensing the unit in a plastic pouch, which also inhibits accidental premature depression of the plunger.

3. *Labeling*

The pharmacist is responsible that all pharmaceuticals in the hospital are labeled in accordance with all legal requirements, professional standards, and the hospital's established policies and procedures for internal standardized labeling. All sterile dosage forms leaving the pharmacy are destined either for floor stock or for specific patients in response to prescriber orders. Floor stock items represent mere transfers from the pharmacy's general inventory to a medication cabinet or closet elsewhere in the hospital. The amount of floor stock in a nursing unit, the emergency room, or the surgical suite is usually that normally required for anticipated clinical needs. Floor stock injectable products usually bear only the manufacturer's original label or, if manufactured or repackaged in the pharmacy, the pharmacy department's stock label. Minimum requirements for departmental stock labels are nonproprietary name of product, dosage form, strength per dose unit, concentration, total contents, special notes, such as refrigerate, expiration date, and control number [28].

Sterile products dispensed for specific patients require additional information. Every dosage unit in a unit-dose system should be labeled as to full product identification, name and location of patient, scheduled administration time for the dosage unit (and sometimes the dosage schedule), and any special instructions for administration or use. A scheduled administration time cannot be included on the label for multiple-dose vials.

For compounded IV admixtures, distinctive, self-adhesive labels are affixed to the LVP container, supplementing the manufacturer's label. Additional labeling information on IV admixtures include the names and amounts of all additives and the LVP solution, the date and time of compounding, compounder identification, and latest time of use. Clarifying information may also be necessary, for example, administration technique, rate and duration of infusion, clinically relevant expressions of concentration (e.g., mOsm/liter or mEq/liter), and the bottle sequence number of the preparation in an order expressed as a series of preparations [29]. Labeling should be clear, unambiguous, precise, and complete and usually should eliminate the need for calculations to be performed by the clinician. The admixture label should provide adequate space for recording the administration starting time and for any additives made during administration.

Considerable opportunity exists for label mix-up in a hospital pharmacy. The average hospital pharmacy prepares and affixes hundreds of unique labels daily. For batch-repackaged items, professional guidelines depict procedural controls, such as isolation of packaging runs and labels, complete removal of all items at the end of a run, including labels, terminal inspection of labeling machines to assure that all labels are removed and that label plates are blanked or removed, and terminal label quantity reconciliation [30]. For extemporaneously compounded items, the label is kept with the order and the other compounding supplies until affixed, then labeling accuracy should be checked during the postcompounding inspection (see the Appendix) prior to issuing the medication. Each label on batch-repackaged items should be spot-checked. Computer-printed labels have become very popular in hospital pharmacies, resulting in more accuracy and simplicity in label production. Computerization still requires personal care and accuracy in label setup and diligent checking of labeling accuracy.

V. CLINICAL SUPPLY AND USE OF STERILE PRODUCTS

The pharmacy department is accountable for the quality of all drug products throughout the institution, regardless of location. Improper handling or the use of incorrect techniques during transport, storage, and administration can adversely affect product integrity, which must be maintained until the completion of administration. Personnel in other departments are often responsible for carrying out many of the specific activities once the product leaves the pharmacy department. To maintain adequate pharmaceutical control, written policies and procedures for product control outside the pharmacy should be prepared and enforced by the pharmacy department, upon consultation with the nursing service and, if appropriate, courier services. (Ideally, couriers responsible for pharmaceuticals should be employees of the pharmacy department, but this is not always the case.) Administratively sanctioned assignment of duties to nonpharmacy personnel, good interdepartmental relations, pharmacy-conducted inservice training programs, and procedural check systems help in maintaining adequate pharmaceutical control.

A. Transport

The pharmacy department should assure that the package integrity of IV admixtures and prefilled syringes is maintained during transport. Rough or improper handling may dislodge syringe plungers or cause disconnection of assembled administration systems. The proper use of dust covers over containers where required should also be assured. The training program for delivery personnel should instill the motivation and the knowledge that the pharmacist must be notified if any untoward events happen to pharmaceutical products during transport.

B. Storage in Patient Care Areas

Floor stock parenterals are normally stored in accordance with labeled storage requirements in a designated area on the nursing unit, to be withdrawn as needed. They may be retained on the unit until the labeled expiration date. The pharmacy department is responsible for conducting periodic (e.g., monthly) floor stock checks to ascertain that proper storage conditions exist, that all parenterals are being stored properly, and that no expired, deteriorated, or contaminated products are present. Multidose SVP vials are commonly retained on the nursing unit after doses have been withdrawn, and their on-the-floor contamination is well documented. Although refrigeration of in-use vials is common practice in hospitals, the length of time that a used vial may be retained on the nursing unit has been debated. A fixed interval beyond-use time, e.g., 30 days from the first puncture, is in force in many hospitals. However, the variability of conditions to which vials may be subjected, the many variables affecting stability and product integrity, and the unique properties of each injectable result in considerable unpredictability in judging the quality of an in-use vial on a nursing unit.

All IV admixtures and extemporaneously compounded or repackaged sterile products should be issued to specific patients. Even with a unit-dose system, some injectables may be retained on a nursing unit for as long as 24 hr until administration is initiated, depending upon the interval between scheduled deliveries. A 24-hr period is the maximum interval in a unit-dose system, and the interval may be longer in a non-unit-dose system. Adequate procedures should exist to ensure that each product is kept under its proper storage conditions until initiation of administration. Some drugs degrading rapidly after reconstitution may require refrigeration on the unit, holding in a cold pack on a unit-dose cart, or a special delivery just prior to the scheduled administration time.

IV admixtures should be administered as soon as possible after preparation or thawing, preferably within 1 hr. Alternatively, solutions may be refrigerated at 4°C for no more than 24 hr. Injectable products should be at room temperature upon administration.

C. Administration

In addition to product integrity, the pharmacist should be assured that dosing accuracy is not compromised by poor administration technique or by the improper selection and use of sets, catheters, or other administration devices. Although the pharmacist is not usually directly involved in administering parenteral products, he or she could exert influence on product administration as an active participant in the hospital's IV therapy team or its equivalent and can be an advocate for the establishment of an IV therapy team in hospitals without one.

1. *Maintaining Product Integrity*

Causes of compromised integrity include microbial and particulate ingress during administration (discussed in Chap. 2, Vol. 1). A role of the pharmacist is to assure that individual patient monitoring and patient population surveillance for untoward effects from compromised integrity occur routinely and systematically (see Sec. VI.C).

2. *Dosing Accuracy*

Factors associated with containers, administration sets, and the physiology or pathology of the patient may affect the final concentration of a drug in a LVP infusion solution, the rate of administration, or the volume infused.

LVP Containers

The fill volume variance among LVP containers may result in deviation between the actual and expected concentrations in an IV admixture. Furthermore, the calibration marks on the sides of LVP containers represent approximations only. Thus, dosing inaccuracy may occur when a portion of a container's contents is infused for the delivery of a specified dose. Incorporating a total dose in a "mini" LVP container (e.g., 50 ml) minimizes the problem because the entire volume would be infused. A volumetric control device (an IV burette set having an inline metering chamber) may be used to achieve volumetric accuracy for infusions because known accurate drug concentrations and infusion volumes can be achieved.

Administration Sets

The volume of infused fluid may vary from the expected or intended because of the volume required to prime the IV line, the residual volume in a line upon the completion of an infusion, inline filter blockage, and flow rate. The accuracy of the drop orifice calibration, flow control clamp failure, plastic cold flow, and backflow check valve failures influence flow rate accuracy. The drop orifice calibration as specified by the IV set manufacturer (e.g., 10, 15, 20, or 60 drops/ml) is well recognized as an approximation only. A stated calibration is subject to variation from several influences, including solution viscosity (influenced in turn by temperature), surface tension, flow rate, and shunting in the drip chamber.

The flow control clamp regulates the gravity flow of fluid through an IV set by progressive constriction of the IV tubing. However, lumen constriction leads to the cold flow problem encountered with plastic tubing, which is a progressive thickening of the lumen wall to relieve the stress imposed by the clamp. The result is erratic flow rates, usually encountered during the first 15–45 min after establishing a particular flow rate. Flow rate monitoring is therefore important.

Working by gravity and exerting no pressure, electronic infusion controllers electronically count drops to automatically regulate drop rate and increase delivery accuracy over manual devices. Further accuracy may be obtained with the peristaltic or piston-cylinder infusion pumps, which propel or expel fluid under pressure through an IV line. Because of their cost, some hospitals establish protocols for the allocation of pumps on a priority basis. Infusion pump programs, including supply, distribution, maintenance, and the preparation of utilization protocols, have been under the auspices of some pharmacy departments [31].

Needles and Catheters

Back-pressure is inversely proportional to lumen size. Thus, gravity flow rates must be reset after changing any needle or catheter. The "thin-wall" needle has a larger lumen than a regular needle of the same gauge.

3. *Patient Response to Therapy*

A clinical responsibility of the pharmacist is to assess patient response to parenteral therapy. With infusion therapy, monitoring should include state of hydration, electrolyte status, clinical response to therapeutic agents, signs of infusion-associated untoward effects, flow rate, and patency of the infusion system. These activities should be coordinated with the duties and responsibilities of other members of the IV therapy team and the nursing department.

VI. QUALITY ASSURANCE

A. Guiding Principles

Quality assurance for sterile products should encompass the products and their preparation [32], parenteral therapy, and the services involved [5], such as the IV admixture program, an infusion pump program, or a TPN program. The several functions in the parenteral medication cycle can serve as reference points for product-focused quality assurance. The implementation of a quality assurance program should consist of a planned, coordinated, interdisciplinary effort by those departments or groups with decision-making, functional, or evaluative responsibilities involving parenteral products, parenteral therapy, or parenteral services. This would include in most hospitals the pharmacy department, the nursing service, the medical staff, the microbiology laboratory, and the hospital's infections committee. The IV therapy team should also be included in those institutions where it is an organized entity.

The general principles guiding a quality assurance program should include (a) a product must be prepared or a service must be rendered according to plan; (b) standards of quality or descriptions of acceptable performance have been fully specified for the product or service; (c) workable, validated processes are specified unambiguously and used accurately to prepare products or perform services; (d) appropriate surveillance or inspections are conducted according to plan to verify that validated processes are used as specified and that products and services are consistent with specified standards of quality or performance; and (e) documentation exists to show that processes were under control when carried out. In addition, relevant inputs should be verified for operational effectiveness and consistency, for example, the environmental quality of the compounding area and the knowledge, skills, and motivation of the people responsible for performing critical manipulations.

B. Policies and Procedures Manual

The backbone of an effective quality assurance program is the existence of written, current, precise, and specific policies and procedures that have been systematically prepared, compiled into a manual, and used as a basis for practice and training. The American Society of Hospital Pharmacists and the Joint Commission on Accreditation of Hospitals have been advocating for many years that all procedures (including those pertaining to parenteral products and their use) be in writing and in detail.

C. Corrective Action

A quality assurance program must include the capability for initiating planned corrective action in the event that performance deviations or substandard products are detected. At least two levels of action are imperative: (a) detection and correction of the cause of the problem, and (b) seeking and rectifying any adverse patient response resulting from the problem. Detection of product defects may occur through the quality control performed on products in the pharmacy department. However, the first indication of a product defect may be an adverse reaction in a patient. Thus, planned, routine patient monitoring may enhance the capability for detecting product defects. For example, septicemia or phlebitis may be an indication of a contaminated product. Fluid overload, disconnections, kinked tubing, or flow rate device malfunctions are examples of other problems that may be detected during routine monitoring.

Every product defect should be investigated to determine the source of the problem because of the potential magnitude of the population that could be affected. For example, one isolated oversight in procedure would result in a self-limiting problem, but systematic, repetitive procedural breaches may place the hospital's patient population at risk. Intrinsic defects, for example, microbial contamination caused at the manufacturer level, would place patients nationwide at risk. The National Coordinating Committee on Large Volume Parenterals offers guidelines for detecting sources of contamination, for diagnostic and microbiologic methods in cases of suspected septicemia, for treatment, for reporting suspected or confirmed septicemia or contaminated products to the FDA-USP sponsored Drug Product Problem Reporting Program, and for follow-up [27,33]. Any patients having received defective products should be placed under proper medical supervision for subsequent observation and, if needed, appropriate treatment. In recent years, follow-up responsibilities have been advocated as part of the duties and responsibilities of an interdisciplinary IV therapy team of physicians, nurses, and pharmacists.

Procedural changes in compounding or administration of IV infusions may affect the incidence of contaminant-related clinical problems, such as bacteremia and phlebitis. Focused, planned surveillance for a period of time both before and after a change may demonstrate a beneficial or detrimental effect of the change. Ongoing surveillance of selected adverse effects, such as the incidence of infusion-associated nosocomial infection, may provide an early warning that undesirable trends or acute problems may be occurring. The pharmacist should be especially alert to a rise in the rate of any potential contaminant-related problem.

D. Monitoring Product Quality

Several quality control activities or quality audits should be performed routinely to help assure that only defect-free products are issued by the pharmacy department and administered to the patient.

1. *Compounding from Raw Ingredients*

CGMP pertaining to quality control should be followed inasmuch as possible where parenterals are compounded from raw ingredients. The concept of the double-check system for weighed or measured ingredients and final and fill volumes is well accepted in hospital pharmacy. Some hospital pharmacists report the routine use of *Limulus* testing, semiquantitative tests, or identity checks of contents with such instruments as a pH meter, an ion analyzer, or an osmometer. Some hospital pharmacists send samples from every or selected batches to outside organizations for the *Limulus* test, chemical analysis, or other tests.

2. *Physical Inventory Audit*

All pharmaceuticals must be kept under proper conditions of temperature, humidity, light, cleanliness, ventilation, segregation, and security. Pharmaceuticals must not be used beyond their expiration dates. Parenteral products often are kept in locations not under the immediate control or constant scrutiny of the pharmacist. The pharmacy department is then responsible for establishing and maintaining proper security, environmental conditions, and segregation from other dosage forms (especially externals) through the physical design of storage or holding areas, written policies and procedures, and routine periodic inspection. Deteriorated, contaminated, or otherwise defective products detected during inspection should be removed immediately. Inspection reports, including descriptions of findings, any corrective action taken, and any recommendations for improvement, should be maintained. Copies of the reports should be given to and discussed with those persons responsible for the areas where the infractions occurred. A pattern of infractions should result in the pharmacist initiating an inservice training program or seeking administrative sanctions. The hospital's pharmacy and therapeutics committee is expected to provide the administrative support needed by the pharmacy department to rectify such problems.

3. *Visible Defects Inspection*

Parenteral products should be inspected by the hospital pharmacist when goods are received from shipment, just prior to using them for compounding, immediately after compounding, and just prior to delivery. Furthermore, the pharmacist should be assured that nurses inspect products properly just prior to administering them. Written protocols should be prepared for each type of inspection and should include key checks, such as container cracks, chips, or pinholes; cloudiness, discoloration, precipitate, or foreign matter in the contents; intactness of component parts, such as the hanger wire on a glass bottle or the rubber injection port on a plastic container; evidence of leakage, such as wetness or dried solute on the container's exterior surfaces; presence of filth; and, where applicable, consistency of the information on the immediate label with other identification marks, such as on the seal or outer carton. Complete, thorough inspection of each container should be performed for each type of inspection except when receiving goods, in which case representative units may be spot checked. If a potential intrinsic defect is noted, the inventory on hand of the same lot number should also be checked. Nurses should be instructed to notify the pharmacy of any potential defects in products.

4. *Clarity Inspection*

Every parenteral product compounded in the pharmacy department should be inspected for clarity by visually observing the contents before well-lit white and black backgrounds. Units containing visible foreign matter should not be issued. The counting and sizing of particulates in LVPs is not common practice in the hospital pharmacy.

5. *Checking Compounding Accuracy*

Prior to release, every compounded parenteral product should be double-checked for accuracy, preferably by another pharmacist. Checkpoints for extemporaneously compounded IV admixtures include labeling accuracy, the additives used, and their volumes. Containers from which the additives have been drawn should be quarantined together with the finished product until the final compounding check. The volume of an addition usually must be surmised from observing the volume remaining in the additive container. The reliability of the volume check can be improved by having the operator also quarantine the syringe with its plunger drawn back to the volume mark actually used. Some hospital pharmacies may do a rapid instrumental check, such as pH or osmoticity on selected admixtures, but this is not common. Any instrumental analysis would probably be on a sampling basis for the retrospective evaluation of compounding accuracy in general rather than for making a release/do not release decision for a specific product.

6. *Pyrogen Testing*

Microbial contamination during compounding may lead to pyrogen formation if unrefrigerated delays between compounding and administration occur. Thus, the pharmacist should be alert to any pyrogenic responses in patients. Potential pyrogen reactions from compounded IV admixtures should prompt the pharmacist to confirm the pyrogenicity of the offending product and to screen appropriate unused products for pyrogenicity. The pharmacist should know where to secure such service or should be able to perform the *Limulus* test. However, caution is advised in interpreting negative results from the *Limulus* test. The test will detect endotoxins only from gram-negative organisms, but most contaminating organisms in IV admixtures will be gram positive [34].

E. Evaluating Processing Effectiveness

Methods for evaluating processing effectiveness in IV admixture compounding include self-reporting checklists, procedural audits, direct observation of critical processing steps, process simulation, and final product testing or inspection. A checklist provides a qualitative indication of regularity of procedural compliance. Examples of the other methods include, respectively, the analysis of completed compounding worksheets or other documentation to determine if procedures of interest had been carried out; the direct observation by a supervisor to determine if a technique is being used properly by an operator; the carrying out of a media fill process using culture medium instead of product to determine if a set of procedures is effective; sterility testing for microbial contamination; microscopic particulate analysis; and 100% inspection for visible particulate matter. A sampling scheme is usually involved when undertaking any of these approaches, except the last one.

For example, with units prepared as a batch process, the population of interest would be the batch, lot, or sublot in which each discreet unit is assumed to be homogeneous with all other units; that is, all units are expected to have been subjected to the same activities and conditions. Extemporaneously compounded IV admixtures represent a stream of unique units, each having been prepared individually in accordance with an order for a particular patient. However, homogeneous groupings (populations) may be declared for all admixtures prepared in accordance with the same set of policies and procedures. Circumscribing units within a frame of reference, such as a 24-hr time span, is usually needed for meaningful data analysis. Trends may be visualized by plotting contamination rates (Y axis) over time (X axis). Cumulative sum control charts [32] have been advanced as an approach to process monitoring in an IV admixture program.

The simple random sampling scheme is normally the method of choice for selecting units for testing. However, when contamination rates are low, for example, less than 1%, the probability of detecting contamination would be low unless large numbers of units are sampled. On this basis, current recommendations from the Center for Infectious Diseases do not include routine culturing of LVP fluids, because good surveillance for problems may be more cost effective than routine monitoring [35]. The method prescribed by the USP provides the accepted basis for the sterility testing of LVPs in hospital pharmacy, although some adaptations have been described in the literature. Reliability in detecting the low level of contamination usually associated with IV admixtures has been shown to vary among different testing methods proposed for hospital pharmacy use [36]. Furthermore, evidence exists that the time interval between compounding and sterility test sampling influences organism recovery [37]. Thus, successful sterility testing in the hospital pharmacy depends upon careful planning with due consideration of several variables in the sampling and in the testing.

The act of data collection may influence operators to perform differently from normal. Even subtle differences may cause misleading results. A method for minimizing sampling influence for extemporaneously compounded IV admixtures is (a) randomly preselect serial numbers of those admixtures to make up the sample; (b) the operator must not know the sampling scheme; (c) draw the sample after compounding; and (d) place the order for the withdrawn unit back among those in line for compounding.

Routine process monitoring may provide an incentive for employee adherence to establish procedures. The results from at least one study indicate that employee awareness of proper aseptic procedures plus procedural audits helped to sustain the improved performance achieved from instituting proper procedures [34].

The expense of routine, continuous process monitoring does not always seem justifiable to hospital pharmacists. A cyclical approach seems to have better acceptance, where an initial audit would be conducted and any noncompliance would be corrected. Periodic short-term follow-up audits of selected procedures or significant determinants of defects would ensue. Each cycle should establish incremental progress toward goals.

F. Evaluating the Compounding Environment

1. *Routine Environmental Monitoring*

Hospital pharmacists should be able to demonstrate that the contamination level in the controlled area (a) is continuously maintained at a low level and

(b) is significantly less than in noncontrolled areas, such as nursing units or the main pharmacy. Hospital pharmacists rely virtually exclusively on the assessment of viable contamination, although the evaluation of particulate loads also should be considered. Accreditation standards require only microbiological monitoring [5]. A basic microbiological monitoring approach should involve at least the planned routine exposure of settling plates for ambient airborne contamination and contact plates (e.g., Rodac plates) for surface contamination.

The steps in establishing a monitoring program include (a) determining the baseline acceptable level of contamination for areas of interest, (b) specifying routine and periodic monitoring procedures, and (c) designing a meaningful data-recording system. Considerable judgment is involved in specifying baseline acceptable contamination levels. There are no published rules. However, since the baseline is for internal comparison, then it should be established within the institution. First, the facility should be designed and operated as well as possible in terms of structure, procedures, personnel codes, and cleaning and disinfection methods. Then, a comprehensive short-term study should be conducted. This would involve a series of tests for airborne and surface contamination of ambient conditions during a rest period and during normal activity levels at representative sites. The sampling plan for the study should include but not be limited to the sampling plan to be specified for routine monitoring, because results from routine monitoring will be compared against the initial results from the baseline study. However, the broader sampling for the study provides a better opportunity to select representative sites for the comparisons to follow. The sampling plan should include specifications of location, frequency, time, and method of sampling. When the method involves settling plates, duration of exposure also must be specified.

Settling plates would be exposed, for example, daily for 20 or 30 min at several buffer area locations, including, but not limited to, the top of the LAFW immediately over the work surface edge, on the outer edge of the work surface, near the entrance to the buffer area, in a corner, and in a relatively highly trafficked area. Once established, the sampling plan must be adhered to for comparability of subsequent data. Data (colony counts per plate) may be recorded on a matrix depicting locations (rows) versus dates (columns) for ready visualization of gradual or abrupt changes across time or variance across locations. Currently collected data may be compared with averaged initial baseline data collected under normal conditions, or significant differences in average colony counts between various locations may be computed for any point or period of time. Aberrant colony counts generally indicate poor environmental control. With surface contact plates, increases in numbers of colonies may signal a need for a different surface disinfectant, more frequent cleaning, or a more effective cleaning procedure. Contact plating is also useful for validating surface cleaning procedures or agents.

Volumetric air sampling or exposure of supplemental settling plates may be used periodically for comparisons between controlled and noncontrolled areas. A volumetric air sampler, for example, a slit sampler, is a particularly useful investigative tool in the planned, intensive follow-up of potential problem areas suspected from the data derived from settling plate exposure. Date derived from volumetric air sampling are more quantifiable, because colony counts can be related to the volume of air sampled per time period. However, the procedures for volumetric sampling are more involved and more time consuming. A hospital pharmacist without the funds to purchase a volumetric sampler may be able to borrow one as needed from the department or person responsible for general environmental microbial monitoring in the hospital.

Hospital pharmacists should consider sampling for airborne particulate matter. Microscopic examination of particulates accumulated on a membrane filter from vacuum air sampling is an approach within the capabilities of many hospital pharmacies.

2. *The Laminar-Flow Workbench*

Each new LAFW should be tested before use and again after a shakedown period, for example, after 30 days of continuous operation. Retesting should occur after relocation of a unit, after installation of a new HEPA filter, and at specified intervals (at least every 12 months, according to the Joint Commission on Accreditation of Hospitals, but some hospitals report more frequent intervals, such as every 6 months). Testing should include (a) a challenge of filter integrity using cold aerosolized dioctylphthalate (DOP) and (b) airflow velocity checks at various locations across the filter face using a velometer or hot-wire anemometer.

In addition, airflow patterns may be checked with a "smoke stick." As a part of the regular testing program, smoke stick checks may help detect, for example, breaches in the work area enclosure and drawing ability of power exhausts, if so equipped. Smoke sticks may be used as an adjunct to training programs, because they help operators visualize dead and turbulent zones to avoid during critical work. For the same reason, any new or significantly modified configurations of work or object placement should be smoke stick checked by operators.

Hospital pharmacists usually have inspections conducted as a contract service. There are no certification or licensure requirements for contract inspectors, so the pharmacist should itemize clearly those inspection services required. Furthermore, the pharmacist should be knowledgeable enough of inspection methods to assess inspector performance. The pharmacist should ascertain the appropriateness of the testing instrumentation used by the inspector and if those instruments are subjected to regular calibration tests by the inspector's firm. Prefilters should be checked frequently by the pharmacist between regular inspections. Prefilters should be replaced as necessary. The cleaner the buffer room, the less frequent will be the need to change prefilters. Clean prefilters, which are inexpensive, protect the expensive HEPA filters from premature fouling.

The pharmacy department (not the contract inspector) is responsible for writing policies and procedures specifying the testing schedule, tests to be performed, and record-keeping requirements. Record keeping should include a chronological log of tests and services performed, a data-recording sheet for each unit, and a test sticker on each unit. The log should include the date, the unit tested or serviced, and who did the work. The data sheet should provide a record of all readings, such as airflow velocity at each filter surface point, photometer measurements, and a detailed description of the test or service, including diagrammed locations and areas ($in.^2$; cm^2) of any applied sealants. A contract inspector would record the data as specified by the pharmacist on a form provided by the inspector or the pharmacist. The completed forms should remain on file in the pharmacy. A summary sticker indicating the date of the test and the next retest date should be affixed to each unit.

G. Assessing Personnel Performance

The NCCLVP recommended guidelines for quality assurance state the need for establishing policies and procedures to ensure the proper selection, education, and training of personnel [32]. IV admixture processes are highly personnel intense, so a major priority of a comprehensive quality assurance program should be the assurance that people are adhering consistently to performance standards and that any performance problems are corrected.

The personnel concern is bidimensional: (a) people shed contamination into the atmosphere of an environment where contamination is not wanted, and (b) people are responsible for carrying out a variety of processes designed to prevent the contamination of the finished product. Personnel-focused objectives, such as the following, should establish the basis for personnel-focused quality assurance efforts:

> My clean room operators, their specific activities, and their overall performance (a) will not contribute to any increase in the contaminant load of the production environment, (b) will not cause any contaminant-related product defects, and (c) will conform to all procedures or protocols specified for contamination control.

Quality assurance activities relevant to achievement of these objectives relate to tasks and to people. For example, compounding and environmental control tasks and their requirements must be studied and their policies and procedures written as discussed previously. This establishes the basis for writing job performance requirements and expectations. These, in turn, provide the basis for writing personnel selection criteria, applicant screening techniques, entry level orientation and training programs, personnel assessment prior to a task assignment, ongoing performance appraisal, and a planned strategy for analyzing and remedying performance deviations. These functions should themselves be a planned, cohesive, coordinated strategy. The pertinent policies and procedures should be included in the hospital pharmacy's policy and procedures manual. Some thoughts about these functions are offered.

1. *Selection Criteria*

Criteria should be designed to discriminate between individuals with high and low potential for contributing significantly to the contaminant load in the environment. Types of criteria include skills and knowledge, physiological factors, and psychological factors. A determination should be made prior to screening candidates as to which specific criteria are true minimum entry level requirements for beginning work or entering a training program and which criteria should be included in a planned, organized training or development program. For the latter, aptitude assessment for success in the training program and future job assignments would be important.

2. *Personnel Assessment Prior to Task Assignment*

Individuals responsible for aseptic compounding, environmental control, and related activities should formally demonstrate their ability to carry out those tasks specified by the written policies and procedures before they use those procedures to prepare products for human use. The assessment technique should be appropriate to the task. For example, the ability to prevent product contamination may be assessed by a media fill technique [38], proper gowning and scrubbing technique by direct observation, predicting incompatibilities or stability problems by a paper-and-pencil test, or attitudes by having the candidate rank or sort a list of attitude-indicating behaviors in reference to would/would not do.

3. *Performance Appraisal*

The quality assurance program should include a planned, organized, ongoing effort to obtain information needed to assess the continuing consistency between actual and expected performance. The effort should also provide a means to convey specific, accurate, objective, and timely feedback to individuals about their performance. The feedback should include indications of acceptable performance as well as deviations.

Implementing a remedy for a performance deviation should be after thoughtful analysis into the possible reasons for the performance problem. Not all performance problems are the result of true knowledge or skill deficiencies, low motivation, or poor attitude. For example, a skills deficiency observed after previously demonstrating ability could be the result of too infrequent use of the skill or from not receiving adequate feedback to sustain the correct performance. Performance deviations without skills deficiencies could be associated with obstacles to, lack of rewards for, or even punishment from expected performance. Occasionally assuring operators that their performance really does matter may sometimes be the only remedy needed to correct performance problems. The Mager-Pipe model [39] is suggested as a way to select cause-associated remedies for performance problems in a manner consistent with the broad perspective of a quality assurance program.

VII. CONCLUSION

Parenteral admixture services are well established within the practice of hospital pharmacy. The predominant issue about the implementation of a new program has moved well beyond the "shall we" phase into the "how to" phase. For those majority of hospitals that have at least some admixture services, the issue would be primarily "how to improve," especially in regard to cost effectiveness, efficiency, quality assurance, and the pharmacist's clinical involvement in parenteral therapy. However, basic technical quality of compounding is questionable in some hospitals. Upgrading in this regard is achieved primarily through education and motivation, because compliance with state-of-the-art standards is voluntary for the most part.

Hospital pharmacists are likely to continue purchasing commercially available products whenever possible rather than compound. When compounding, sterile, ready-to-use products and devices are likely to be used wherever possible. Based on current trends, there is very little reason to expect expanded involvement in the scope of parenteral compounding in the majority of hospital pharmacies beyond IV admixtures and unit-dose repackaging.

The relatively recent introduction of commercially available premixed medications in LVP fluids has provided, according to some hospital pharmacists, decided advantages over the extemporaneous compounding of IV admixtures of the same medications. Documentation has already appeared in the hospital pharmacy literature on the usefulness, cost effectiveness, flexibility, and contribution toward waste reduction provided by premixed admixtures. Hospital pharmacists are likely to welcome the commercially available alternatives to in-house compounding because of imminent budgetary constraints for personnel.

Quality control testing requirements, especially chemical analysis, inhibit many hospital pharmacists from even considering sterile manufacturing. The reasons are complex, including poor undergraduate training in the area of pharmaceutical testing and analysis, lack of self-confidence, and budgetary restrictions on the purchase of expensive analytical instrumentation. The recent clinical direction in pharmacy education and current problems in regard to the financing of health care are not likely to foster more hospital pharmacy involvement in testing and analysis, regardless of need. Rather, the clinical perspective now in pharmacy education is likely to foster enhanced pharmacy involvement in therapeutic decision-making and following patient progress in regard to parenteral therapy. However, these trends in pharmacy education do not alter the fact that the pharmacist is, and undoubtedly will be expected to continue being, that person in the hospital most qualified to evaluate the physical and chemical properties of sterile dosage forms.

Many hospital pharmacists see their clinical role as more exciting and challenging and as a more direct application of their training than their traditional distributive roles. Furthermore, many hospital pharmacists not only dislike the monotonous repetitive nature of IV admixture compounding, but have found compounding by technicians to be more cost effective and sometimes even more accurate. Thus, hospital pharmacists will probably be spending relatively less time in bench work and relatively more time in operational planning and analysis and in quality assurance, especially in regard to the performance of IV admixture technicians, as hospital pharmacists fulfill their responsibilities in assuring that all patients receive only quality drugs.

The Study Commission on Pharmacy has recommended that pharmacists stress the application of their knowledge about drugs as they define and refine professional roles in addition to the effective and efficient development and distribution of drug products [40]. Avenues open to the hospital pharmacist in regard to sterile products are (a) the application of the pharmacist's knowledge about the advantages and limitations of the several dosage forms to therapeutic decision-making, (b) the formulation of a product not commercially available for the special needs of a particular patient, (c) the design and provision of educational programs to health professionals, paraprofessionals, and patients, and (d) purchasing of sterile products.

Much can be learned by the hospital pharmacist from the industry for the fulfillment of the several roles and responsibilities noted above. Hospital pharmacists should keep abreast of advances in sterile pharmaceutical processing through the current industrial pharmacy literature and by attending professional meetings, such as those of the Parenteral Drug Association. Hospital pharmacy organizations should plan continuing education programs around topics to be presented by invited industrial pharmacists. Further, hospital pharmacists can learn much from plant tours. After the initial needs of the hospital pharmacy have been addressed, continued liaison between hospital pharmacy and the pharmaceutical industry may lead to mutual efforts toward common problem resolution in matters pertaining to quality parenteral products and therapy for better patient care.

VIII. APPENDIX: ABBREVIATED SEQUENCE FOR PREPARING A SERIES OF EXTEMPORANEOUSLY COMPOUNDED IV ADMIXTURES

1. *Assembly*

All components needed for an admixture are selected, cleaned, and placed in a cleaned tray. Paperwork (e.g., worksheet, profile card, and label) is kept with, but not inside, the tray. The prescribed precompounding inspection of the large volume parenteral (LVP) container should be carried out prior to traying.

Comment

Use of the tray is a control procedure to minimize chance of mix-ups from occurring before, during, and after preparation through the effective segregation of components for different orders. Trays also facilitate the final quality control inspection. Items in a tray would consist usually of the LVP containers, the small volume parenteral (SVP) containers of additives, and the transfer devices, such as syringes, needles, and membrane filter units.

2. *Staging*

Line up a convenient number of assembled trays next to the laminar-airflow workbench (LAFW).

Comment

There should be a staging counter next to the LAFW within easy reach of the operator working at the unit. The size of the counter should be of adequate size and dimensions to accommodate a reasonable number of trays in an orderly and uncluttered manner.

3. *Compounding*

All paper work for the next order is clipped to the outside of the LAFW, easily visible to the operator. Supply items are removed from the tray, sanitized, and introduced into the LAFW. The tray is moved to the inspection counter on the other side of the LAFW. The admixture is compounded using aseptic technique.

Comment

Only one order should be compounded at a time. The LAFW should be cleaned of the previous order before this step is begun. The work surface should be resanitized as needed. Sanitization refers to an appropriate, validated procedure involving, for example, thorough wiping using a clean, nonlinting pad saturated with 70% alcohol. There should be an inspection counter next to the LAFW work space, at the opposite end from the staging counter.

4. *Finishing*

The completed admixture, the SVP containers, selected devices, and the paperwork are placed in the empty tray on the inspection counter. The next order may then be compounded.

Comment

All items needed to help verify the additives and the quantities added should be retained for the postcompounding checker to see. For example, empty or partially filled SVP containers and used devices can be partial evidence of quantities used in that any remaining contents would be consistent or not consistent with the order.

5. Postcompounding Inspection

The completed admixture is checked against the order and the worksheet. Particular attention is given to visual inspection of container integrity, contents appearance, label accuracy and completeness, calculations, final fluid level of the finished product, and residual contents of SVP containers. Finally, the label is affixed.

Comment

A pharmacist other than the compounder should perform the inspection. If this is not possible, the operator should compound a series of admixtures then inspect them, which should provide some degree of dissociation between the compounding and checking steps. Remaining at the LAFW to do several orders in sequence reduces in-and-out activity, providing for better environmental control. When workload warrants it, two pharmacists can alternate between assembly/staging inspection and compounding. Thus, one person carries out a supportive role to the other operator, who is at the LAFW.

6. Consignment

The finished, inspected product is placed in the designated holding area. Expended materials are discarded in appropriate receptacles. Paperwork is properly filed.

Comment

There should be standard operating procedures designating holding areas for use in conjunction with various categories of orders, for example, delivery carts addressed to specific nursing units (set up for the next regularly scheduled delivery), a "stat-hold" area for early pickup by a nurse or courier, or a refrigerator for later delivery schedules.

REFERENCES

1. C. H. Deiner, Editor, Lilly Hospital Pharmacy Survey 1983, Eli Lilly and Company, Indianapolis, 1983, pp. 15, 24.
2. V. S. Crane, *Hosp. Pharm.*, 19:625–628 (1984).
3. National Coordinating Committee on Large Volume Parenterals, *Am. J. Hosp. Pharm.*, 37:660–663 (1980).
4. National Coordinating Committee on Large Volume Parenterals, *Am. J. Hosp. Pharm.*, 32:261–270 (1975).
5. Joint Commission on Accreditation of Hospitals, Accreditation Manual for Hospitals, Pharmaceutical Services, Chicago, 1984, pp. 101–102, 133–142.
6. American Society of Hospital Pharmacists, *Am. J. Hosp. Pharm.*, 31: 1198–1207 (1974).

7. T. C. Eickhoff, *N. Engl. J. Med.*, 306:1545–1546 (1982).
8. L. A. Trissel, *Handbook on Injectable Drugs*, 3rd Ed. American Society of Hospital Pharmacists, Bethesda, MD, 1983.
9. J. C. King, *Guide to Parenteral Admixtures*. Cutter Laboratories Publishers, St. Louis, looseleaf current service.
10. American Society of Hospital Pharmacists, *Am. J. Hosp. Pharm.*, 37:1097–1103 (1980).
11. J. A. Syverson, *Bull. Parent. Drug Assoc.*, 26:239–246 (1972).
12. S. J. Turco, *Am. J. Intravenous Ther. Clin. Nutr.*, 9(9):9–10 (1982).
13. C. J. Holmes, R. K. Ausman, R. B. Kundsin, and C. W. Walter, *Am. J. Hosp. Pharm.*, 39:104–108 (1982).
14. S. J. Turco, *Parenterals*, 2(2):1, 6–7 (1984).
15. K. E. Avis and J. W. Levchuk, *Am. J. Hosp. Pharm.*, 41:81–87 (1984).
16. S. Rosenstein and P. P. Lamy, *Am. J. Hosp. Pharm.*, 30:800–804 (1973).
17. W. R. Frieben, *Am. J. Hosp. Pharm.*, 40:1928–1935 (1983).
18. K. E. Avis and M. J. Akers, *Sterile Preparation for the Hospital Pharmacist*. Ann Arbor Science, Ann Arbor, MI, 1981.
19. National Sanitation Foundation, Standard Number 49, Class II (Laminar Flow) Biohazard Cabinetry, Ann Arbor, MI, 1983.
20. National Study Commission on Cytoxic Agents, *Cancer Chemother. Update*, 1(1):4–7 (1983).
21. J. L. Laidlaw, T. H. Connor, J. C. Theiss, R. W. Anderson, and T. S. Matney, *Am. J. Hosp. Pharm.*, 41:2618–2623 (1984).
22. M. H. Stolar, L. A. Power, and C. S. Viele, *Am. J. Hosp. Pharm.*, 40:1163–1171 (1983).
23. P. L. Vaccari, K. Tonat, R. DeChristoforo, J. F. Gallelli, and P. F. Zimmerman, *Am. J. Hosp. Pharm.*, 41:87–93 (1984).
24. N. A. Mason, S. Cline, M. L. Hyneck, R. R. Berardi, N. F. H. Ho, and G. L. Flynn, *Am. J. Hosp. Pharm.*, 38:1449–1454 (1981).
25. R. F. Chaney and M. R. Summerfield, *Am. J. Hosp. Pharm.*, 41: 1150–1152 (1984).
26. B. Weiner, D. J. McNeely, R. M. Kluge, and R. B. Stewart, *Am. J. Hosp. Pharm.*, 33:1254–1259 (1976).
27. National Coordinating Committee on Large Volume Parenterals, *Am. J. Hosp. Pharm.*, 32:1251–1253 (1975).
28. American Society of Hospital Pharmacists, *Am. J. Hosp. Pharm.*, 34: 613–614 (1977).
29. National Coordinating Committee on Large Volume Parenterals, *Am. J. Hosp. Pharm.*, 35:49–51 (1978).
30. American Society of Hospital Pharmacists, *Am. J. Hosp. Pharm.*, 40:451–452 (1983).
31. L. A. Robinson and T. W. Vanderveen, *Am. J. Hosp. Pharm.*, 34: 697–705 (1977).
32. National Coordinating Committee on Large Volume Parenterals, *Am. J. Hosp. Pharm.*, 37:645–655 (1980).
33. National Coordinating Committee on Large Volume Parenterals, *Am. J. Hosp. Pharm.*, 35:678–682 (1978).
34. L. H. Sanders, S. A. Mabadeje, K. E. Avis, C. A. Cruze, III, and D. R. Martinez, *Am. J. Hosp. Pharm.*, 35:531–536 (1978).
35. W. W. Williams, *Am. J. Hosp. Pharm.*, 41:258–259 (1984).

36. K. H. Hoffman, F. M. Smith, H. N. Godwin, L. C. Hogan, and D. Furtado, *Am. J. Hosp. Pharm.*, 39:1299–1302 (1982).
37. R. L. DeChant, D. Furtado, F. M. Smith, H. N. Godwin, and D. E. Domann, *Am. J. Hosp. Pharm.*, 39:1305–1308 (1982).
38. B. G. Morris, K. E. Avis, and G. C. Bowles, *Am. J. Hosp. Pharm.*, 37:668–672 (1980).
39. R. F. Mager and P. Pipe, *Analyzing Performance Problems.*, 2nd Ed. Pitman Learning, Belmont, CA, 1984.
40. J. S. Millis, Chairman, *Pharmacists for the Future: The Report of the Study Commission on Pharmacy*. Health Administration Press, Ann Arbor, MI, 1975, p. 140.

Index

A

D

G

H

T

U

V

W

Y

Z